Signing With Your Clients

A Practical Manual for Audiologists and Speech/Language Pathologists

Florence C. Vold
Mary Ann Kinsella-Meier
Mary C. Hughes Hilley

Illustrated by Lois Lehman-Lenderman

Clerc Books Gallaudet University Press Washington, D.C.

Clerc Books
An imprint of Gallaudet University Press
Washington, DC 20002

Published 1990.
Printed in the United States of America

03 02 01 4 3 2

Library of Congress Cataloging in Publication Data

Vold, Florence C.
Signing with your clients : a practical manual for audiologists and speech/language pathologists / Florence C. Vold, Mary Ann Kinsella-Meier, Mary C. Hughes Hilley.
p. cm.
"Clerc books."
Includes glossary.
ISBN 0-930323-53-X
1. Sign language—Handbooks, manuals, etc. 2. Audiologists–Handbooks, manuals, etc. 3. Speech therapists—Handbooks, manuals, etc. I. Kinsella-Meier, Mary Ann. II. Hilley, Mary C. Hughes, 1996- . III. Title.
[DNLM: 1. Deafness–rehabilitation–handbooks. 2. Manual Communication–handbooks. 3. Referral and Consultation–handbooks.
HV 2474 V914s]
HV 2474.V65 1990
419–dc20
DNLM/DLC
for Library of Congress 90-13968
CIP

ISBN 1-56368-111-0 (pbk.)

Dedication

To the Gallaudet University Audiology and Speech-Language Pathology former and future graduate students for giving us the impetus and encouragement for writing this book.

Contents

Chapter 1

How To Use This Book

Book Format and Design

Technical signs related to our profession are included in sentences that cover a full range of services commonly offered to deaf clients at Gallaudet University. Because signing is fluid, or "coarticulated," we have chosen a sentence format to illustrate the continuous nature of sign communication. The sentences originated from actual diagnostic and rehabilitative sessions. The drawings in the book show appropriate facial expressions for each sentence. This will help you to see the importance of using facial expressions when you sign. The arrows in the drawings indicate the movement of the sign, and the symbol RM in a circle means that the movement is repeated.

Notes to the Reader

We have purposely limited the client's length of response to questions you might ask. Yes/no questions have been used whenever appropriate, as opposed to open-ended questions. This sentence structure will allow the novice signer to understand the client's response. Sentences were chosen to show signs in context, not to show every sentence to be used in a particular rehabilitative or diagnostic procedure.

This book was not designed to be used as a "cookbook" or "script." Instead, it is a reference for expressive sign language. It is strongly recommended that in conjunction with using this book, you enroll in a course of sign communication. A sign language course will help you develop the necessary aspects of receptive sign language as well as the nuances of expressive sign communication. In addition, a course on sign language may also expose you to information regarding the unique qualities of Deaf culture. As your signing ability improves, we would recommend that you move away from this format and make use of the glossary. The glossary will assist you in producing individual signs for original sentence creation. This will lead to a greater exchange and flow of information between clinician and client.

We hope that you will find this book informative, worthwhile, and productive.

Rationale

Working at Gallaudet University, particularly in the Audiology and Speech-Language Pathology Graduate Program, we saw the need to improve our graduate students' signing skills. We were frustrated to find that the sign books on the market did not include the professional signs we needed for everyday clinical work. Several years ago, in an effort to meet the needs of our students, we established a "Graduate Student Orientation Program" at Gallaudet for our incoming graduates. We began by cutting, pasting, revising, and drawing signs related to our field. We gave these "books" to our students and found that even this minimal attempt improved both their confidence and their skills. We decided that we should approach Gallaudet University Press with our idea to publish a sign book designed specifically for our profession. Their support has been tremendous over the past four years that our work has been in progress. We hope that you will enjoy the format of this manual, and that you too will feel more confident and better skilled as your sign language skills grow.

Purpose

This book is intended to prepare speech-language-hearing and other allied professionals to communicate with clients who are deaf. The use of the term *deaf* refers to those individuals who are "culturally deaf." These individuals, regardless of their degree of hearing loss, use sign language as their primary mode of communication.

This manual includes signs related to the oral/aural diagnostic, rehabilitative, and counseling process. You should be aware that many times you will encounter regional signs. What we have attempted to do here is to provide the most often seen signs at Gallaudet University and the most conceptually correct signs. You yourself may sign some of these words slightly differently; that is fine, as long as they are conceptually correct and your client understands you.

In addition, special binding has been chosen to allow you to have both hands free for producing signs. The intent was to write a book that would be easy to manipulate and convenient for you, the reader, while practicing your signs.

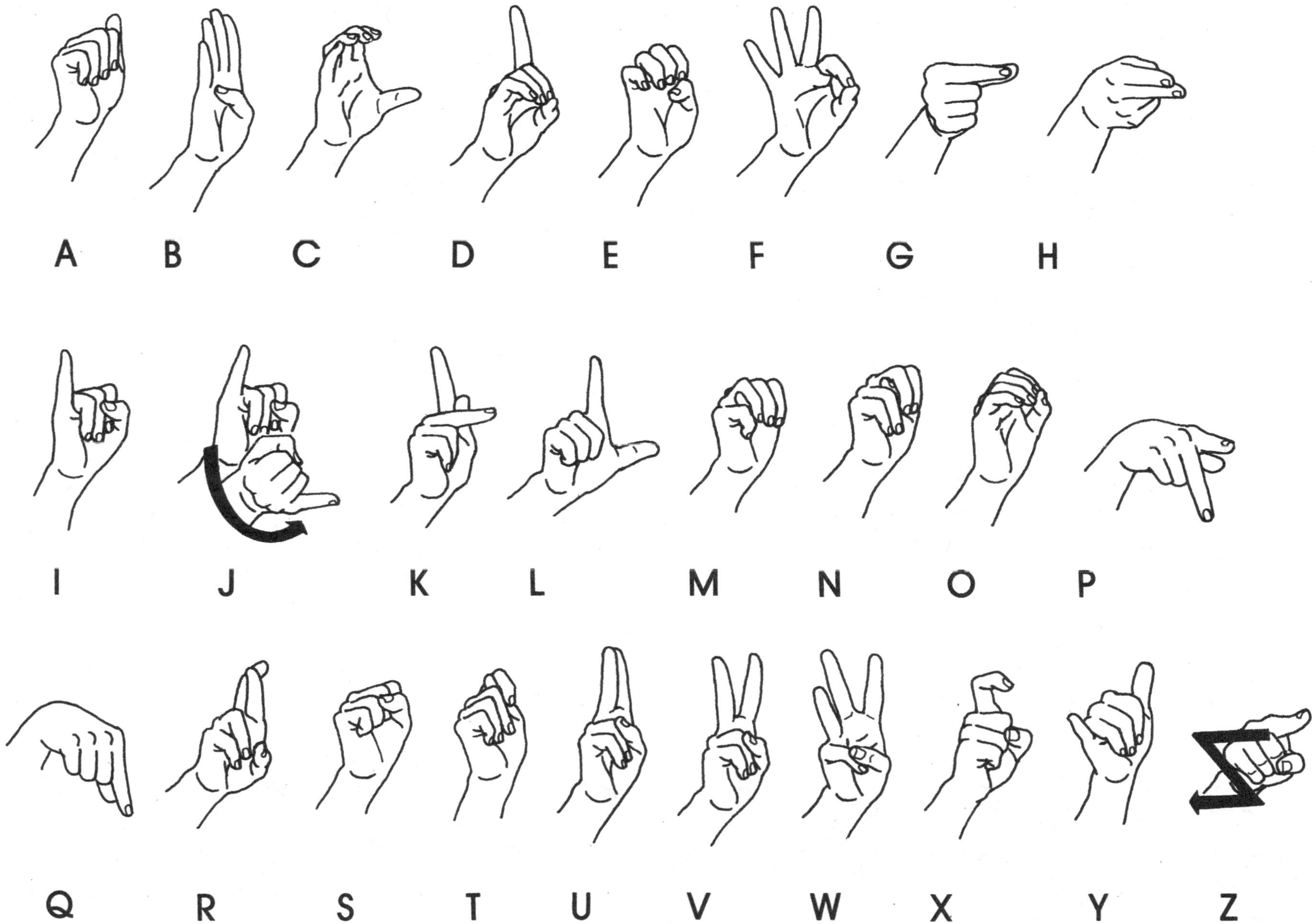
A B C D E F G H
I J K L M N O P
Q R S T U V W X Y Z

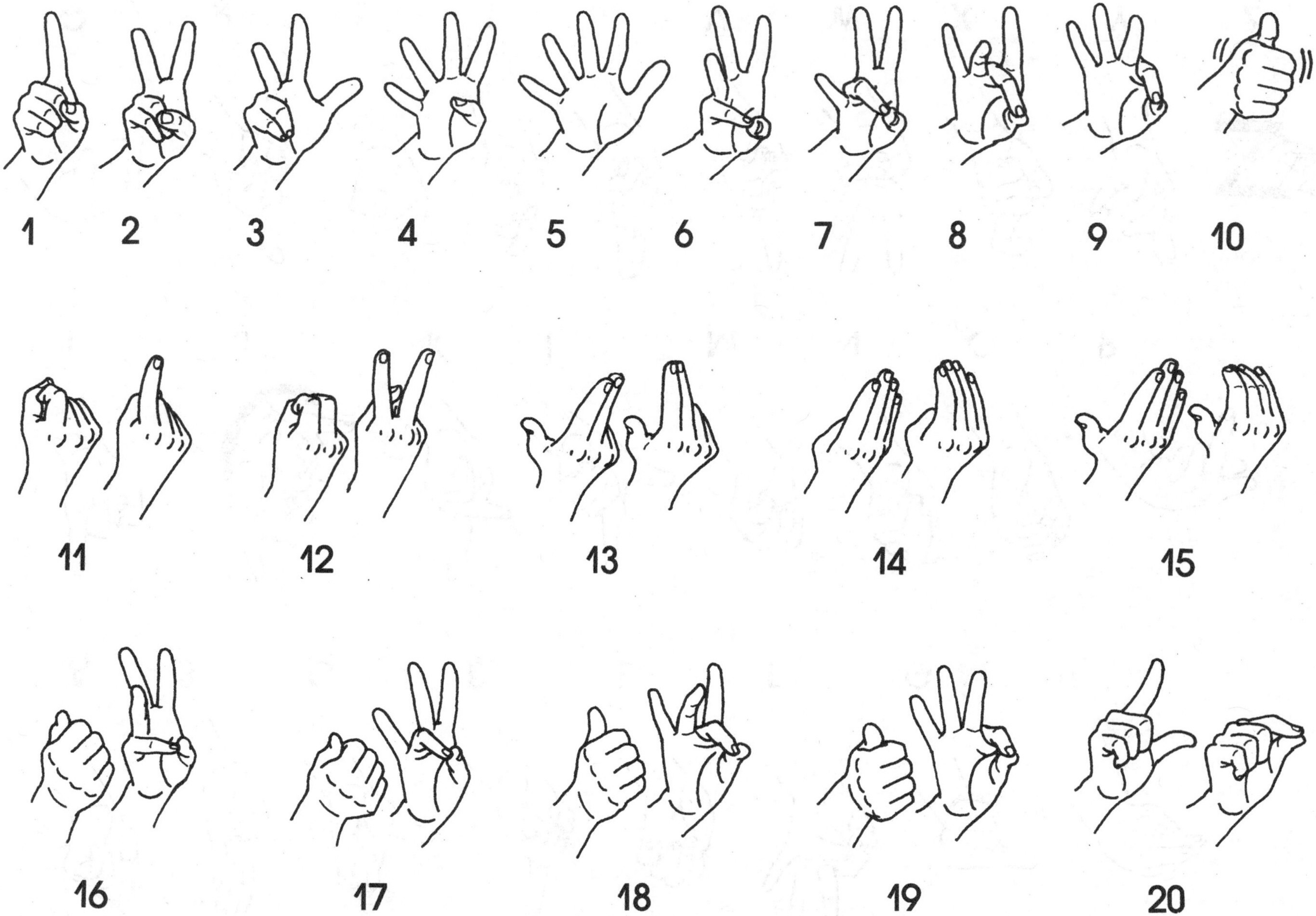
1
2
3
4
5
6
7
8
9
10
11
12
13
14
15
16
17
18
19
20

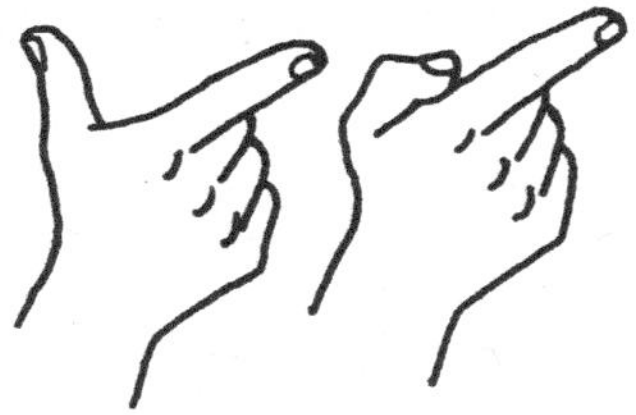

21

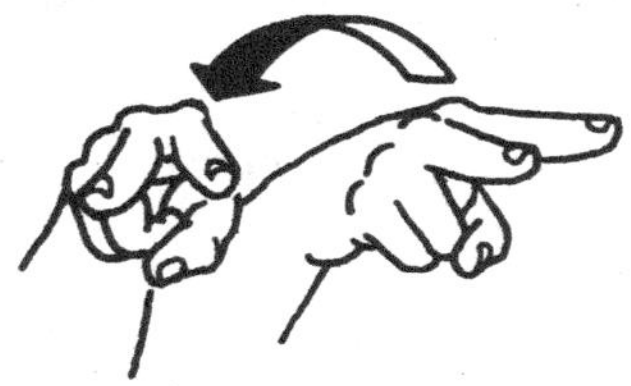

22

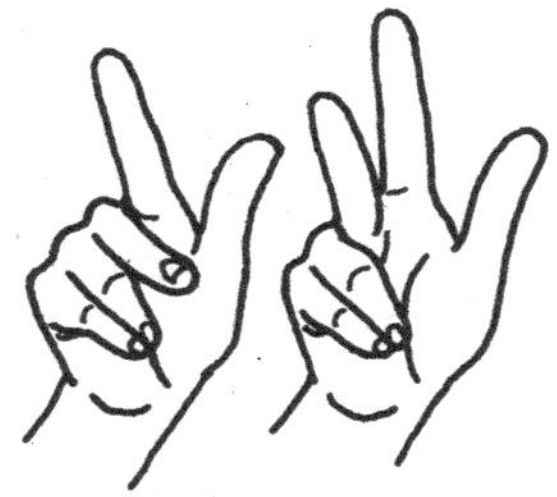

23

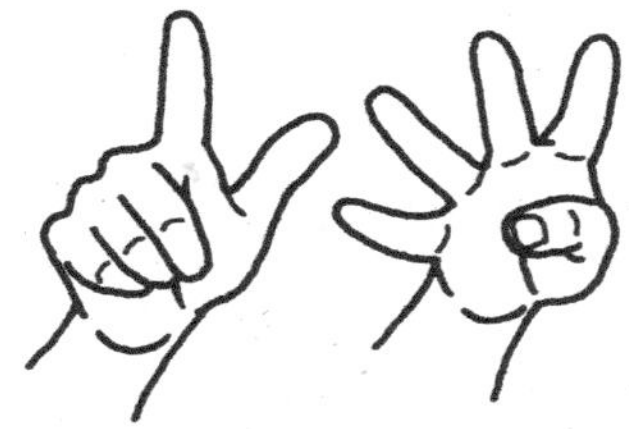

24

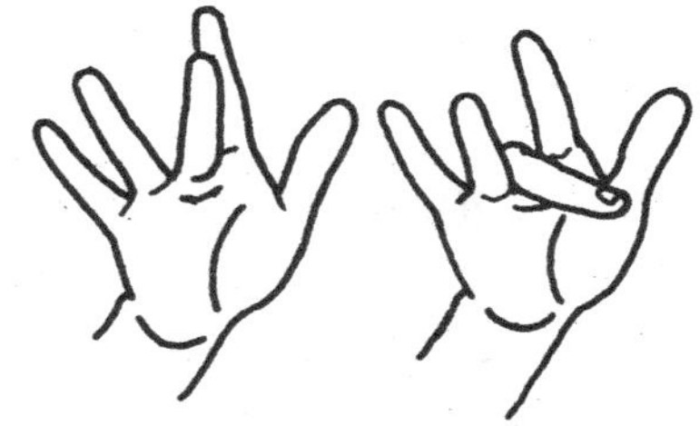

25

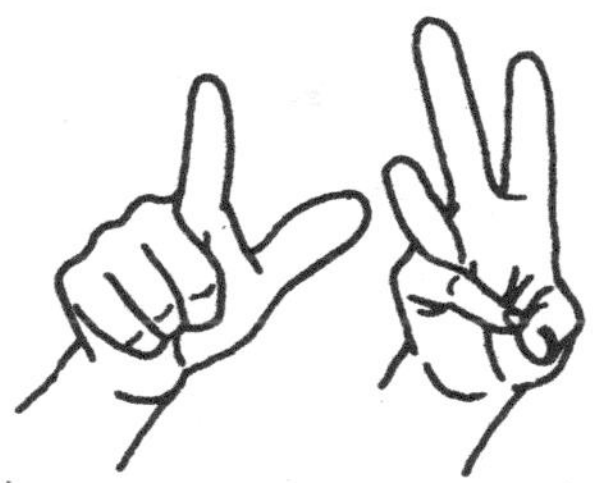

26

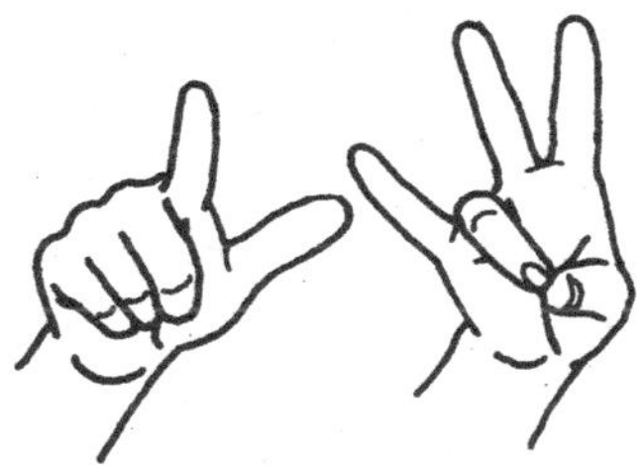

27

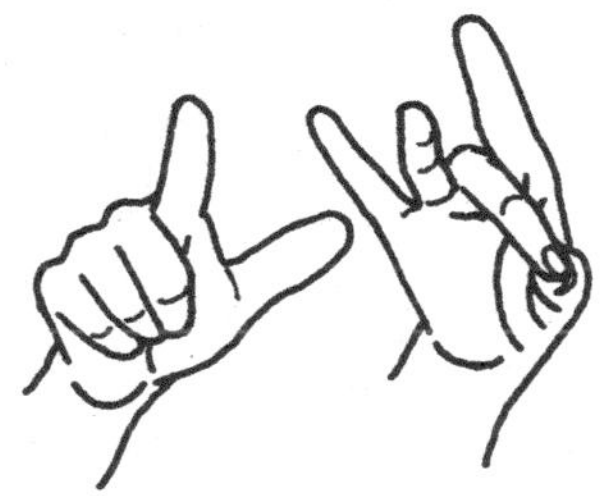

28

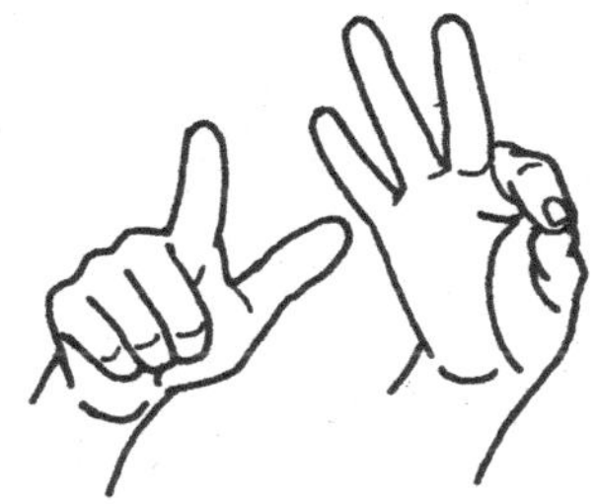

29

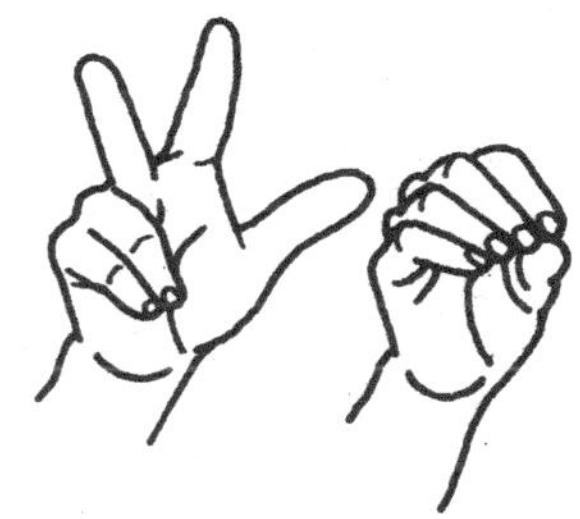

30

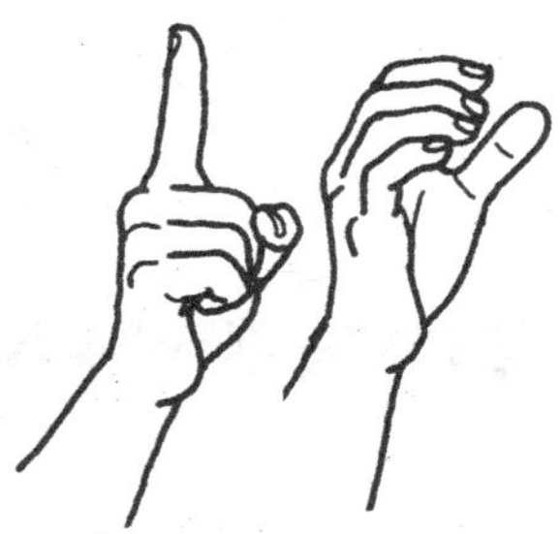

100

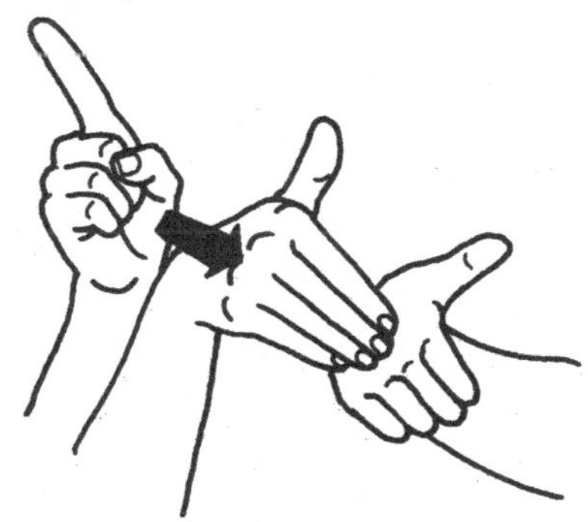

1000

Chapter 2

Interview of Deaf Parents with a Deaf Infant

Audiologic History

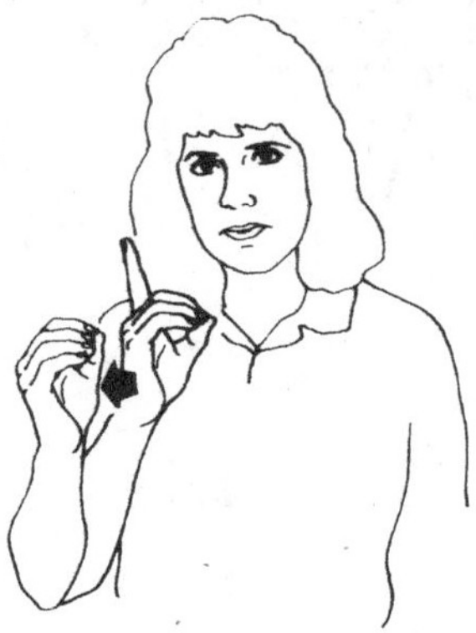

D-O

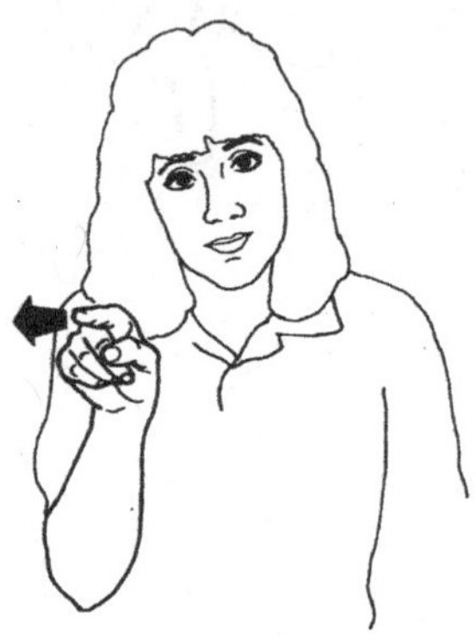

YOU

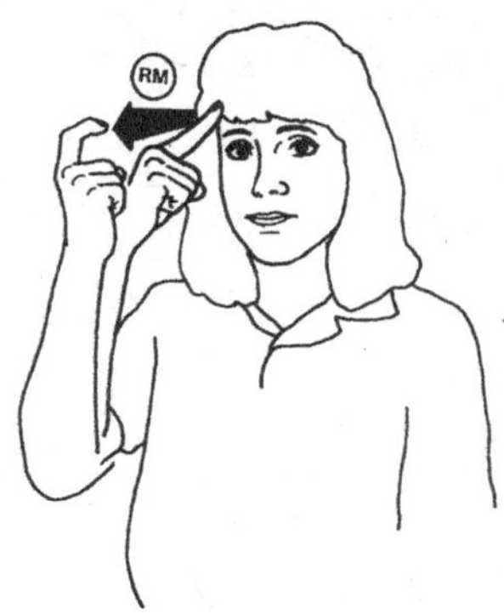

SUSPECT

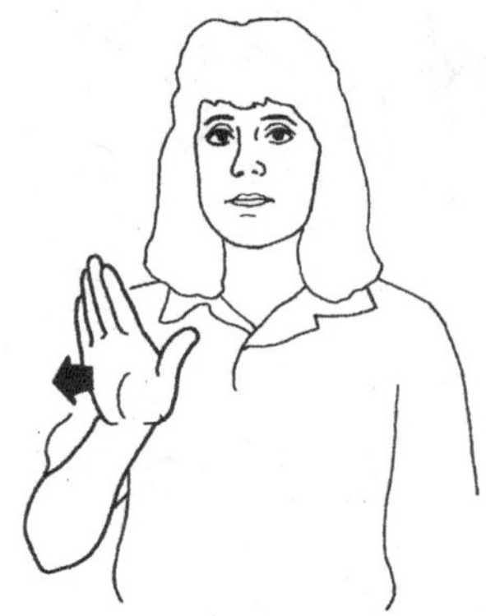

YOUR

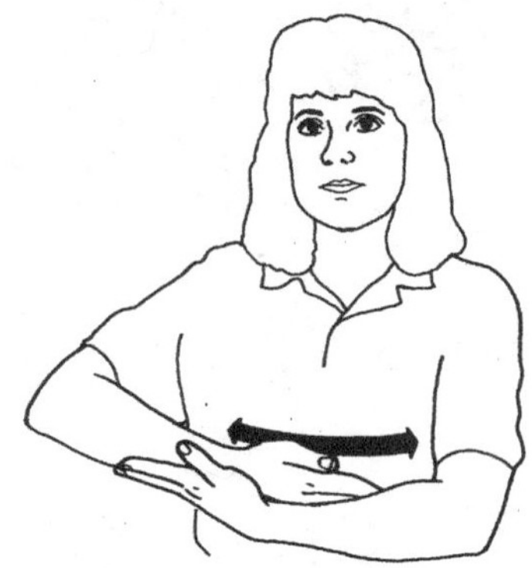

BABY

Do you suspect your baby has a hearing problem?

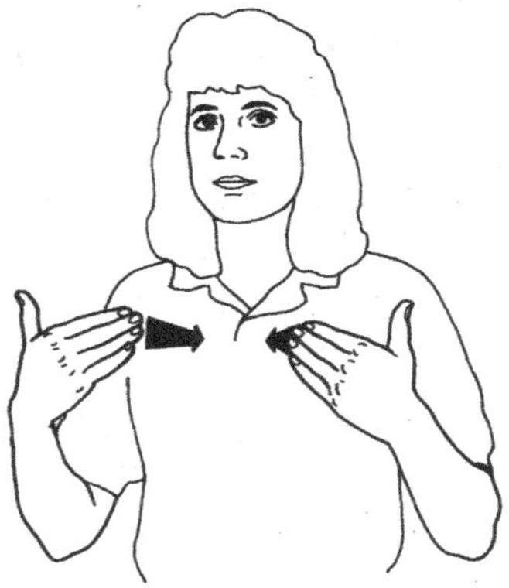

HAVE

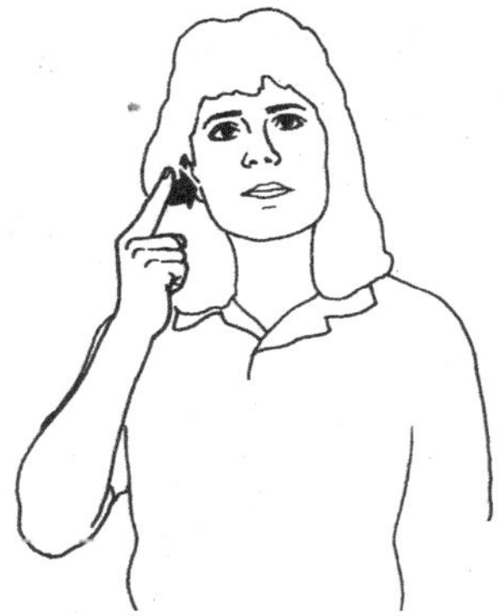

HEAR

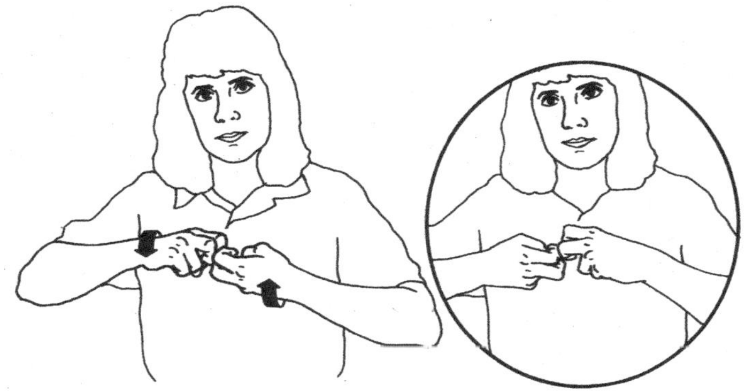

PROBLEM?

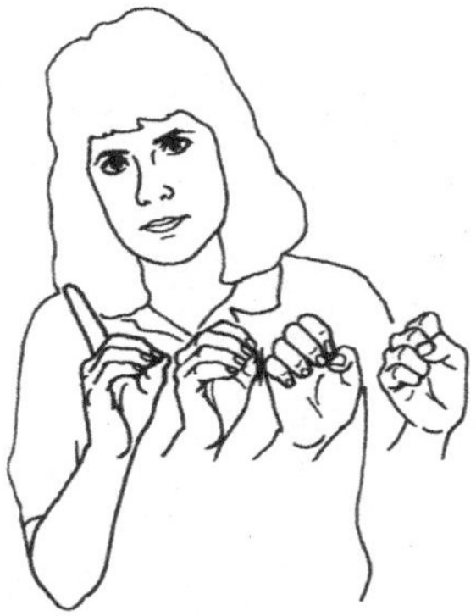

D-O-E-S

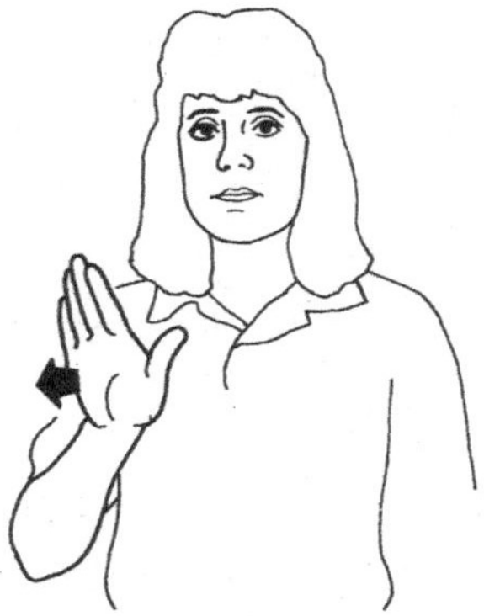

YOUR

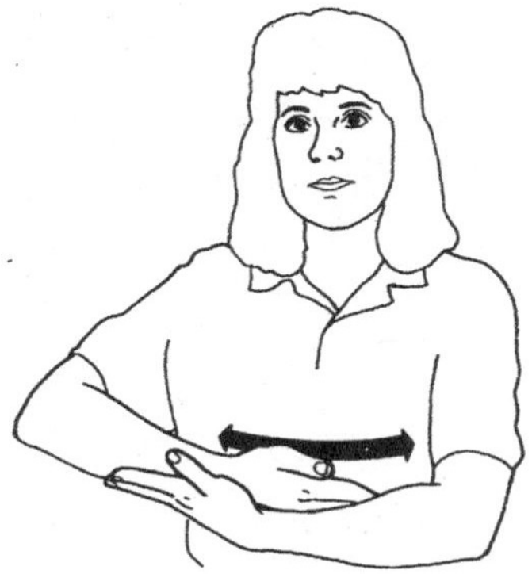

BABY

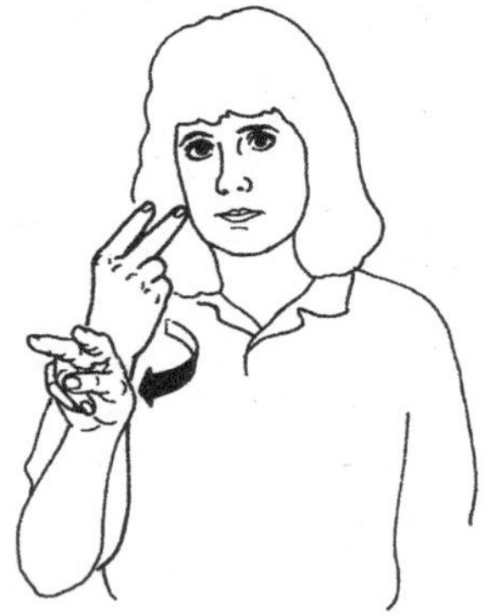

LOOK-AT-YOU

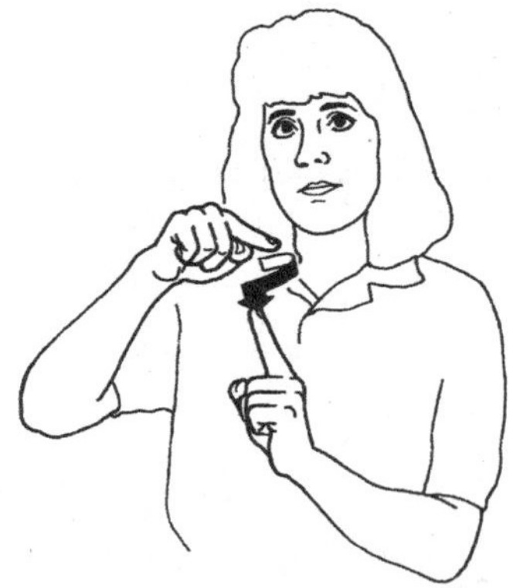

WHEN

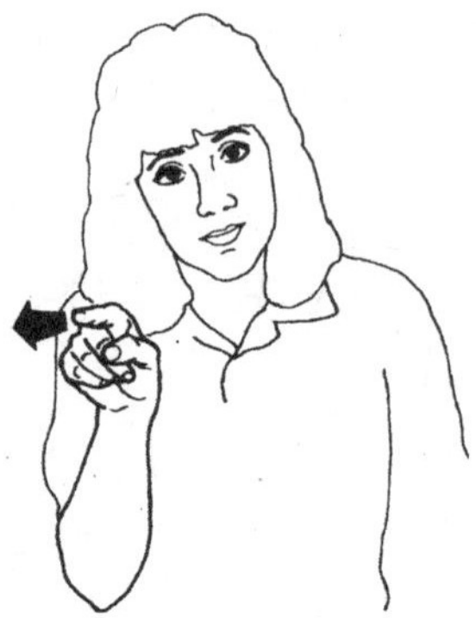

YOU

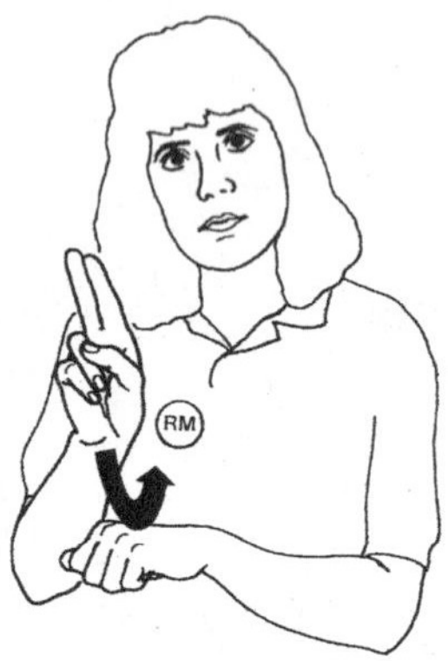

USE

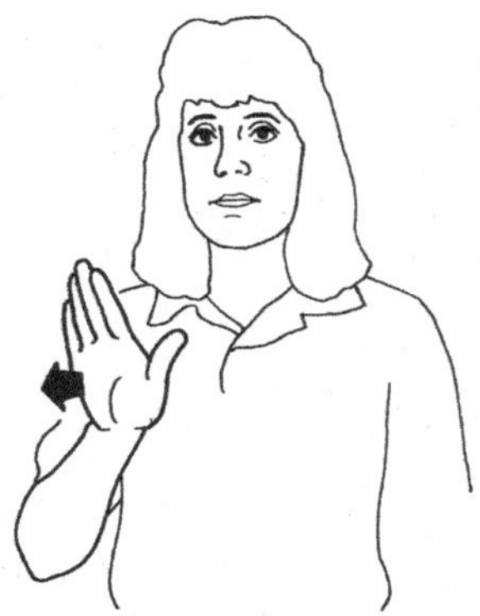

YOUR

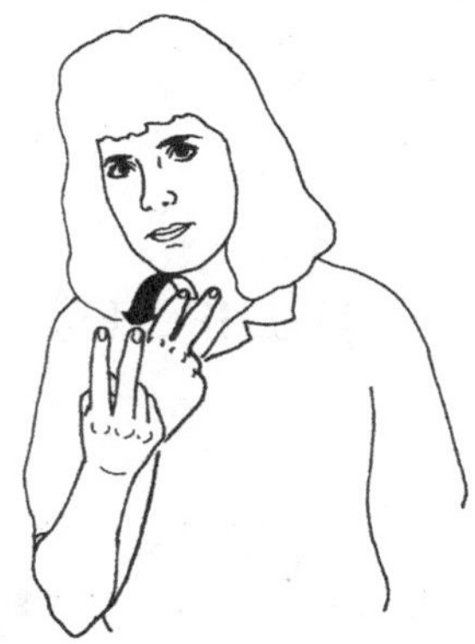

VOICE?

Does your baby look at you when you use your voice?

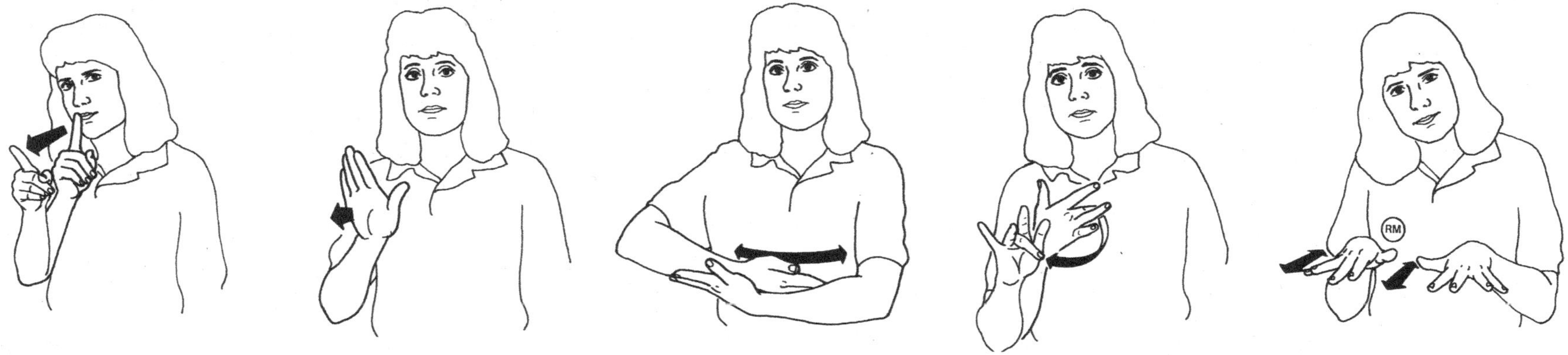

IS YOUR BABY SENSITIVE VIBRATION?

Is your baby sensitive to vibrations?

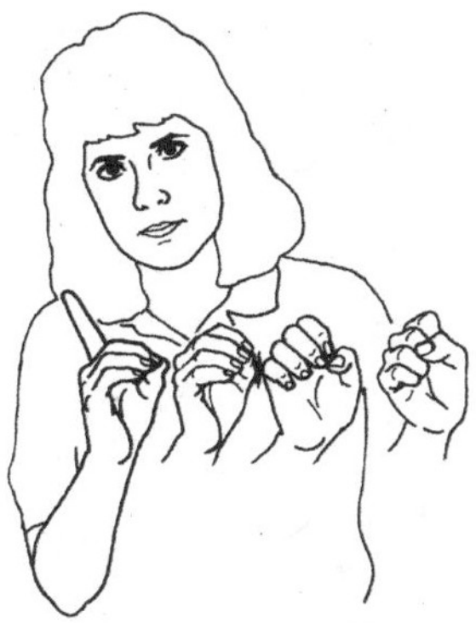

D-O-E-S

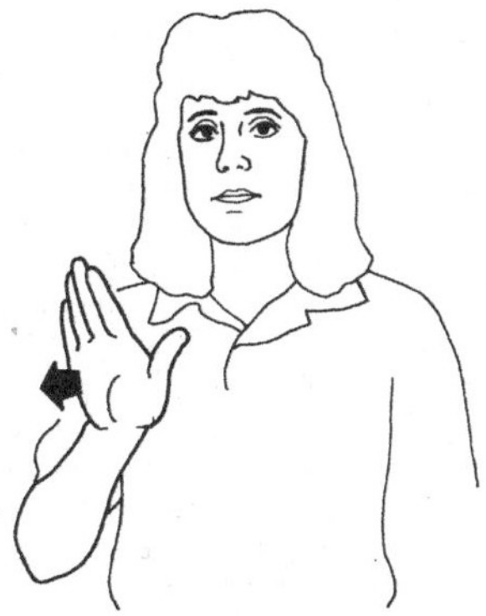

YOUR

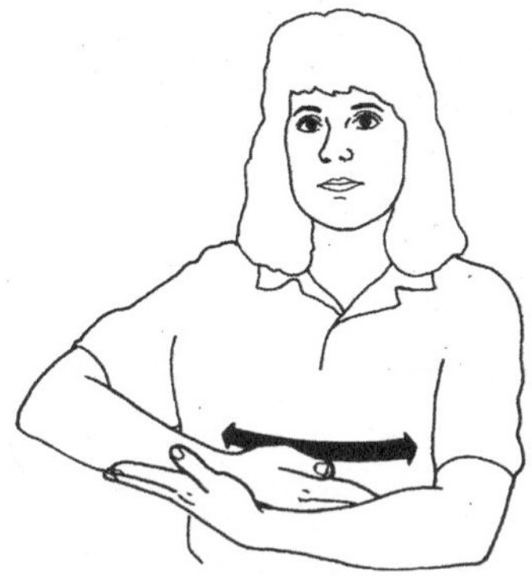

BABY

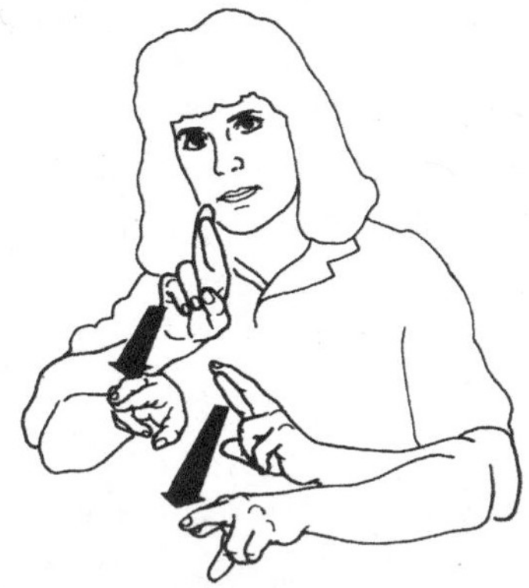

RESPOND

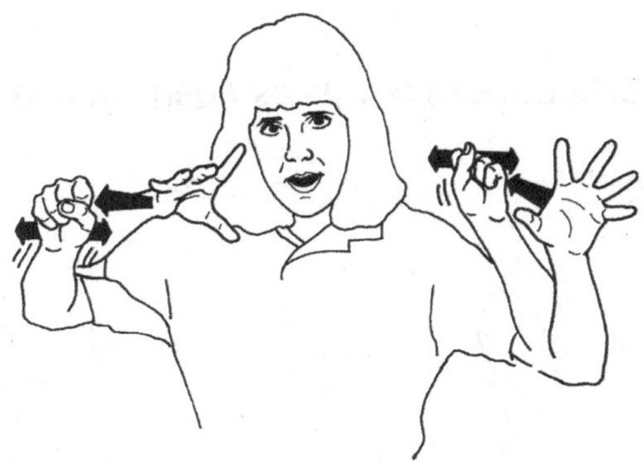

LOUD

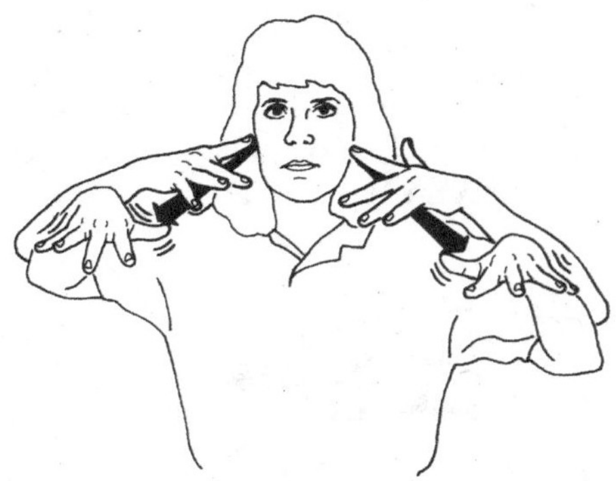

NOISE?

Does your baby respond to loud noises? For example, an ambulance, a dog barking, a telephone ringing, etc.

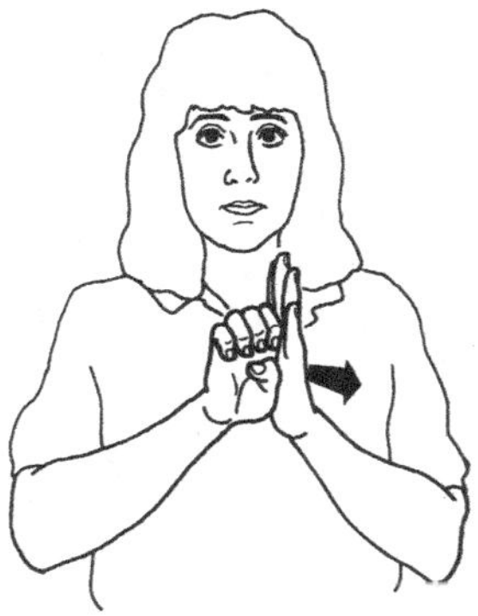

FOR-EXAMPLE

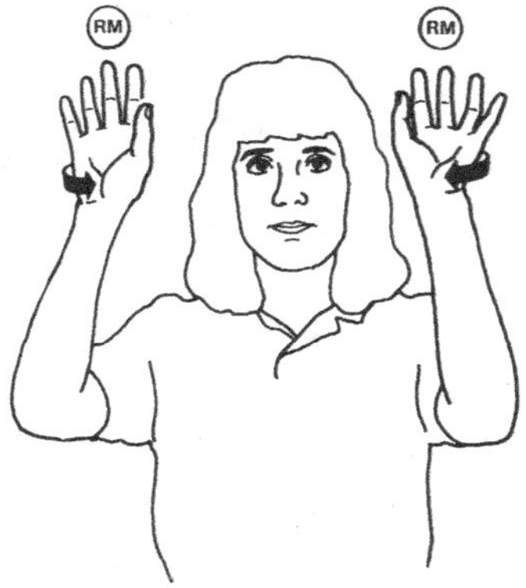

AMBULANCE

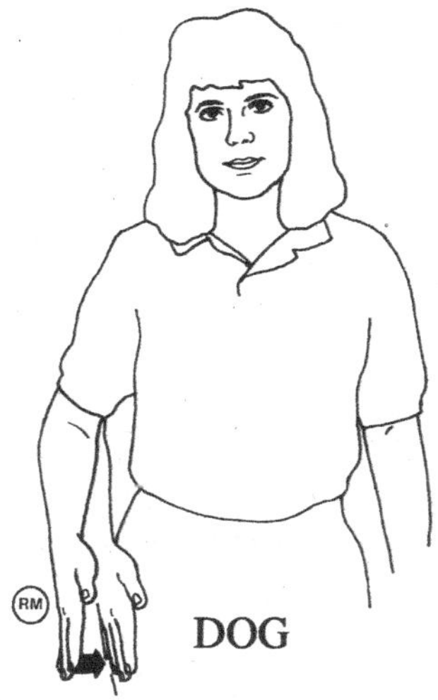

DOG

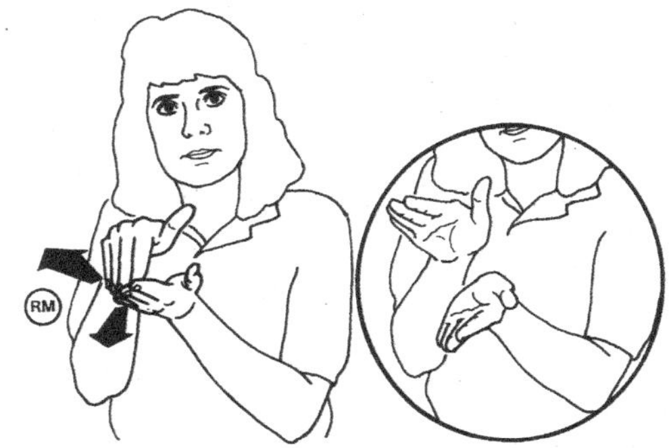

BARK

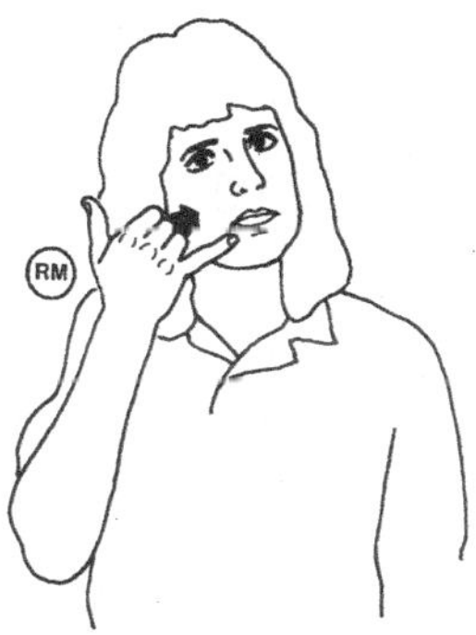

TELEPHONE

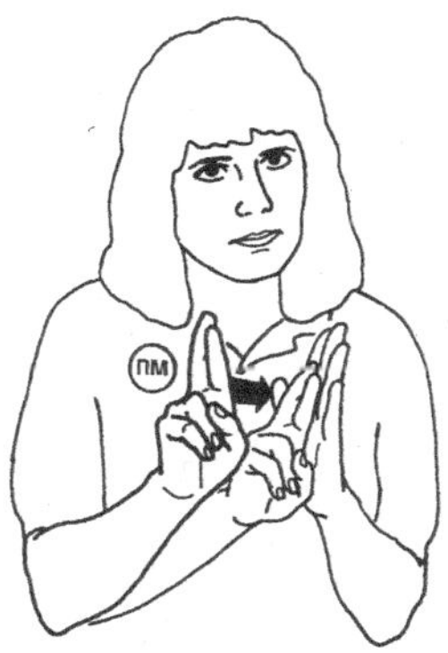

RING,

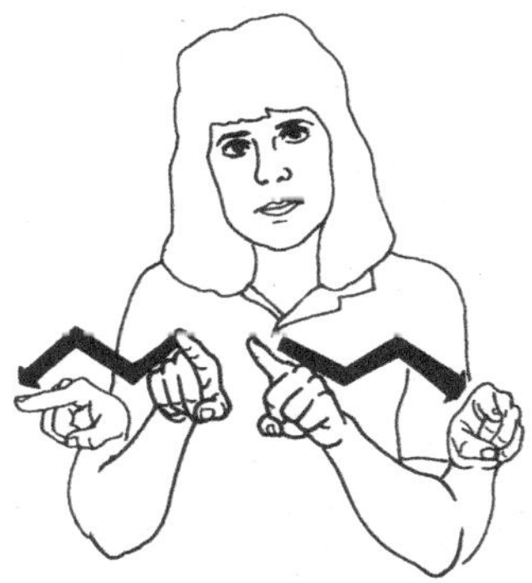

ETC.

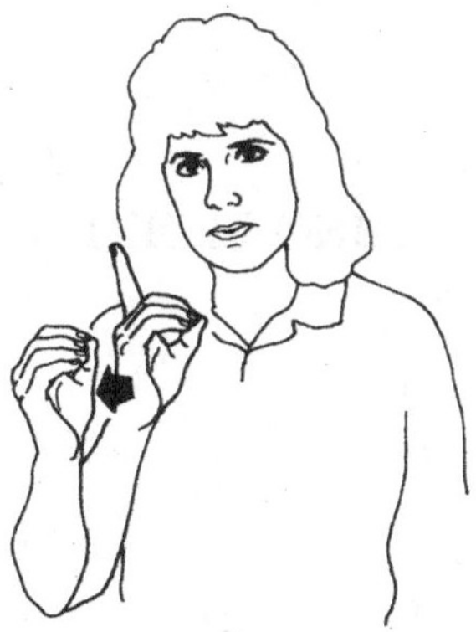

D-O

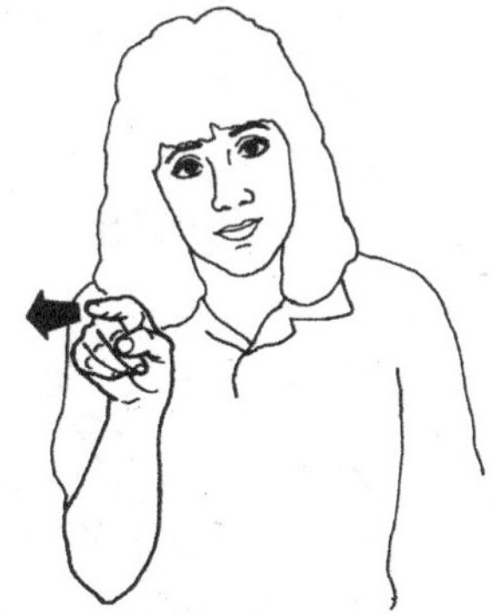

YOU

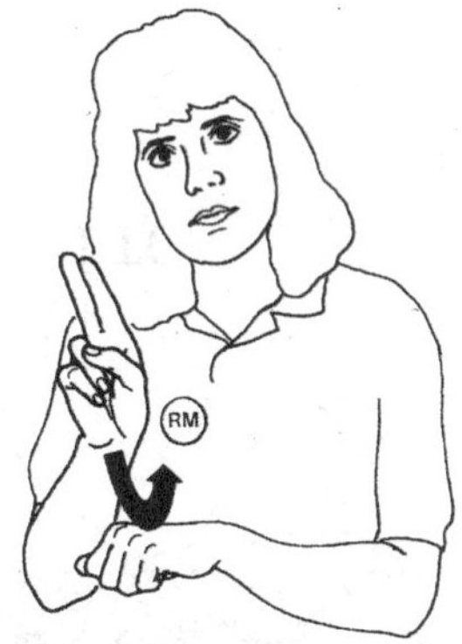

USE

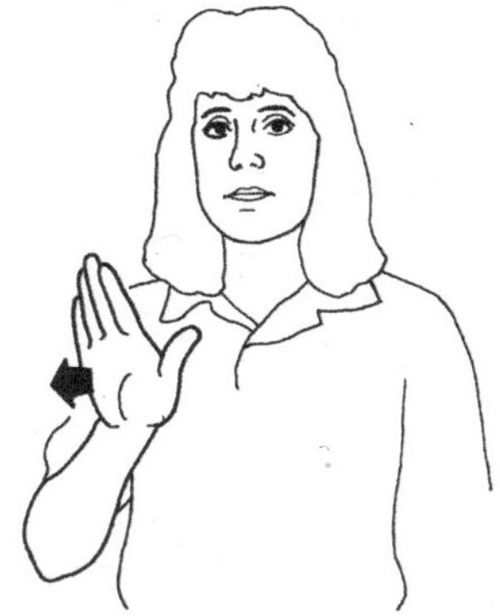

YOUR

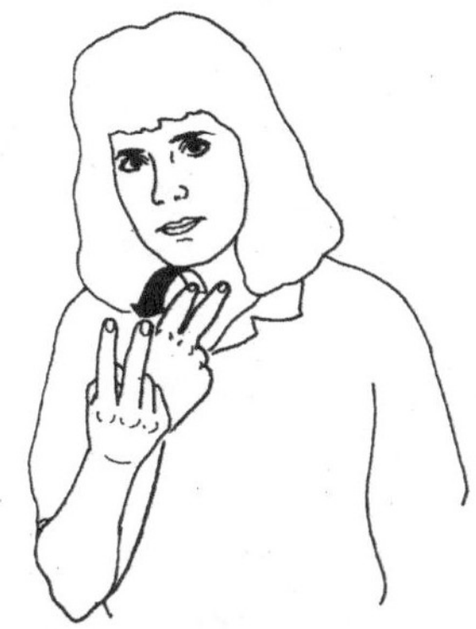

VOICE

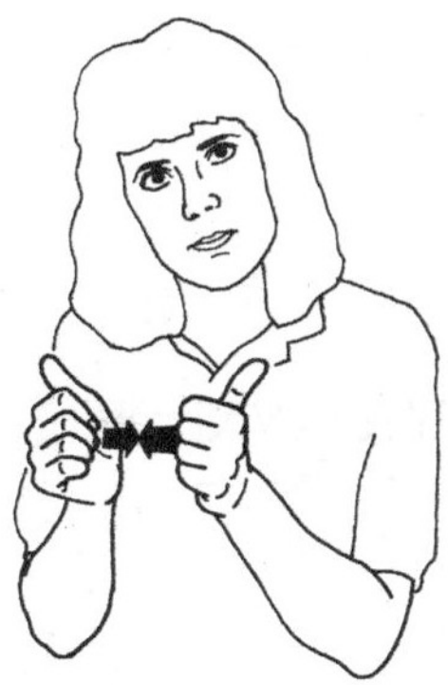

WITH

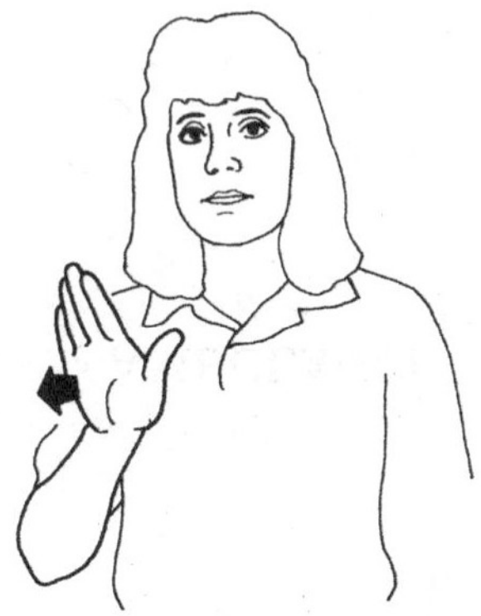

YOUR

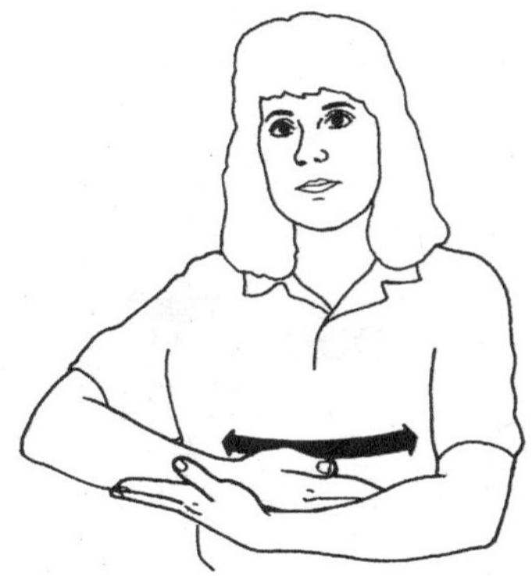

BABY?

Do you use your voice with your baby?

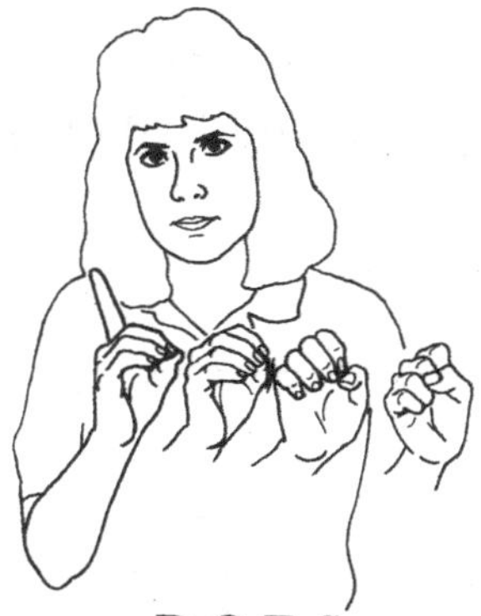

D-O-E-S

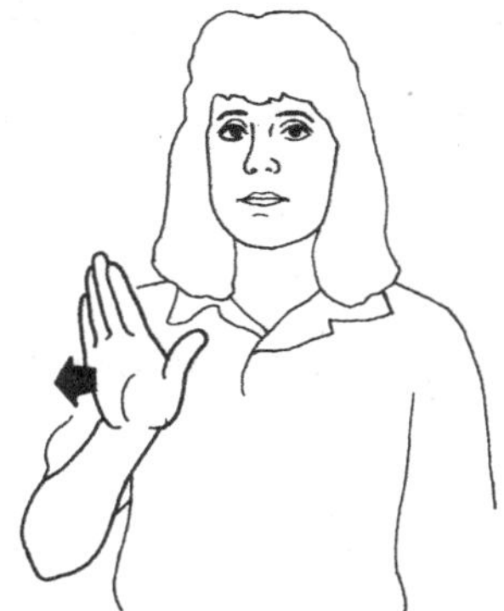

YOUR

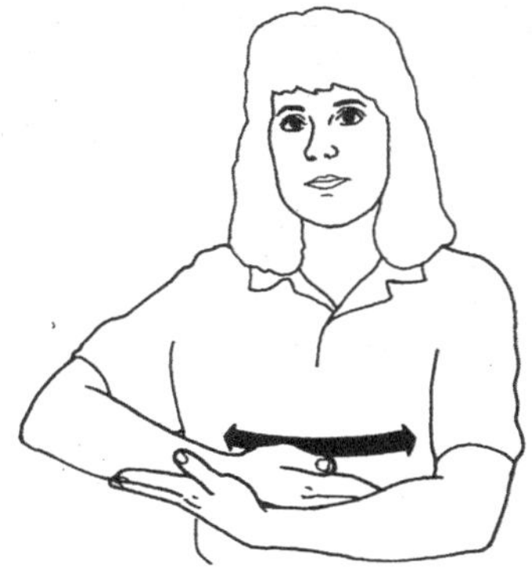

BABY

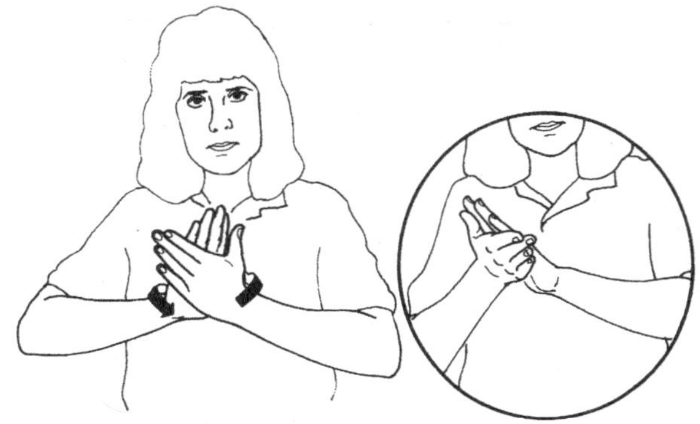

BECOME

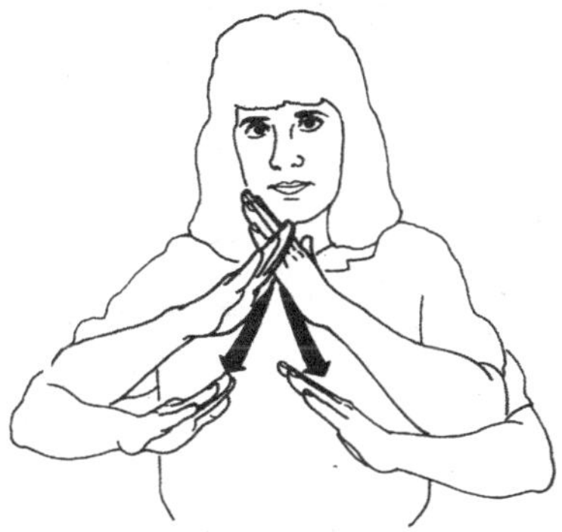

QUIET

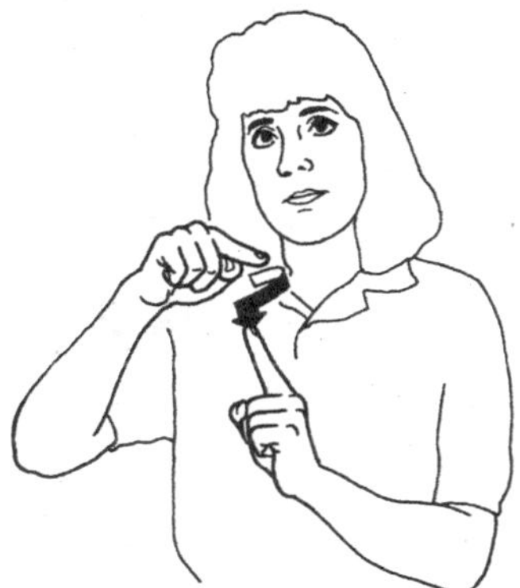

WHEN

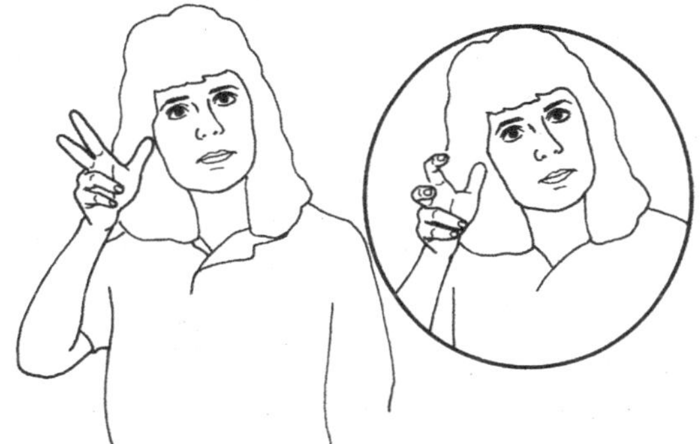

LISTEN

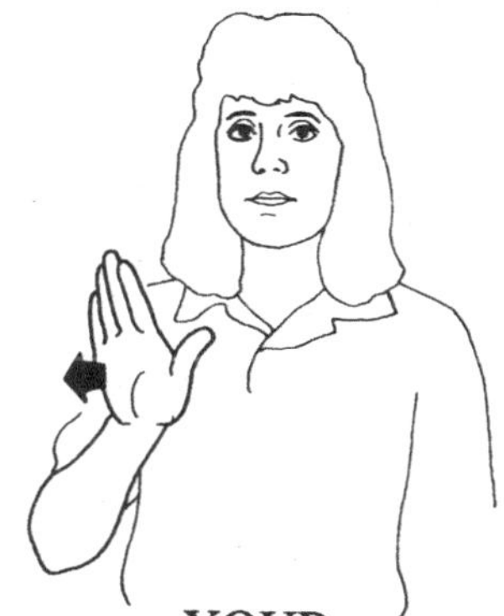

YOUR

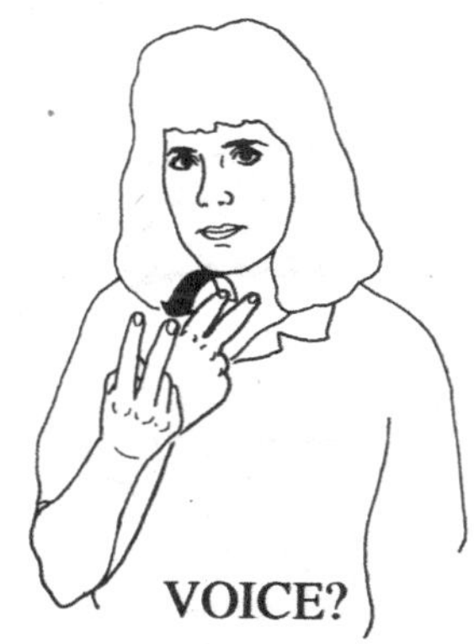

VOICE?

Does your baby become quiet when listening to your voice?

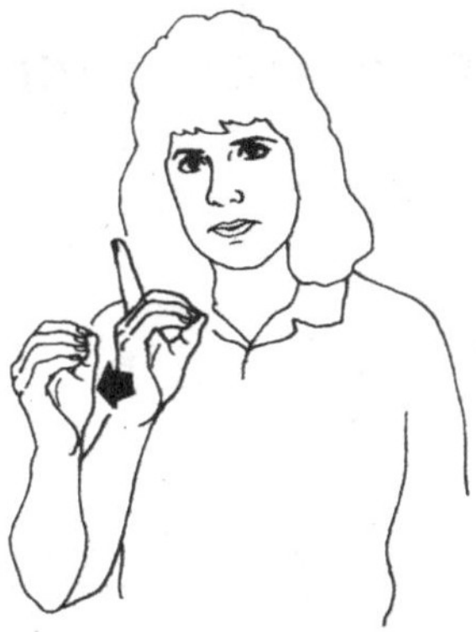

D-O

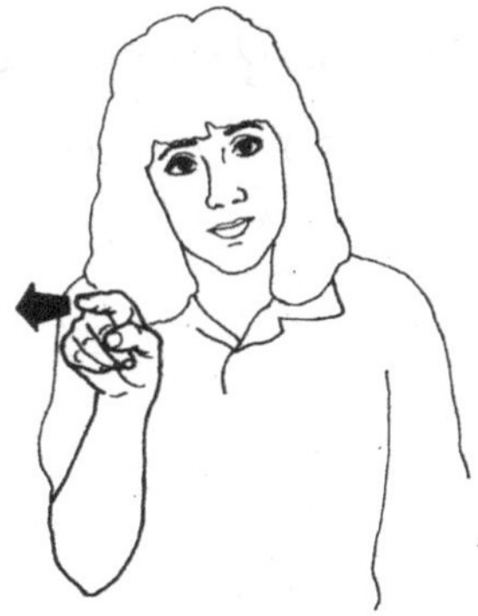

YOU

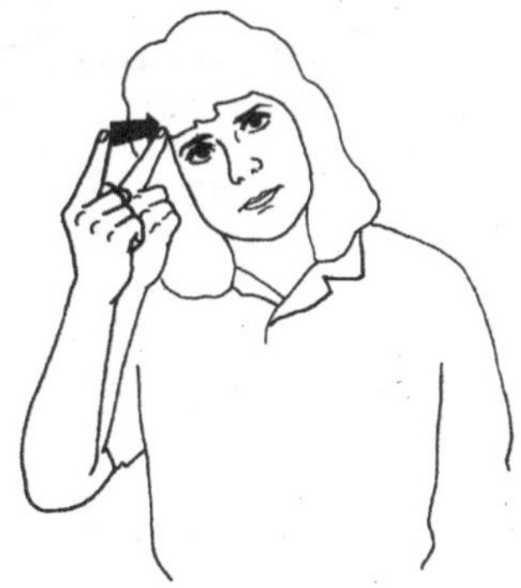

THINK

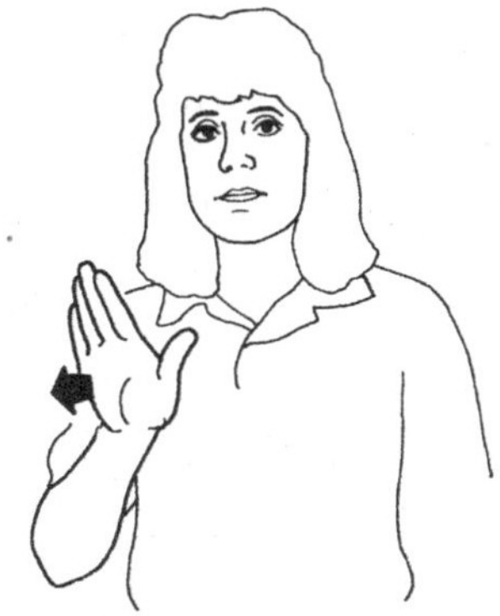

YOUR

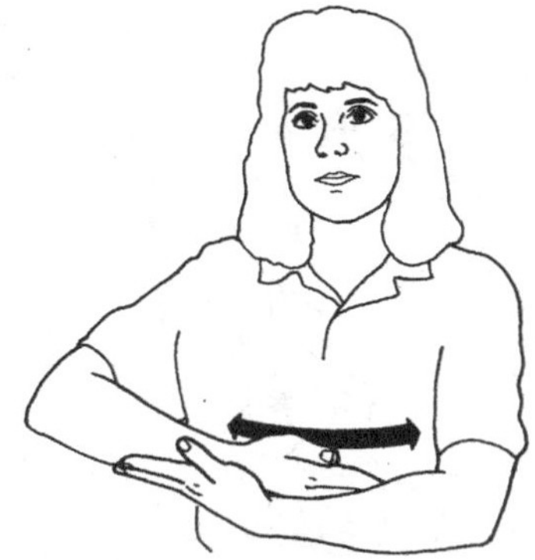

BABY

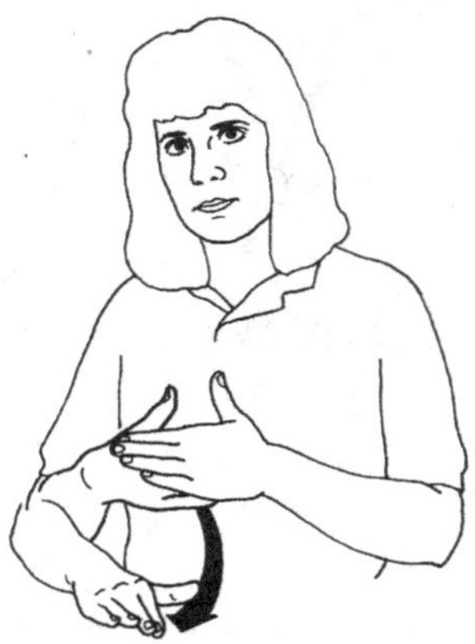

BORN

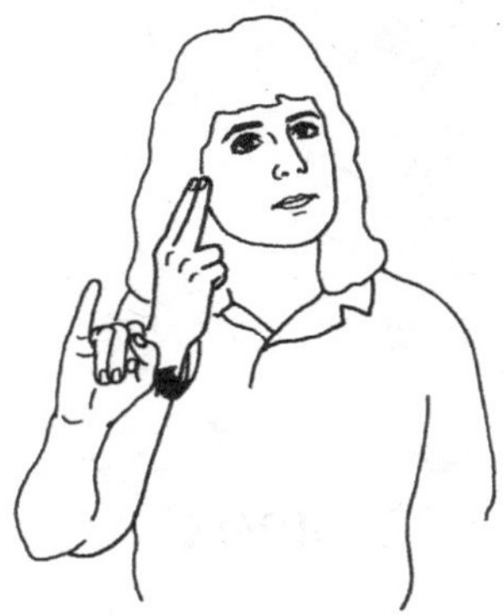

HEARING IMPAIRED?

Do you think your baby was born hearing impaired?

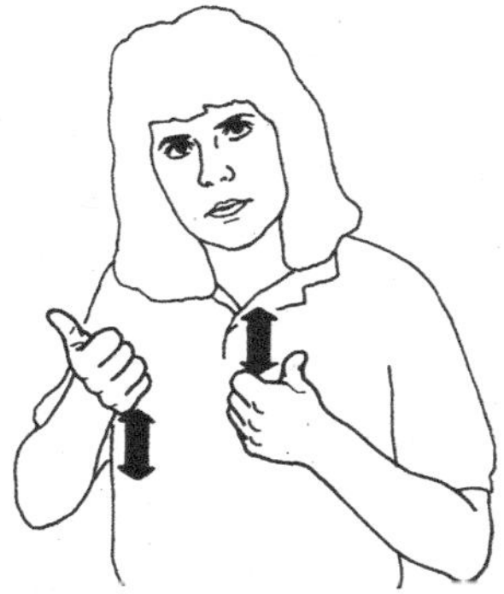

WHICH

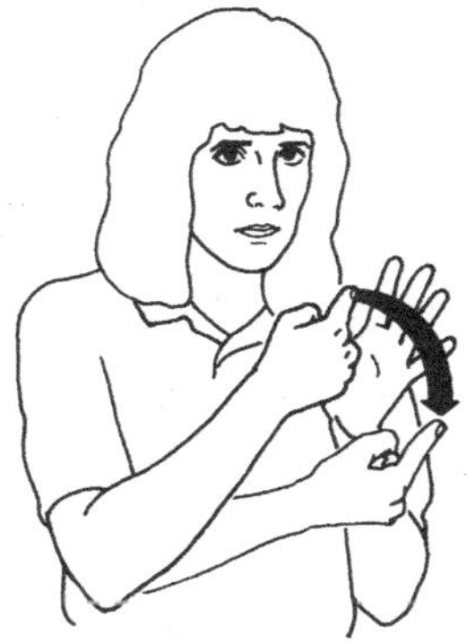

OF-THESE

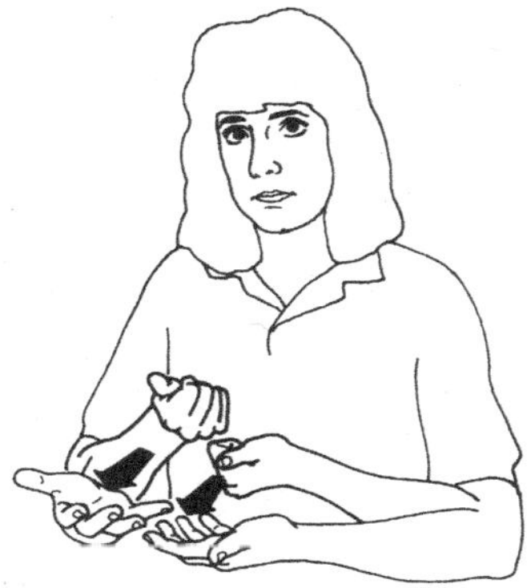

CAUSE

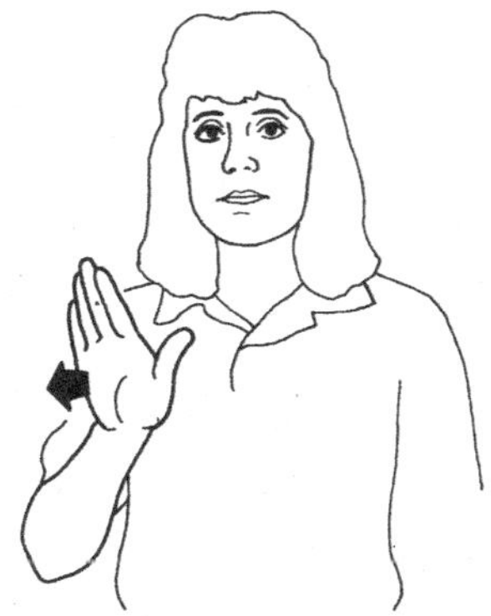

YOUR

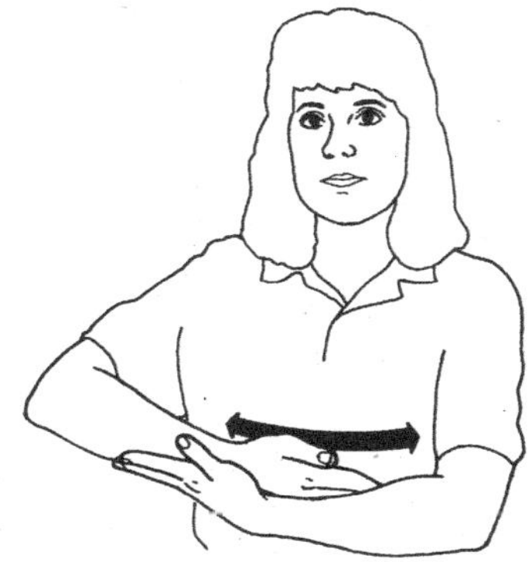

BABY

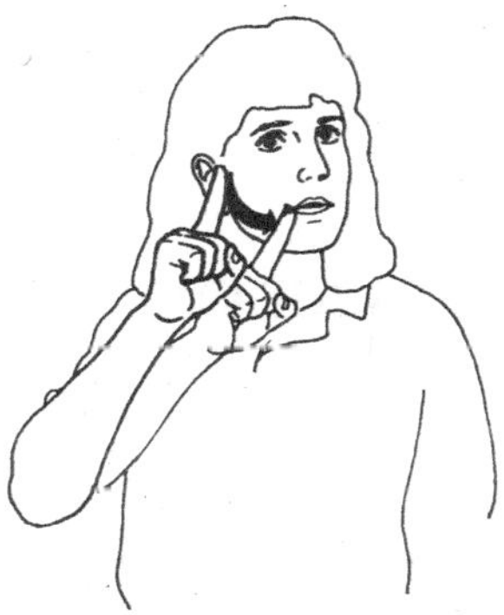

DEAF

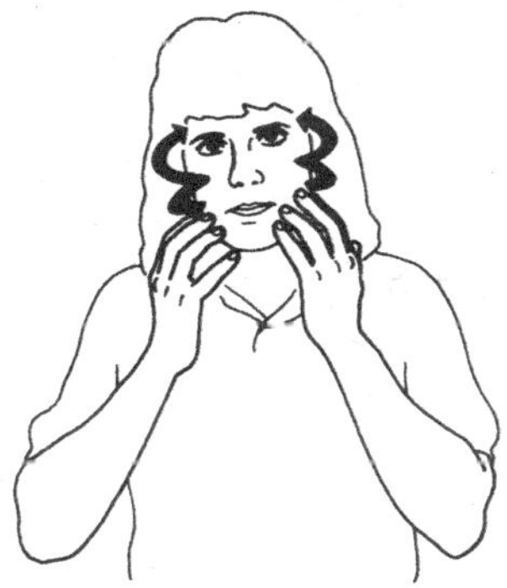

RUBELLA

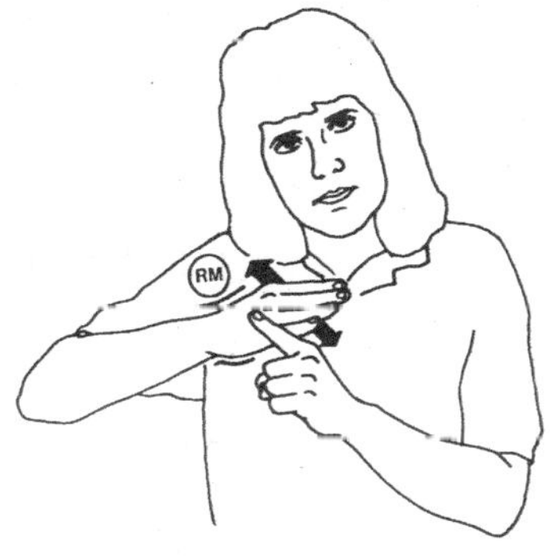

FEVER

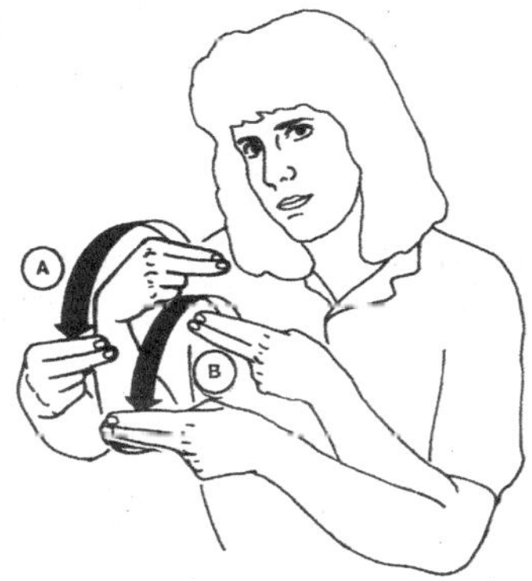

HEREDITY

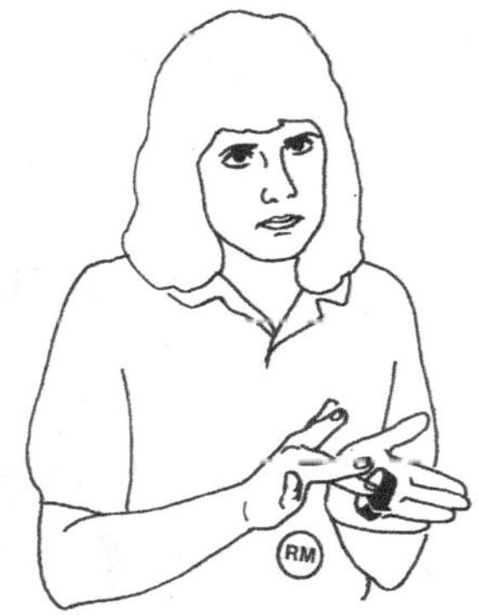

MEDICATION

Which of the following caused your baby's deafness: rubella, fever, heredity, medication, accident, Rh-factor, prematurity, or unknown causes.

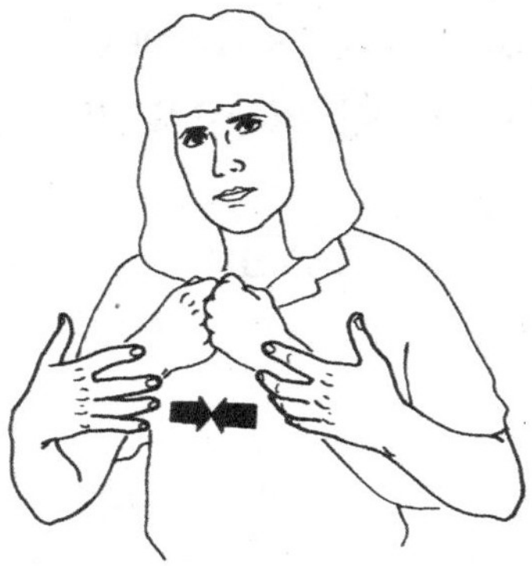

ACCIDENT

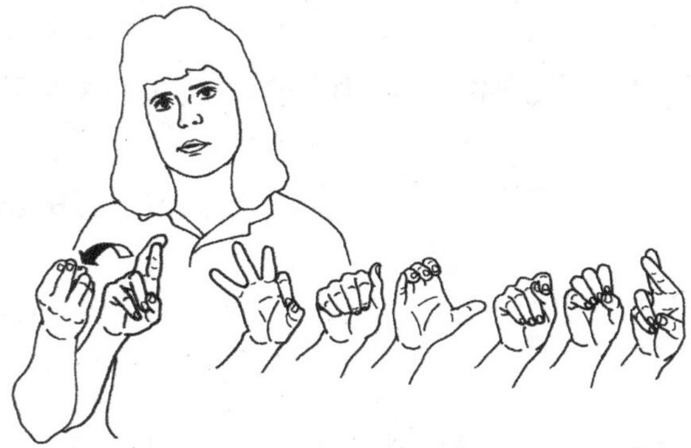

R-H F-A-C-T-O-R

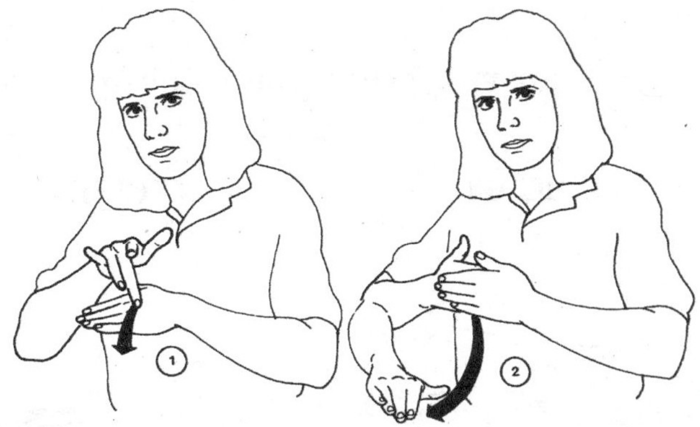

PREMATURITY

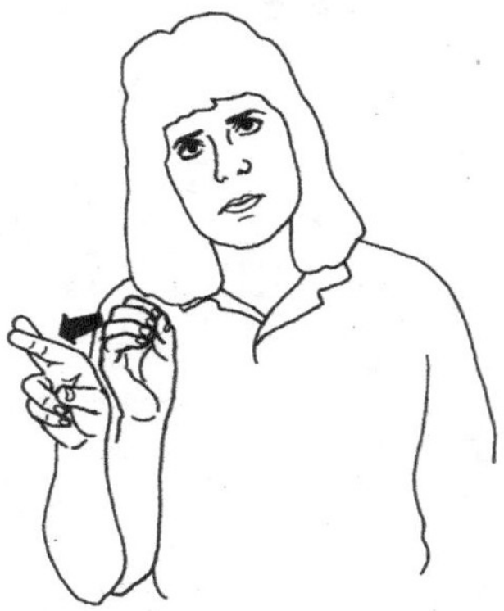

OR

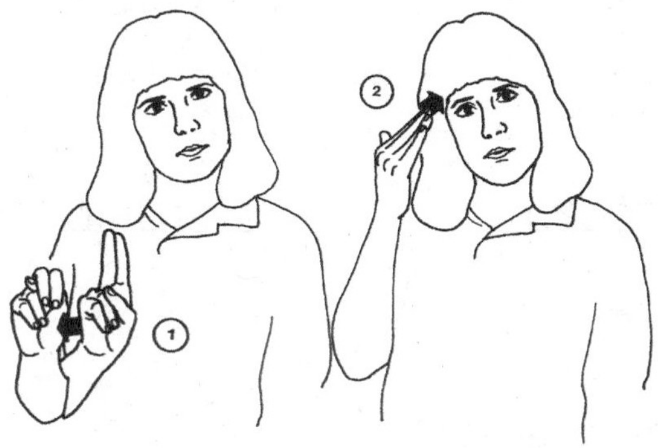

UNKNOWN?

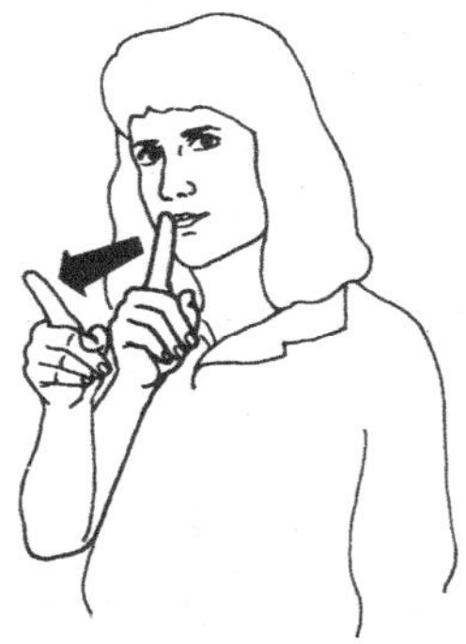

WAS

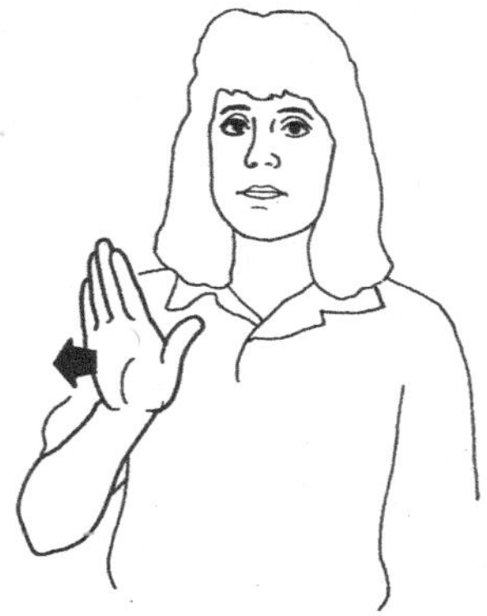

YOUR

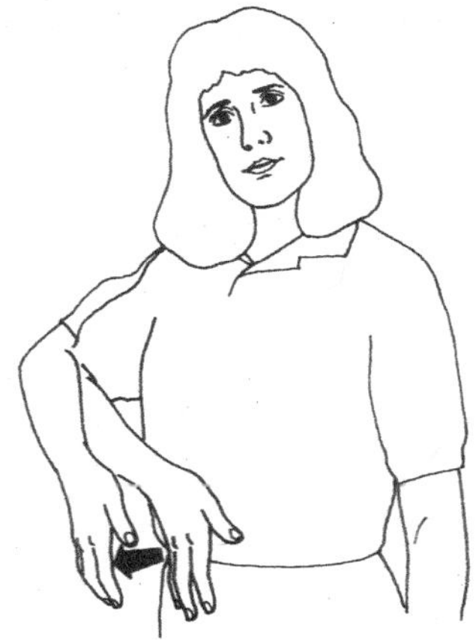

PREGNANT

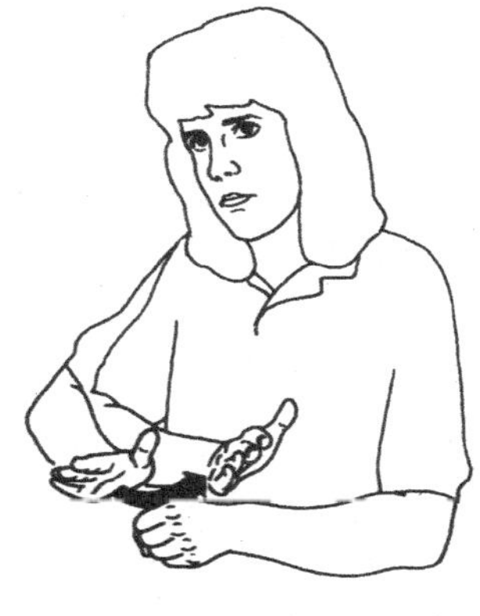

FULL

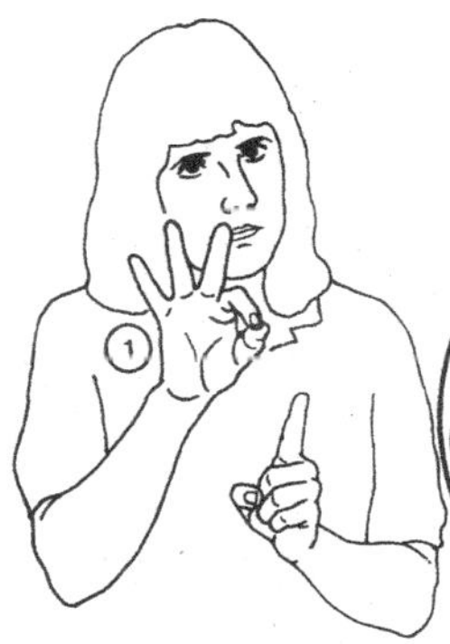

NINE

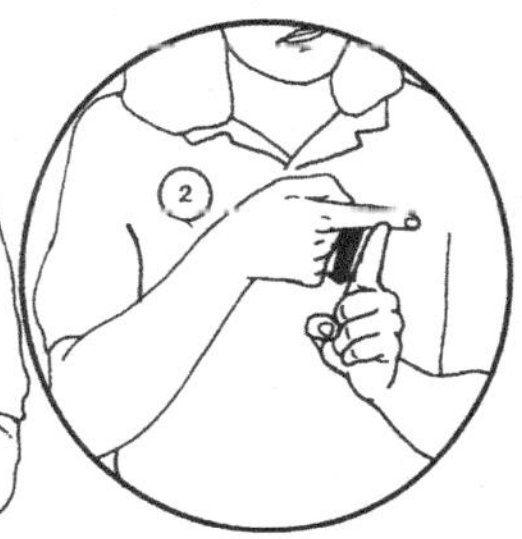

MONTH?

Was your pregnancy full term (nine months)?

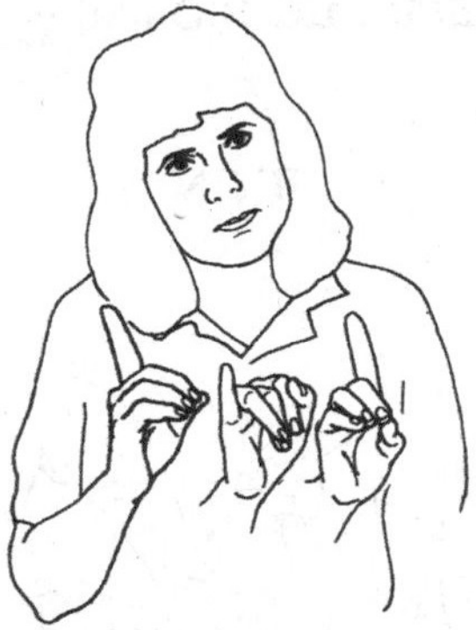

D-I-D

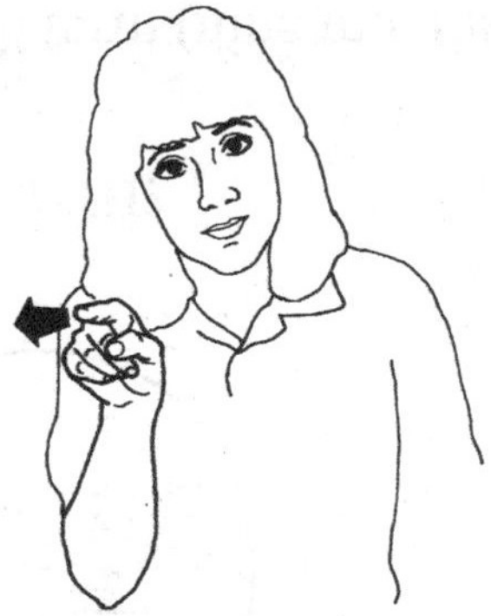

YOU

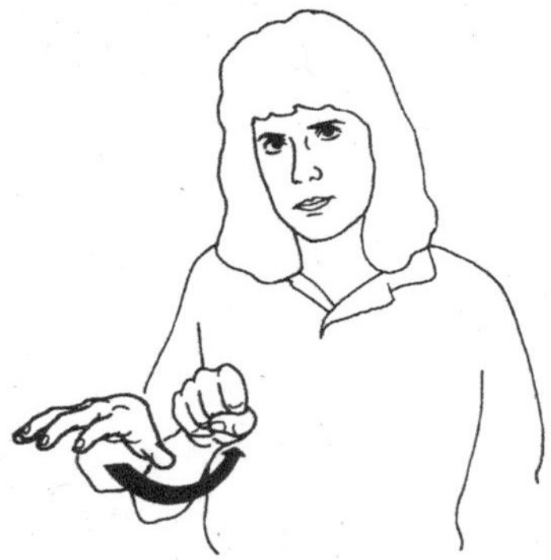

TAKE

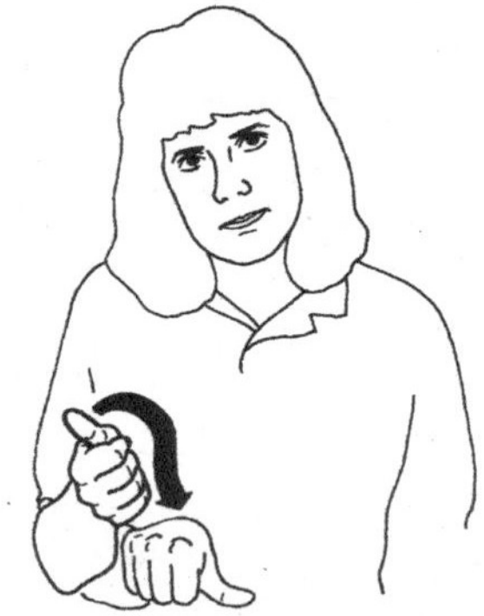

ANY

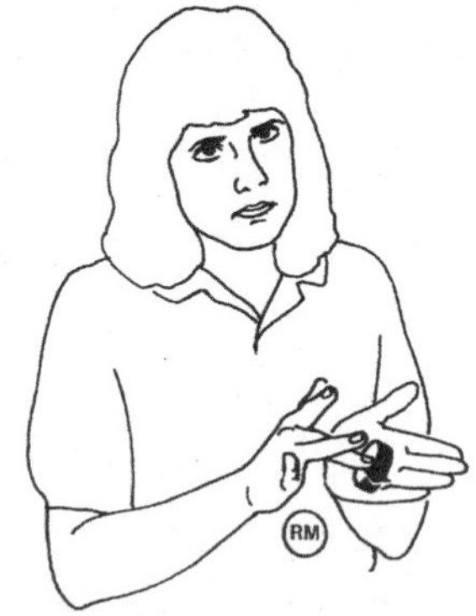

MEDICINE

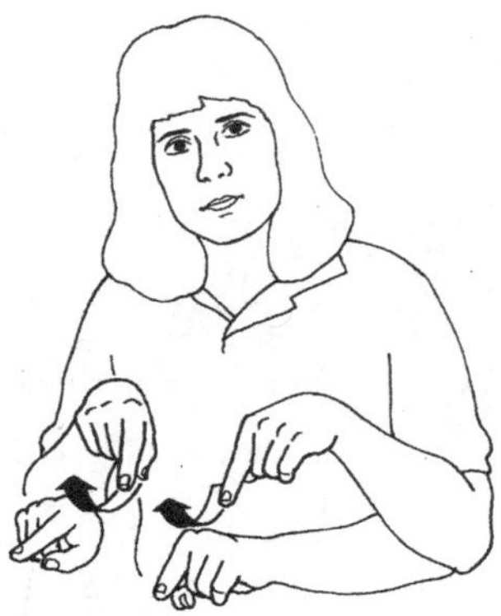

DURING

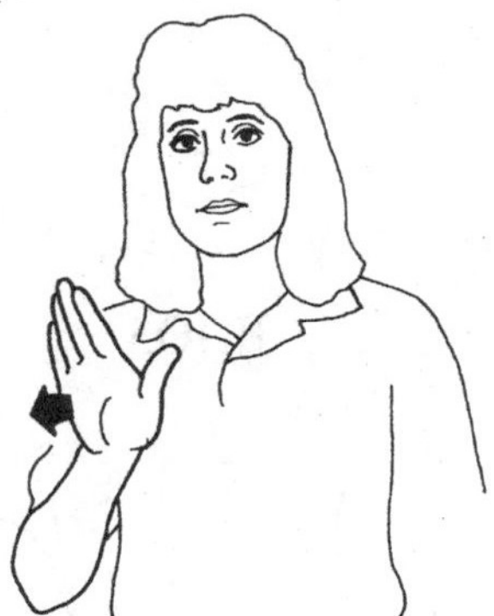

YOUR

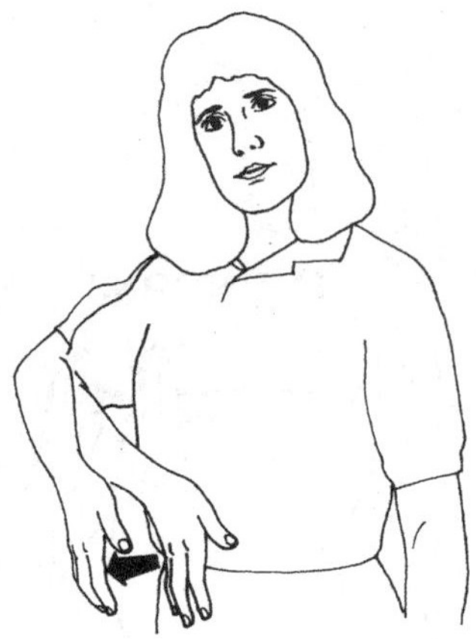

PREGNANT?

Did you take any medications during your pregnancy?

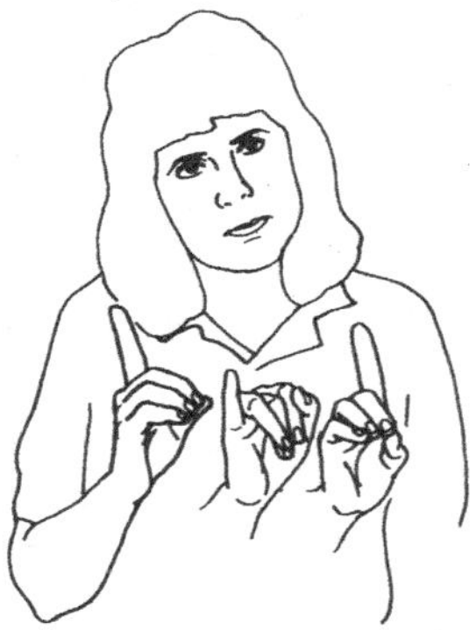

D-I-D

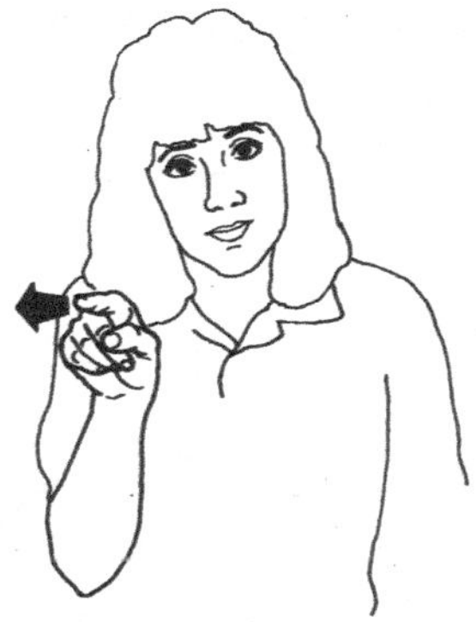

YOU

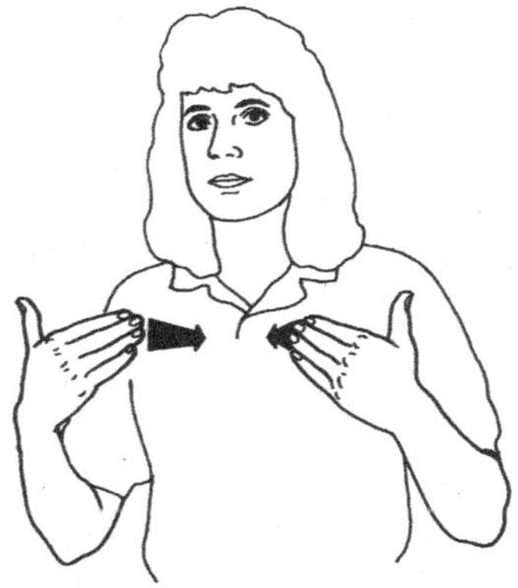

HAVE

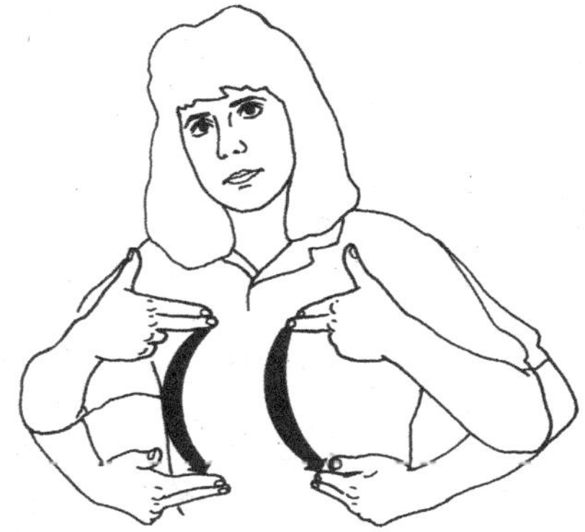

HEALTH

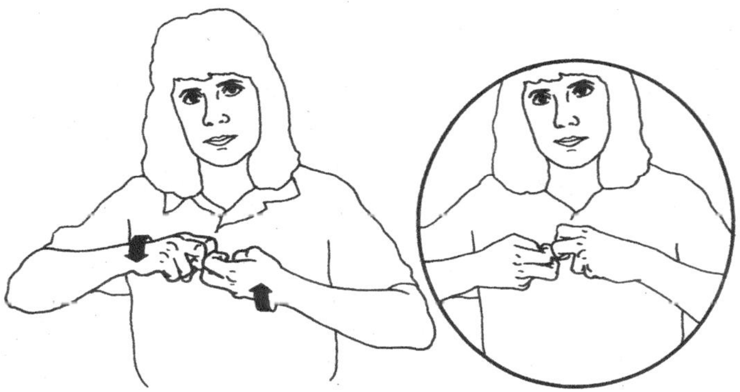

PROBLEM

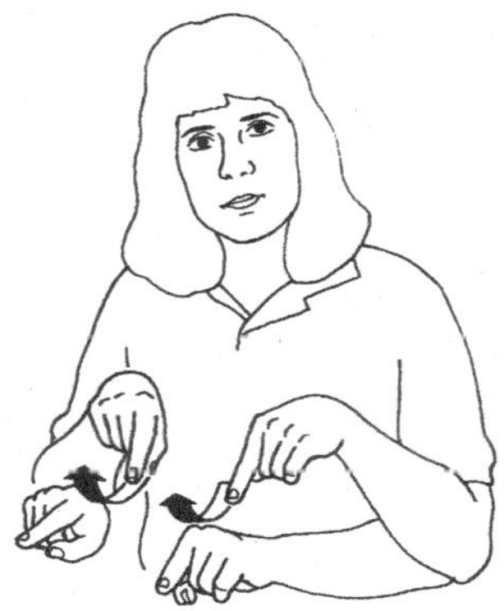

DURING

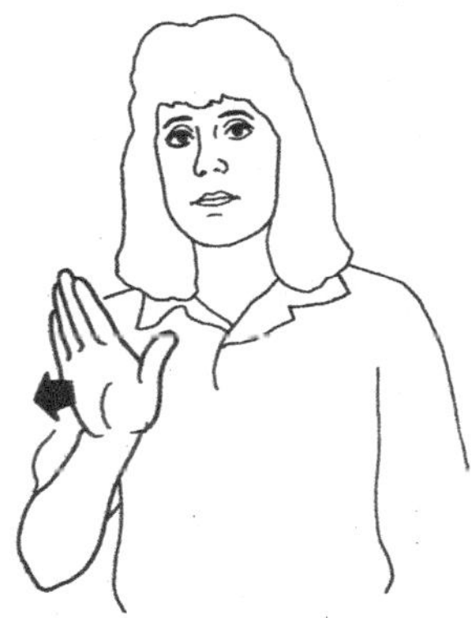

YOUR

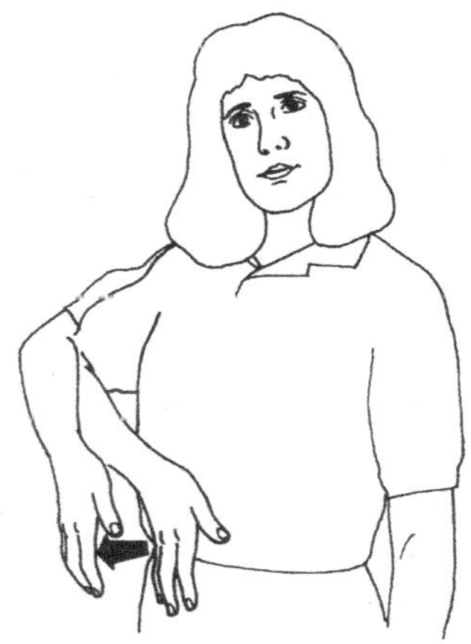

PREGNANT?

Did you have health problems during your pregnancy?

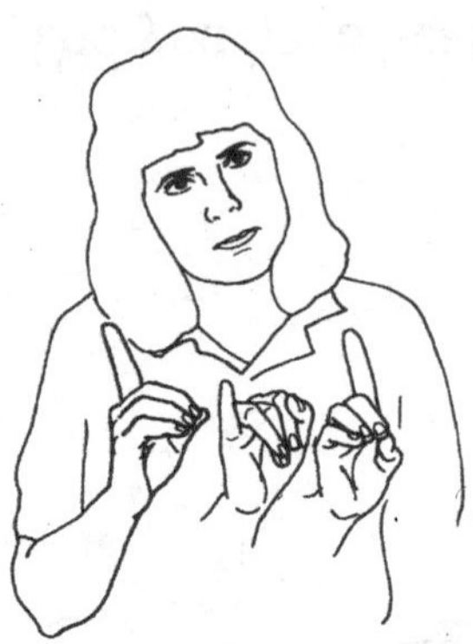

D-I-D

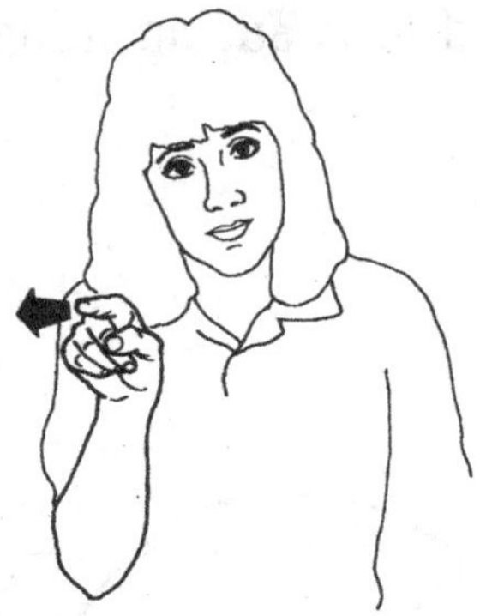

YOU

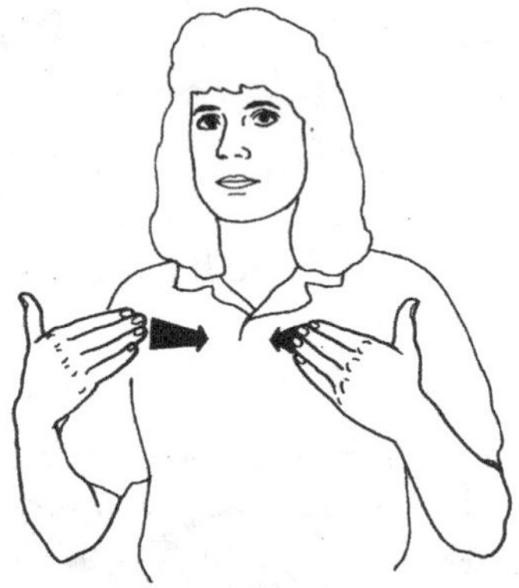

HAVE

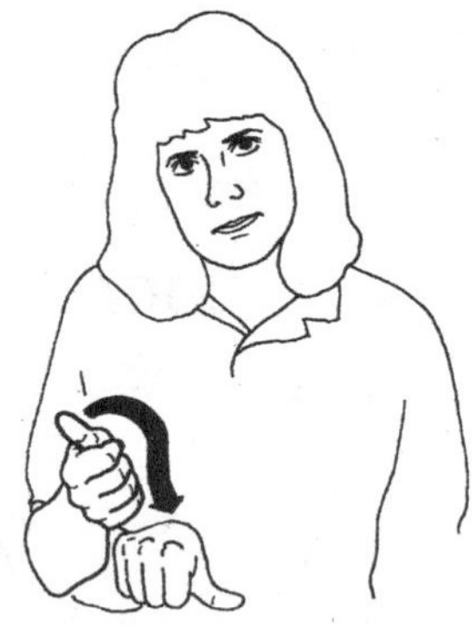

ANY

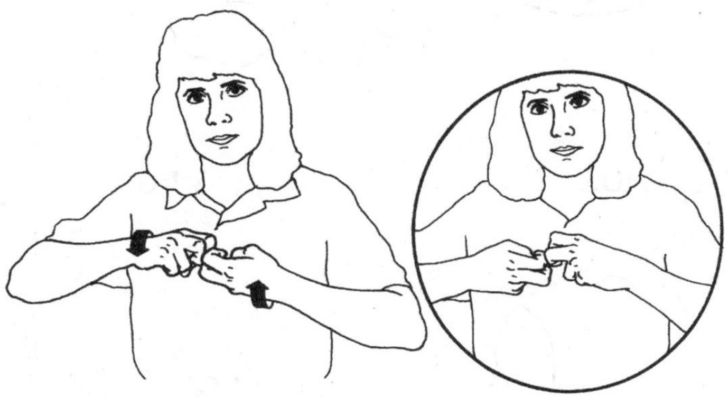

PROBLEM

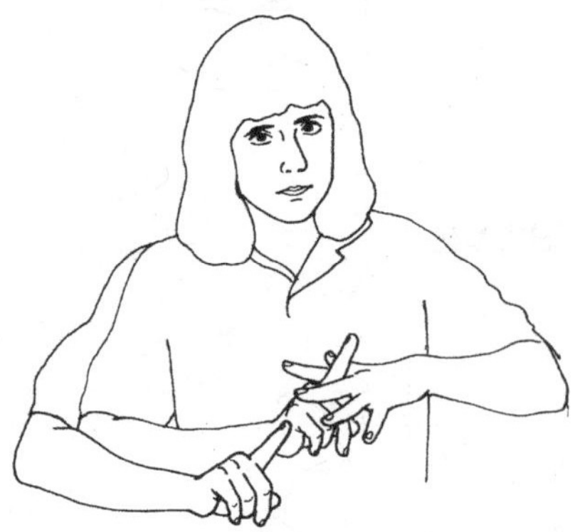

ARISE

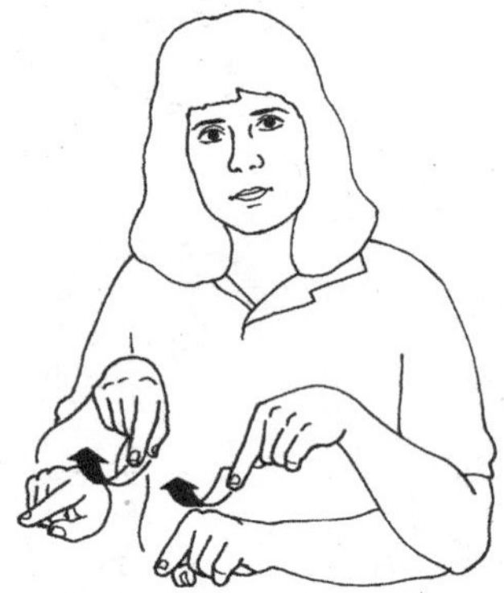

DURING

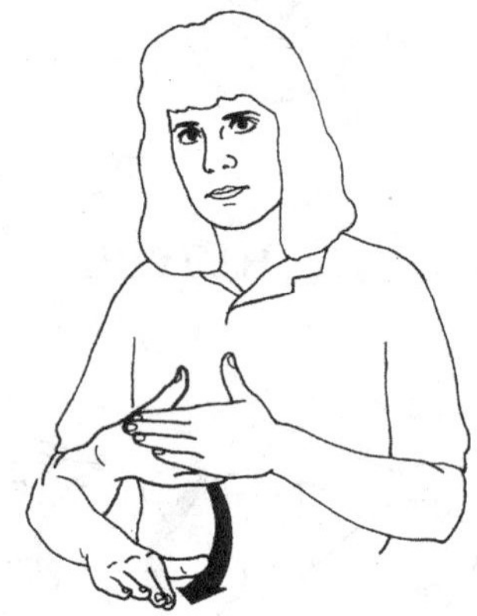

BIRTH?

Did you have any problems arise during the birth?

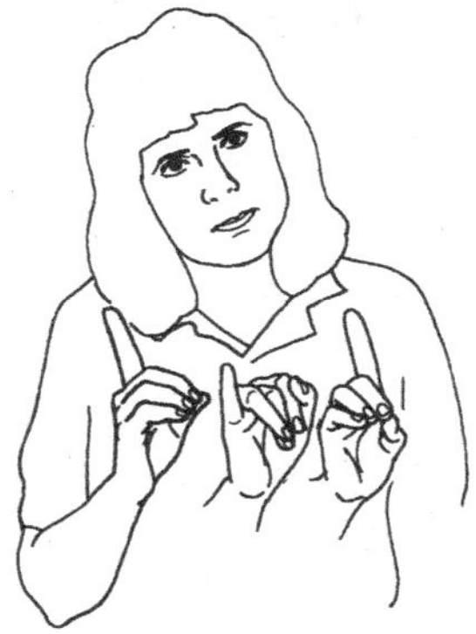

D-I-D

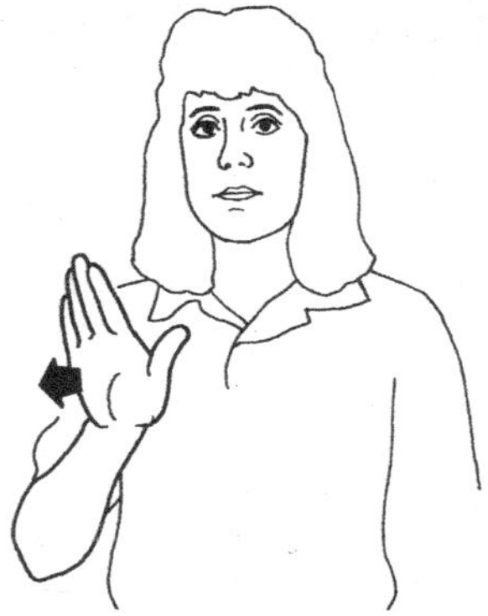

YOUR

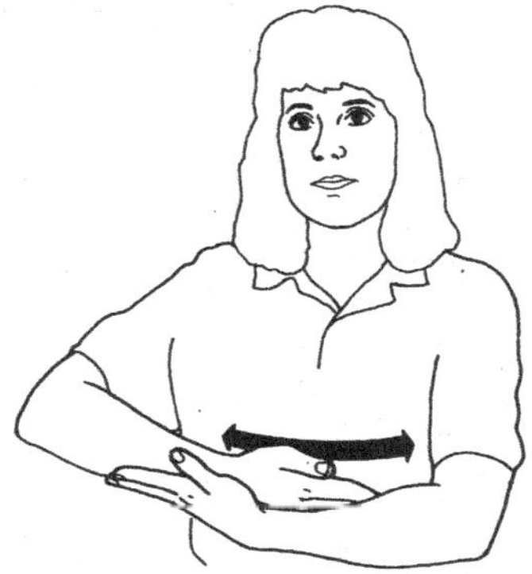

BABY

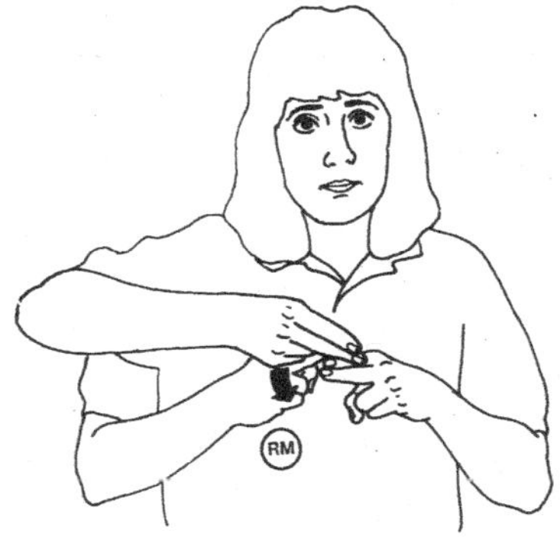

WEIGH

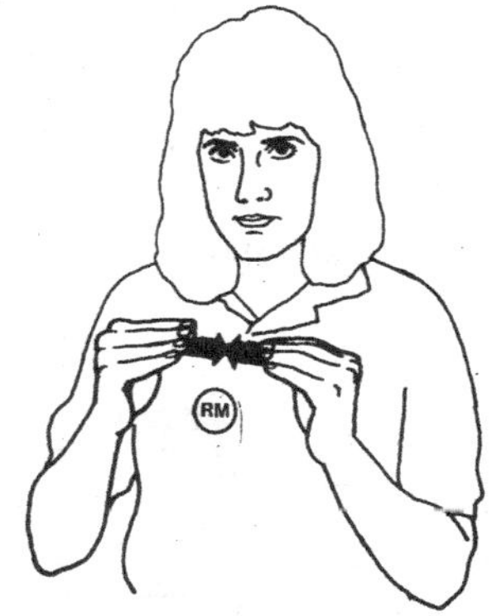

MORE

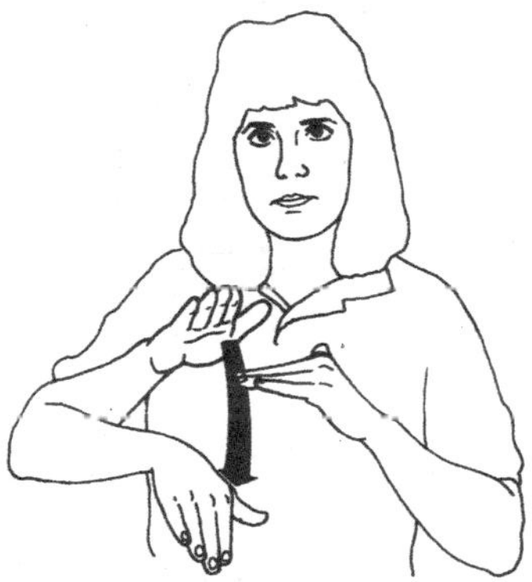

THAN

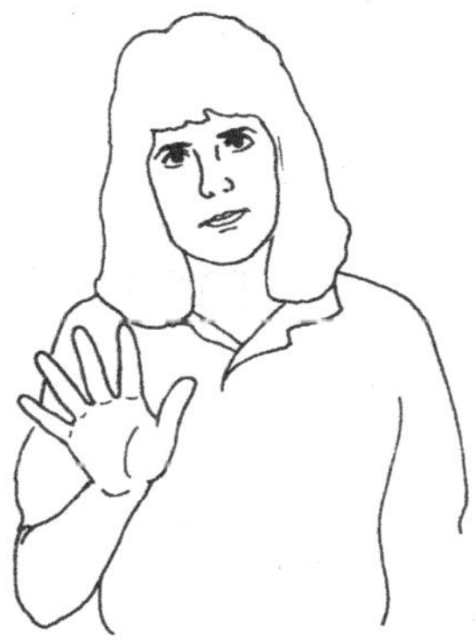

FIVE

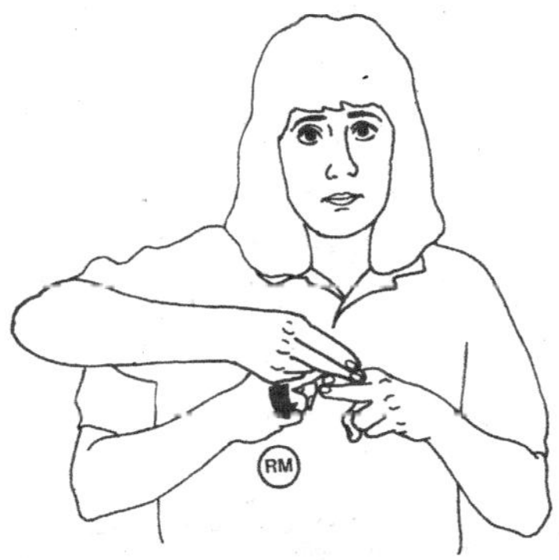

POUND

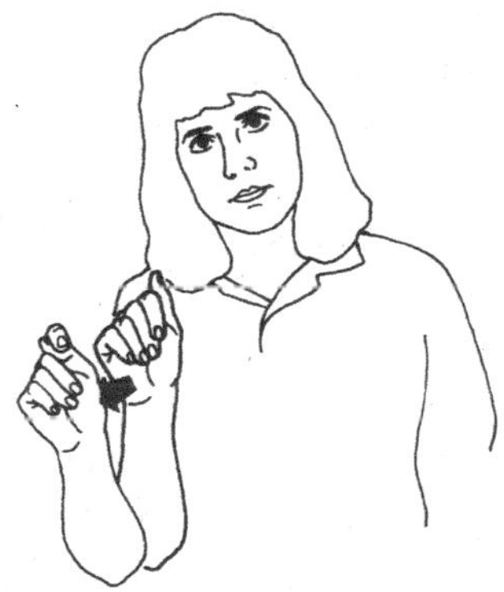

A-T

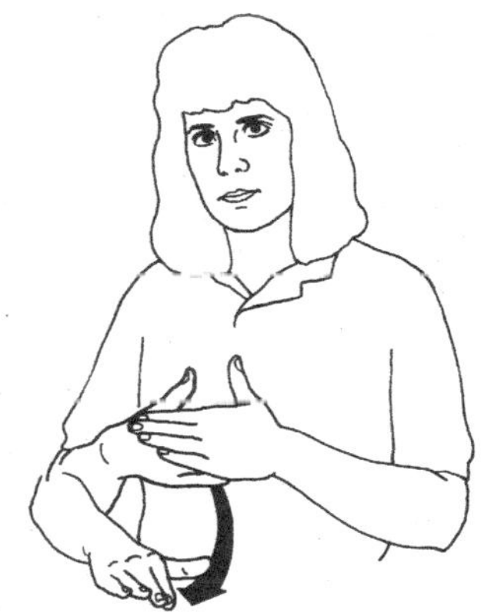

BIRTH?

Did your baby weigh more than five pounds at birth?

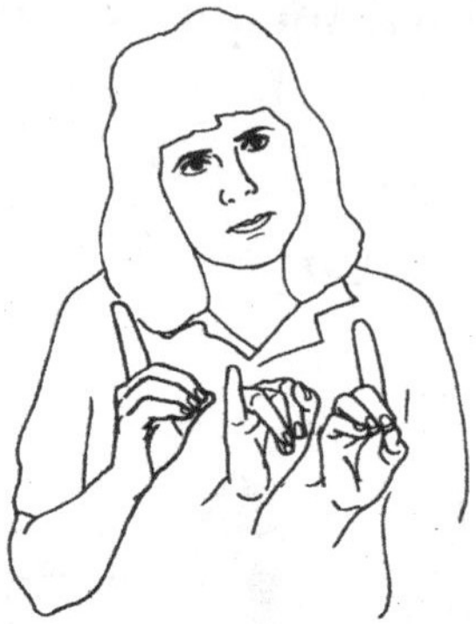

D-I-D

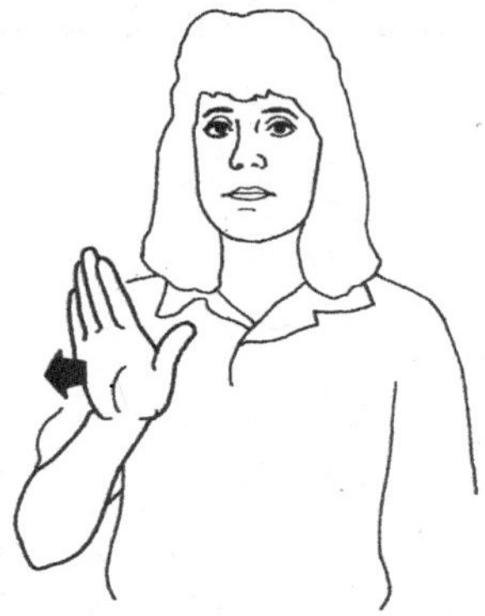

YOUR

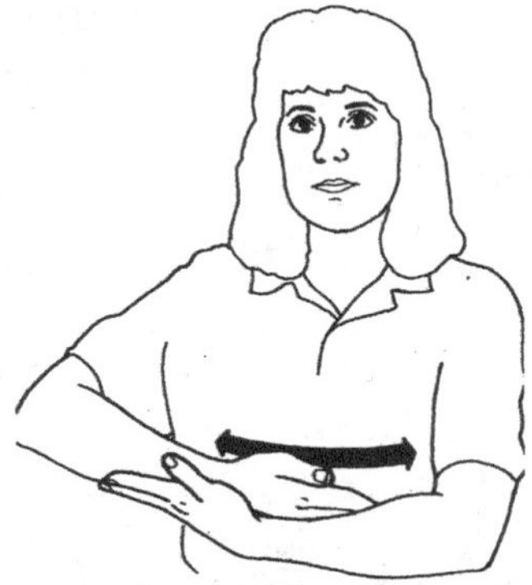

BABY

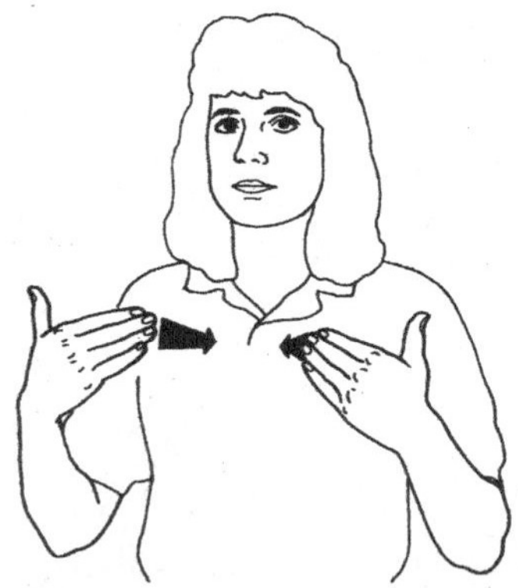

HAVE

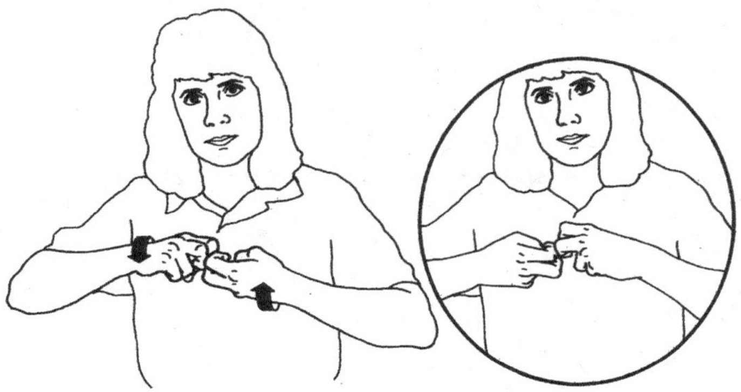

DIFFICULT

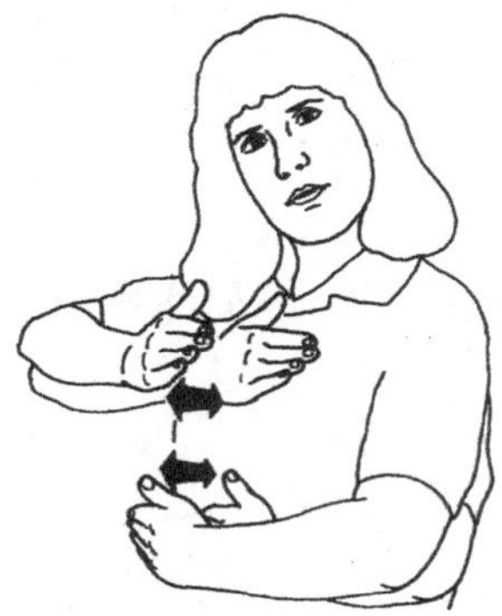

BREATHE

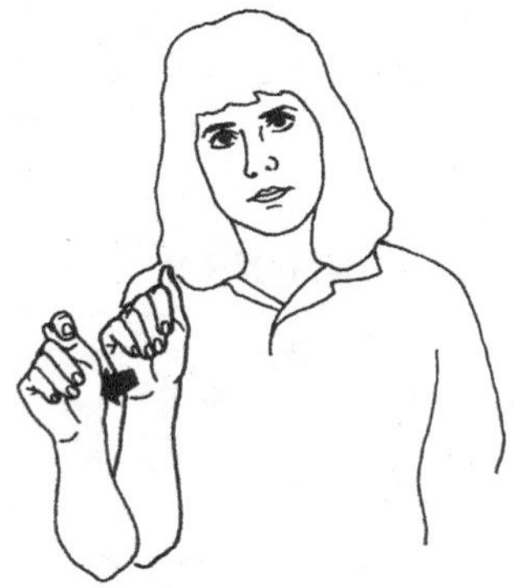

A-T

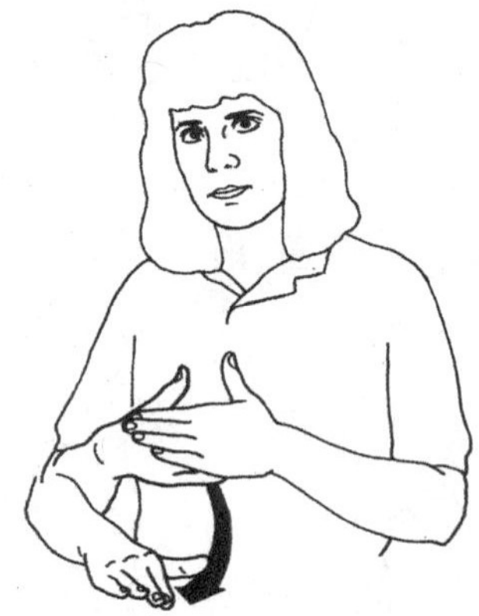

BIRTH?

Did your baby have difficulty breathing at birth?

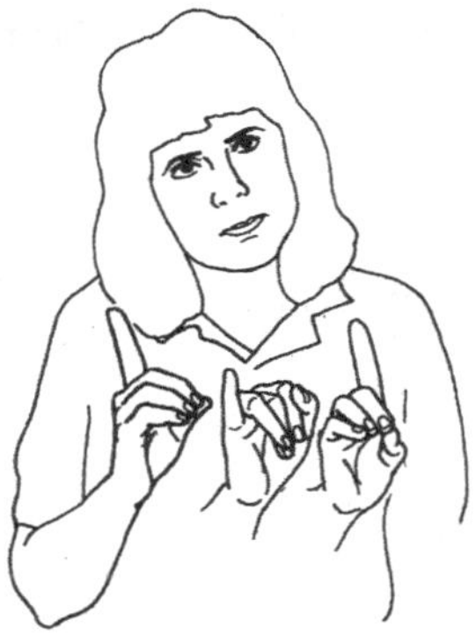

D-I-D

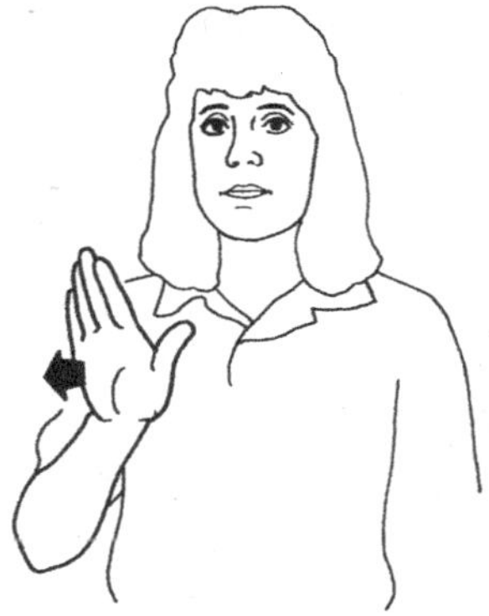

YOUR

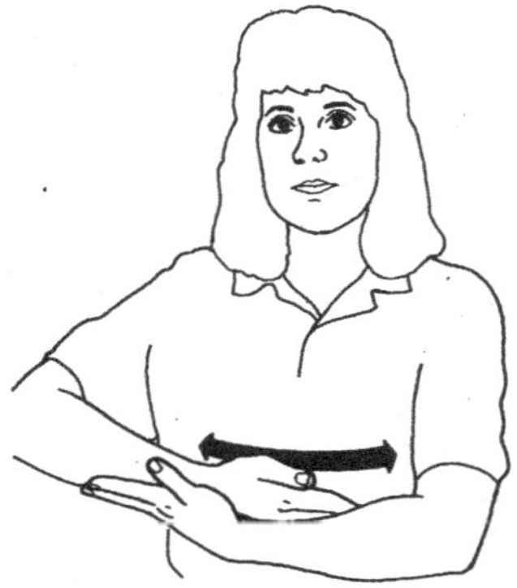

BABY

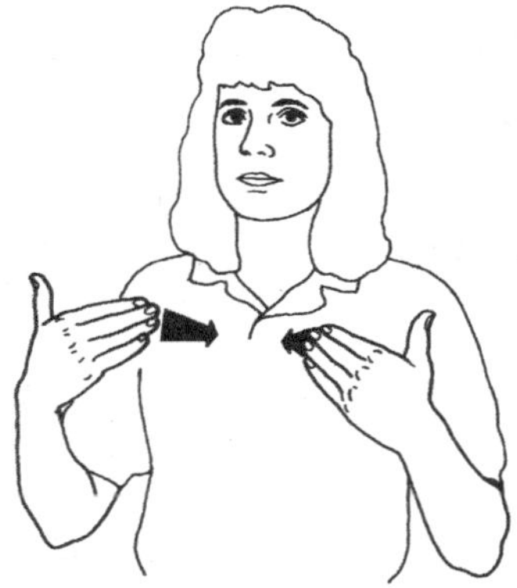

HAVE

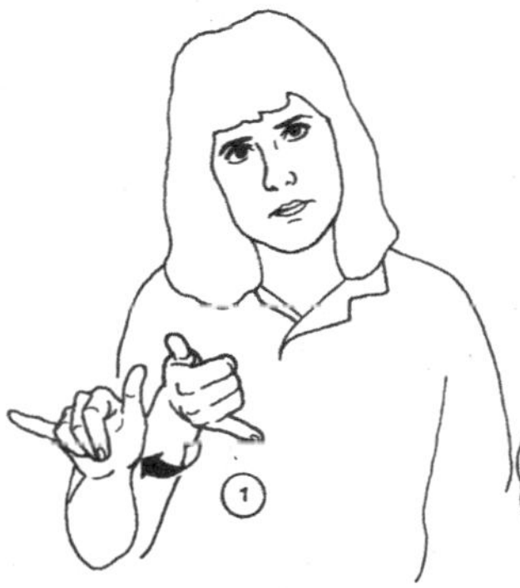

YELLOW

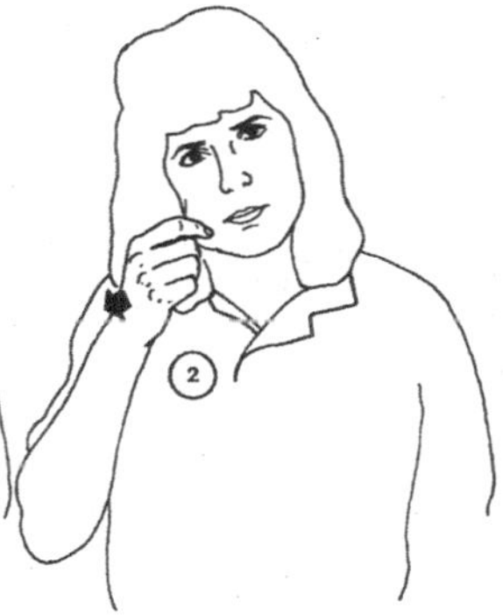

SKIN

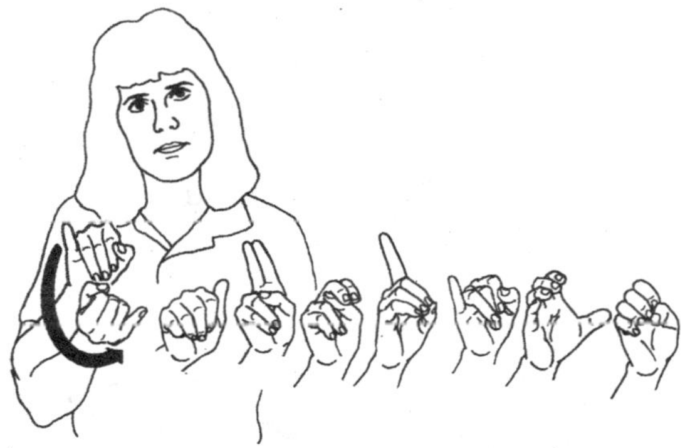

J-A-U-N-D-I-C-E?

Did your baby have jaundice?

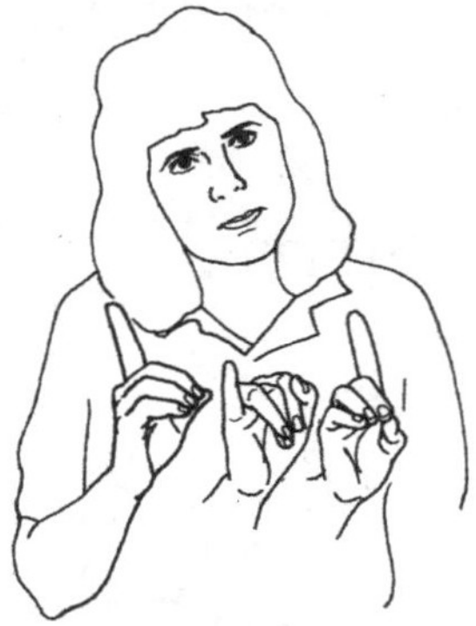

D-I-D

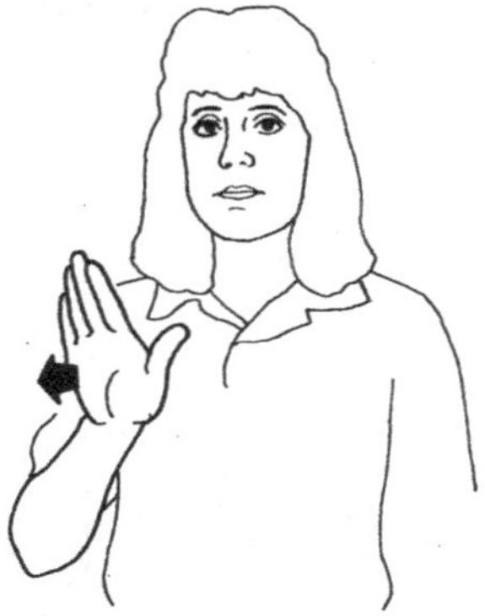

YOUR

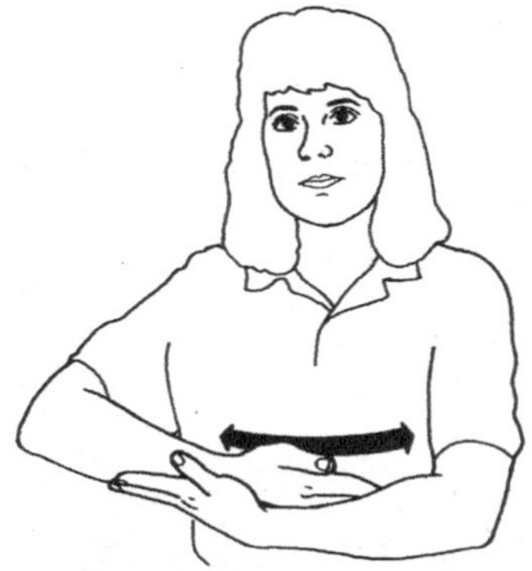

BABY

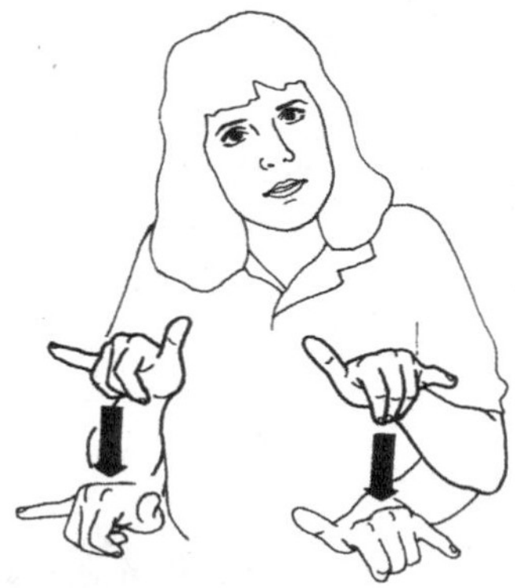

STAY

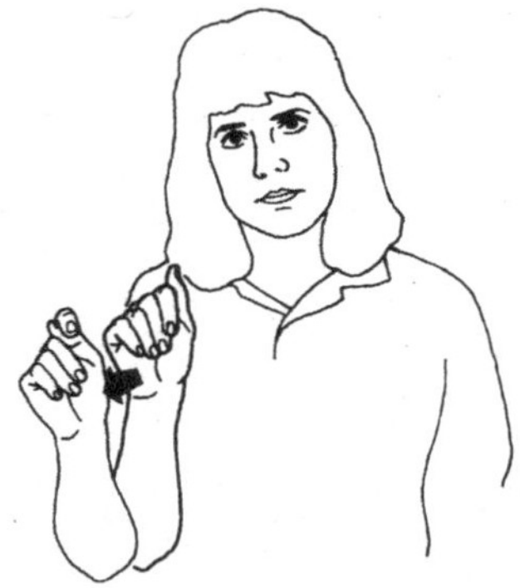

A-T

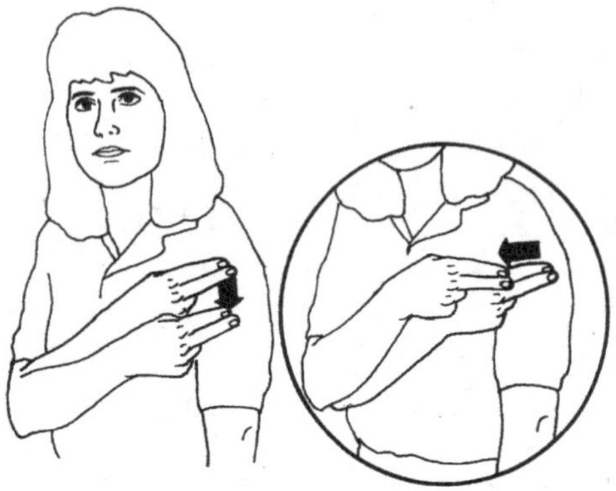

HOSPITAL

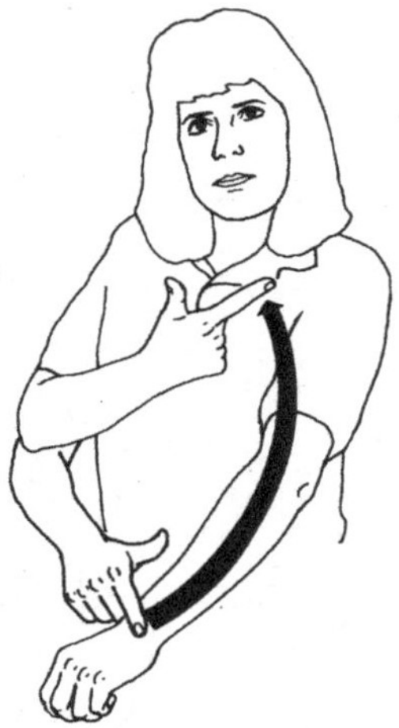

LONG

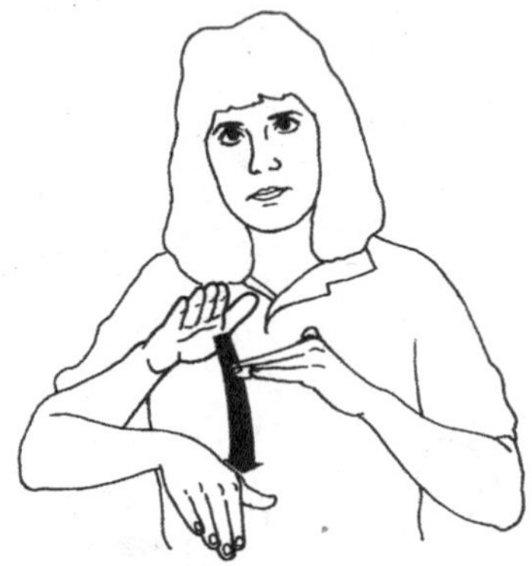

THAN

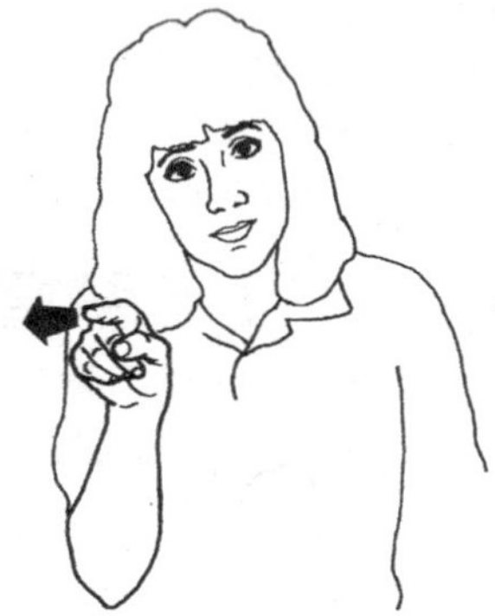

YOU?

Did your baby stay in the hospital longer than you?

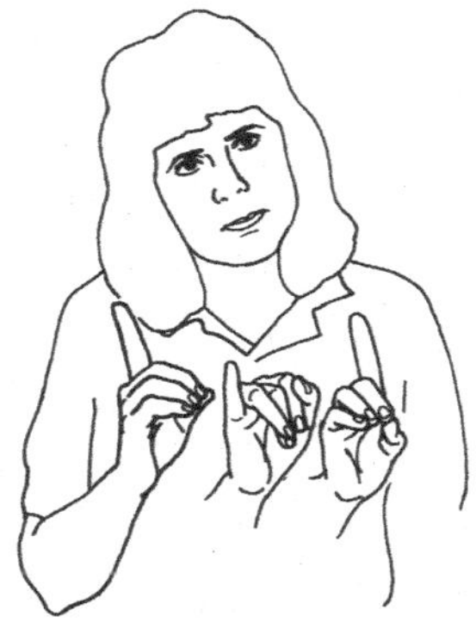

D-I-D

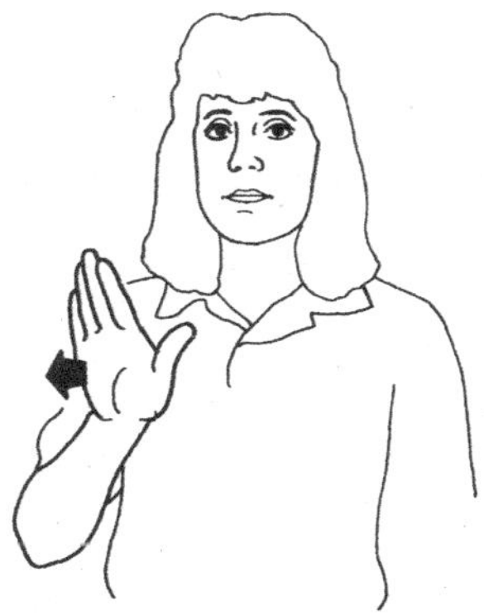

YOUR

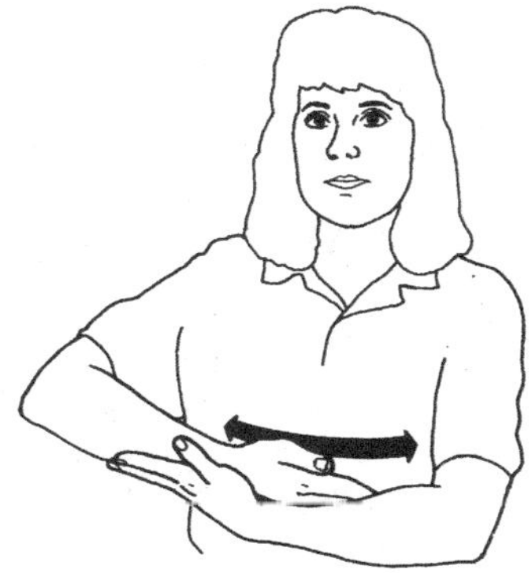

BABY

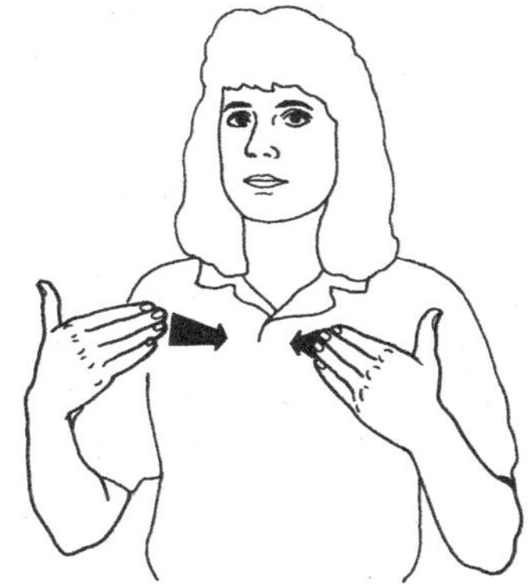

HAVE

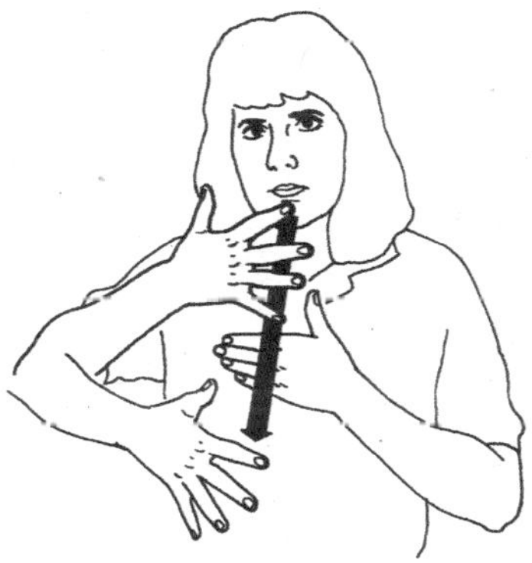

BLOOD

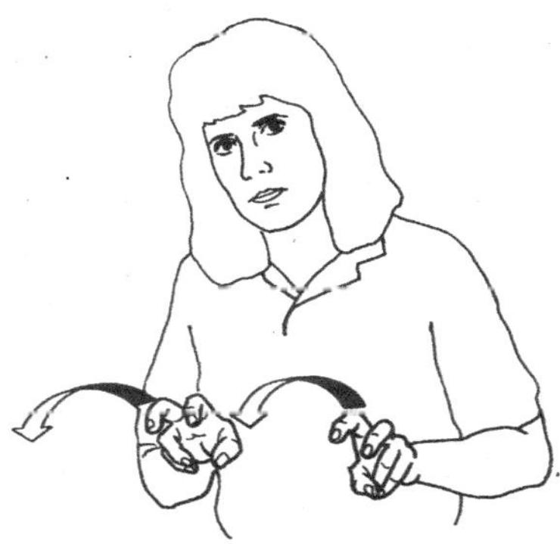

TRANSFUSION?

Did your baby have blood transfusions?

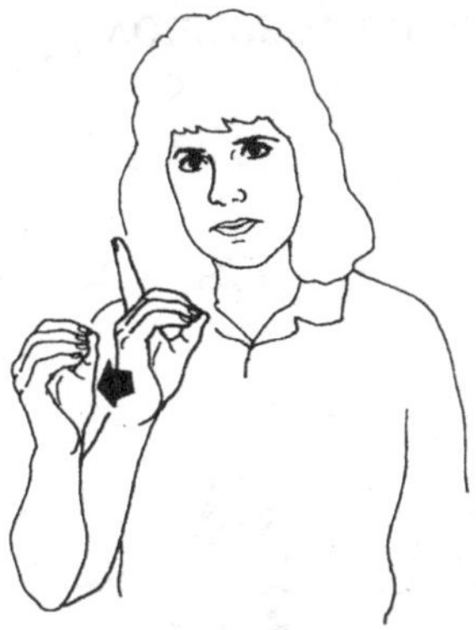

D-O

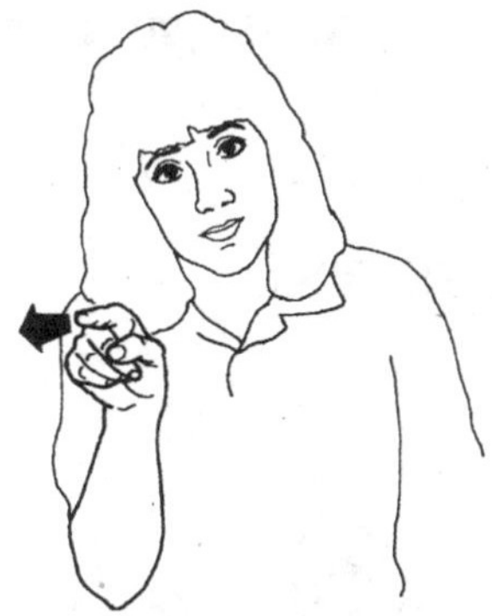

YOU

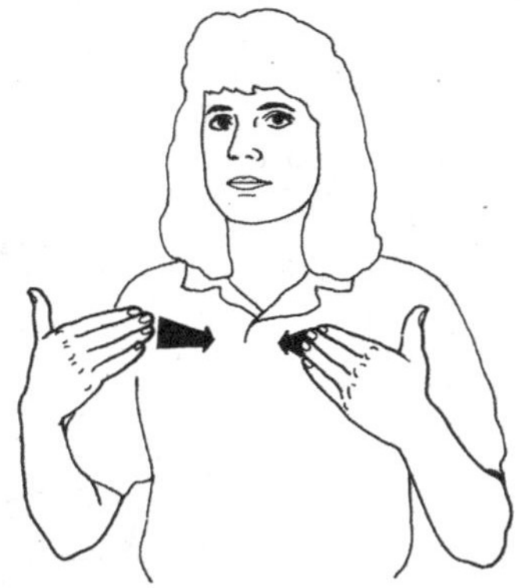

HAVE

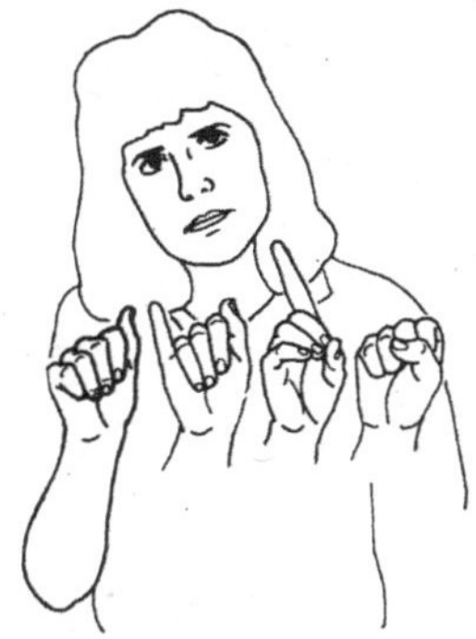

A-I-D-S?

Do you have AIDS?

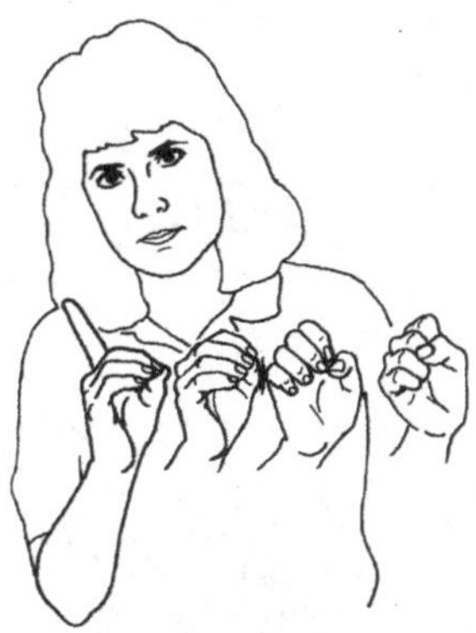

D-O-E-S

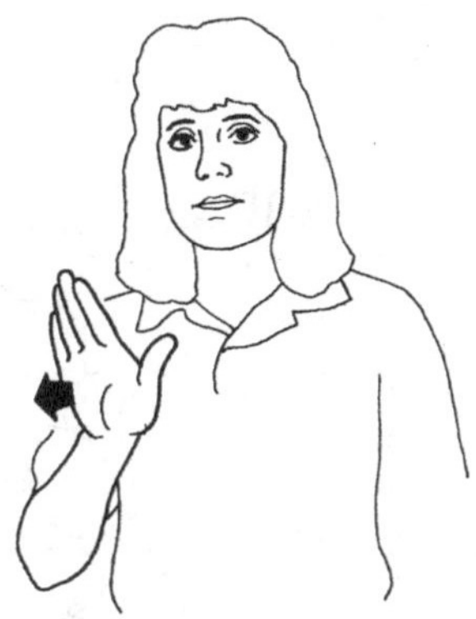

YOUR

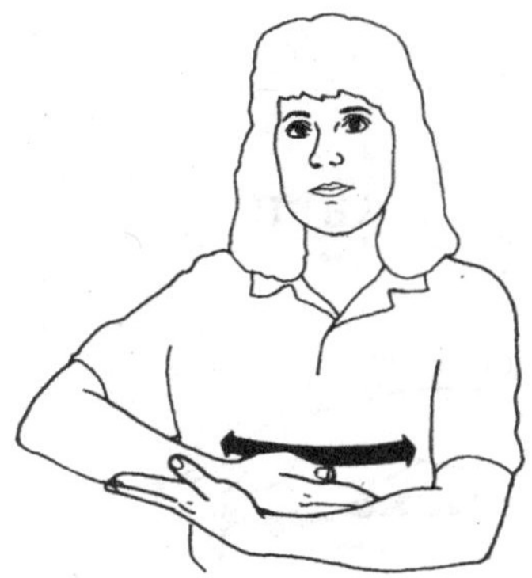

BABY

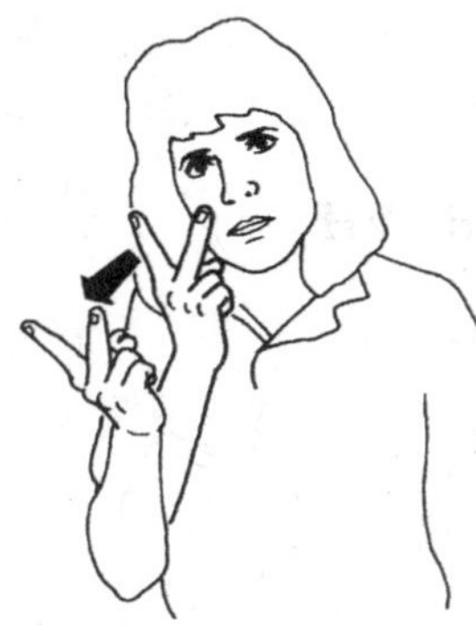

SEE

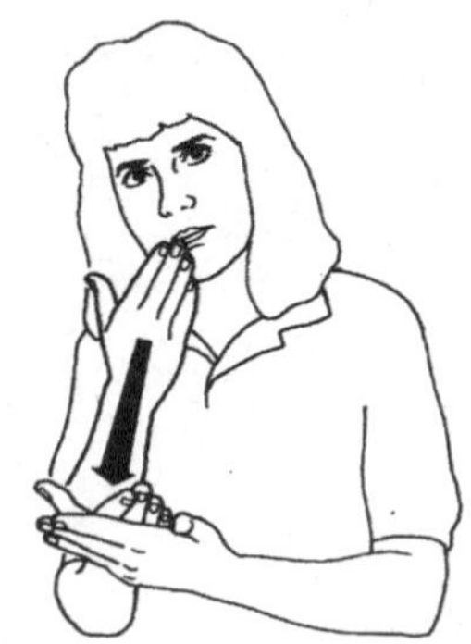

WELL?

Does your baby see well?

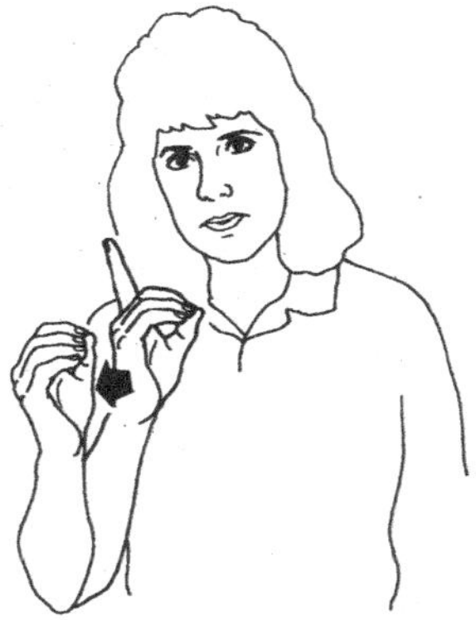

D-O

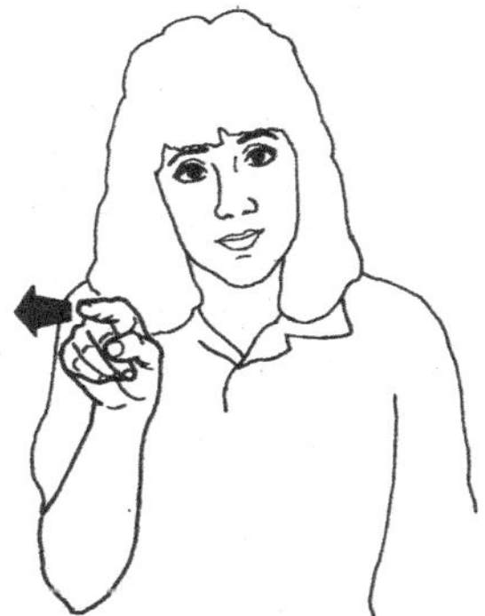

YOU

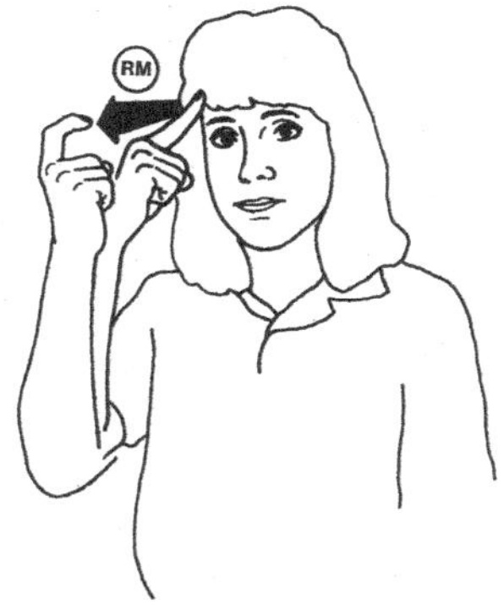

SUSPECT

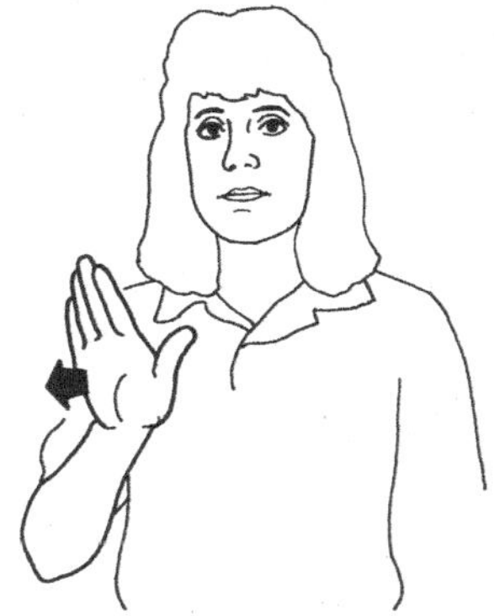

YOUR

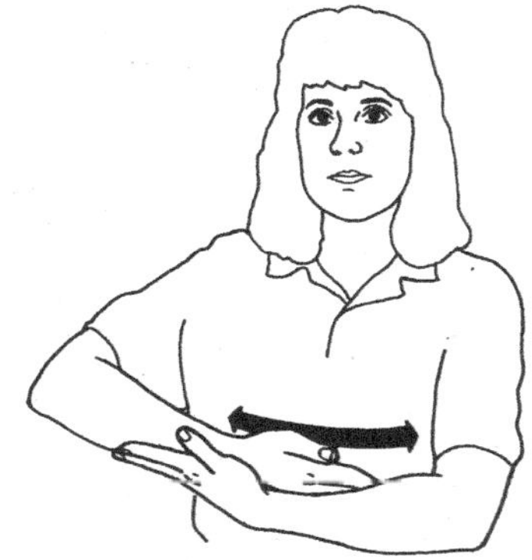

BABY

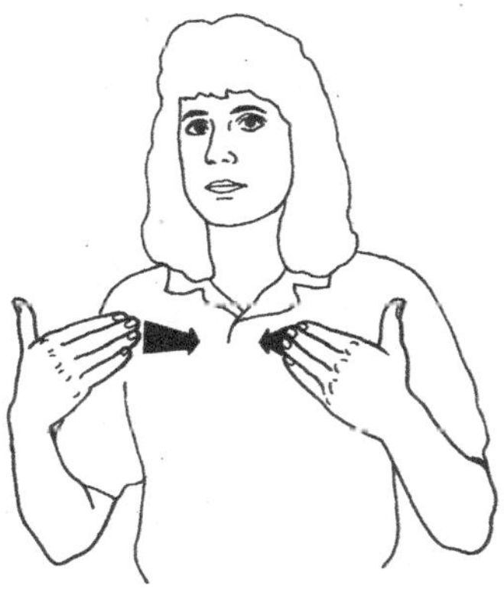

HAVE

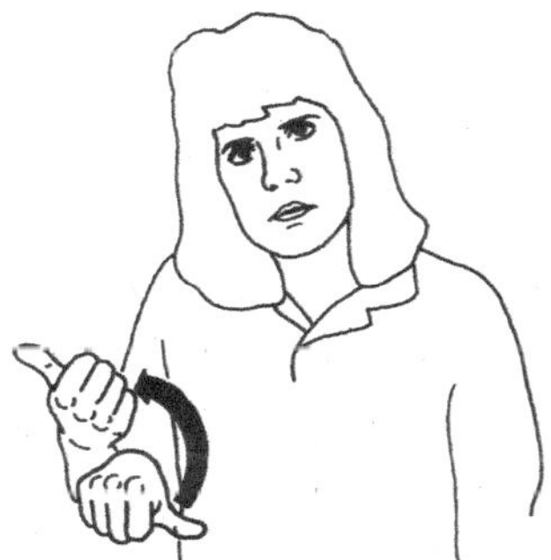

OTHER

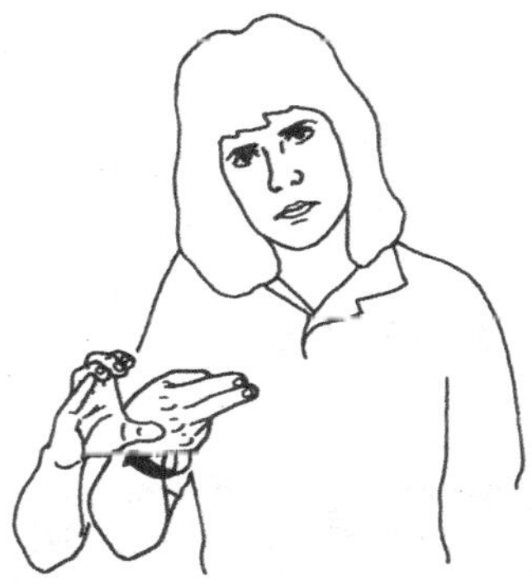

H-C

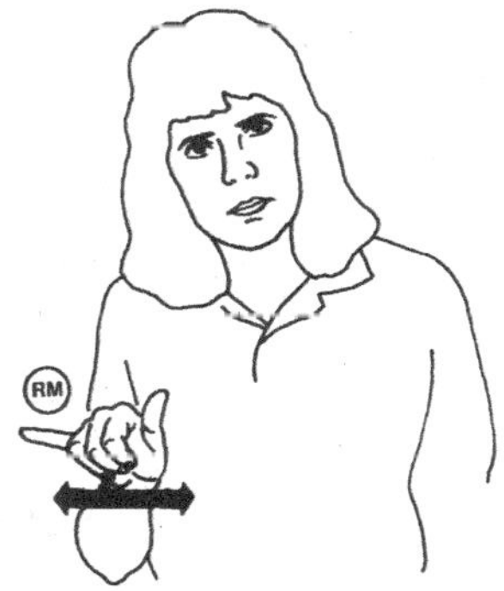

LIKE

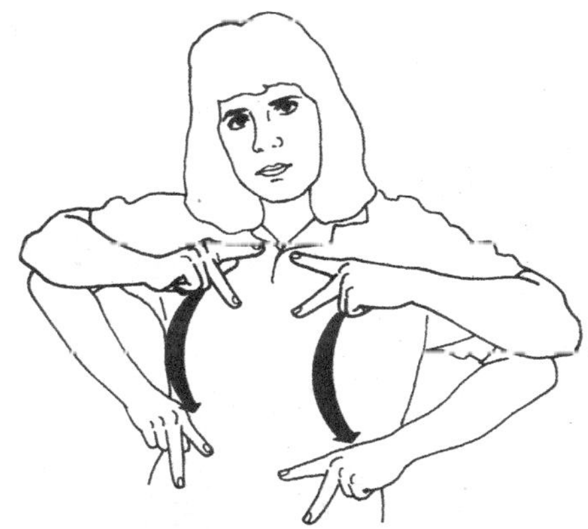

PHYSICAL

Do you suspect your baby has other handicaps, like physical, mental, or behavior problems?

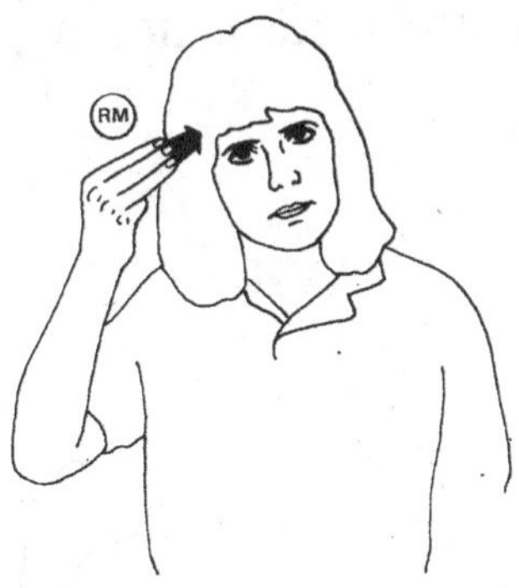

MENTAL

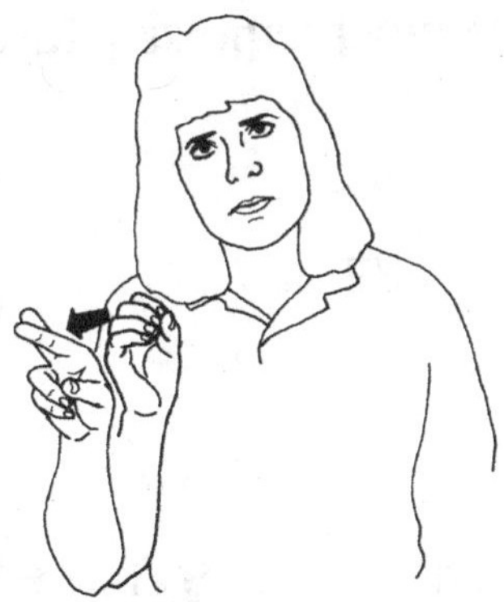

O-R

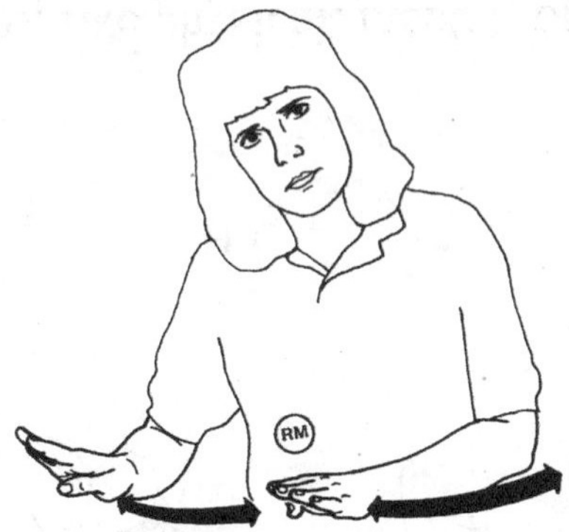

BEHAVIOR

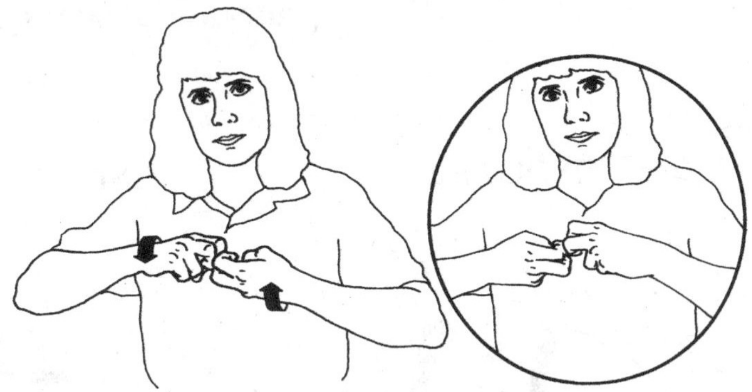

PROBLEM?

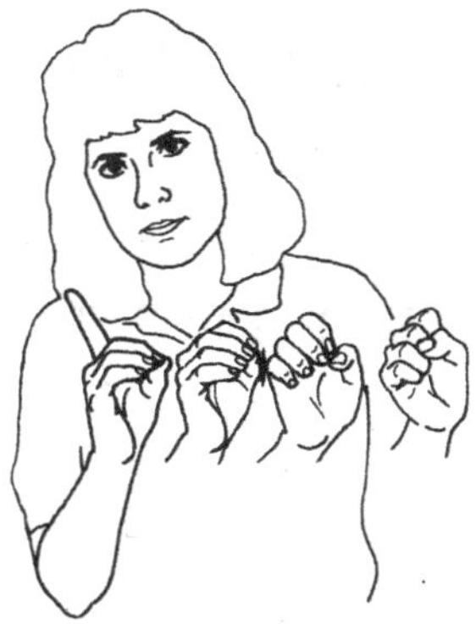

D-O-E-S

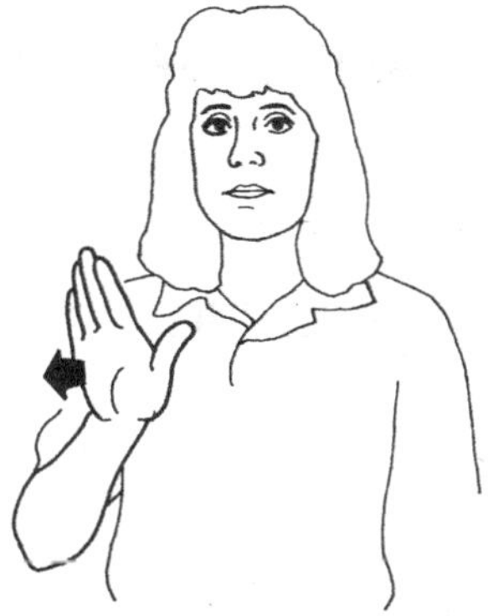

YOUR

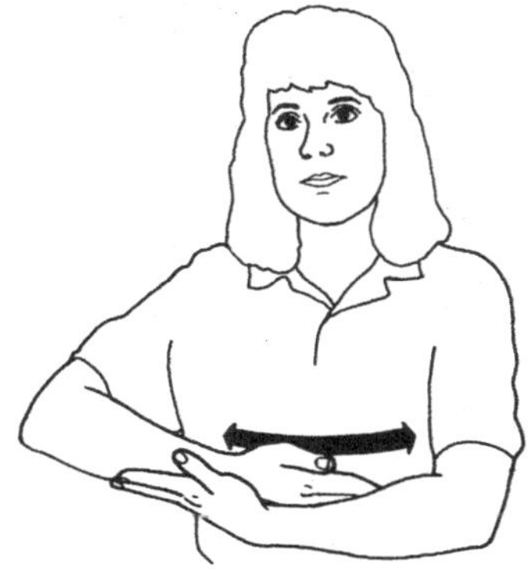

BABY

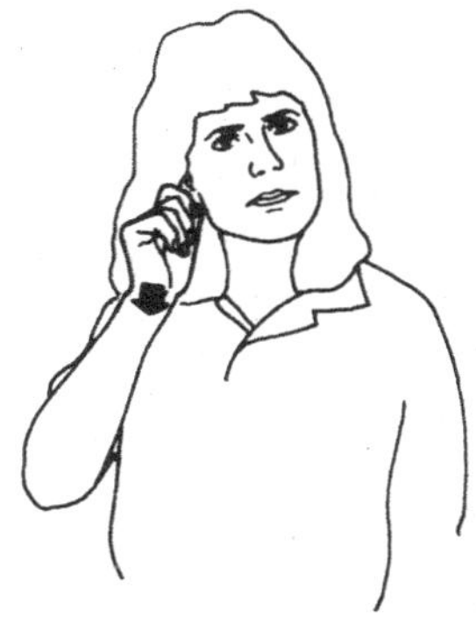

PULL-EAR

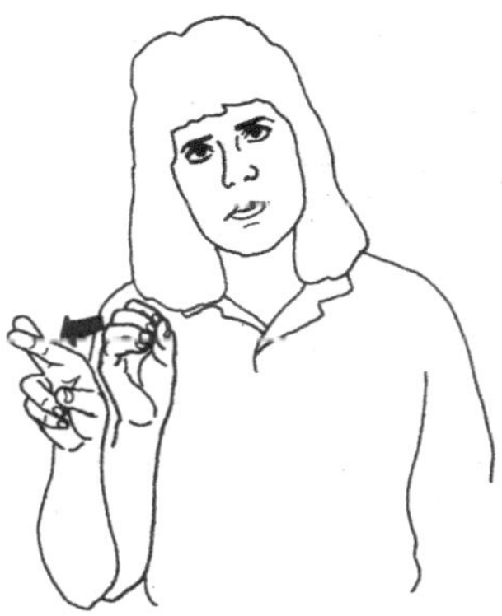

O-R

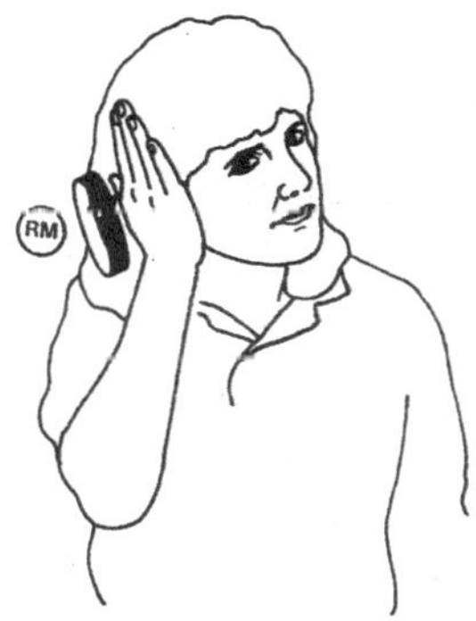

RUB-EAR?

Does your baby pull or rub his or her ears?

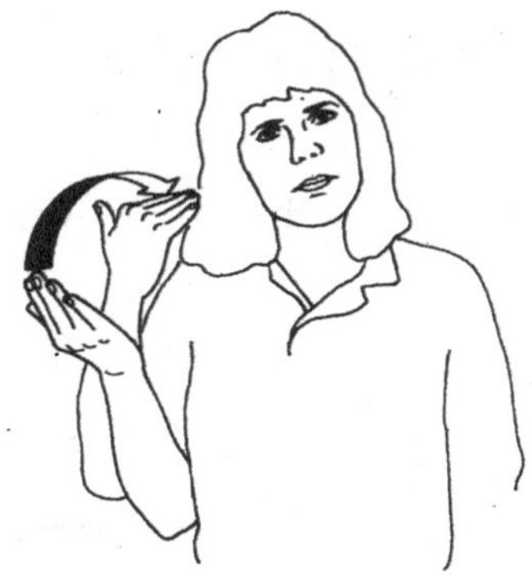

PAST

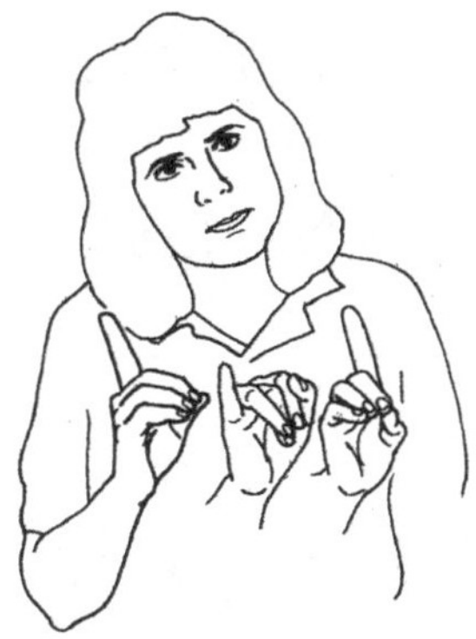

D-I-D

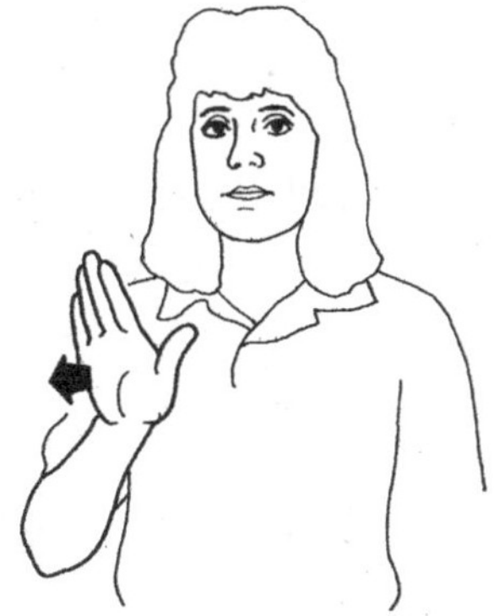

YOUR

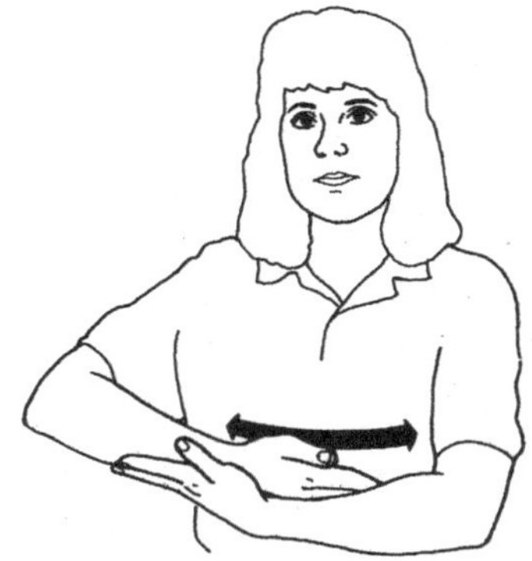

BABY

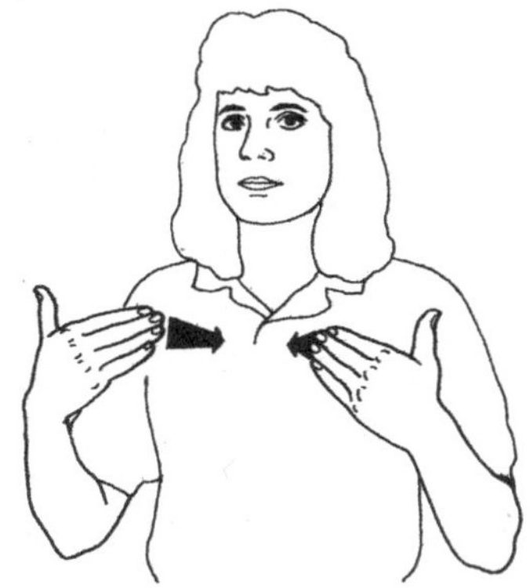

HAVE

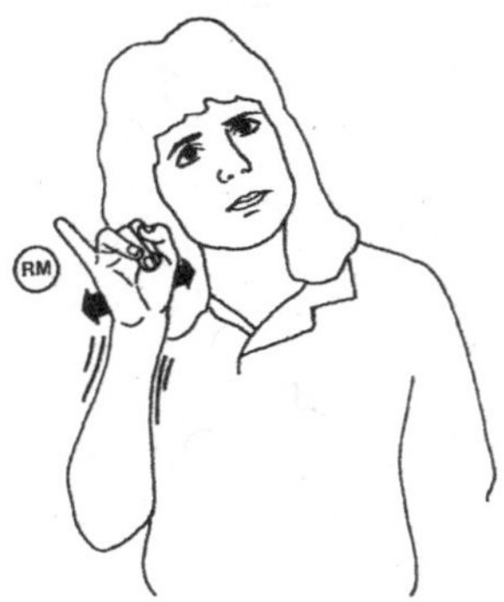

EAR-INFECTION

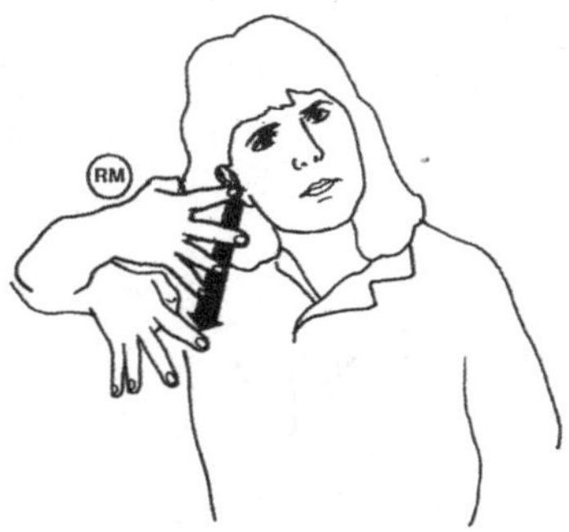

DRAINAGE?

In the past did your baby have ear infections/drainage?

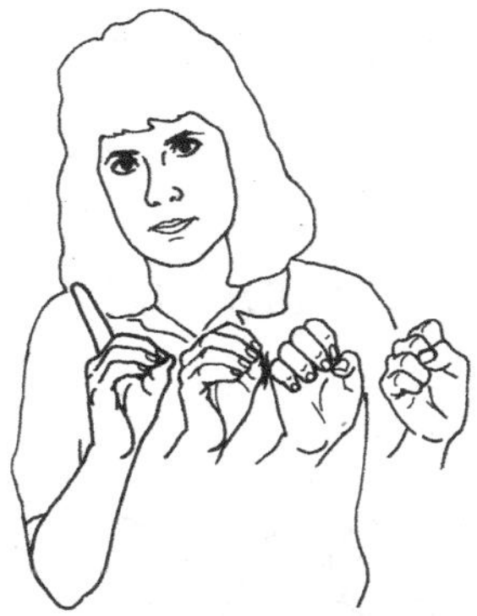

D-O-E-S

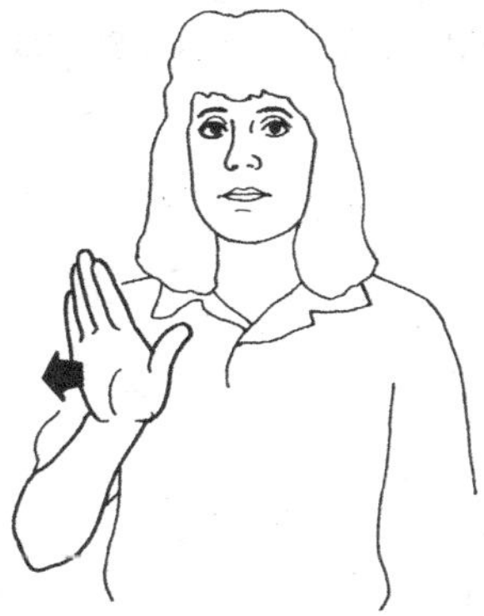

YOUR

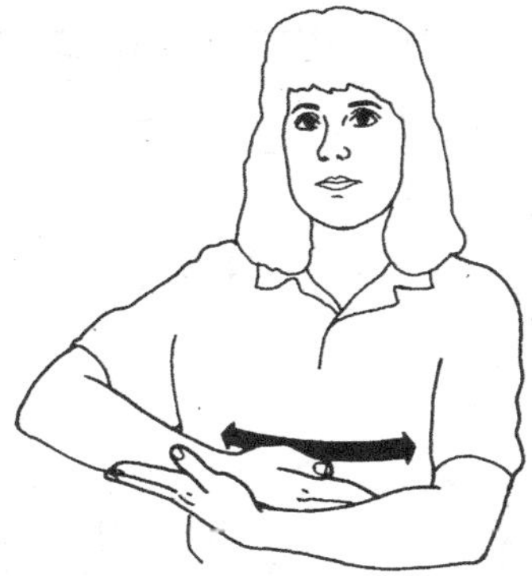

BABY

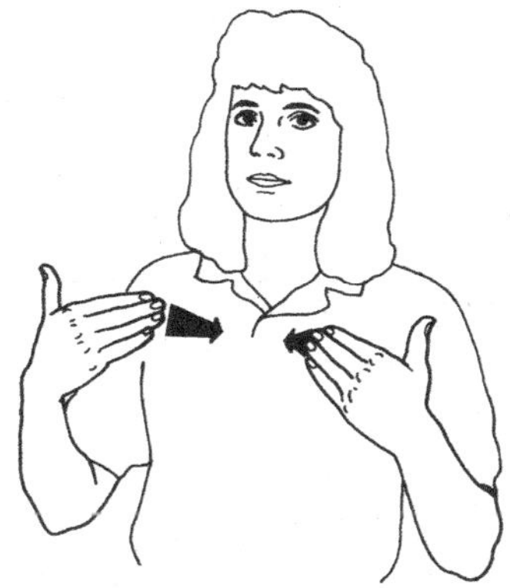

HAVE

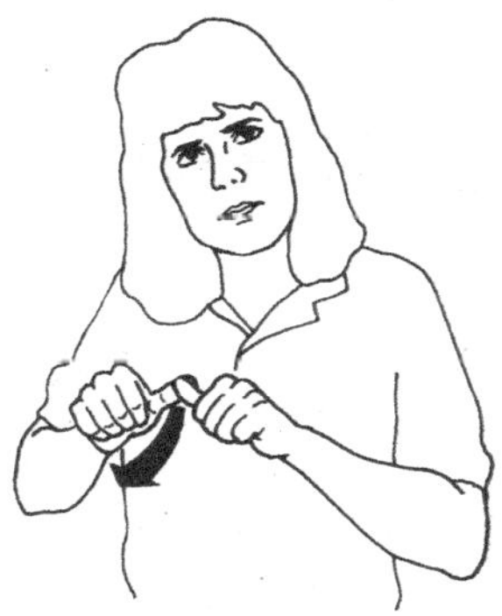

CONSTANT

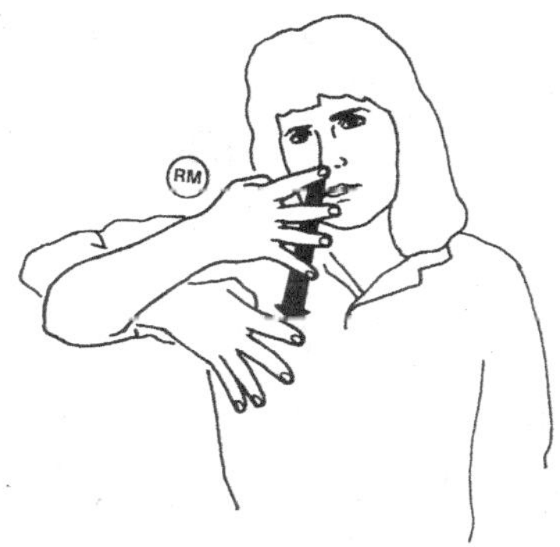

RUNNY-NOSE?

Does your baby have a constant runny nose?

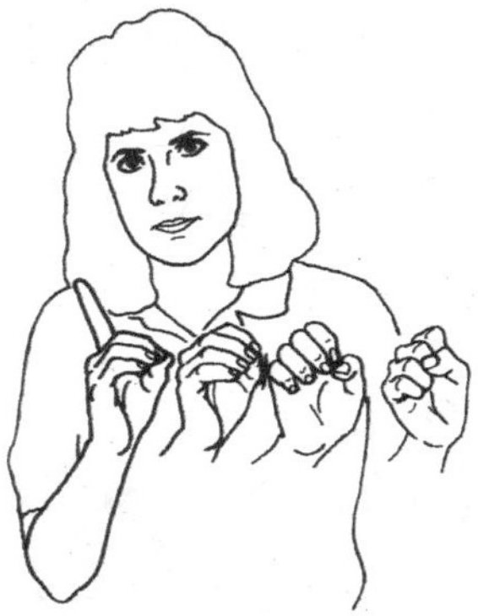

D-O-E-S

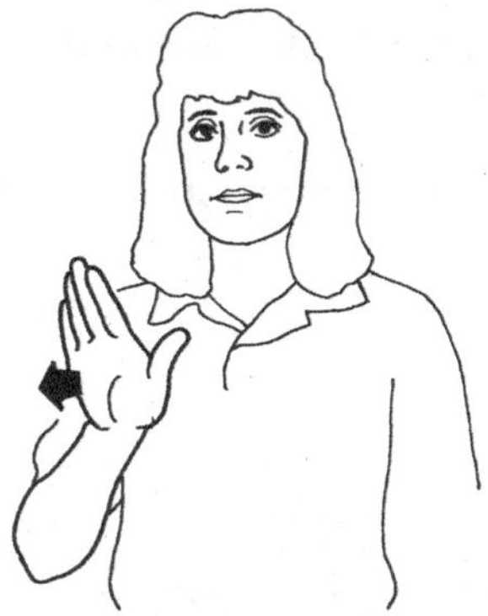

YOUR

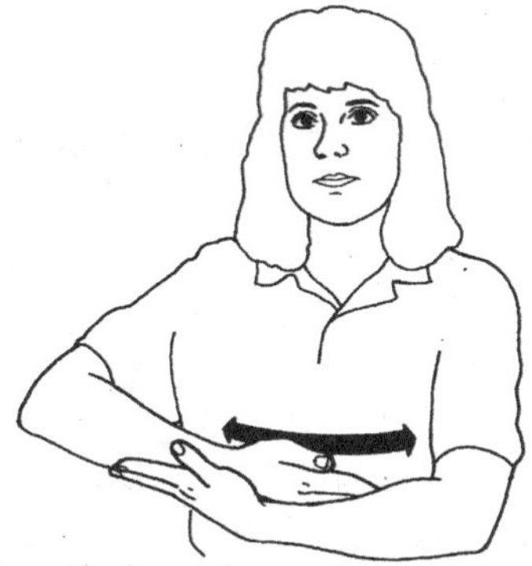

BABY

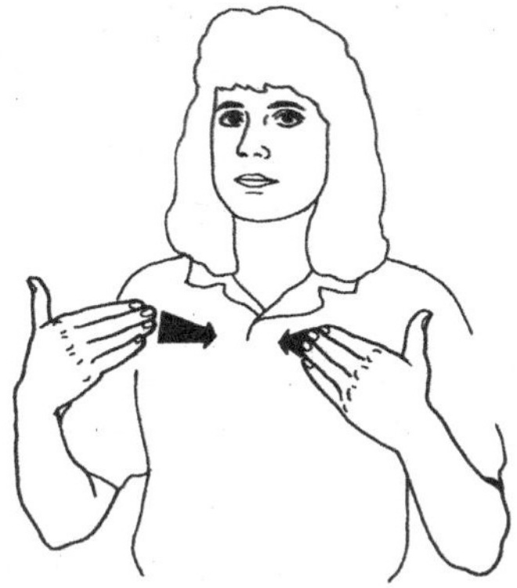

HAVE

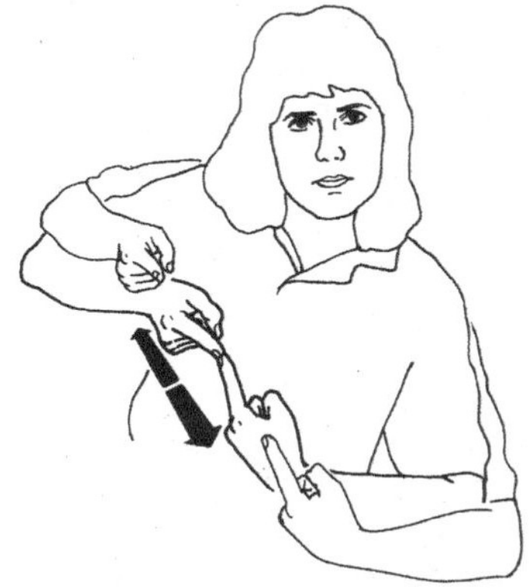

ALLERGY

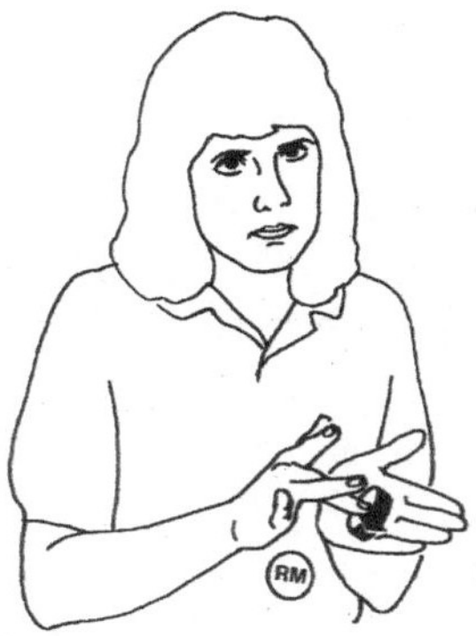

MEDICINE

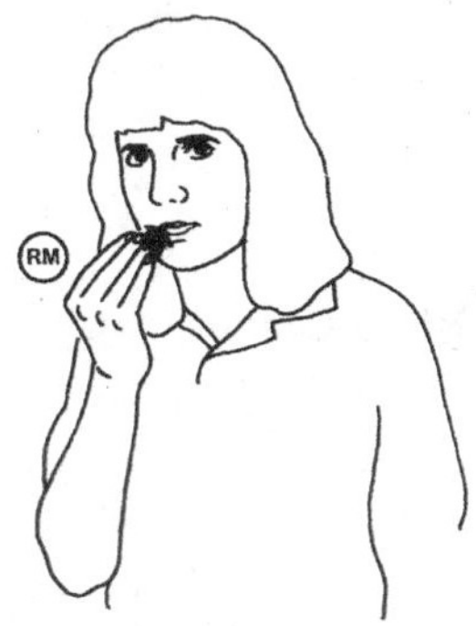

FOOD

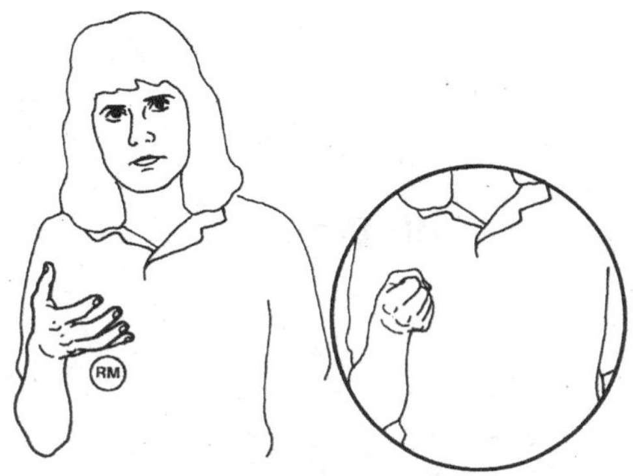

MILK

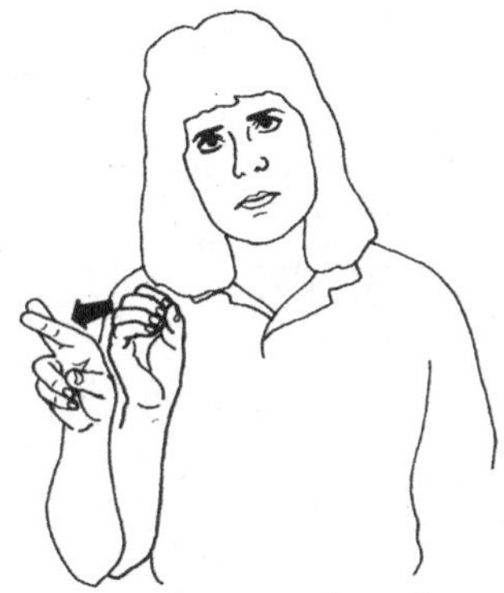

O-R

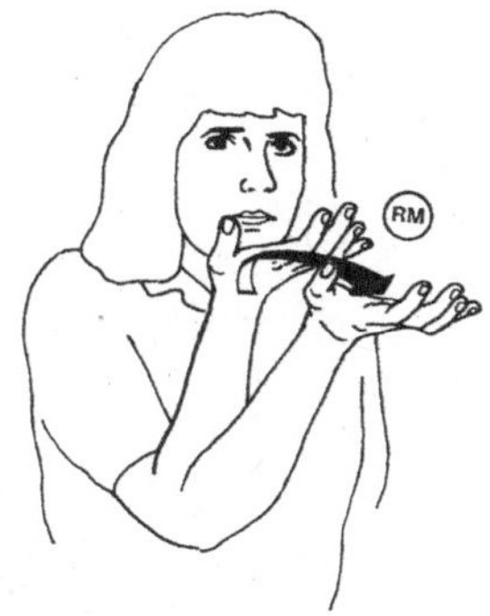

GRASS?

Does your baby have allergies to medications, food, milk, or grasses?

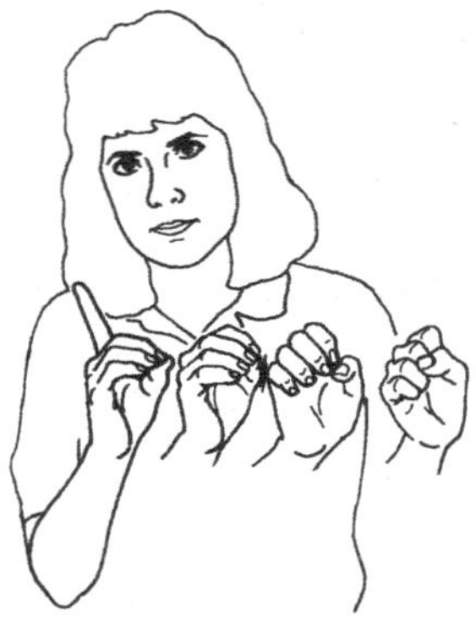

D-O-E-S

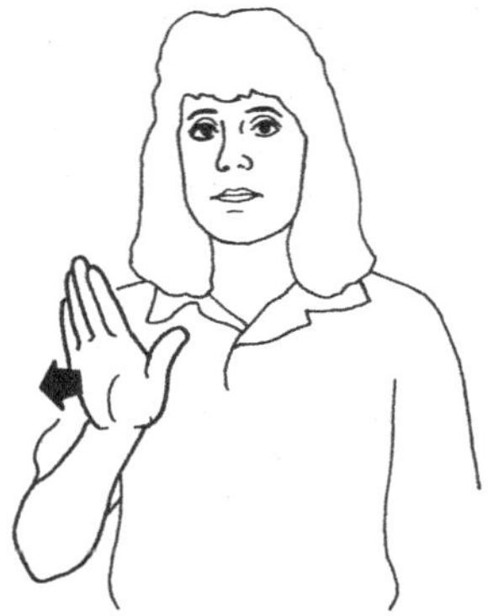

YOUR

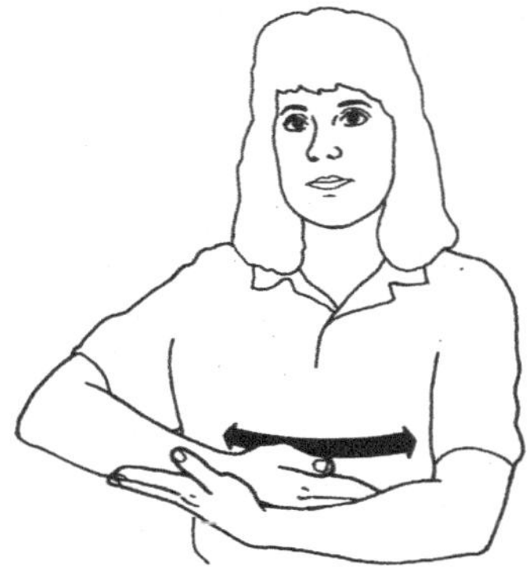

BABY

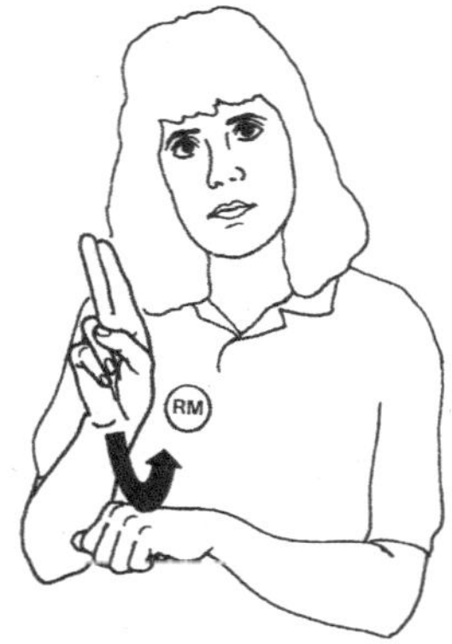

USE

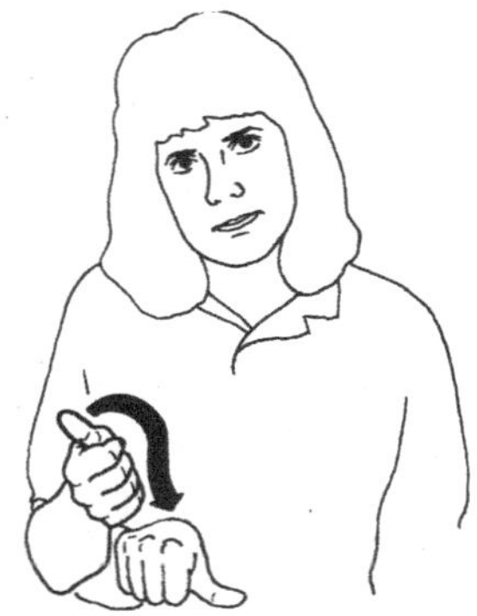

ANY

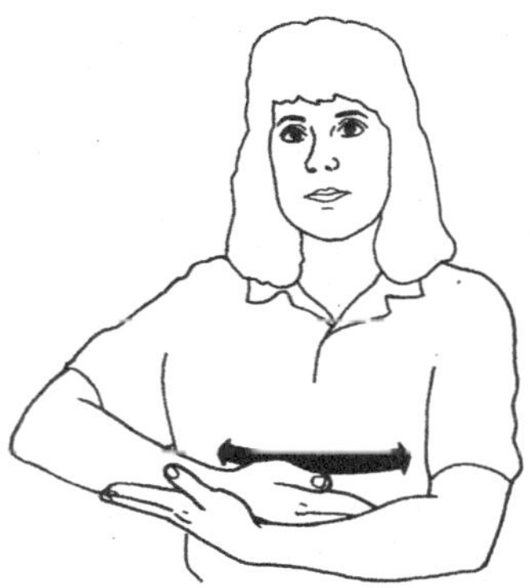

BABY

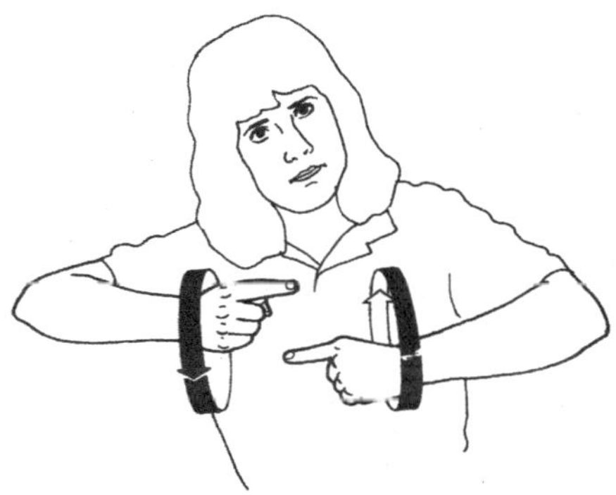

SIGN?

Does your baby use any baby sign?

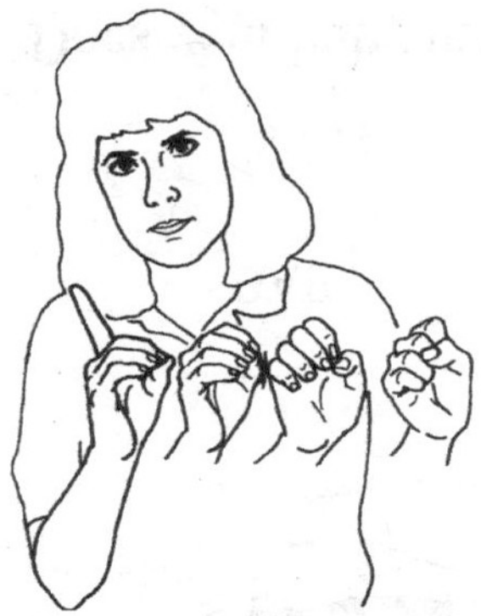

D-O-E-S

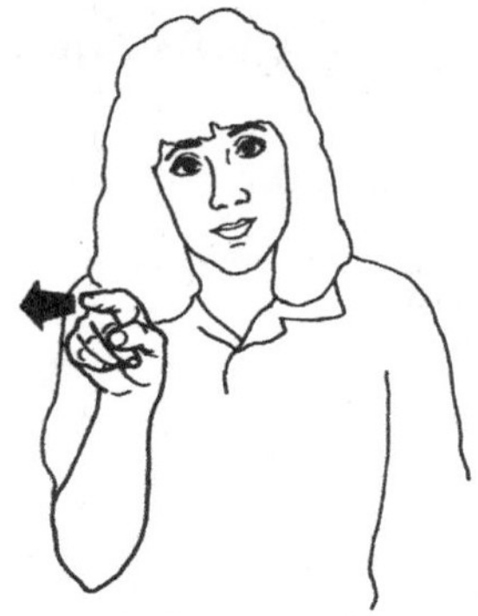

SHE

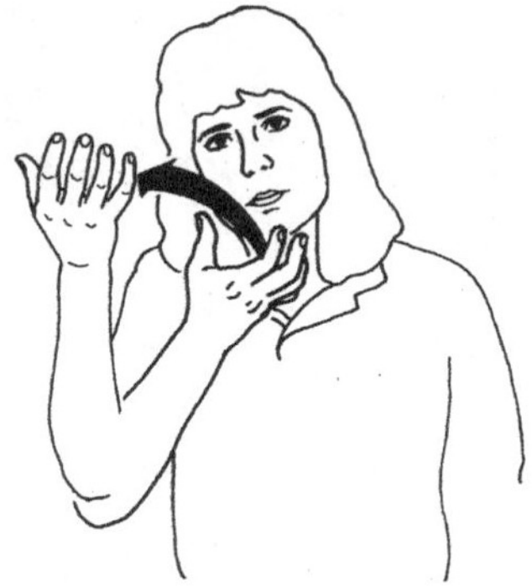

SCREAM

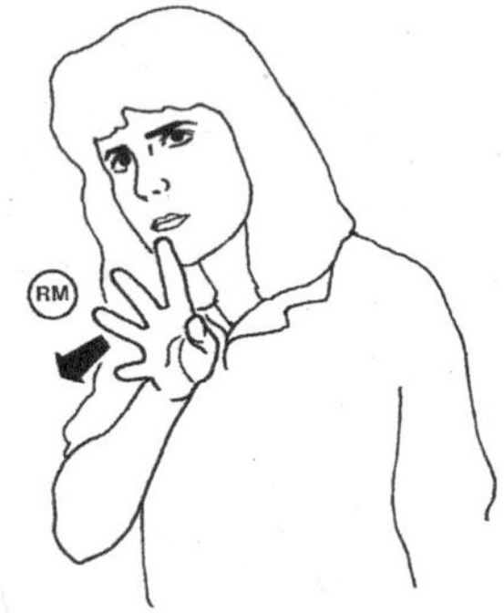

TALK

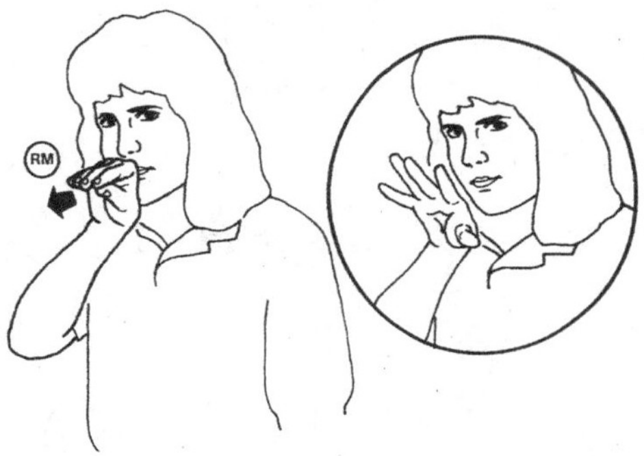

BABBLE

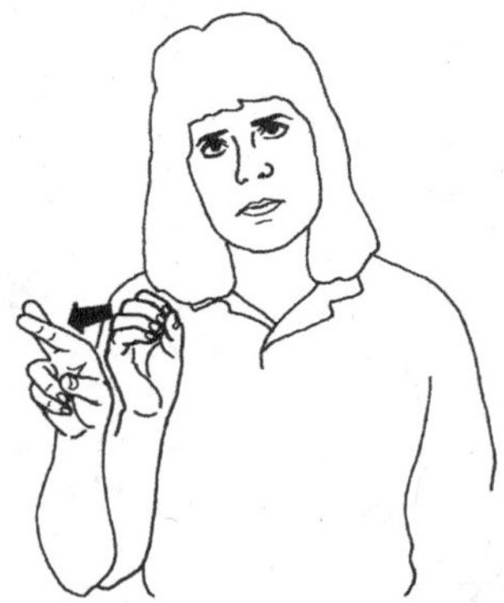

O-R

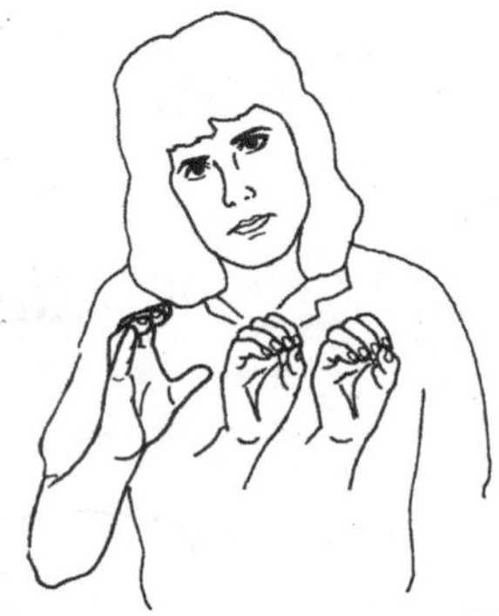

C-O-O?

Does she or he scream, talk, babble, or coo?

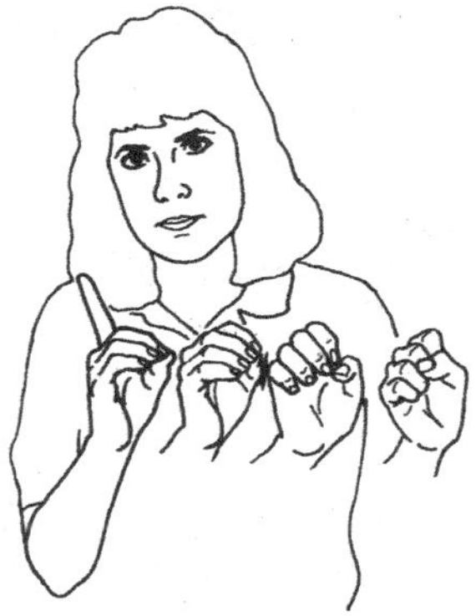

D-O-E-S

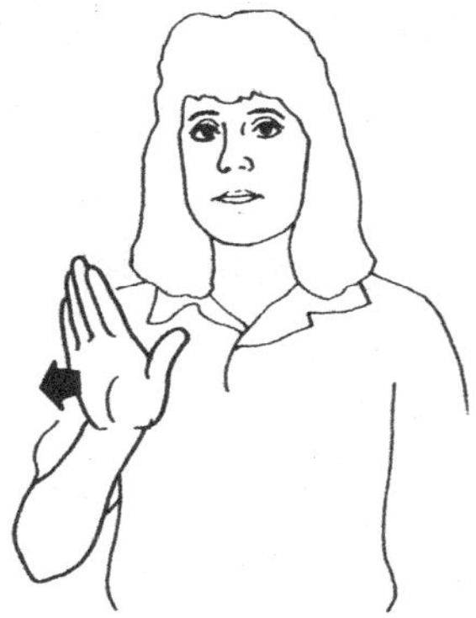

YOUR

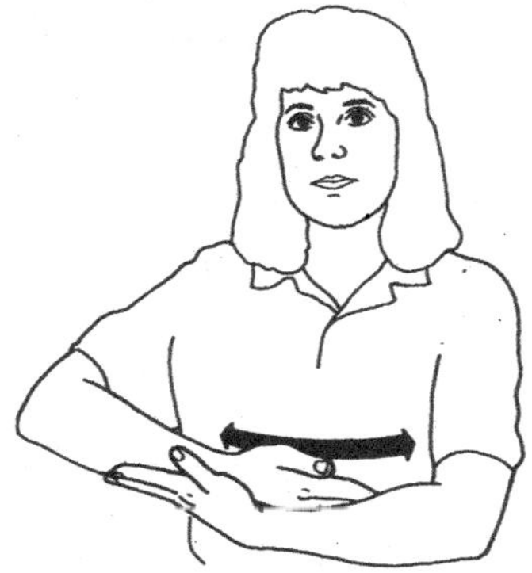

BABY

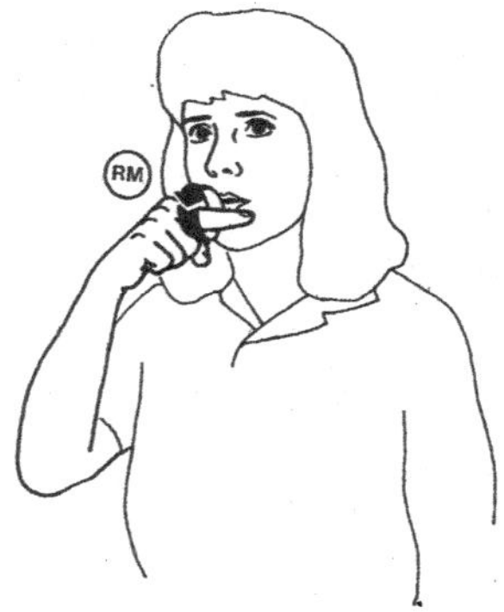

SAY

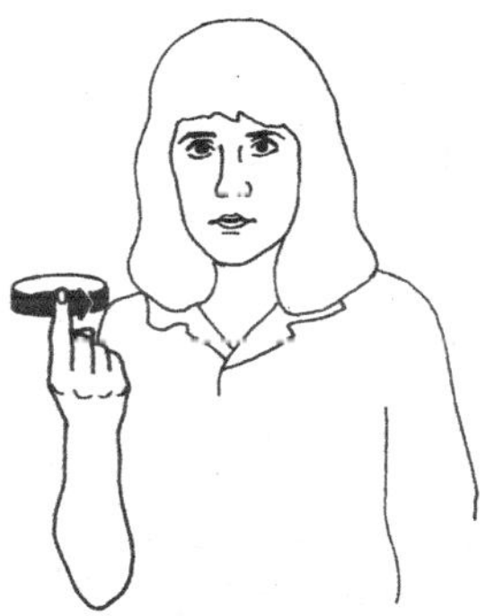

SINGLE

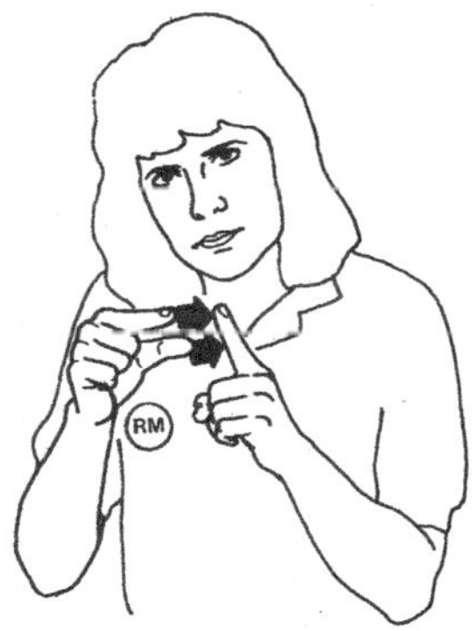

WORD?

Does your baby say single words?

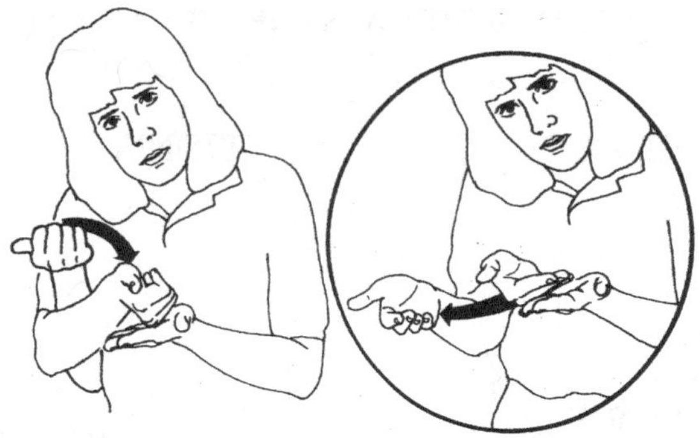

ANYTHING

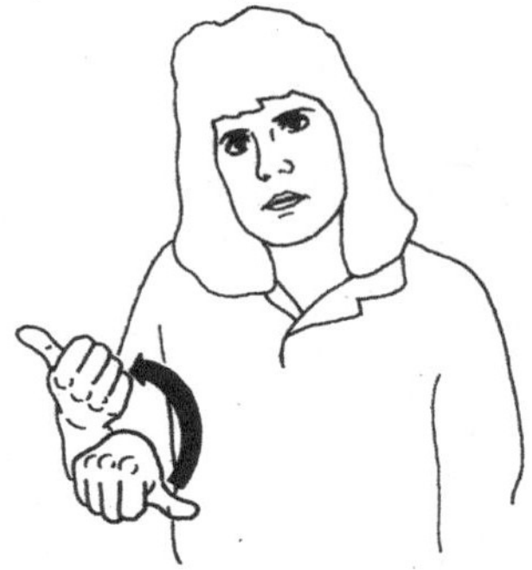

ELSE

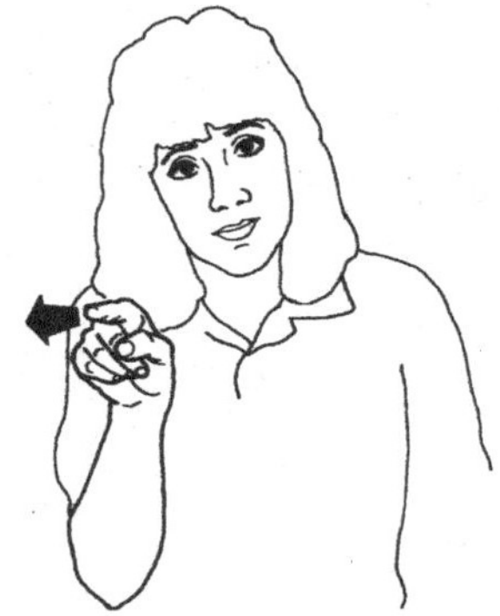

YOU

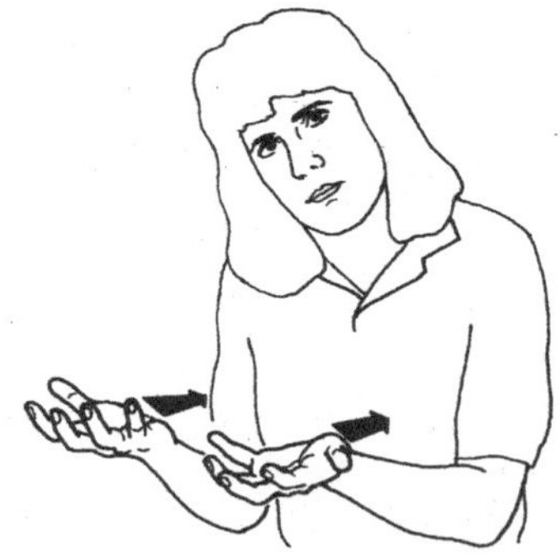

WANT

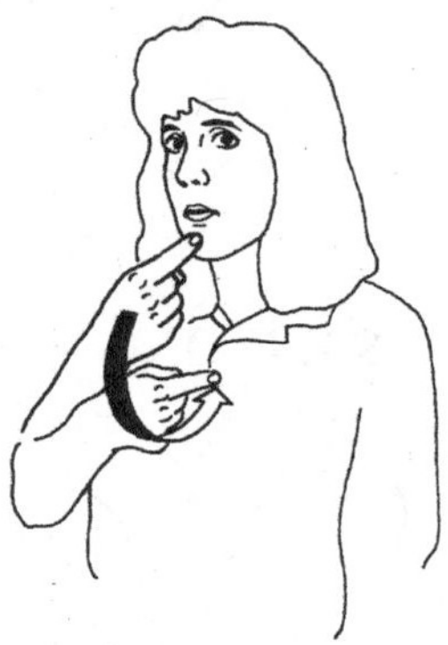

TELL-ME

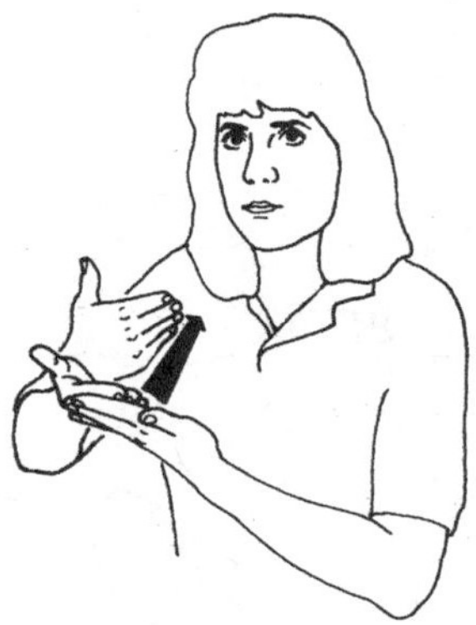

BEFORE

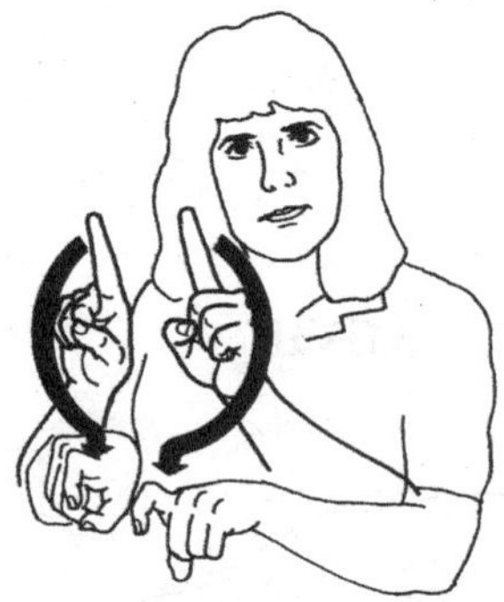

TEST

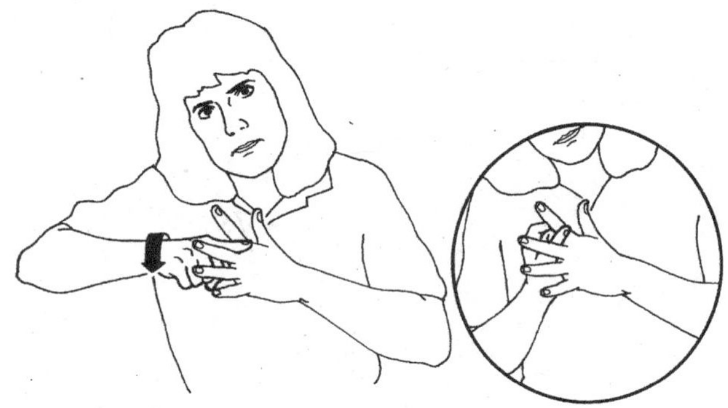

BEGIN?

Is there anything else you want to tell me before testing begins?

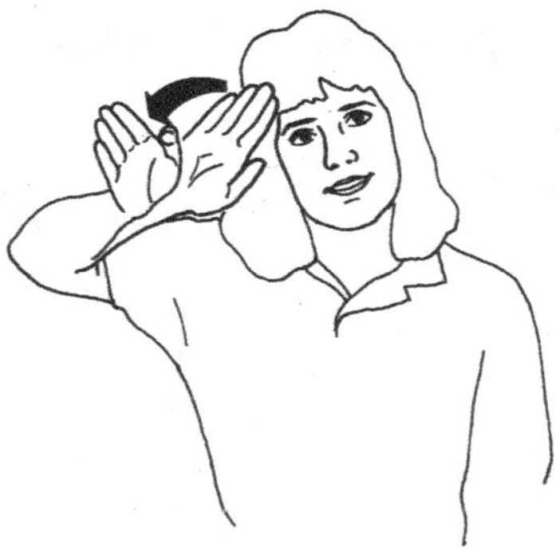

HELLO.

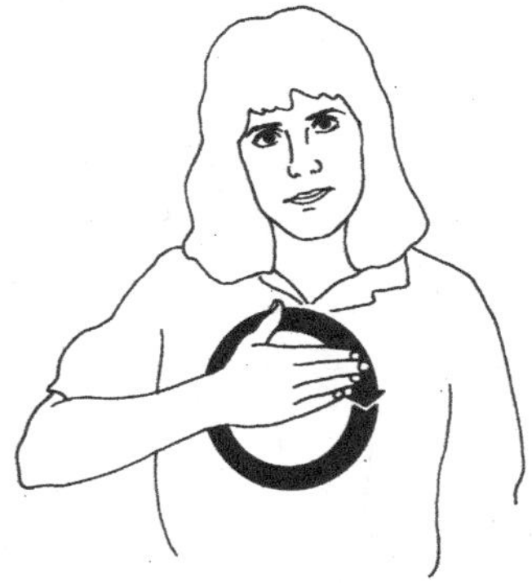

PLEASE

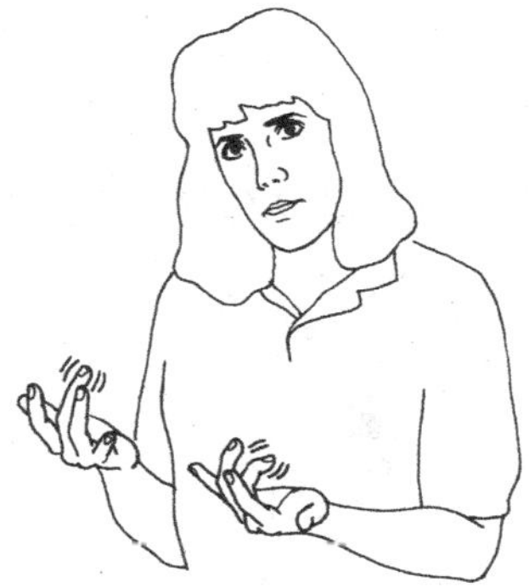

WAIT

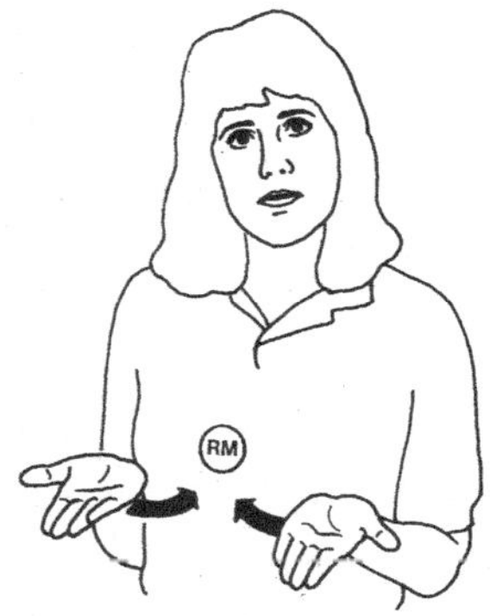

HERE

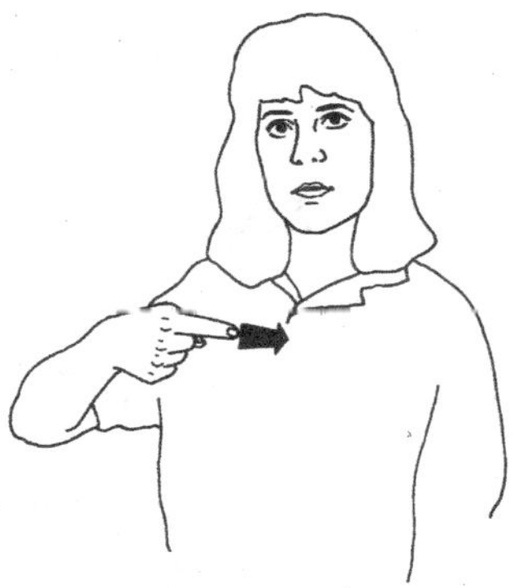

I

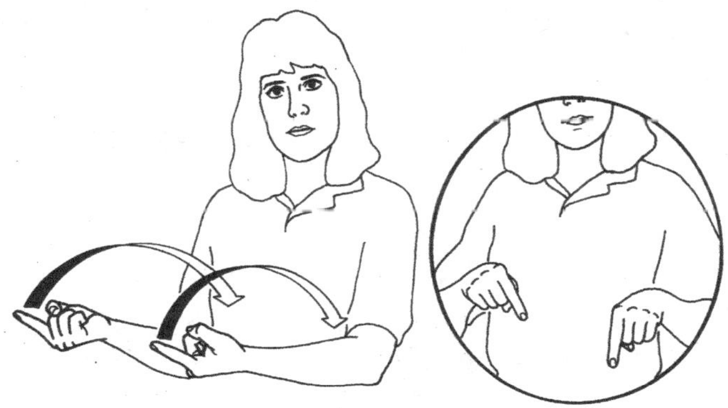

COME-BACK

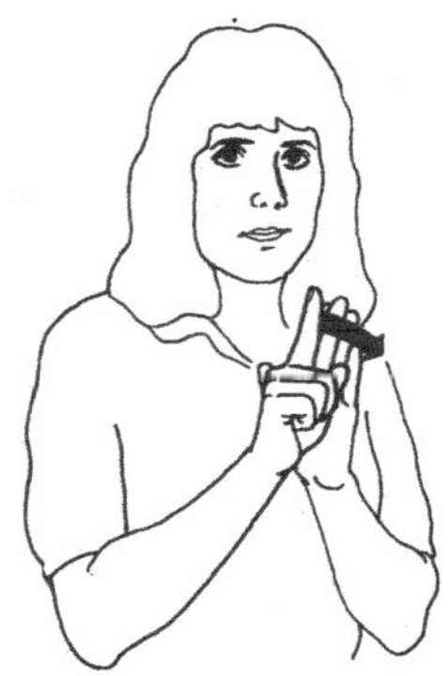

MINUTE.

Hello. Please wait here, I'll come back in a minute.

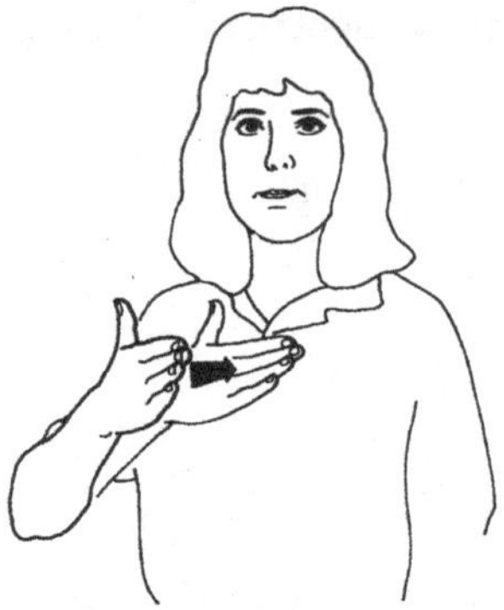

MY

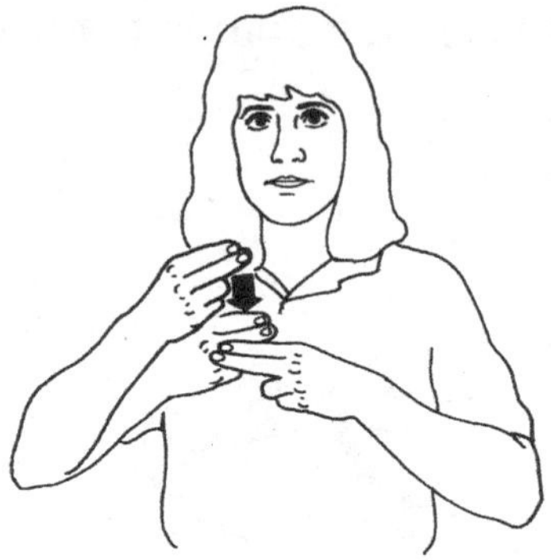

NAME

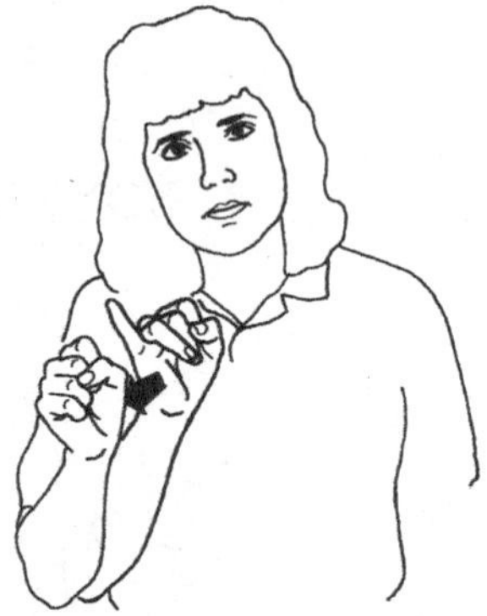

IS

My name is ____

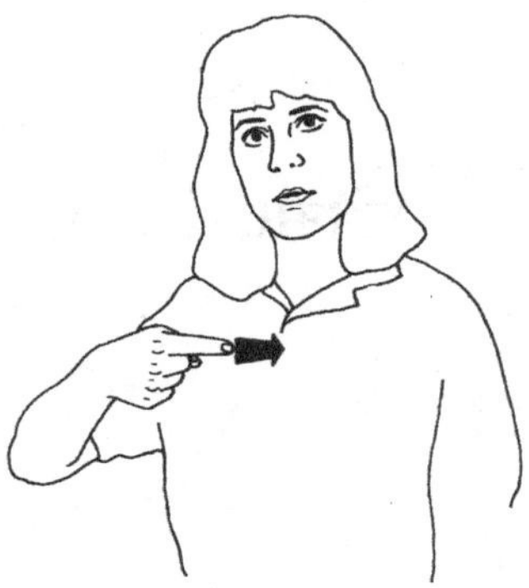

I

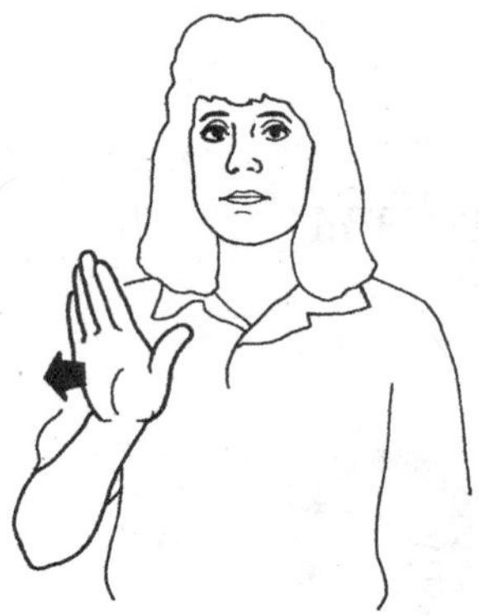

YOUR

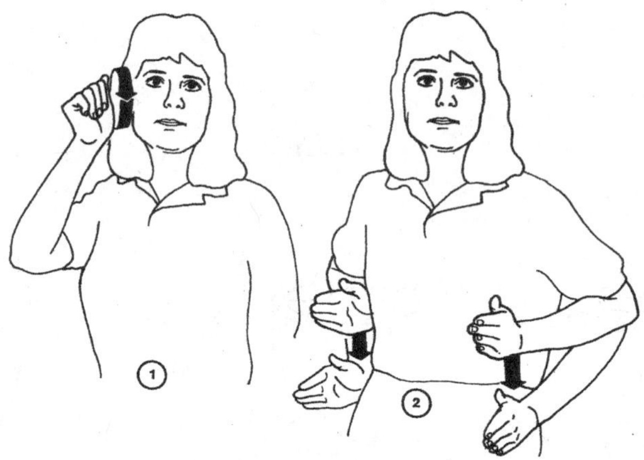

AUDIOLOGY-PERSON.

I am your audiologist.

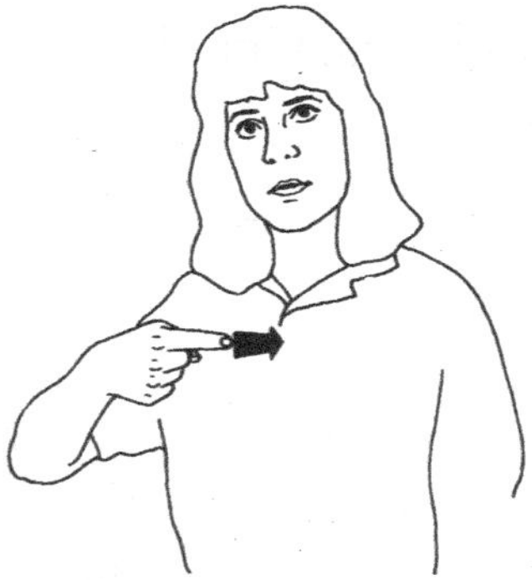

I

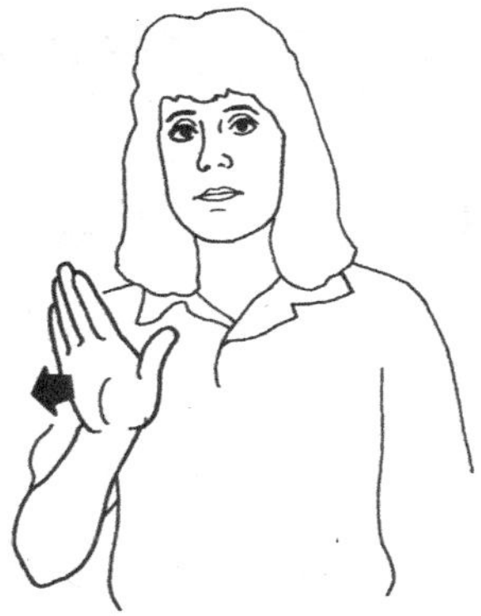

YOUR

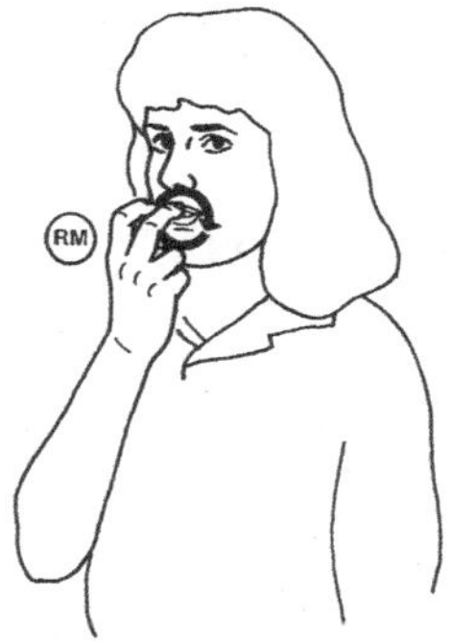

SPEECH

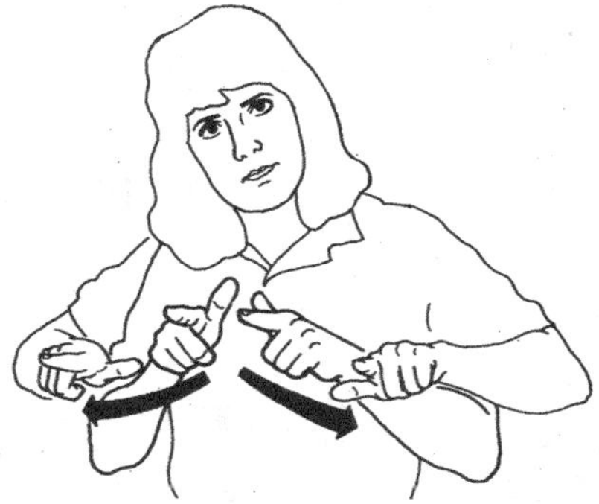

LANGUAGE

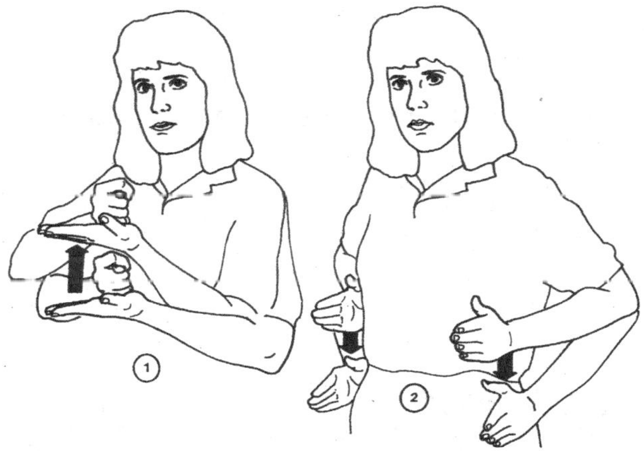

THERAPY-PERSON.

I am your speech/language pathologist.

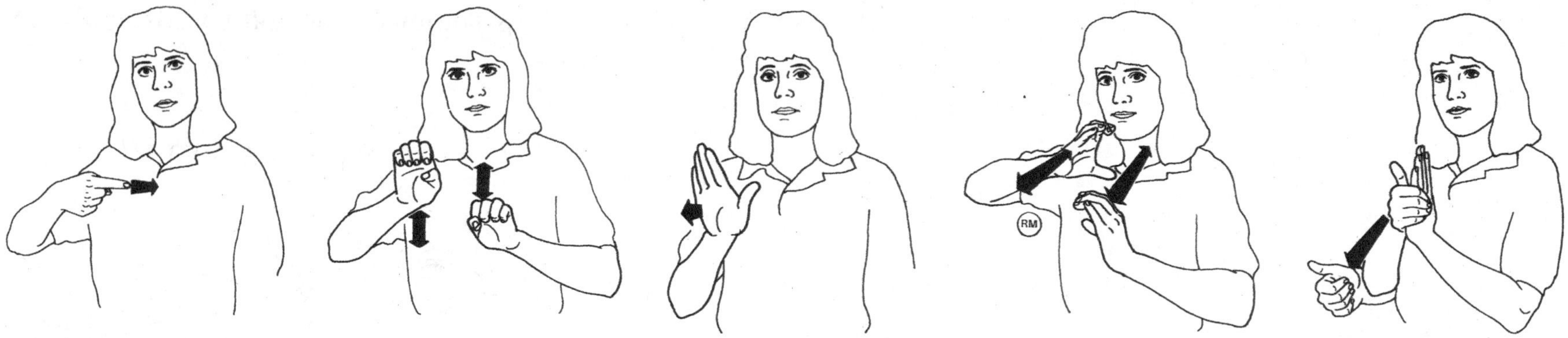

I EVALUATE YOUR COMMUNICATION SKILL.

I'll evaluate your communication skills.

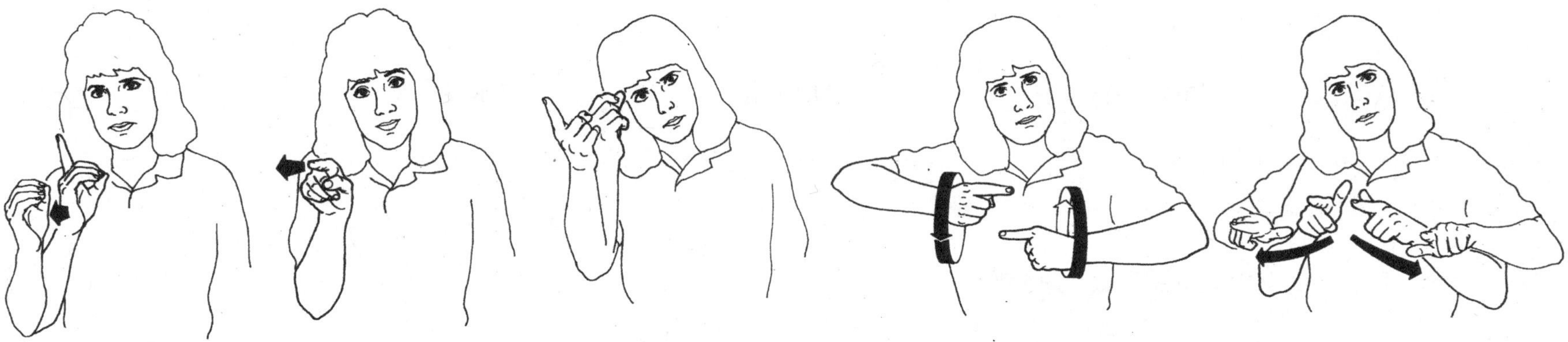

D-O YOU UNDERSTAND SIGN LANGUAGE?

Do you understand sign language?

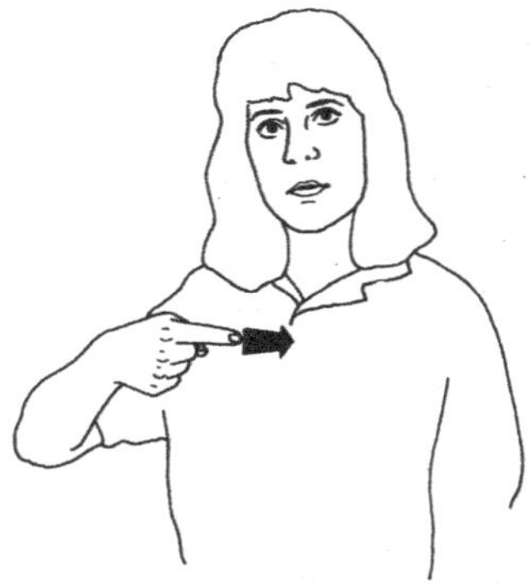

I

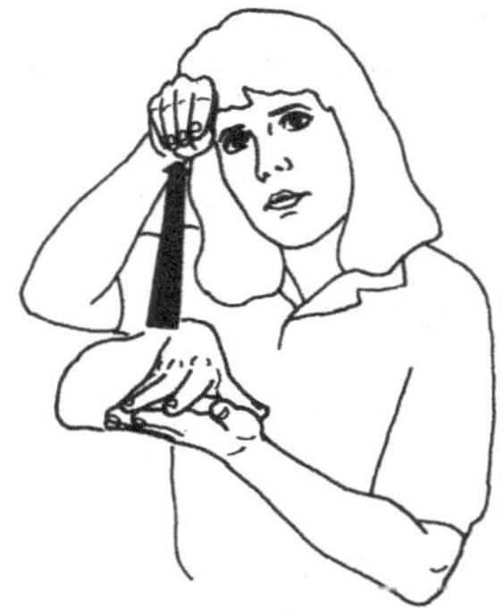

LEARN

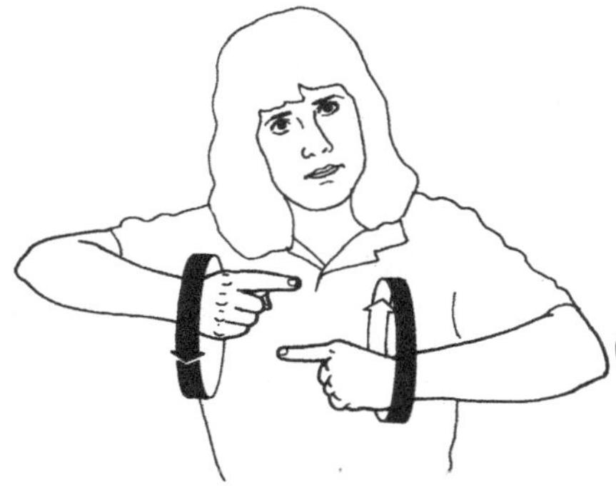

SIGN

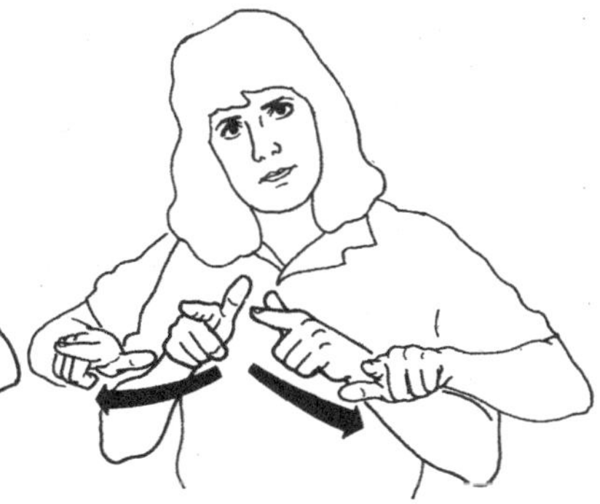

LANGUAGE

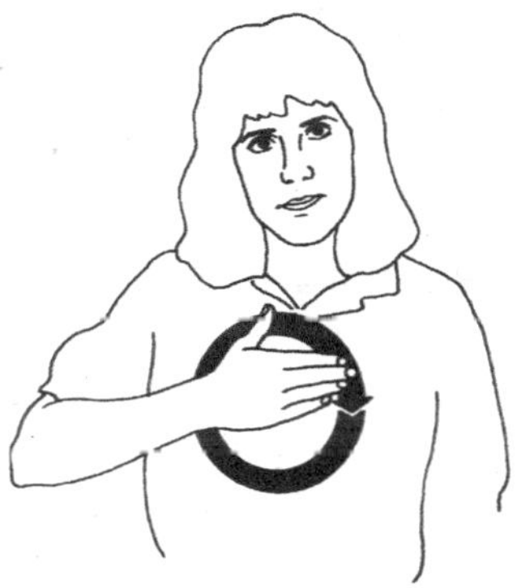

PLEASE

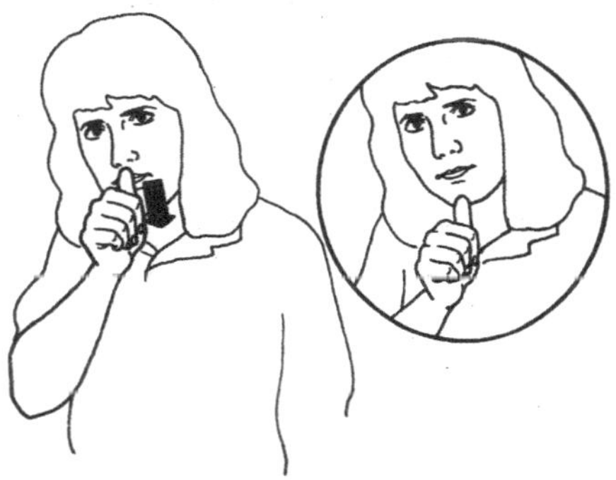

PATIENT.

I'm learning sign language; please be patient.

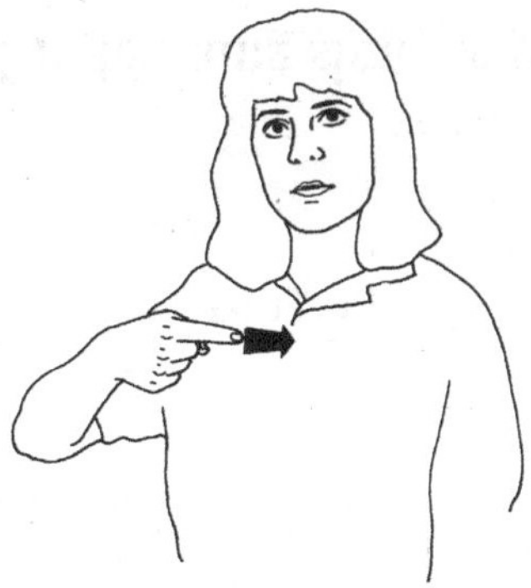

I

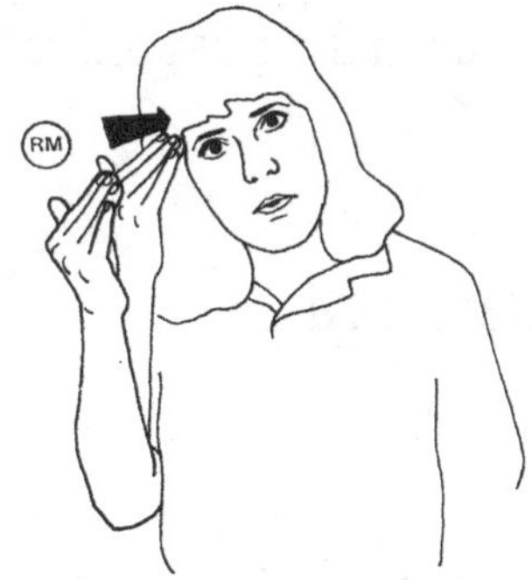

KNOW

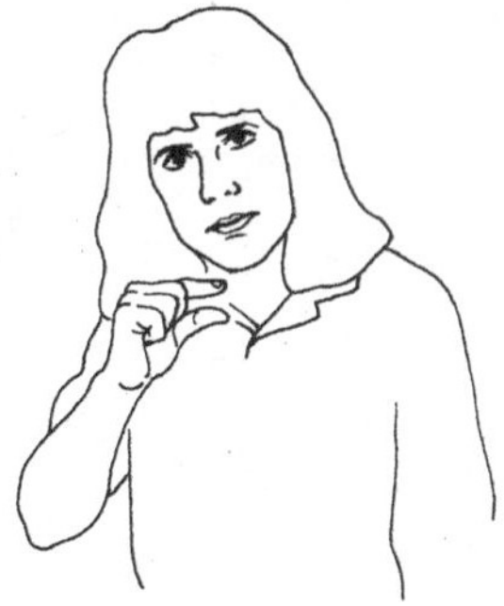

LITTLE-BIT

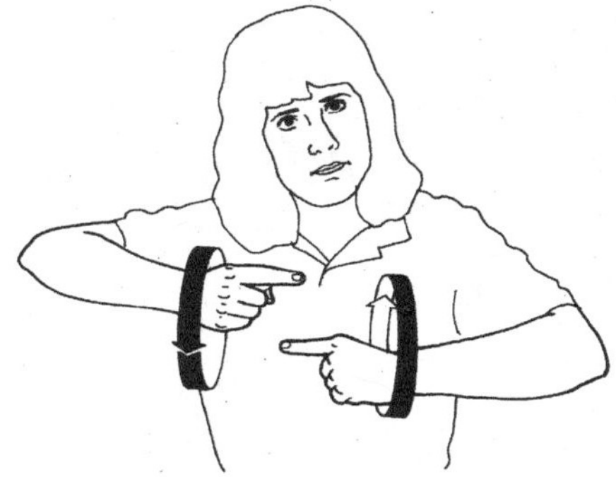

SIGN

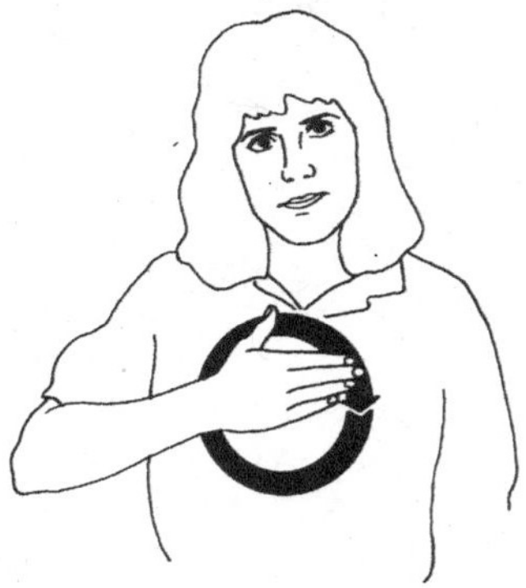

PLEASE

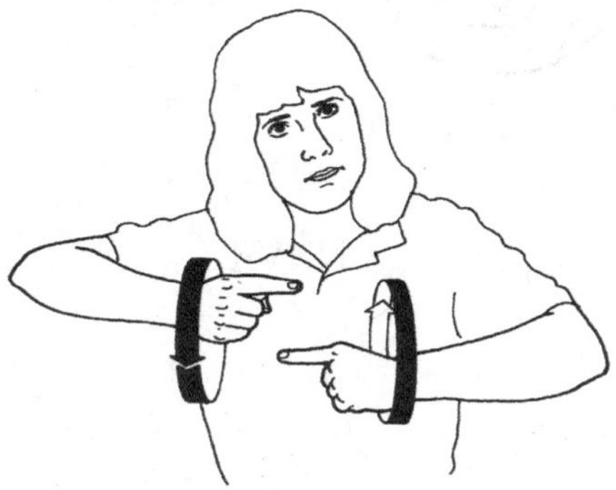

SIGN

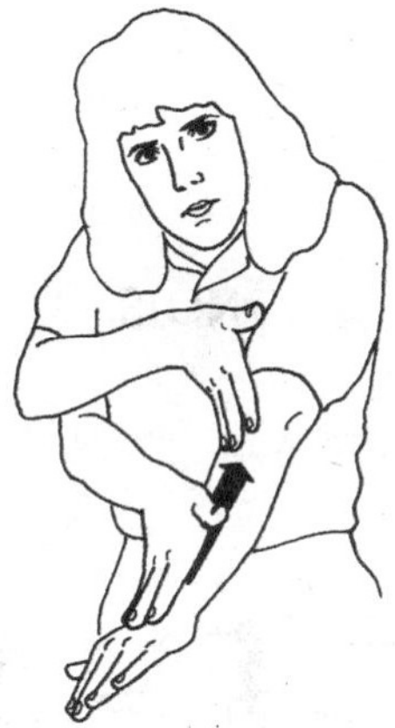

SLOW.

I know a little bit of sign; please sign slowly.

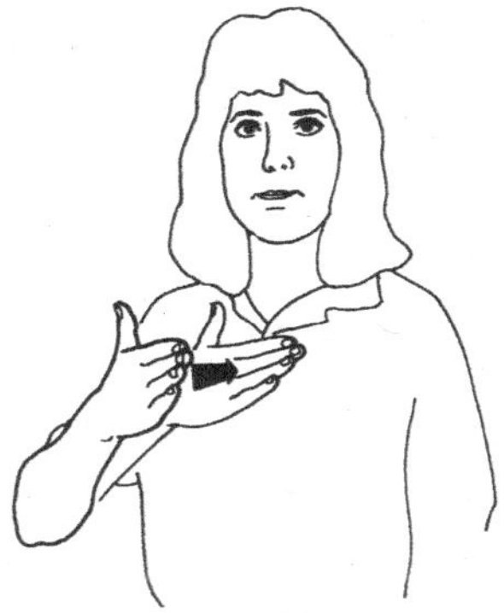

MY

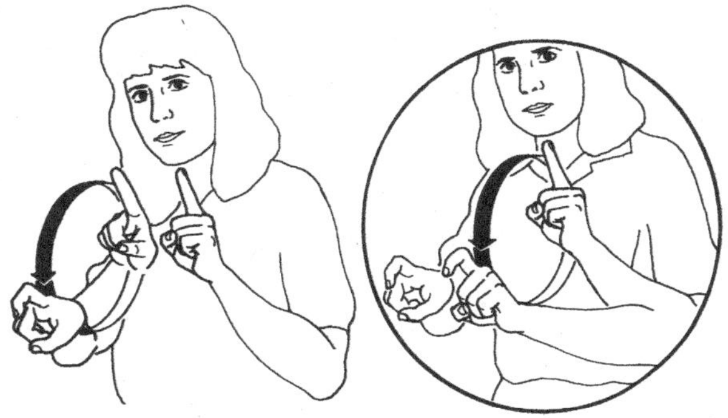

QUESTION

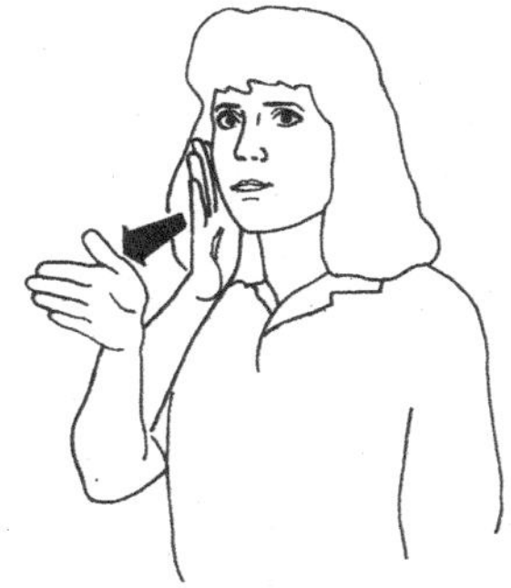

WILL

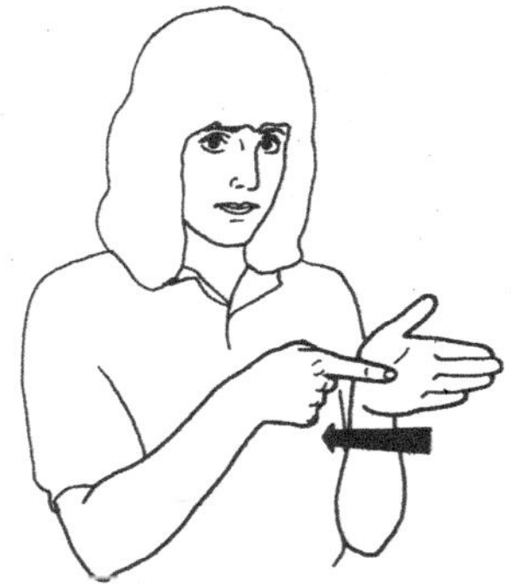

REQUIRE

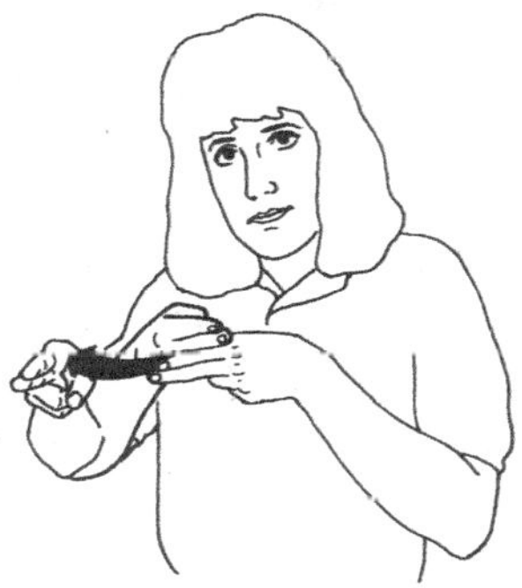

BRIEF

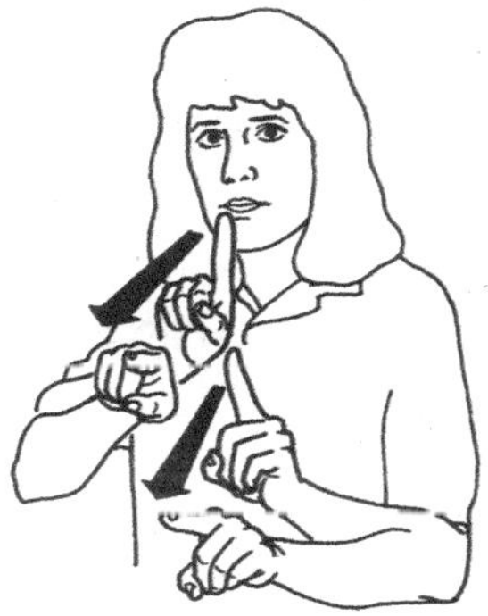

ANSWER.

My questions will require brief answers.

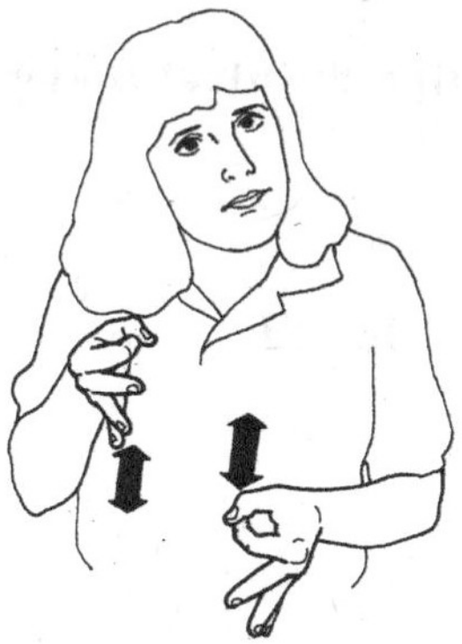

IF

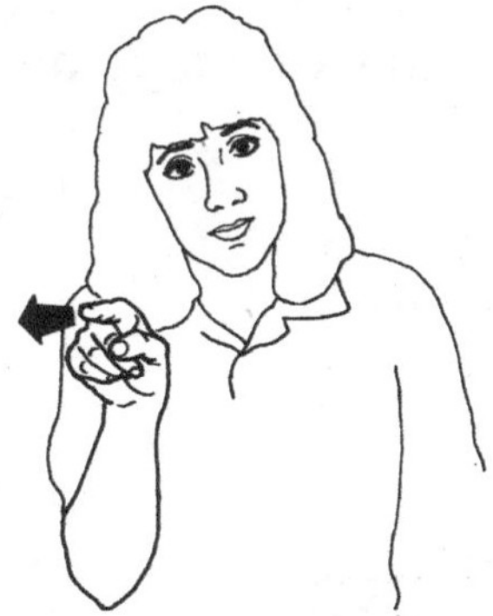

YOU

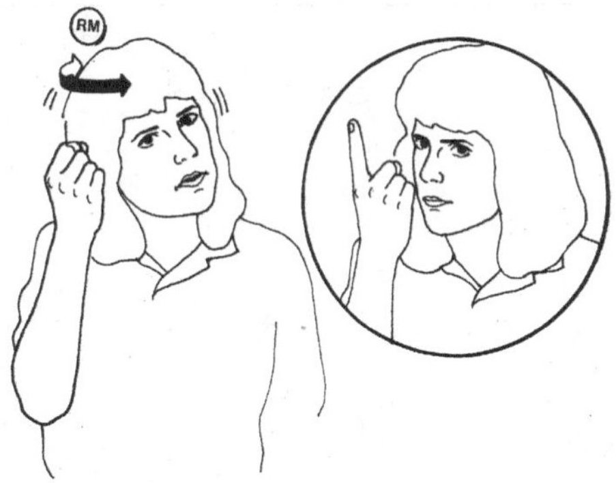

DON'T-UNDERSTAND

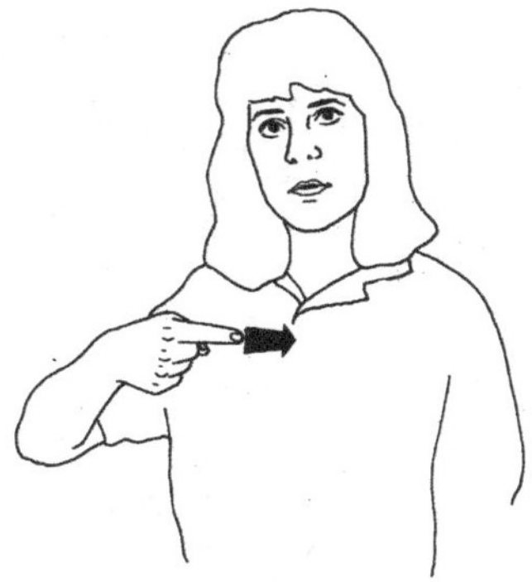

ME

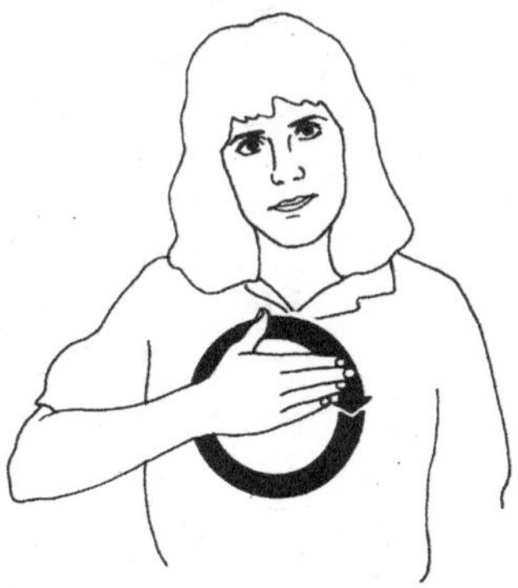

PLEASE

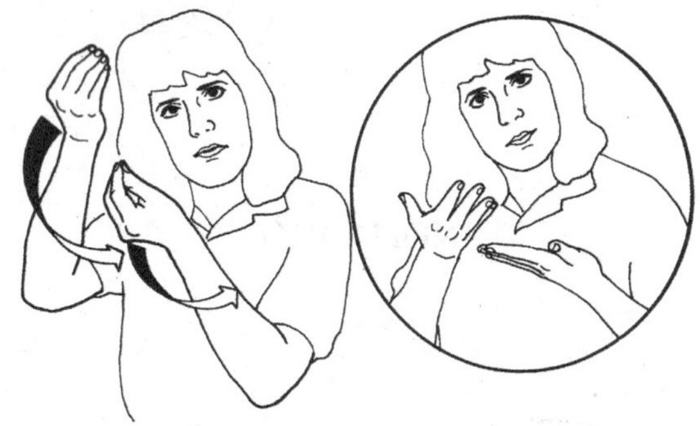

LET-ME-KNOW.

If you don't understand me, please let me know.

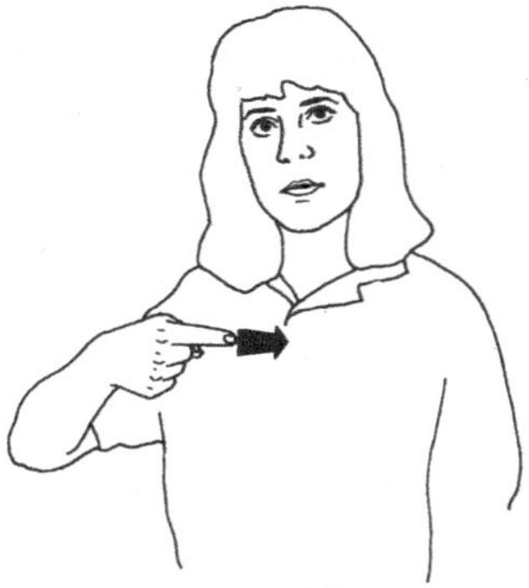

I

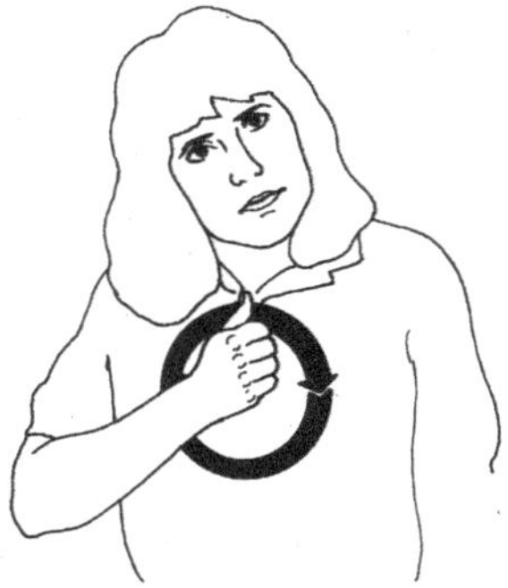

SORRY

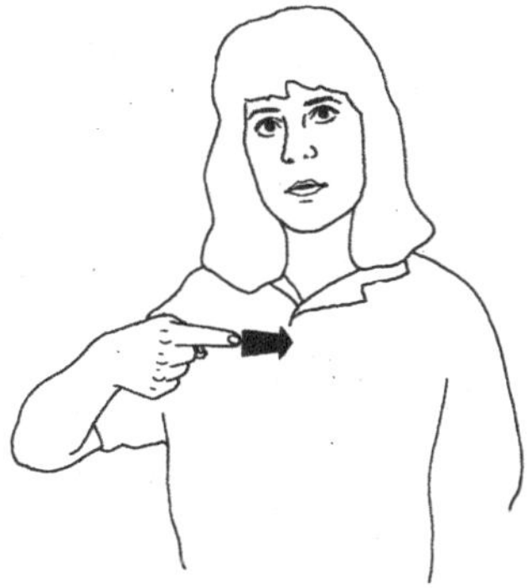

I

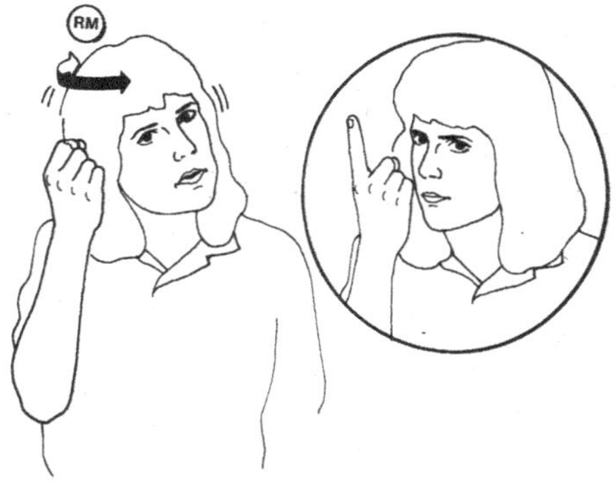

DON'T-UNDERSTAND

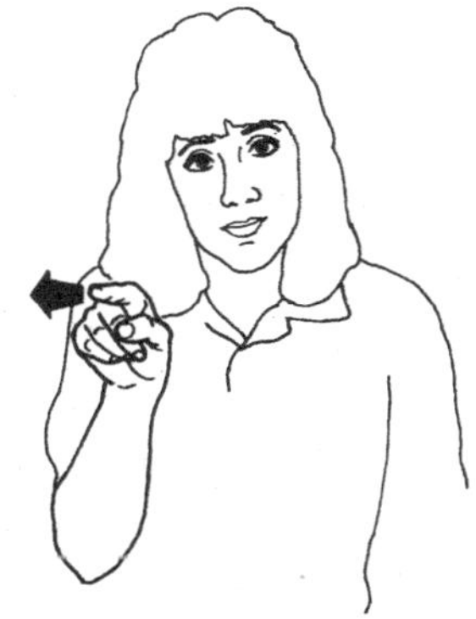

YOU.

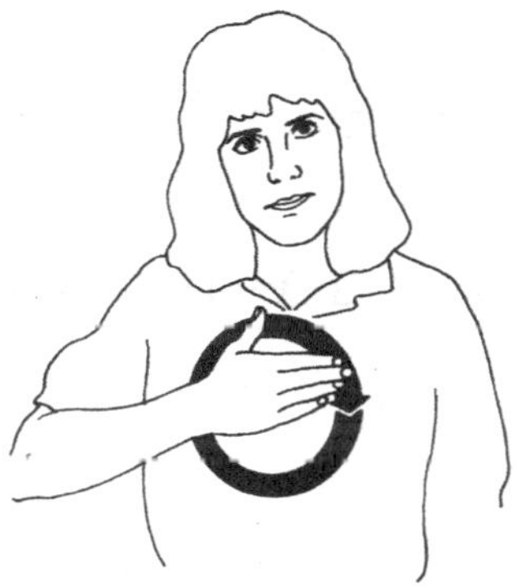

PLEASE

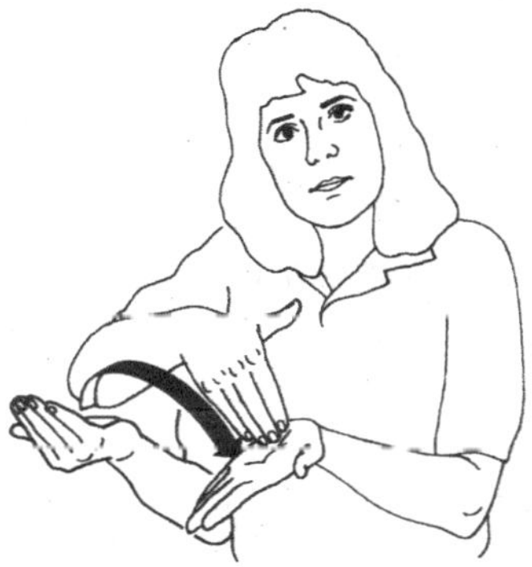

REPEAT.

I'm sorry I don't understand you. Please repeat.

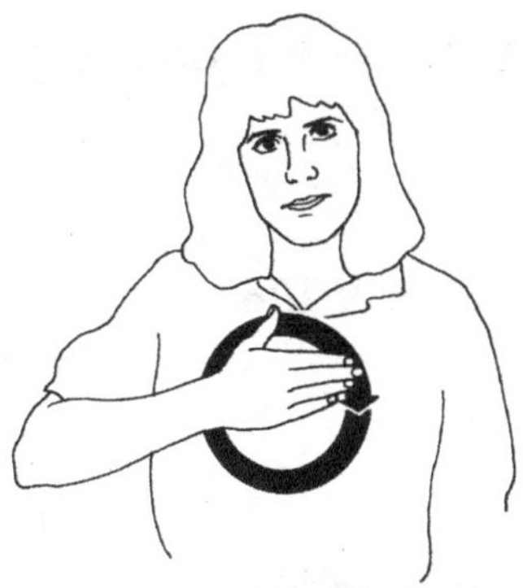

PLEASE

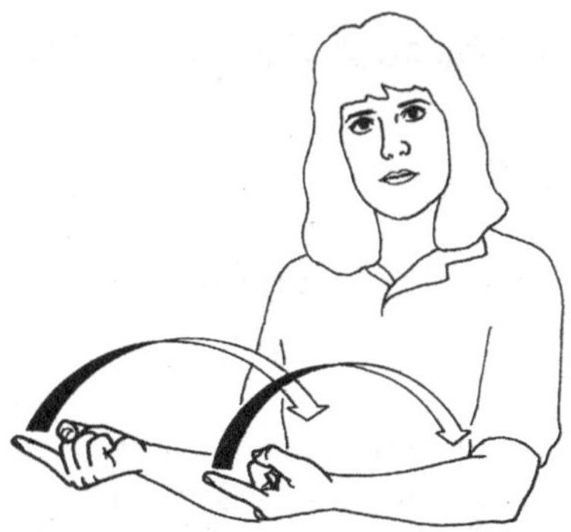

COME

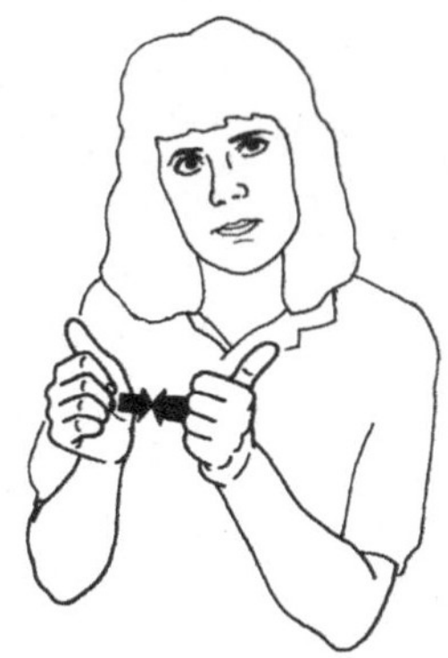

WITH

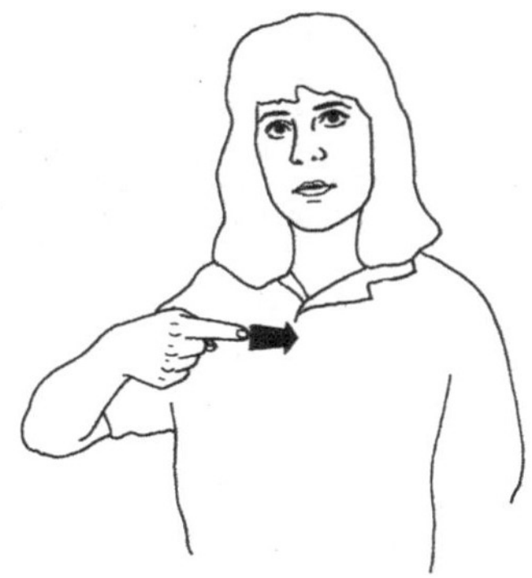

ME.

Please come with me.

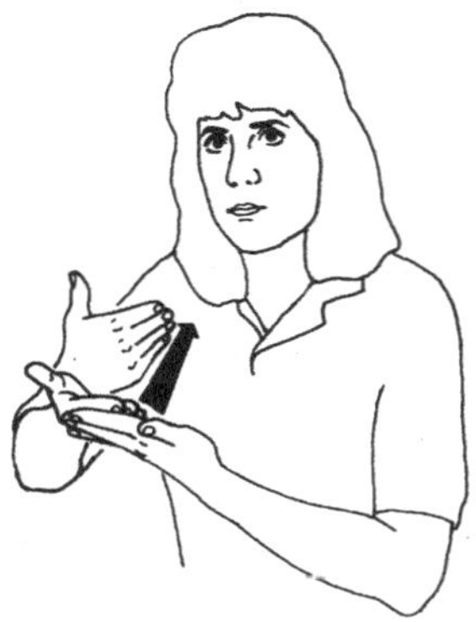

BEFORE

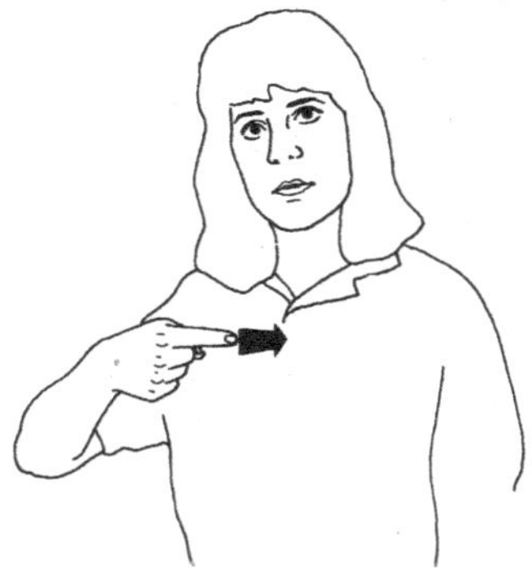

I

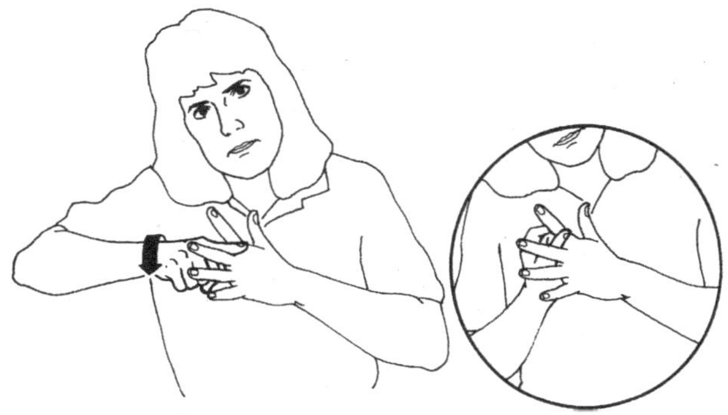

START

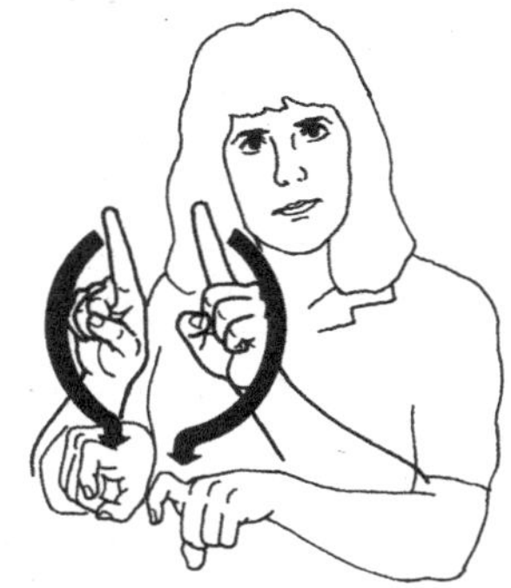

TEST

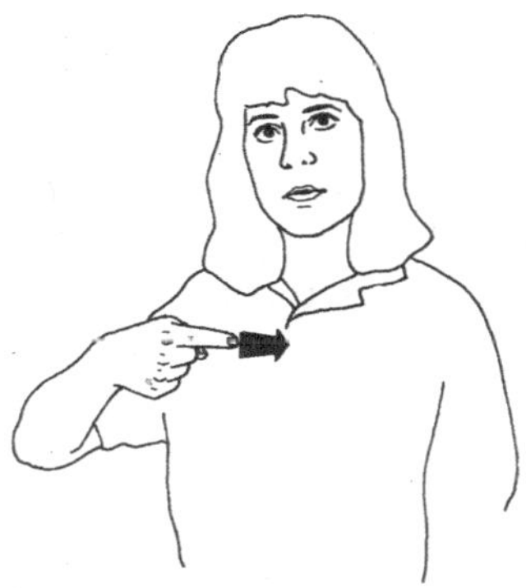

I

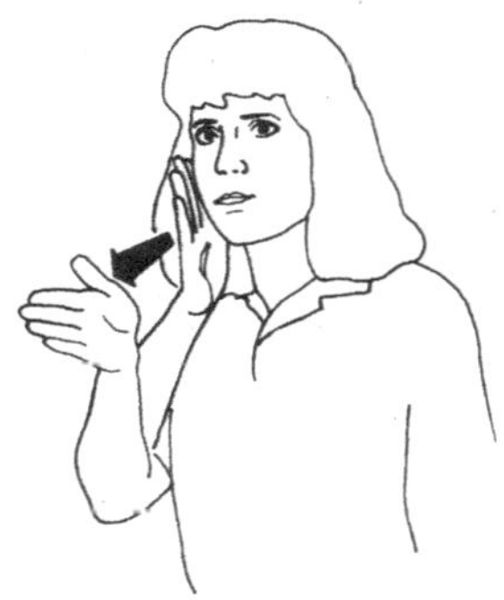

WILL

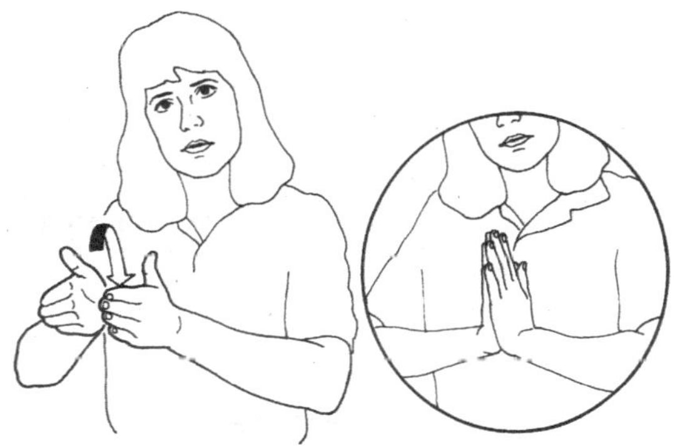

ASK

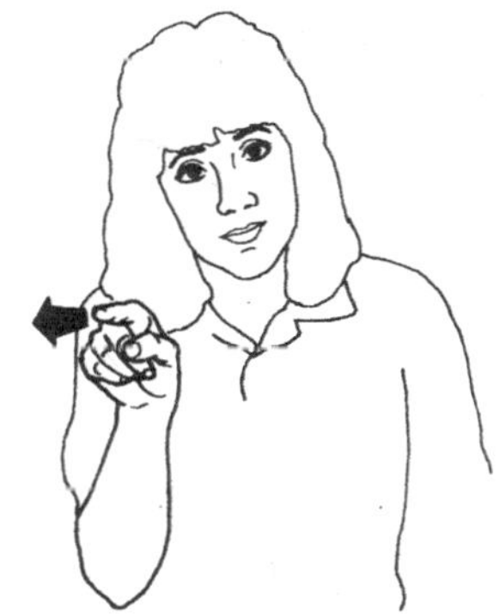

YOU

Before I start testing, I will ask you a few questions.

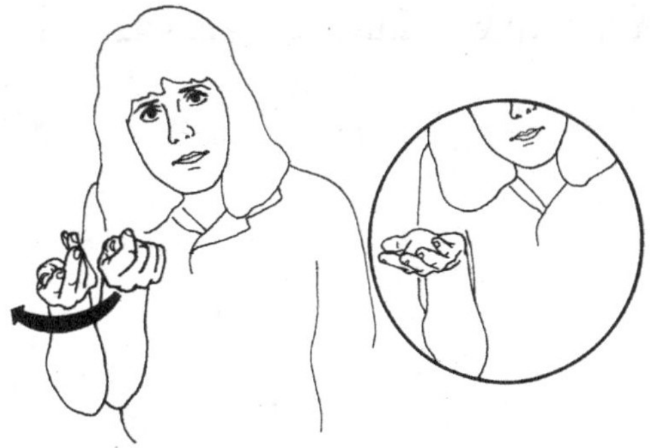

FEW

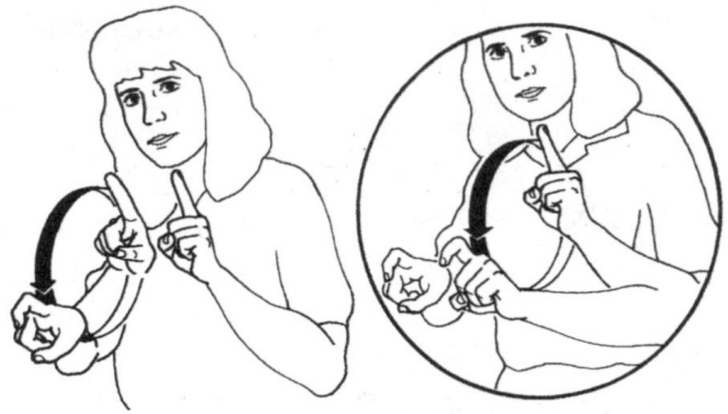

QUESTION.

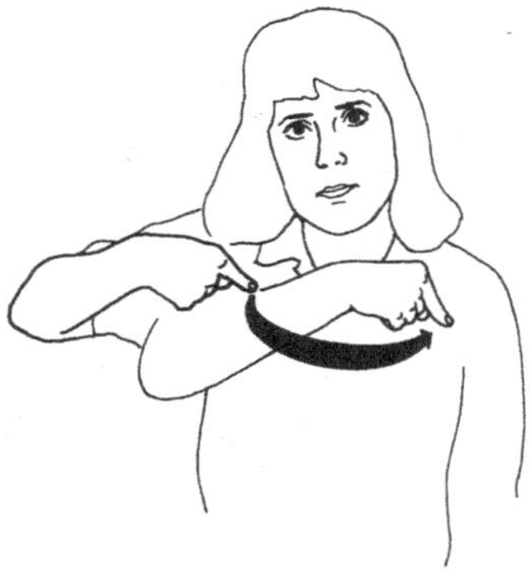

WE

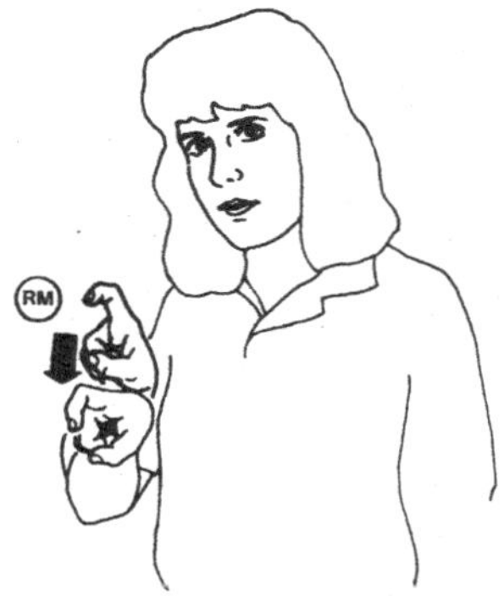

NEED

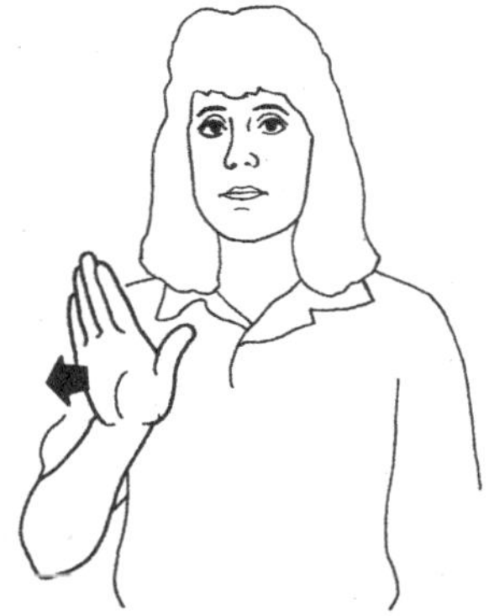

YOUR

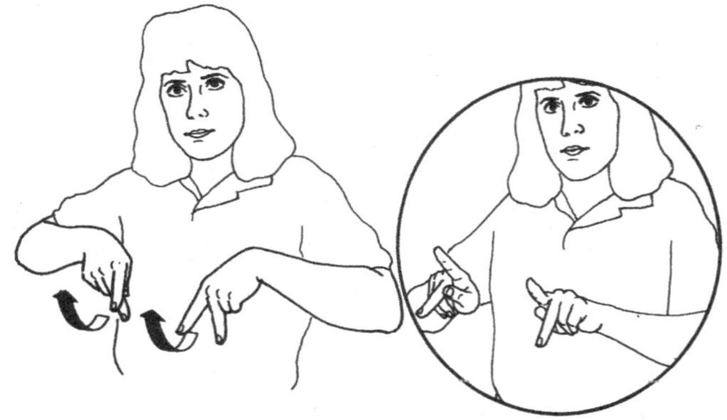

PERMISSION

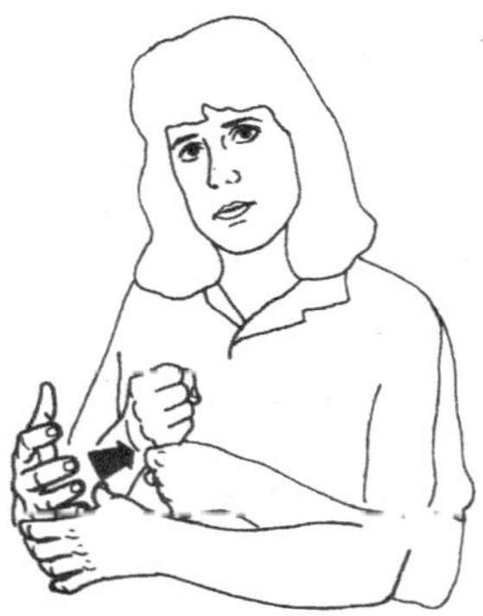

OBTAIN

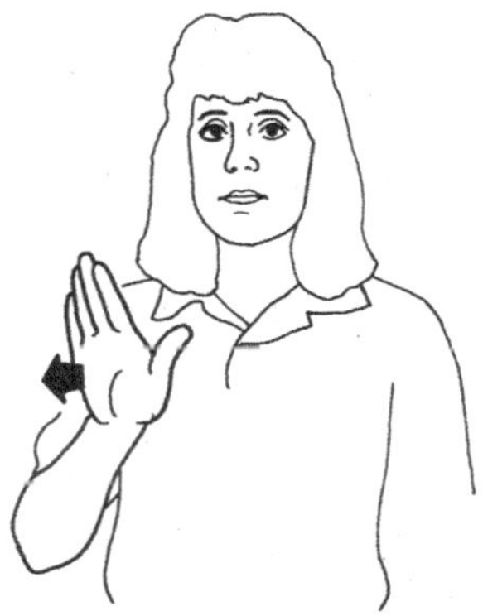

YOUR

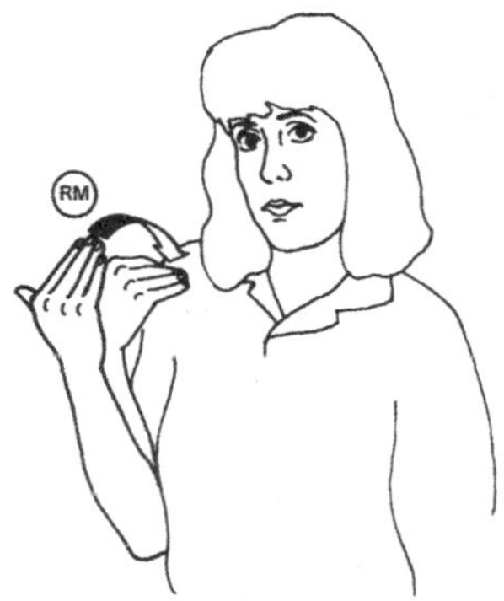

PREVIOUS

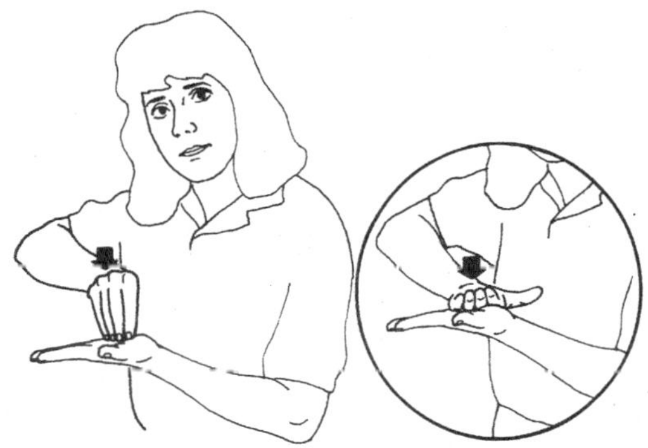

RECORDS.

We need your permission to obtain your previous records.

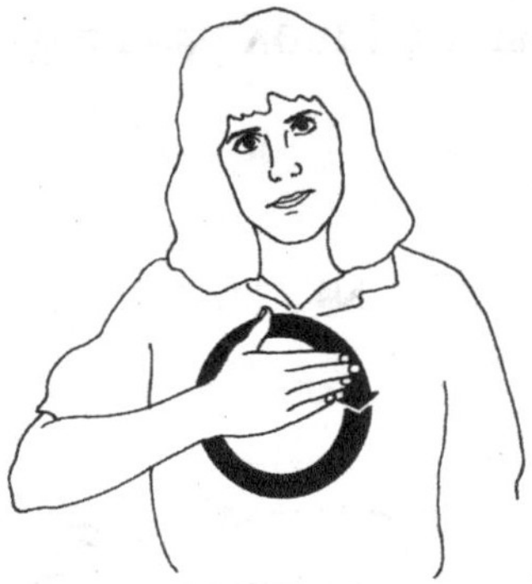

PLEASE

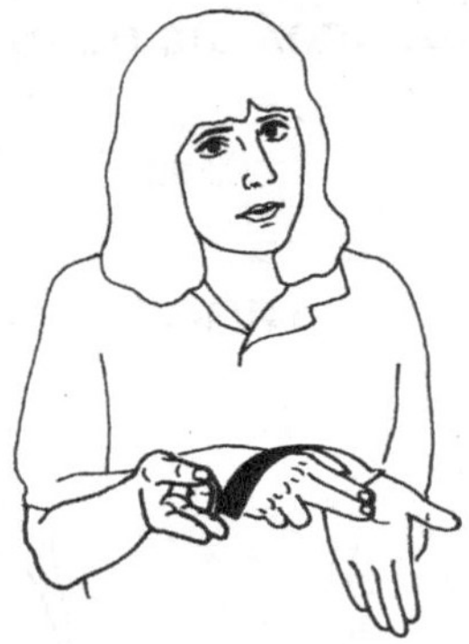

SIGN

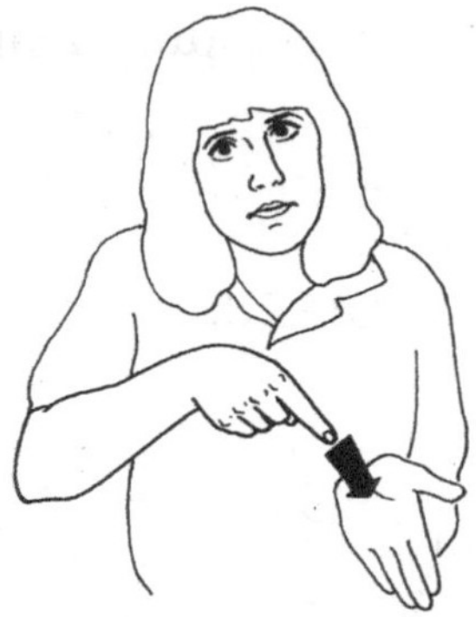

THIS

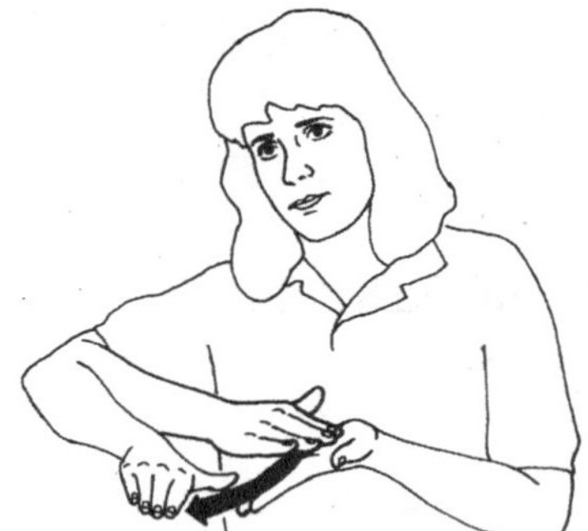

RELEASE

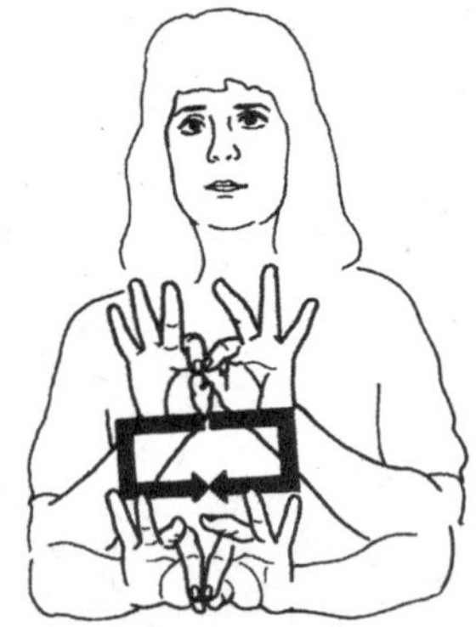

FORM.

Please sign this release form.

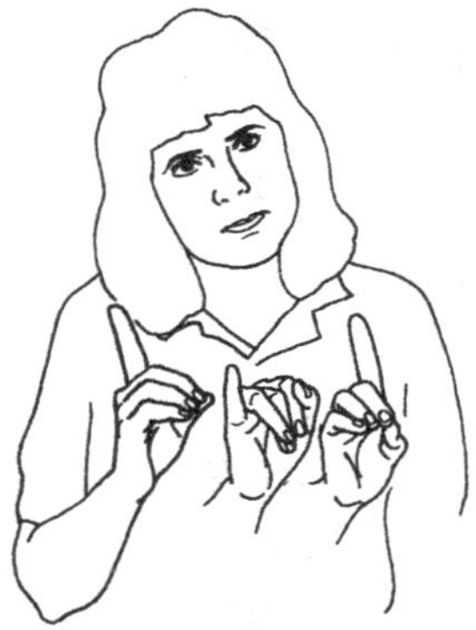

D-I-D

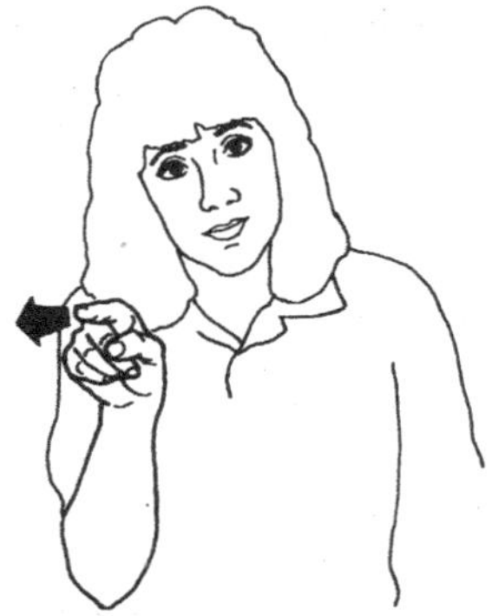

YOU

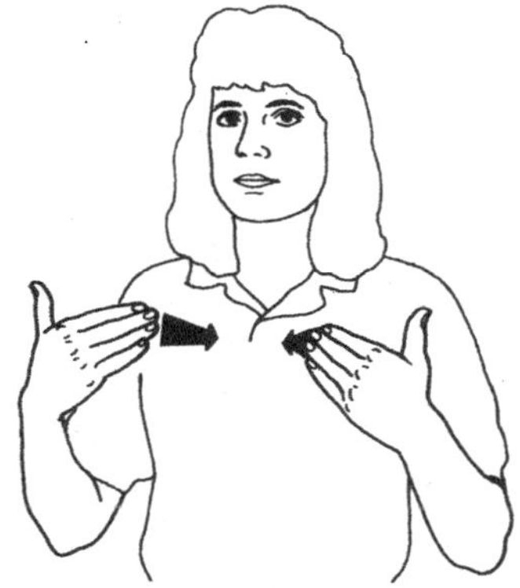

HAVE

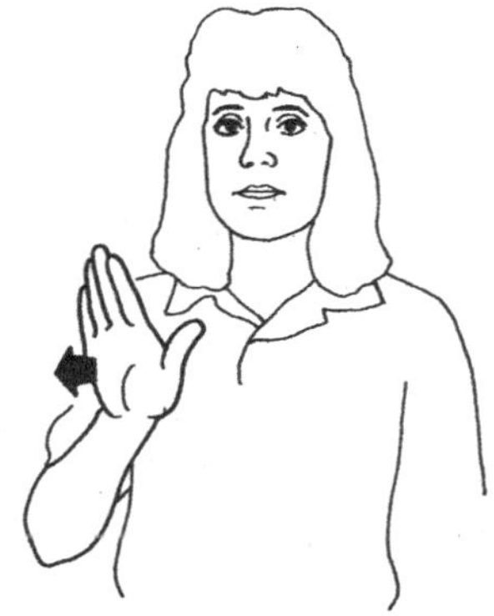

YOUR

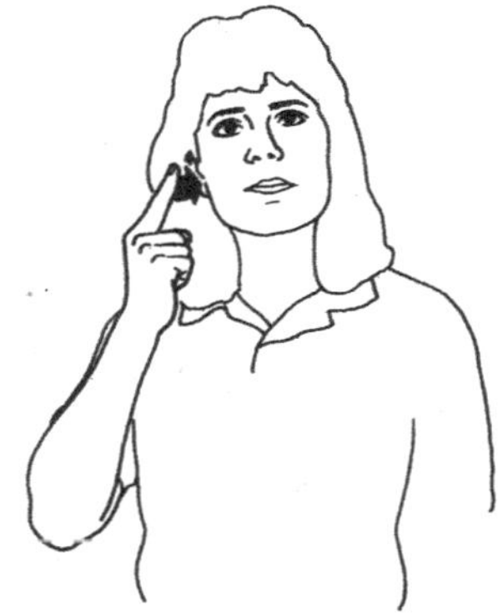

HEAR

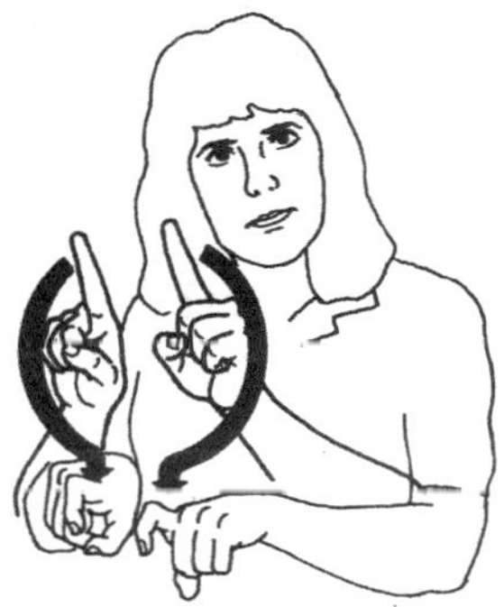

TEST

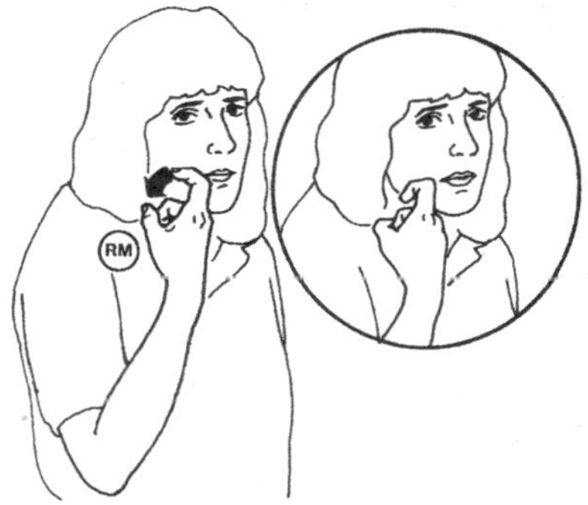

RECENT?

Did you have your hearing tested recently?

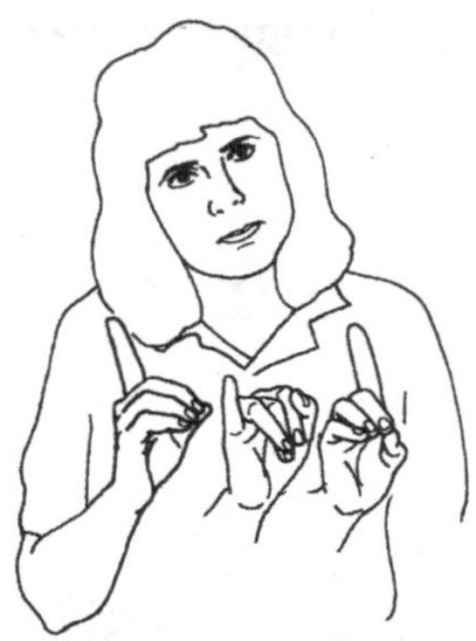

D-I-D

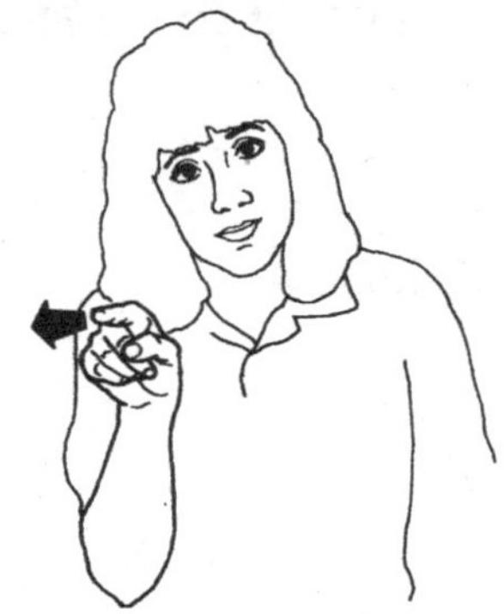

YOU

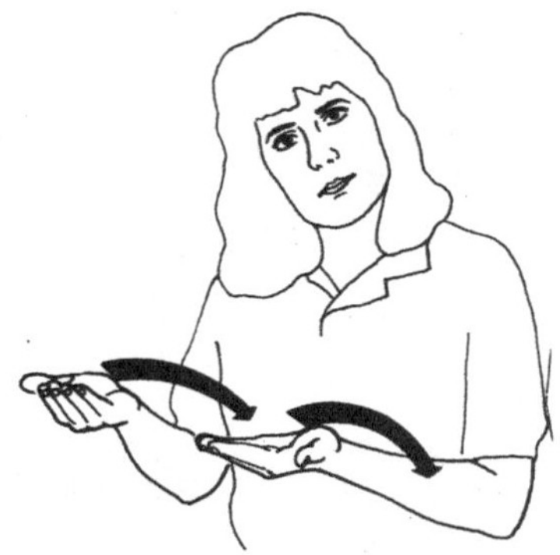

BRING

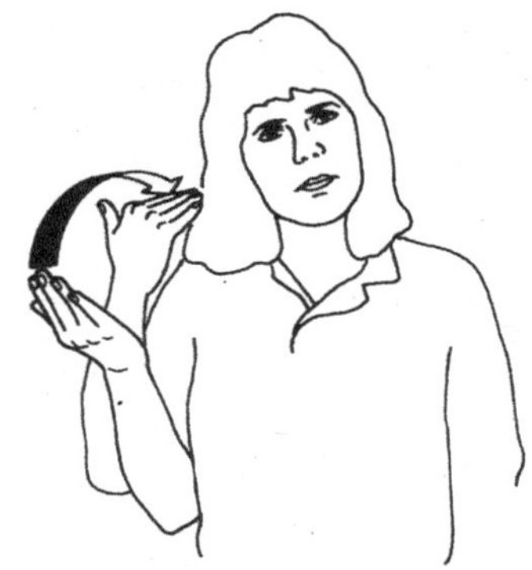

PAST

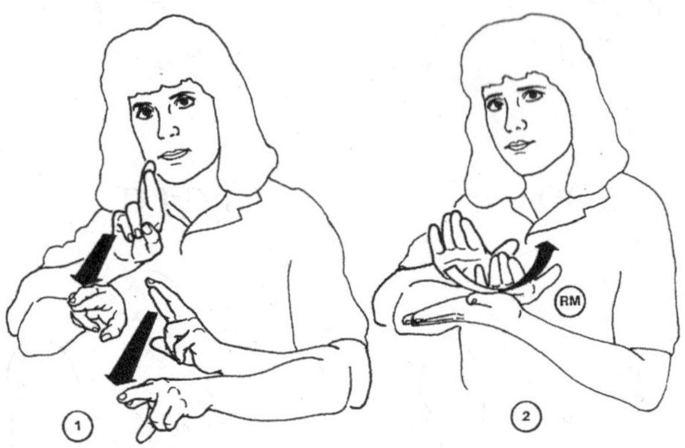

REPORT

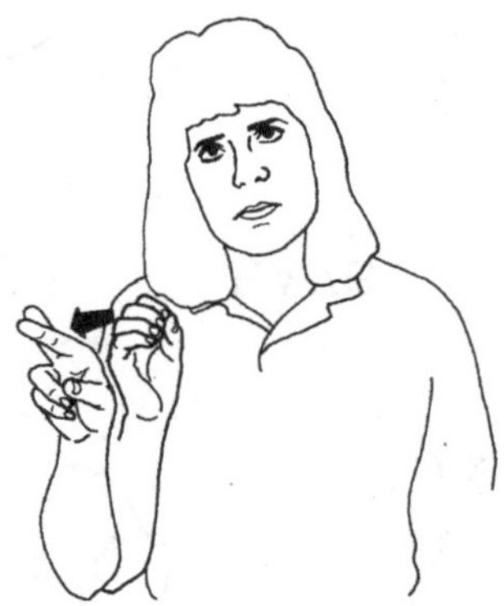

O-R

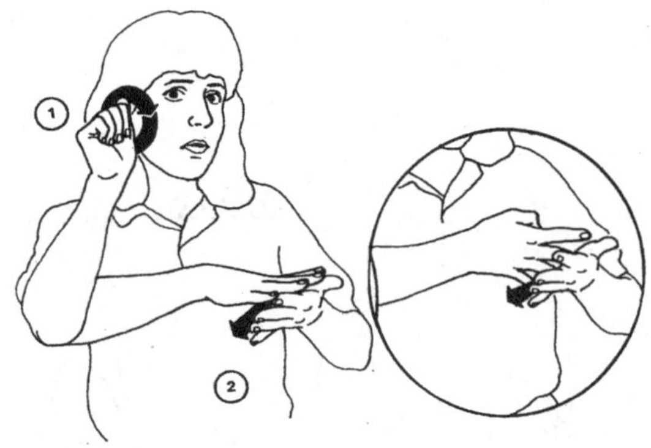

AUDIOGRAM?

Did you bring past reports or audiograms?

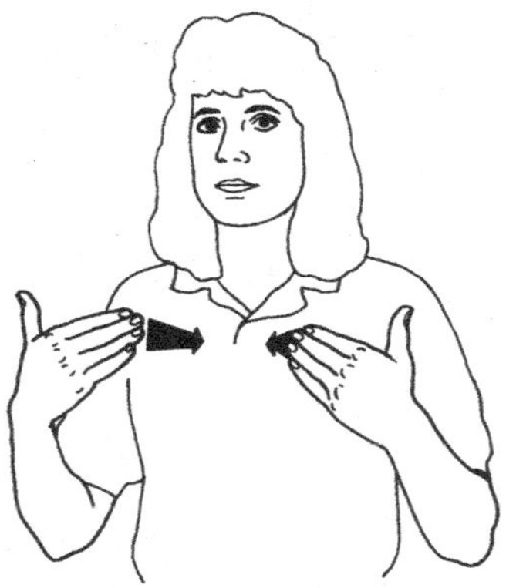

HAVE

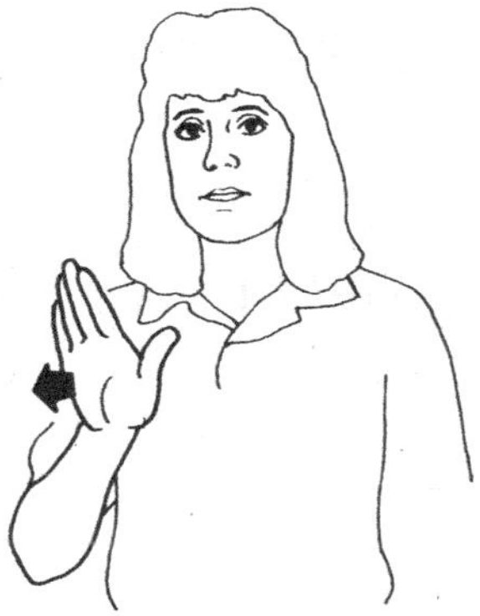

YOUR

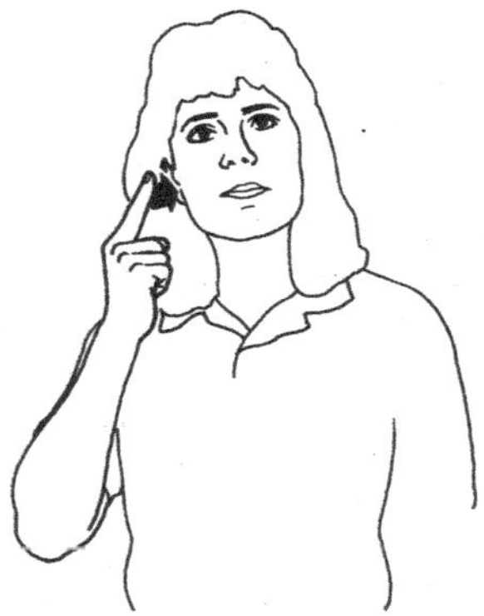

HEAR

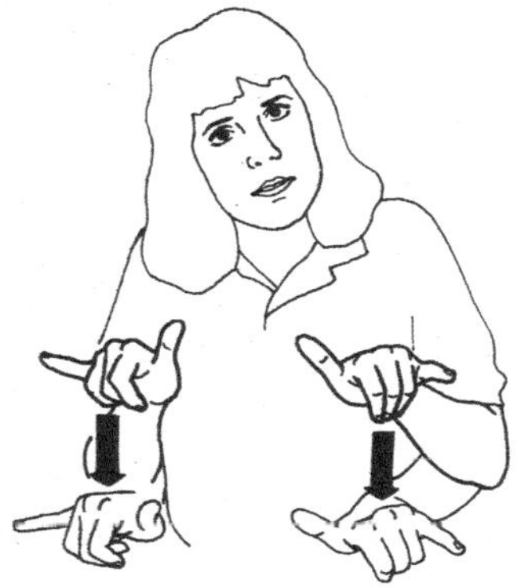

STAY

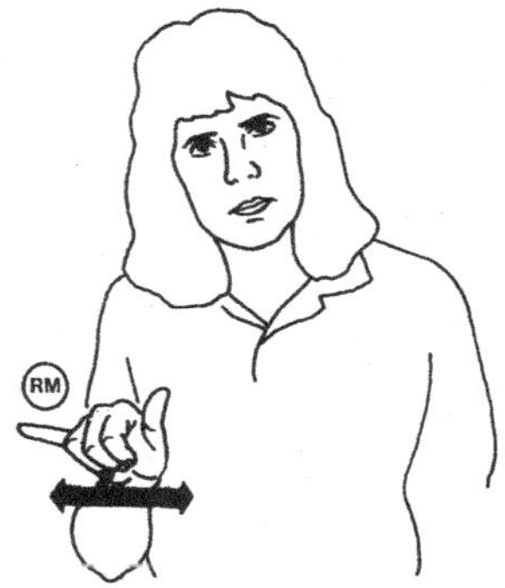

SAME

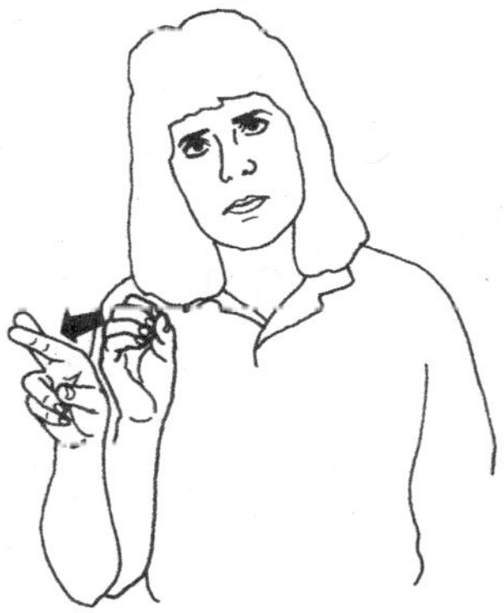

O-R

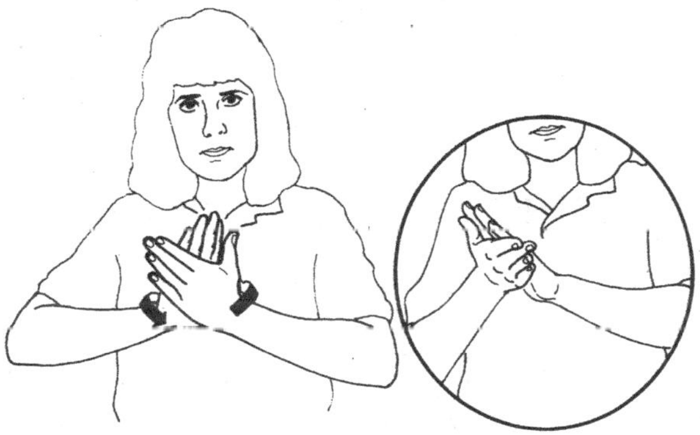

BECOME

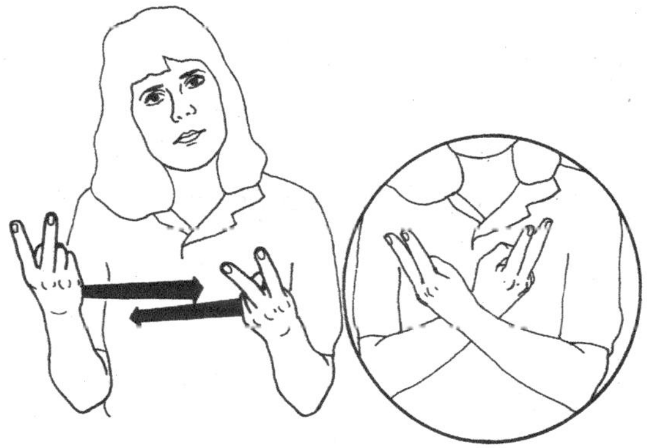

WORSE?

Has your hearing stayed the same or become worse?

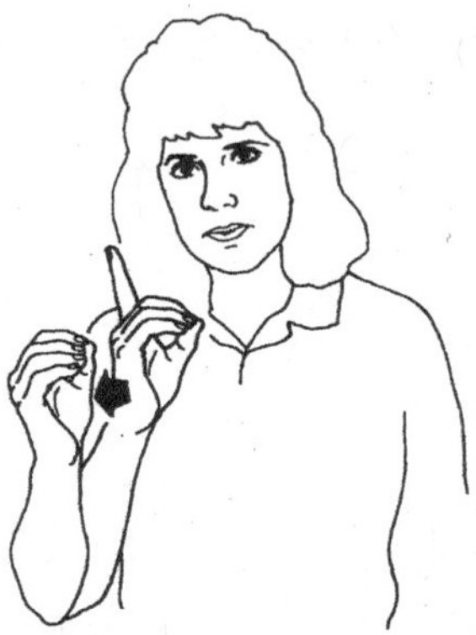

D-O

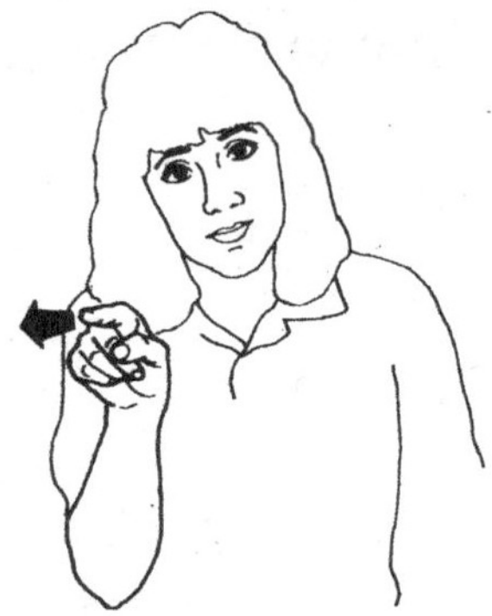

YOU

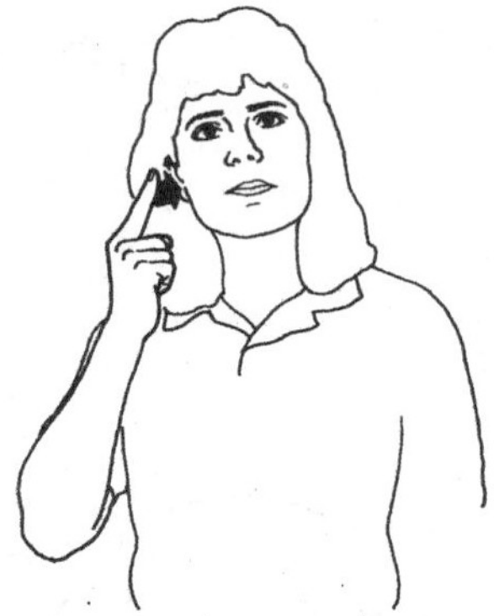

HEAR

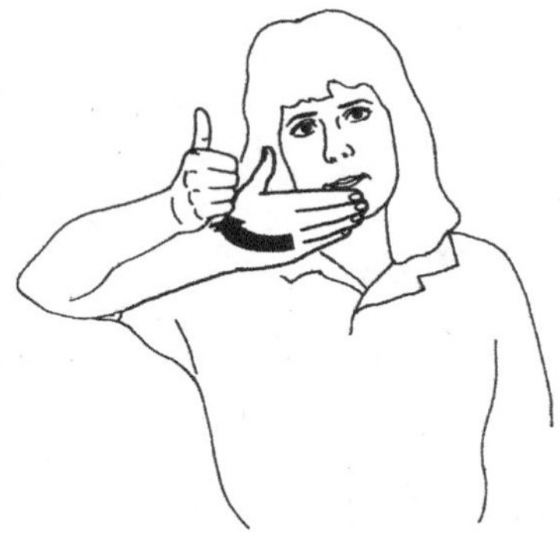

BETTER

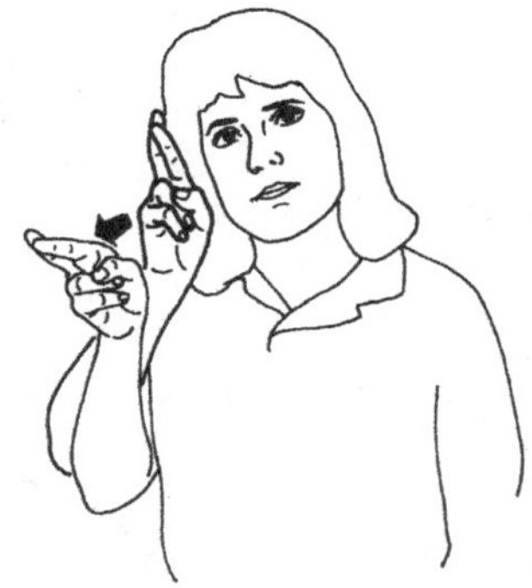

RIGHT-EAR

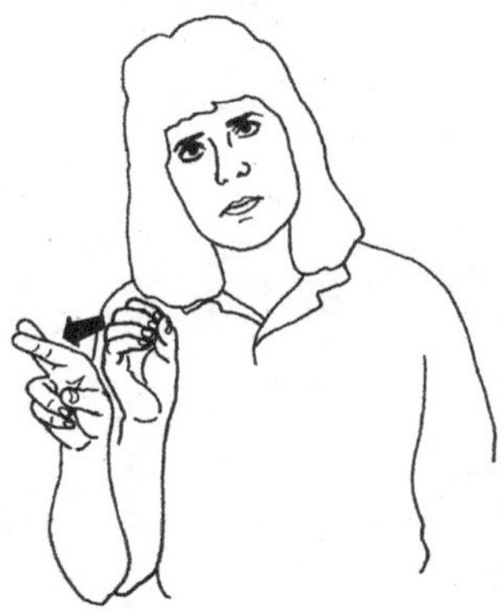

O-R

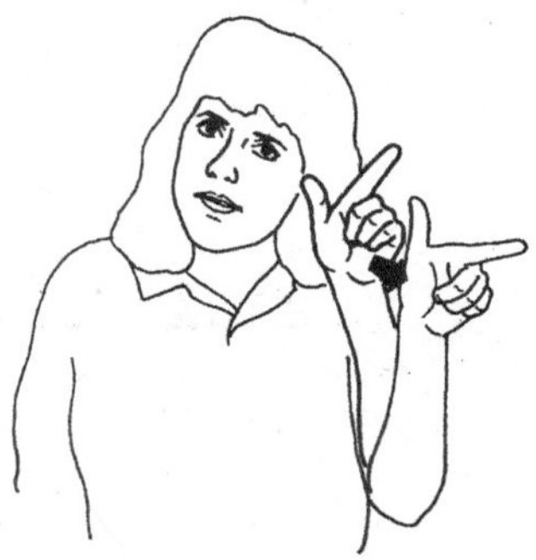

LEFT-EAR?

Do you hear better in your right or left ear?

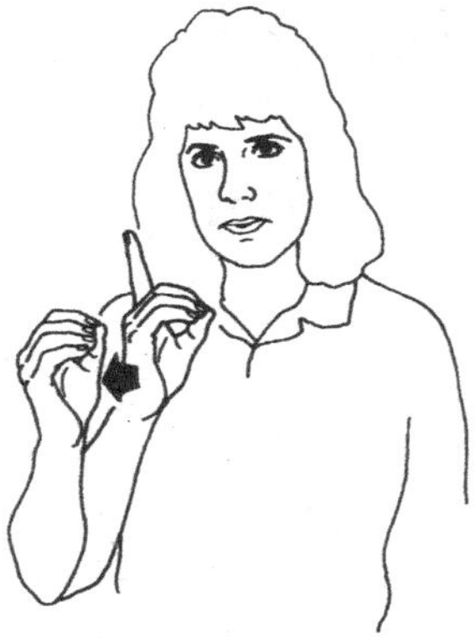

D-O

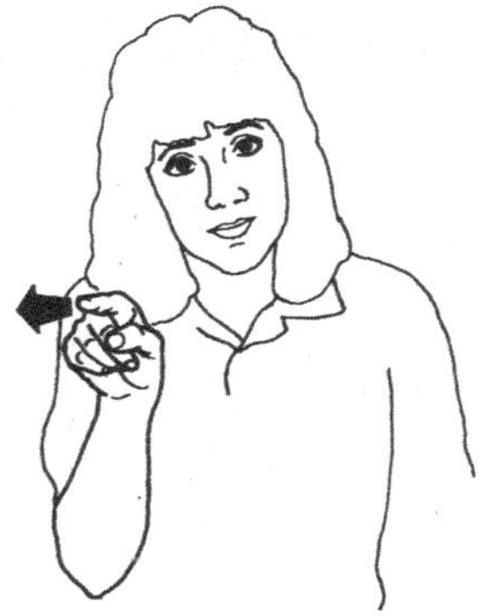

YOU

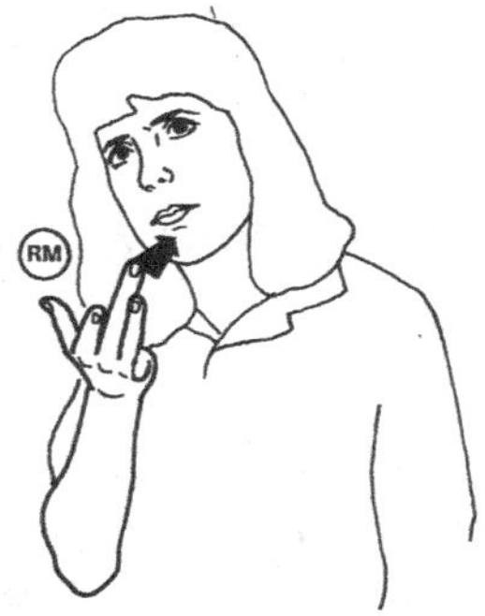

PREFER

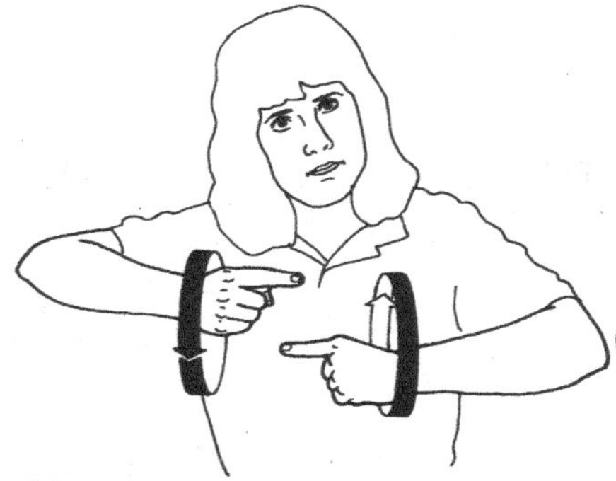

SIGN

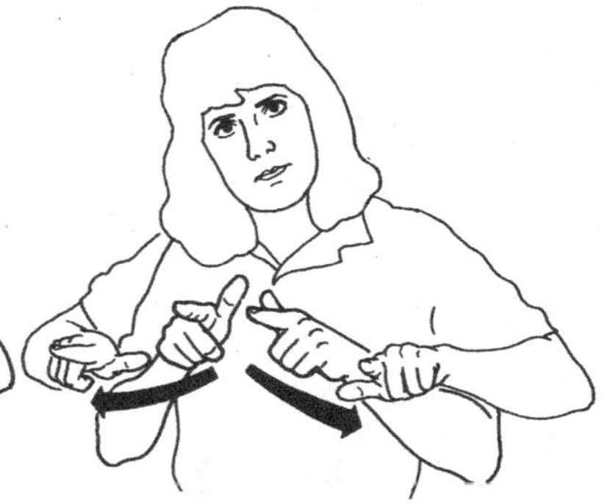

LANGUAGE

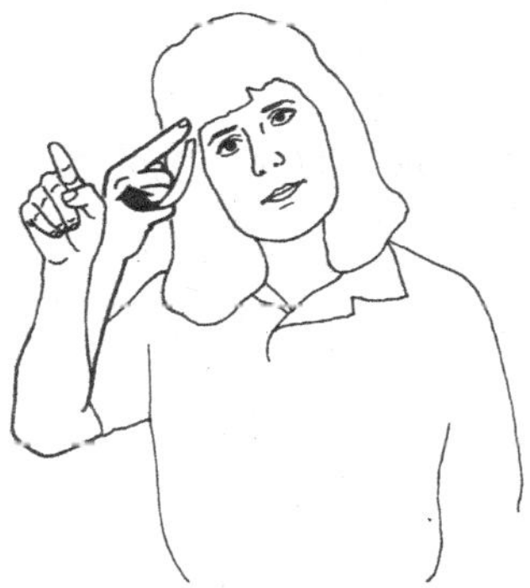

FOR

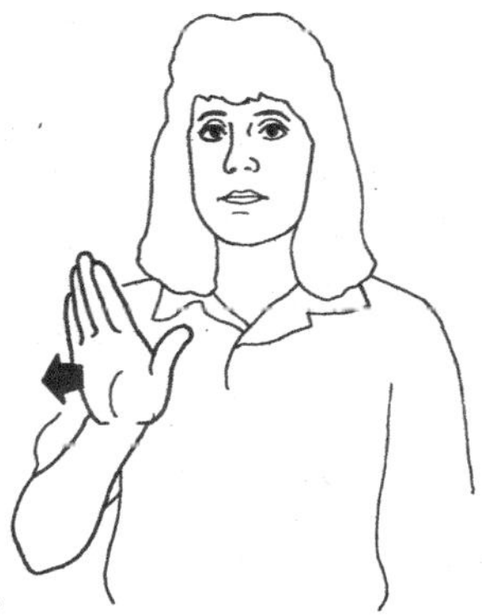

YOUR

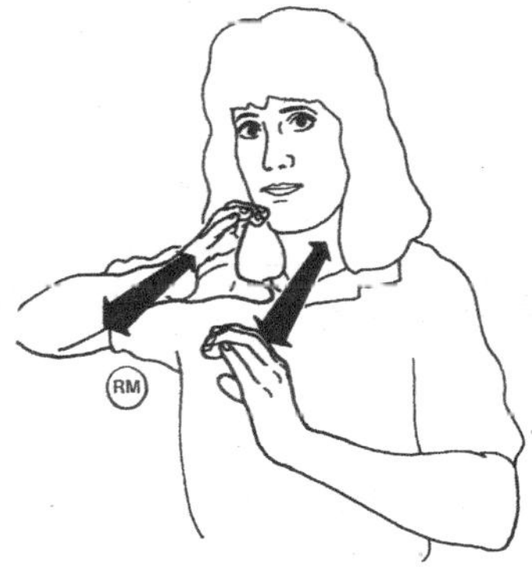

COMMUNICATION?

Do you prefer sign language for your communication?

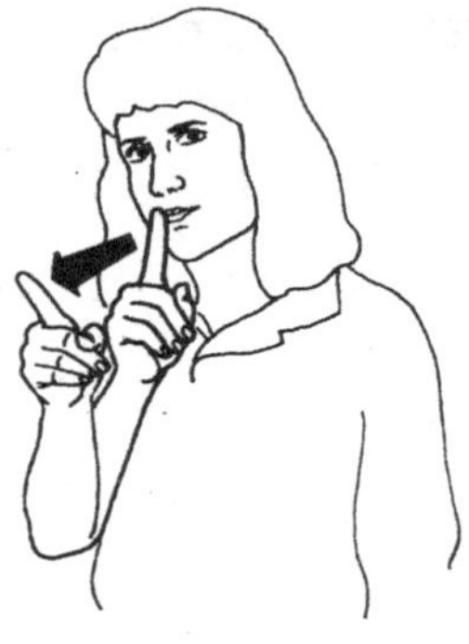

ARE

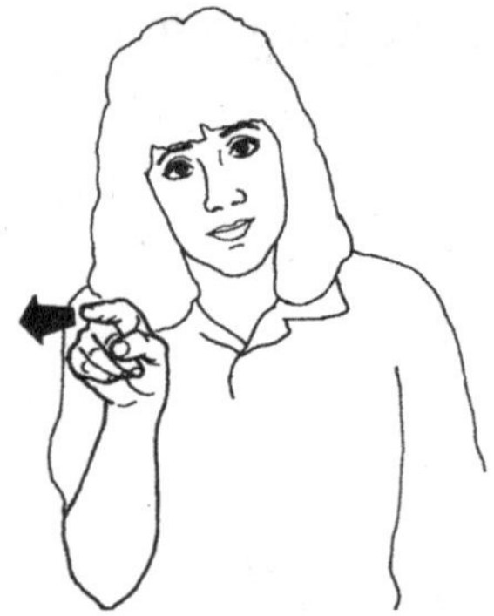

YOU

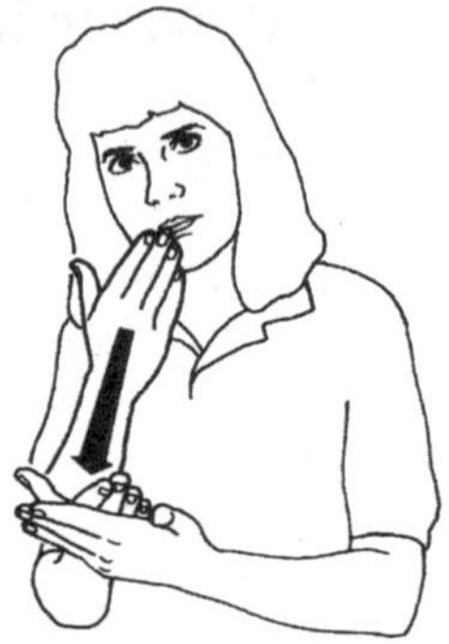

GOOD

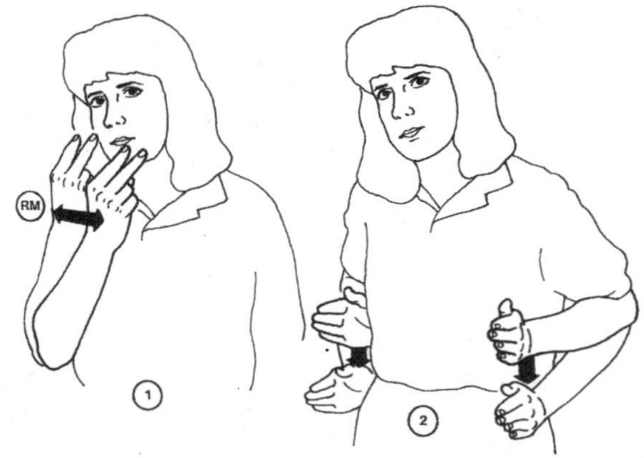

SPEECHREAD-PERSON?

Are you a good speechreader?

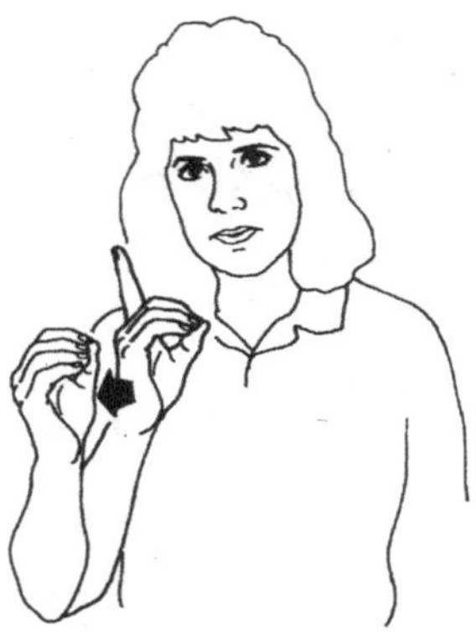

D-O

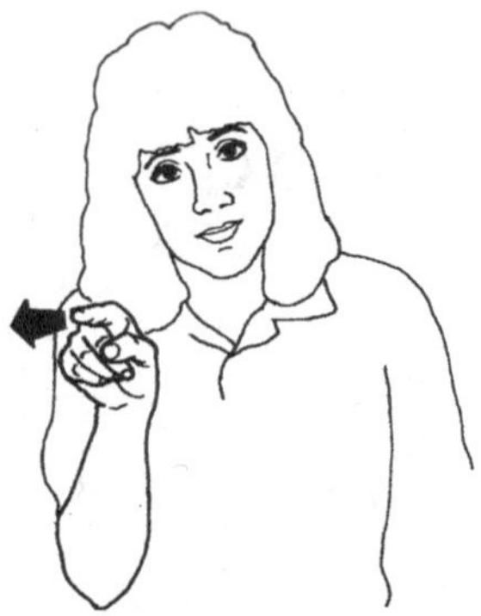

YOU

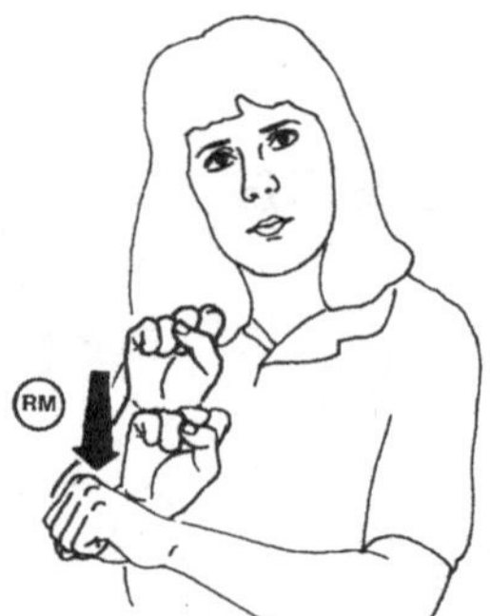

WORK

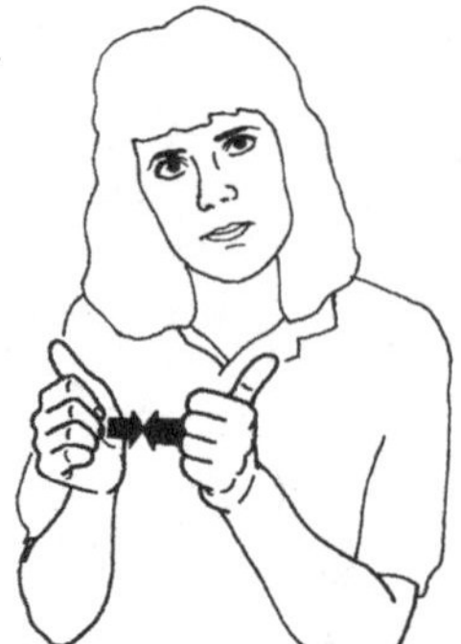

WITH

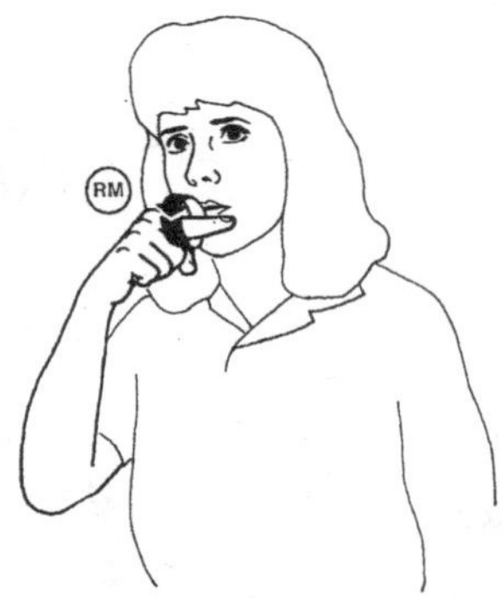

HEARING

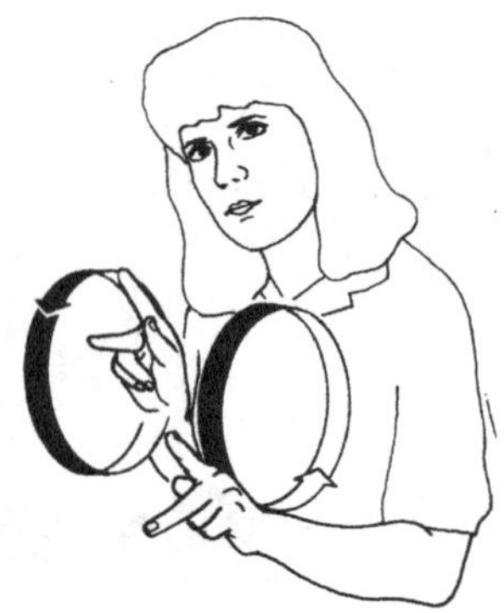

PEOPLE?

Do you work with hearing people?

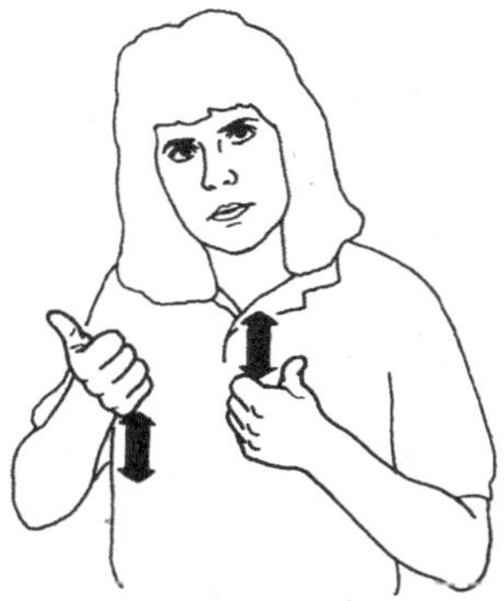

WHICH

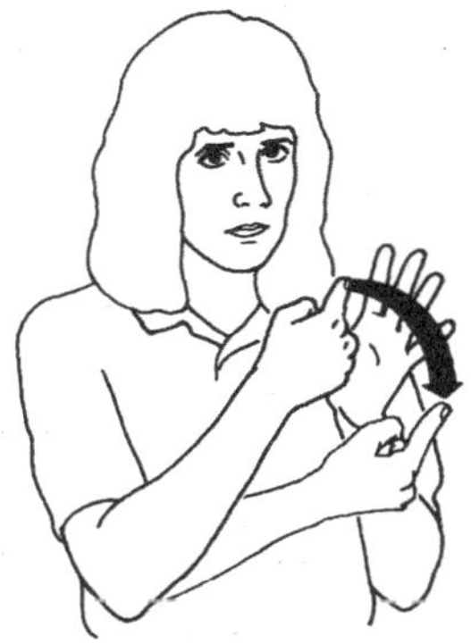

OF-THESE

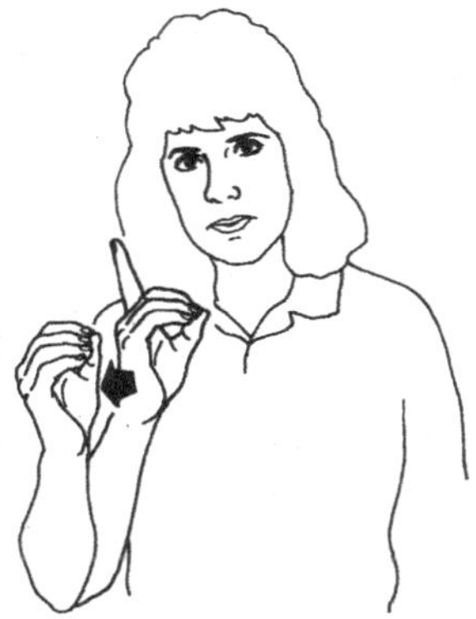

D-O

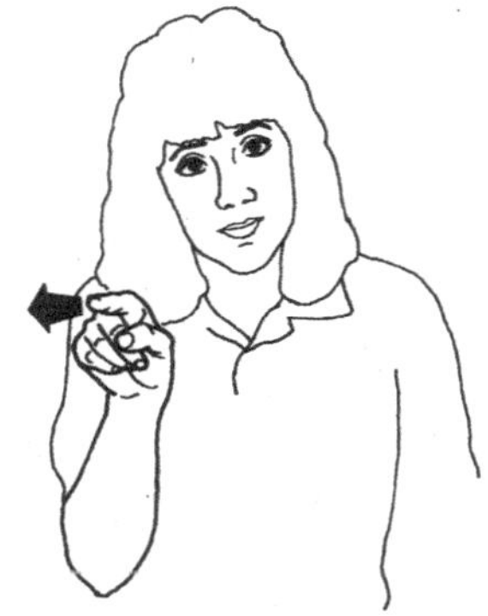

YOU

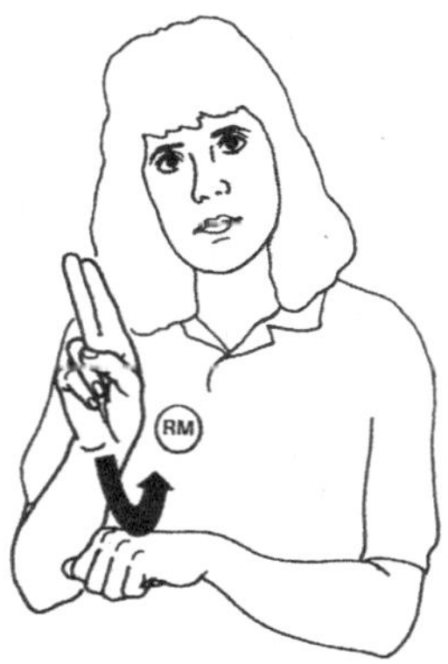

USE

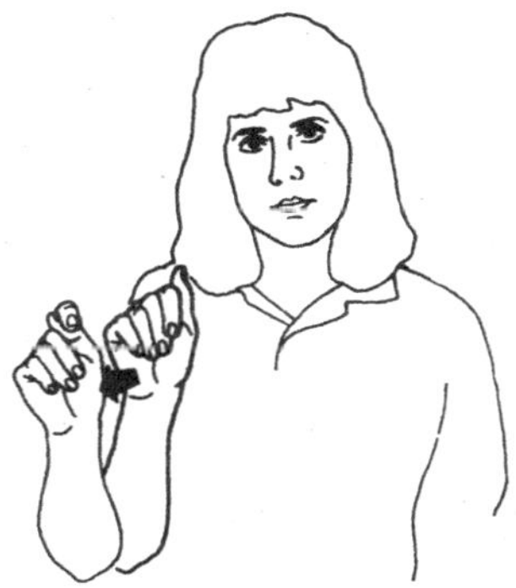

A-T

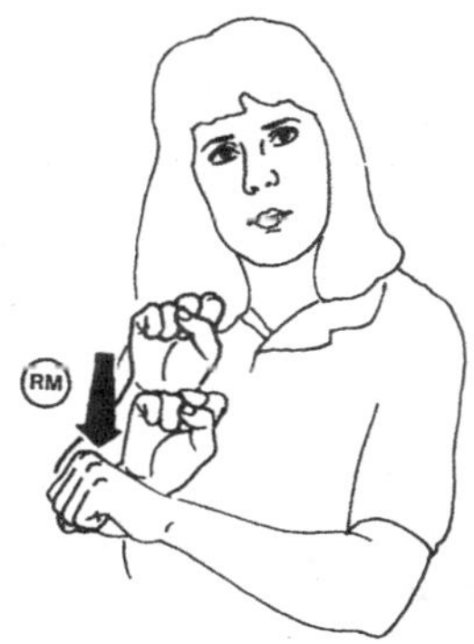

WORK

Which of the following do you use at work: talking, signing, fingerspelling, gesturing, or writing?

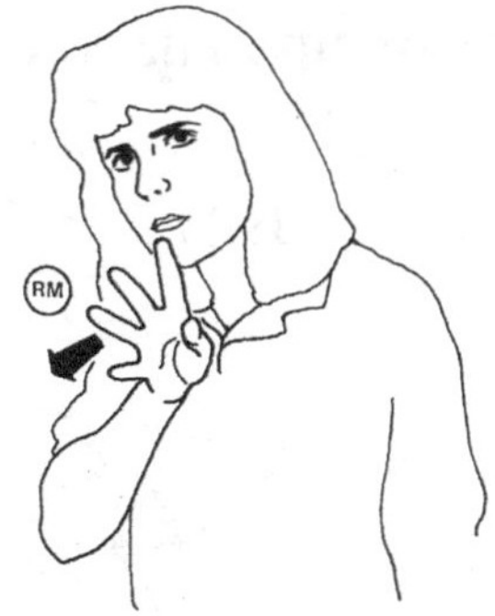

TALK

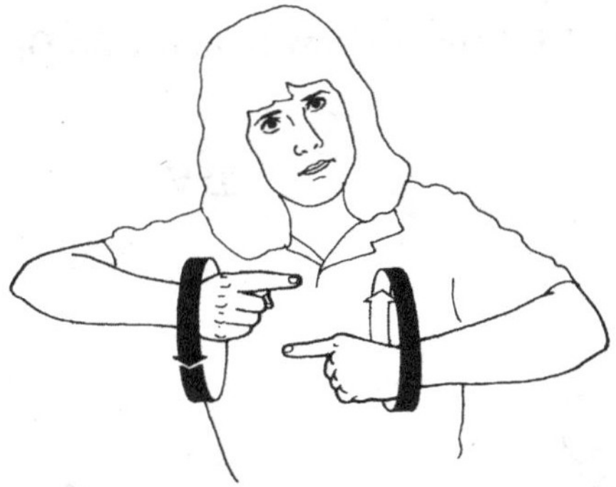

SIGN

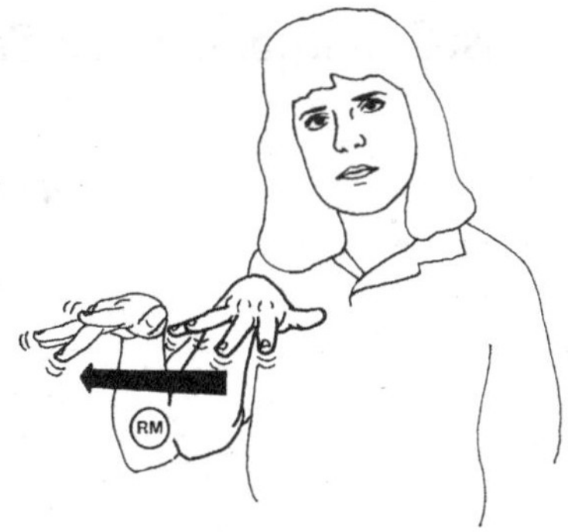

FINGERSPELL

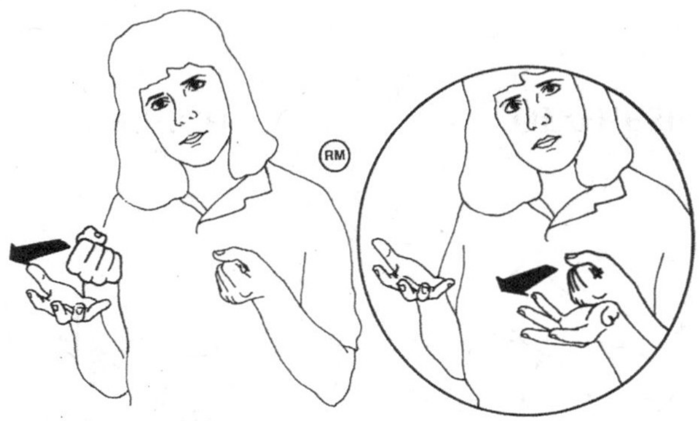

GESTURE

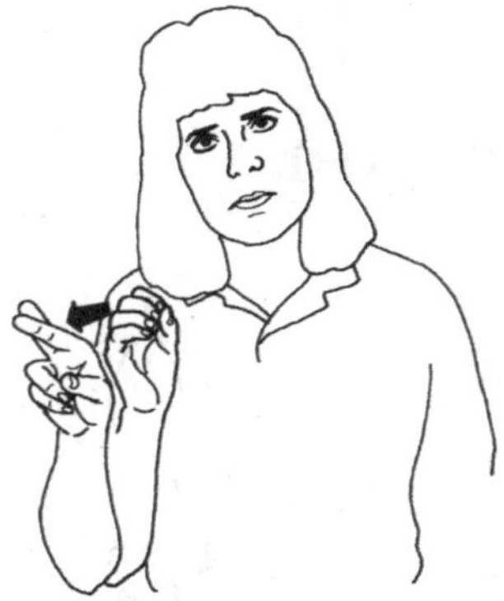

O-R

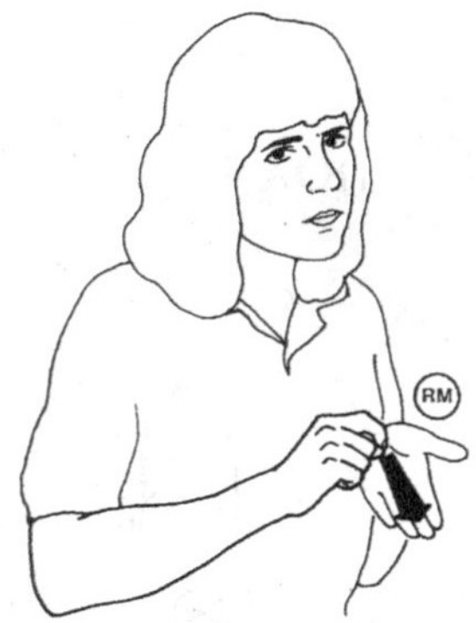

WRITE?

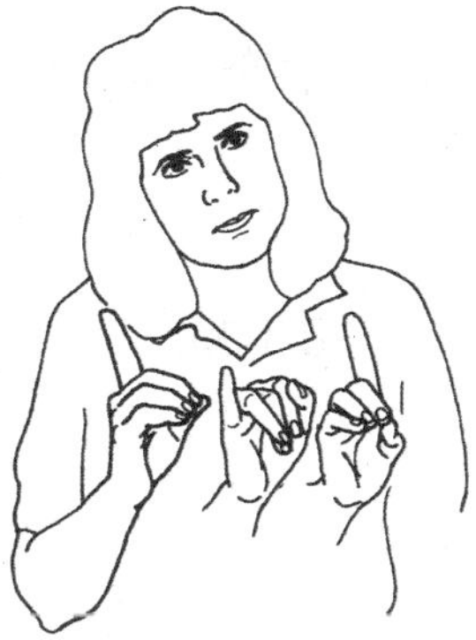

D-I-D

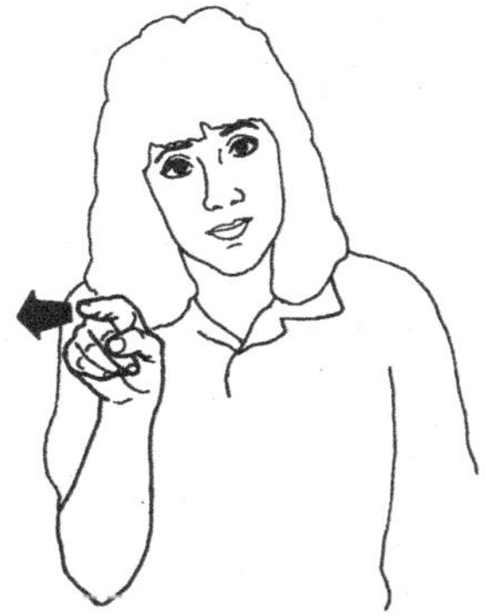

YOU

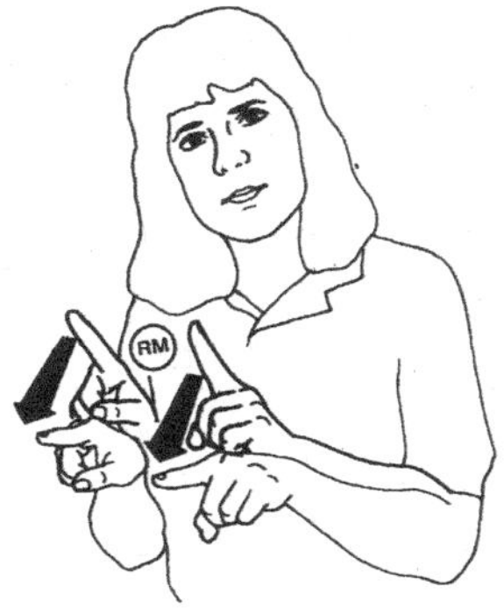

ATTEND

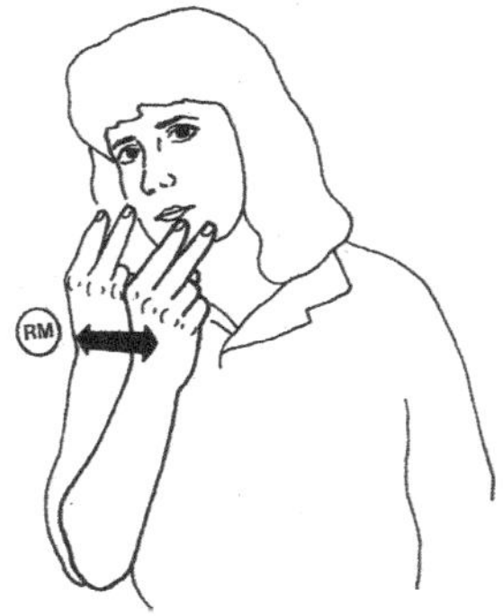

SPEECHREAD

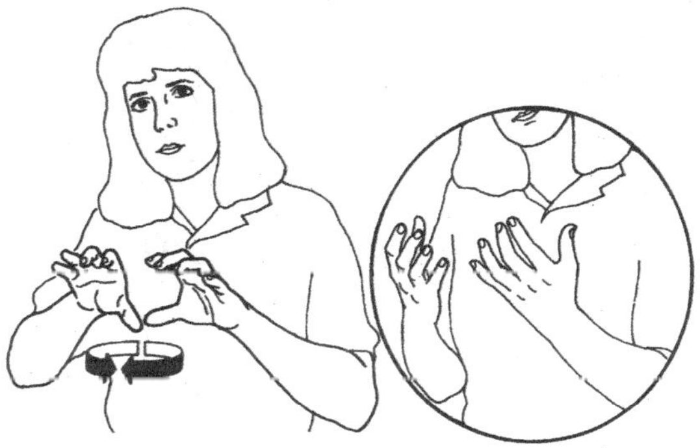

CLASS

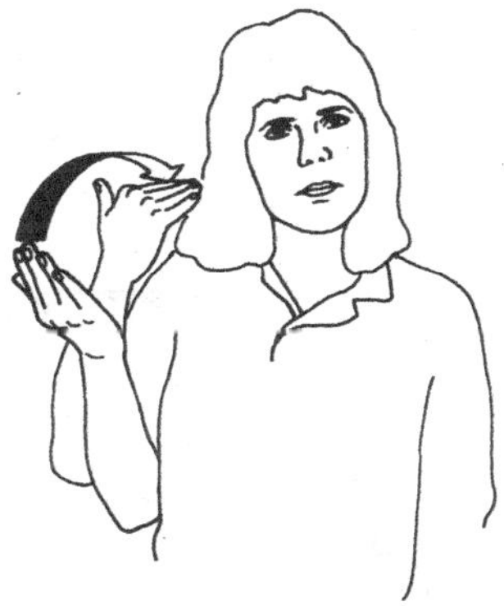

PAST?

Did you attend a speechreading class in the past?

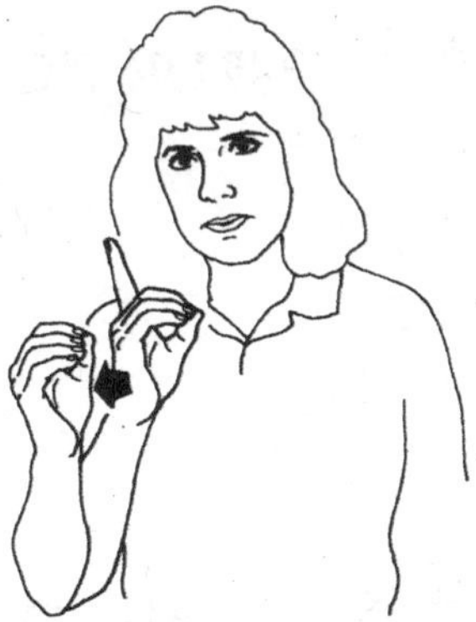

D-O

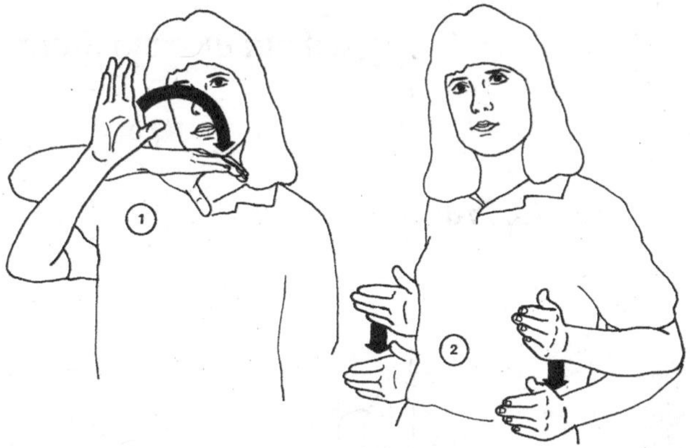

STRANGER

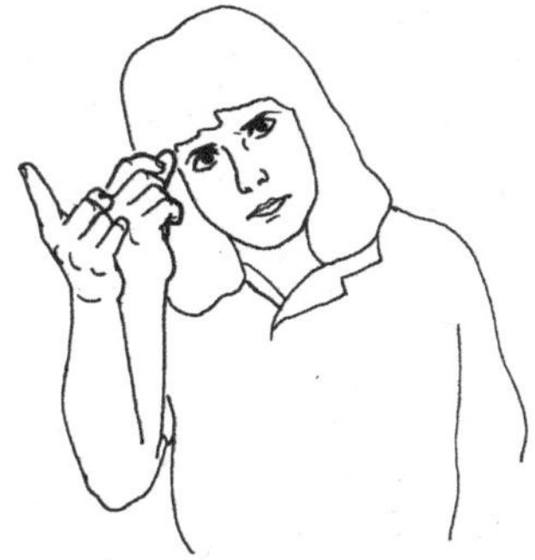

UNDERSTAND

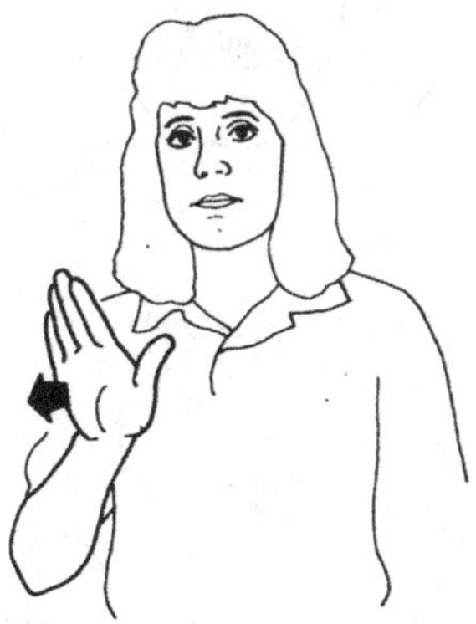

YOUR

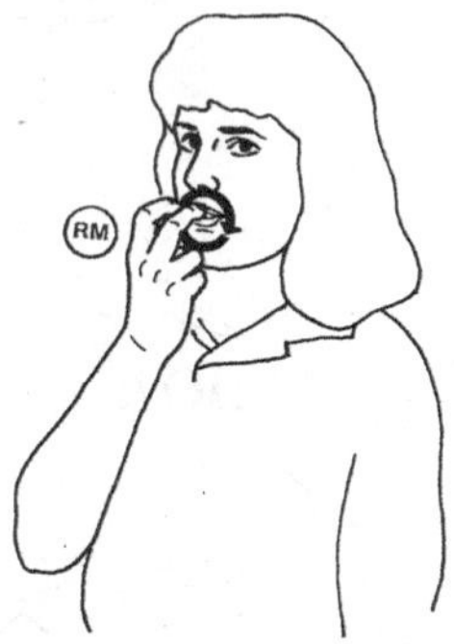

SPEECH?

Do strangers understand your speech?

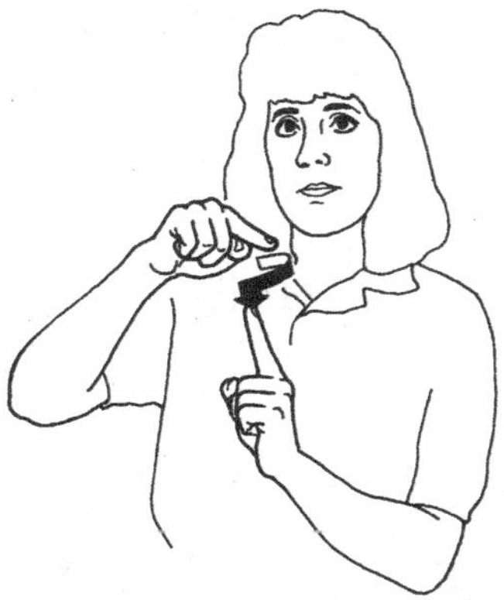

WHEN

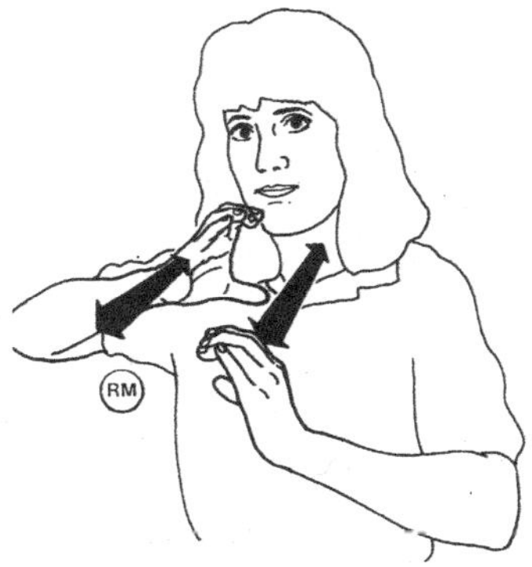

COMMUNICATION

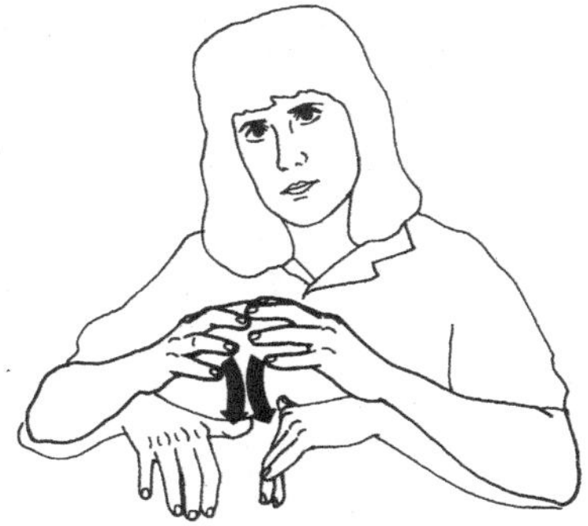

BREAKDOWN

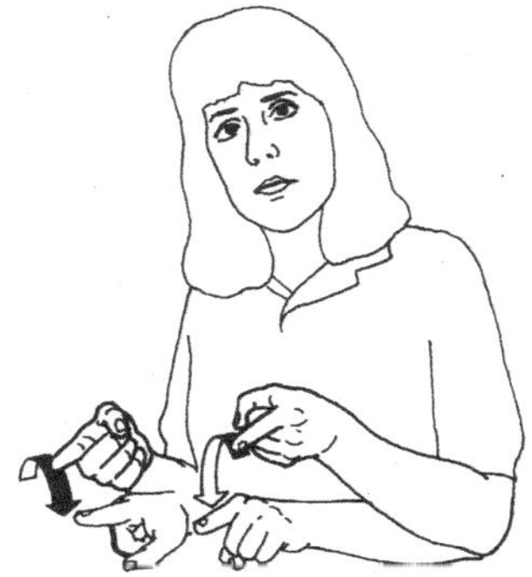

HAPPEN

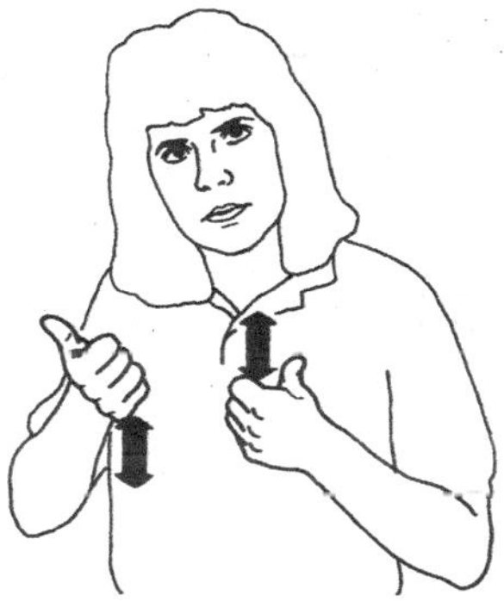

WHICH

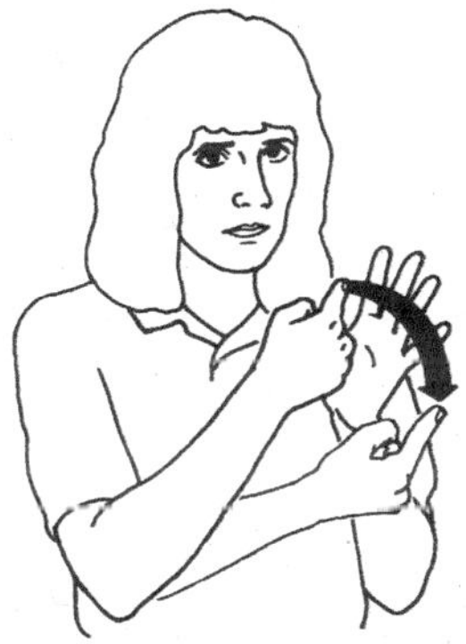

OF-THESE

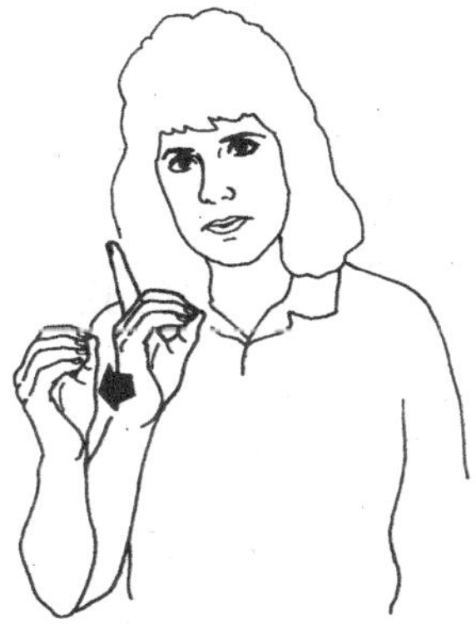

D-O

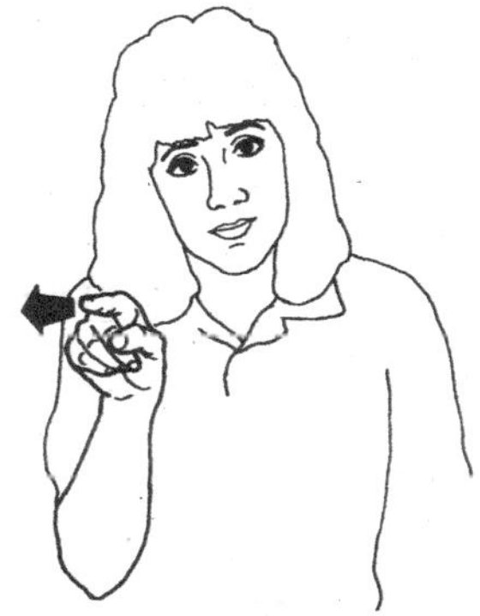

YOU

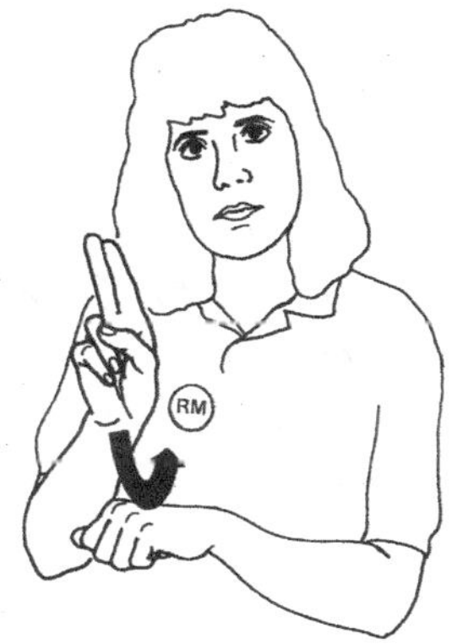

USE

When communication breakdown happens, which of these do you use: revise, repeat, write, or give-up?

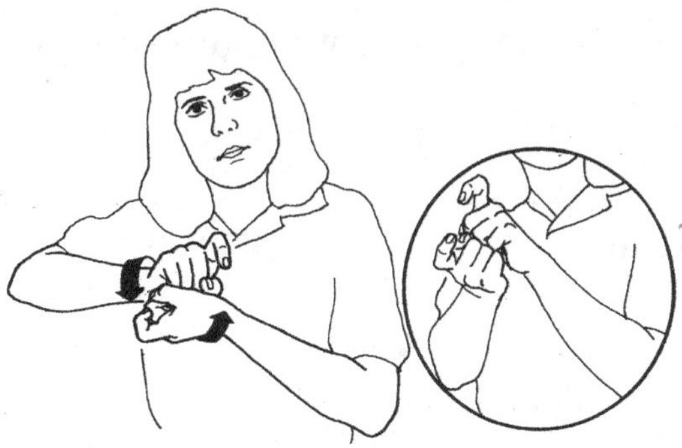

REVISE

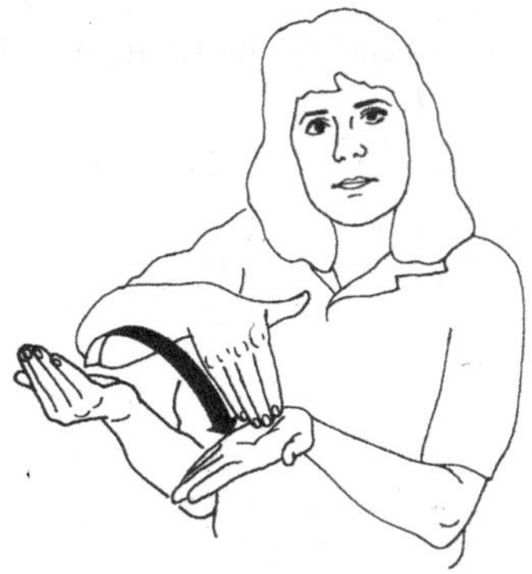

REPEAT

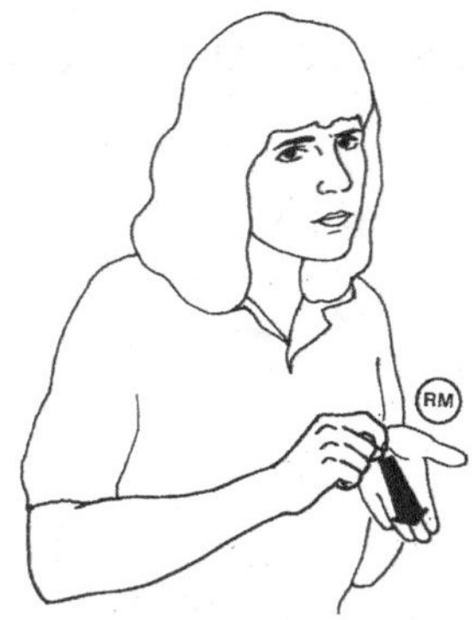

WRITE

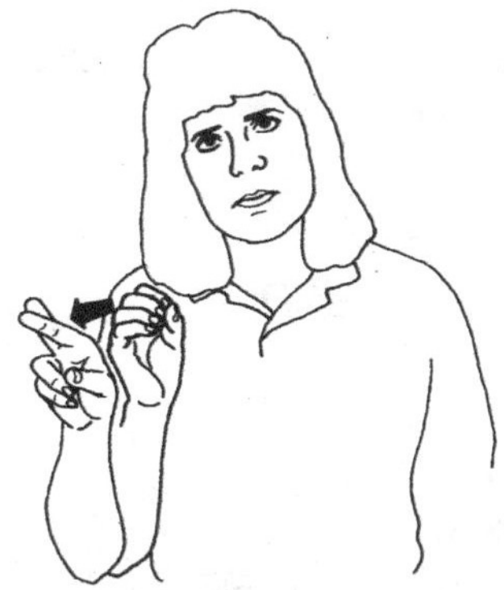

O-R

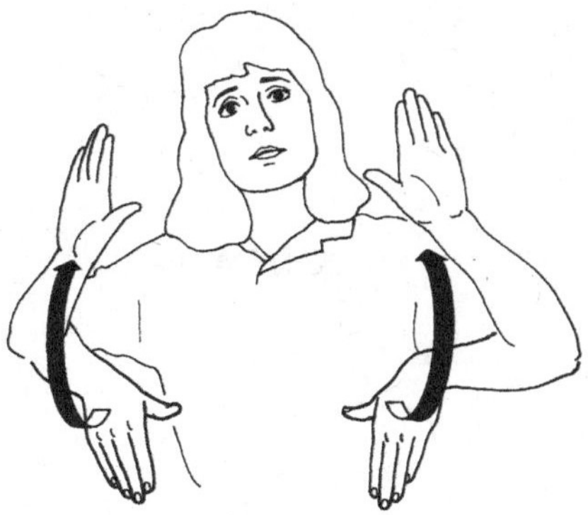

GIVE-UP?

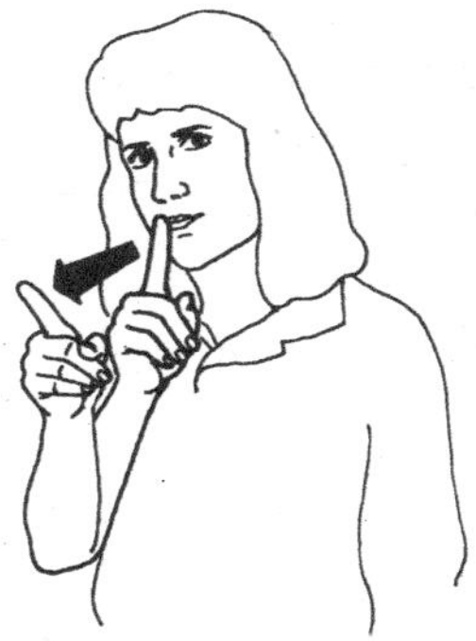

ARE

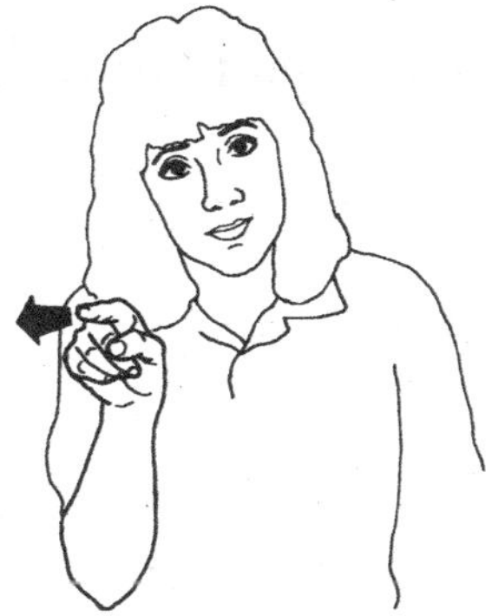

YOU

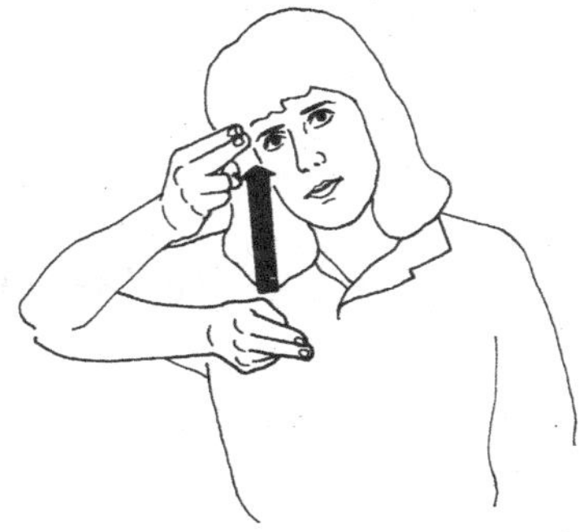

HIGH

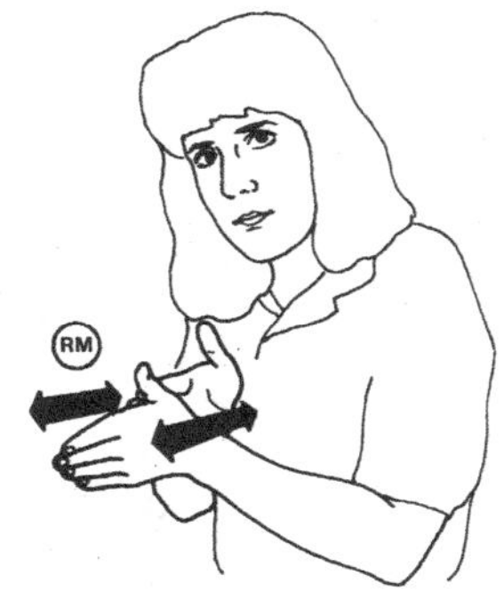

MOTIVATE

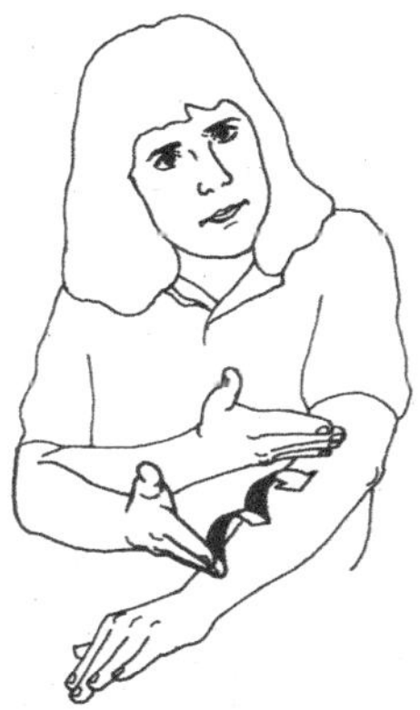

IMPROVE

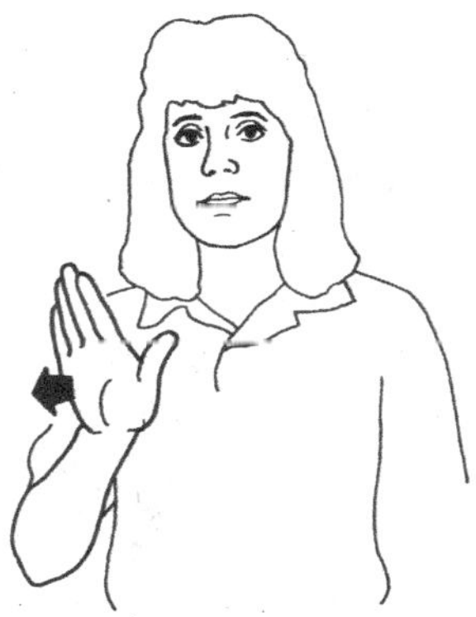

YOUR

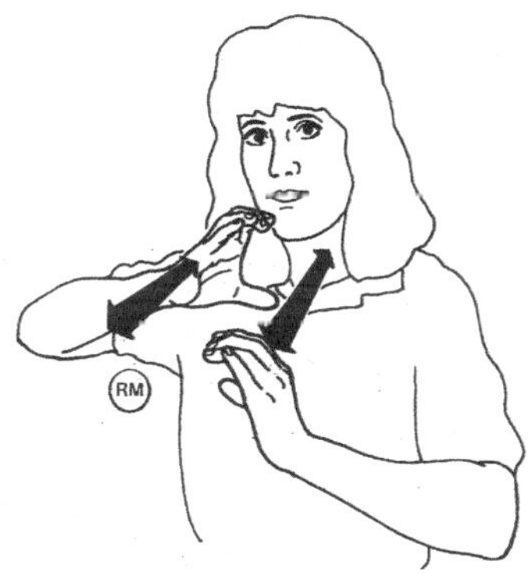

COMMUNICATION?

Are you highly motivated to improve your communication?

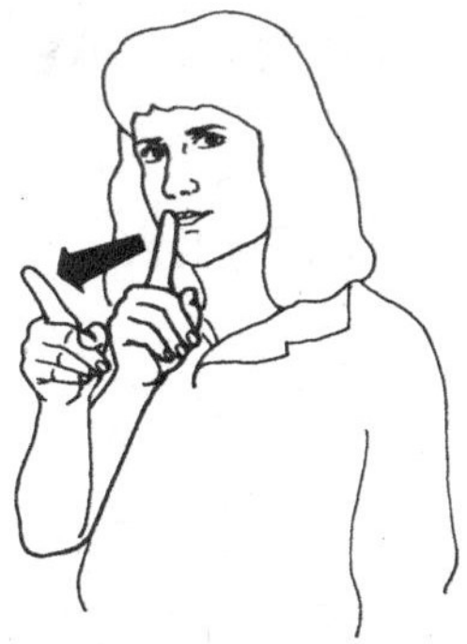

IS

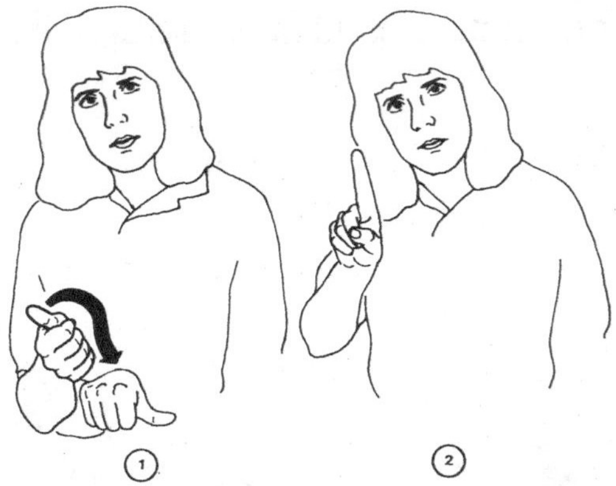

ANYONE

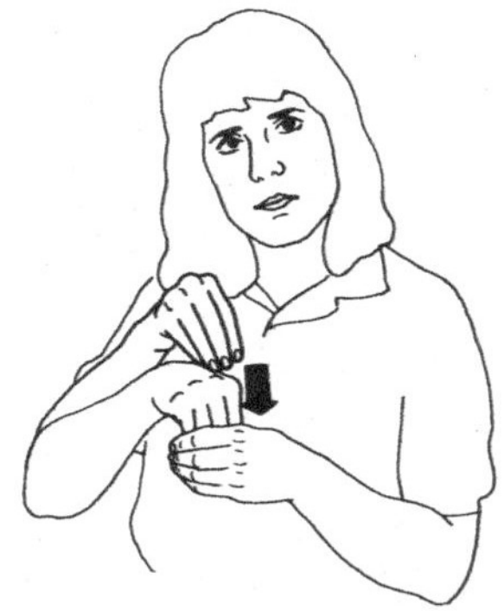

IN

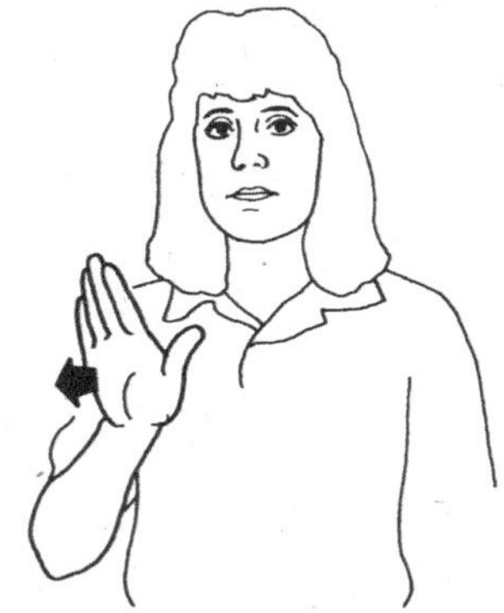

YOUR

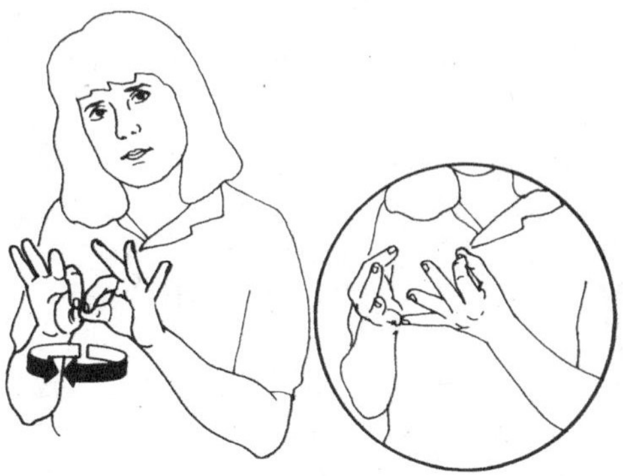

FAMILY

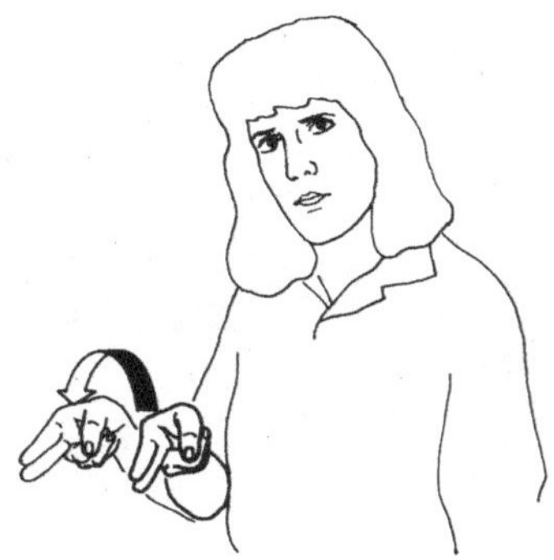

HARD-OF-HEARING

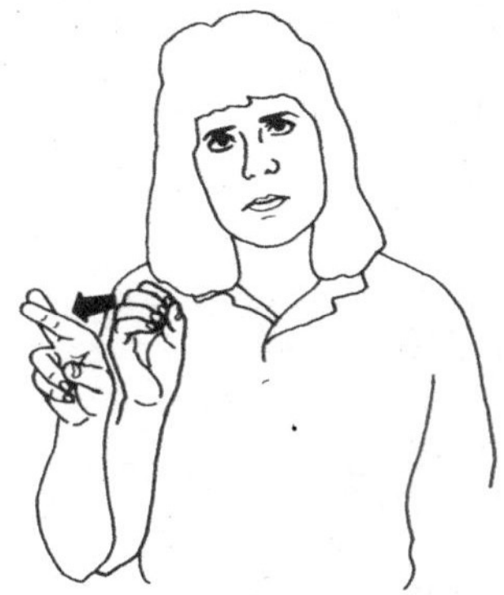

O-R

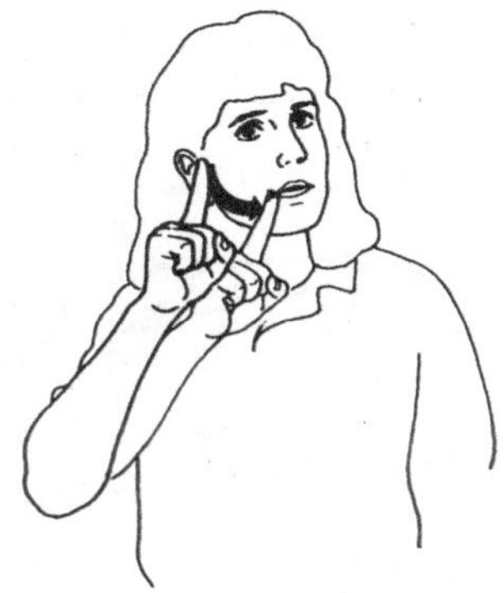

DEAF?

Is anyone in your family hard of hearing or deaf?

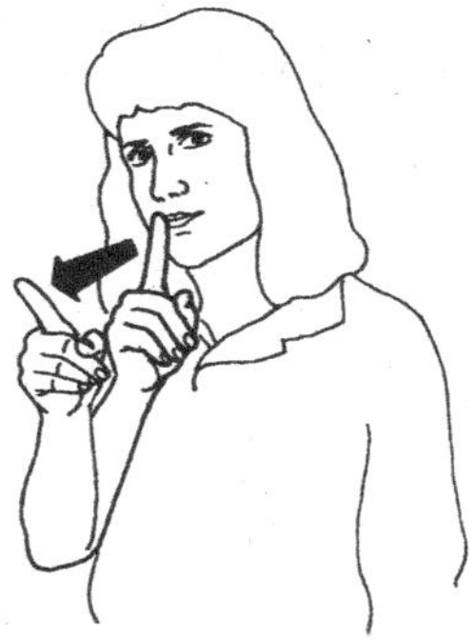

IS

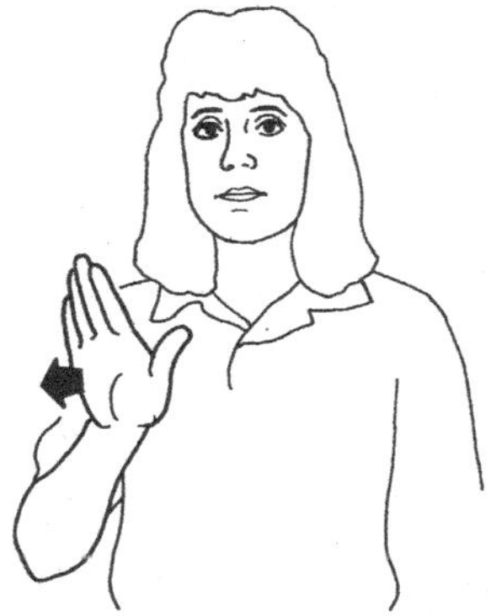

YOUR

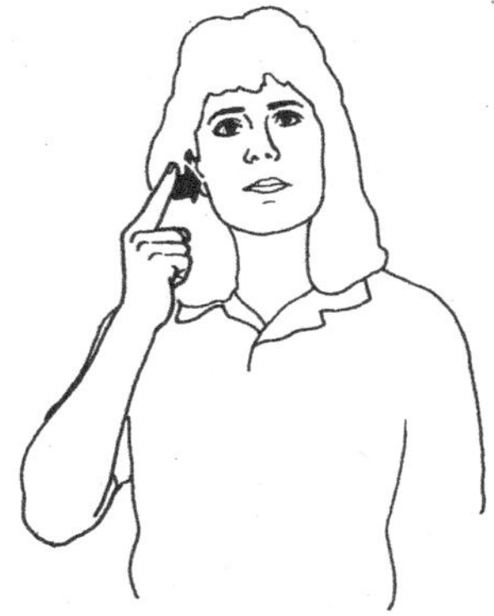

HEARING

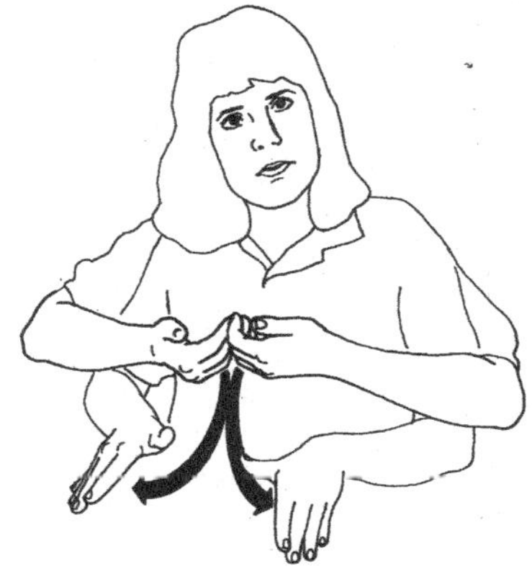

LOSS

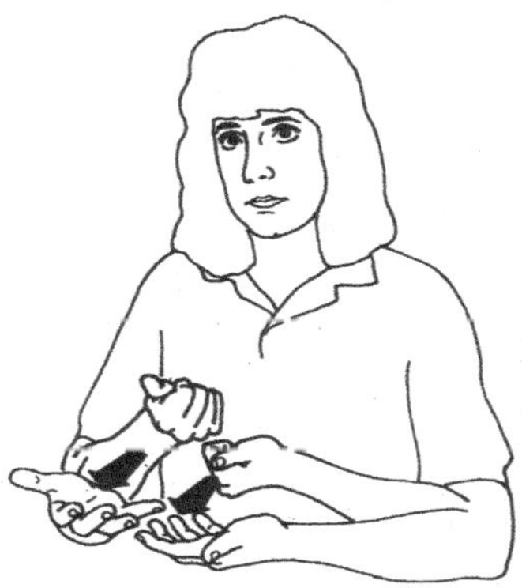

CAUSE

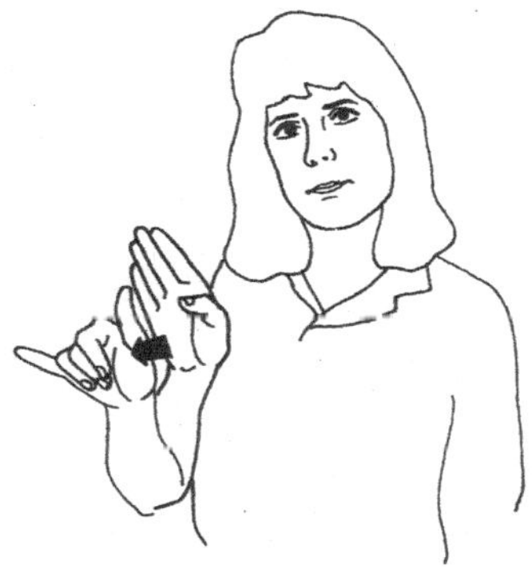

B-Y

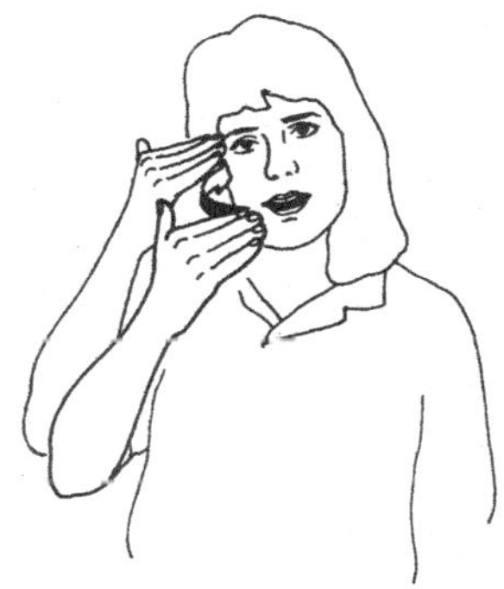

HEAD

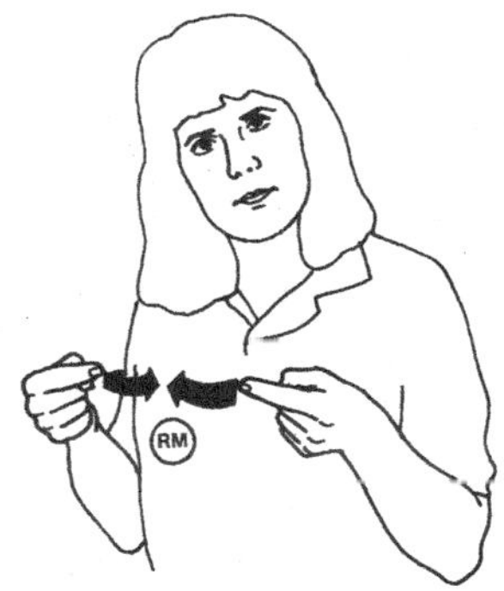

INJURY?

Is your hearing loss caused by a head injury?

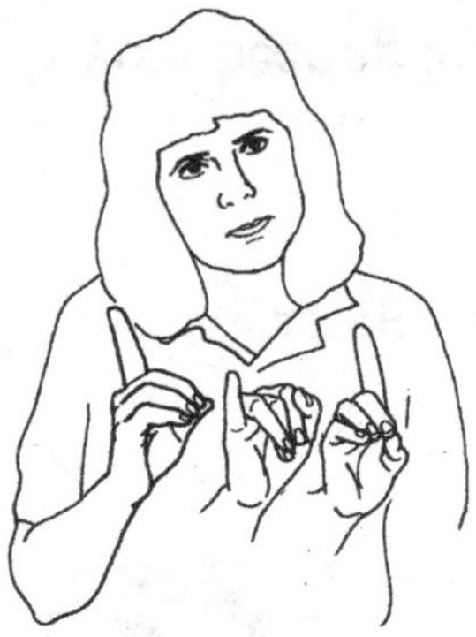

D-I-D

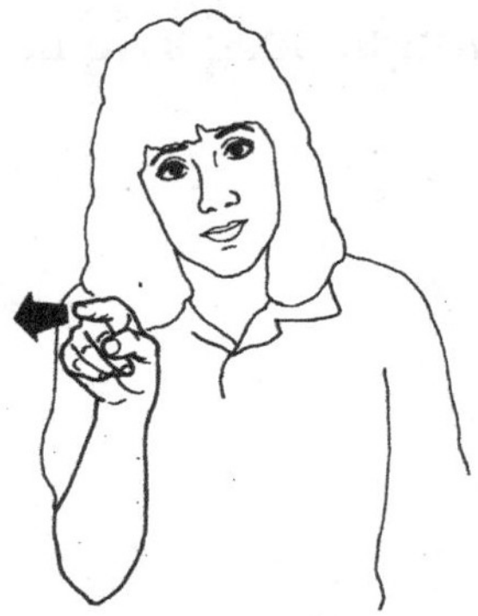

YOU

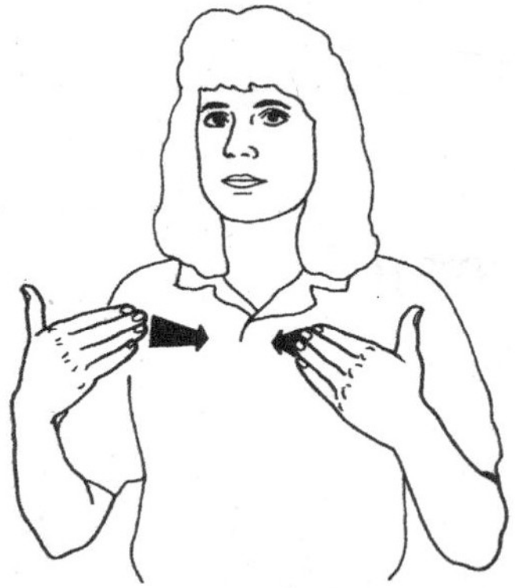

HAVE

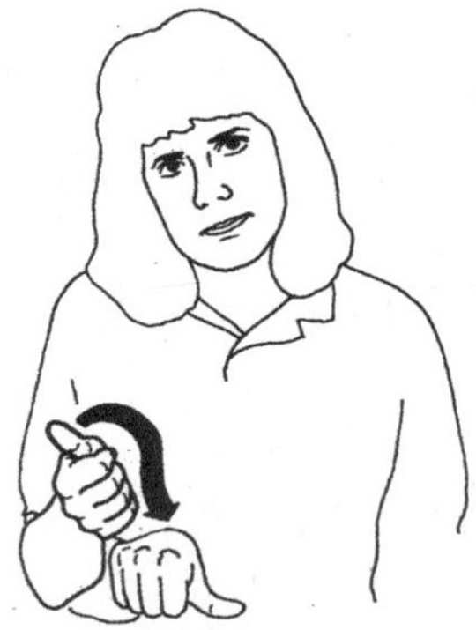

ANY

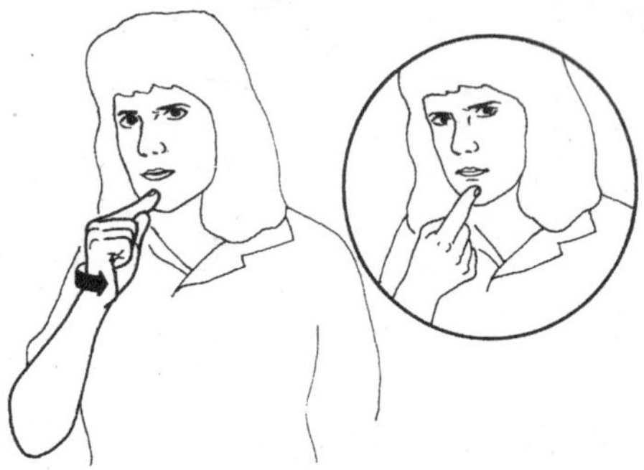

SERIOUS

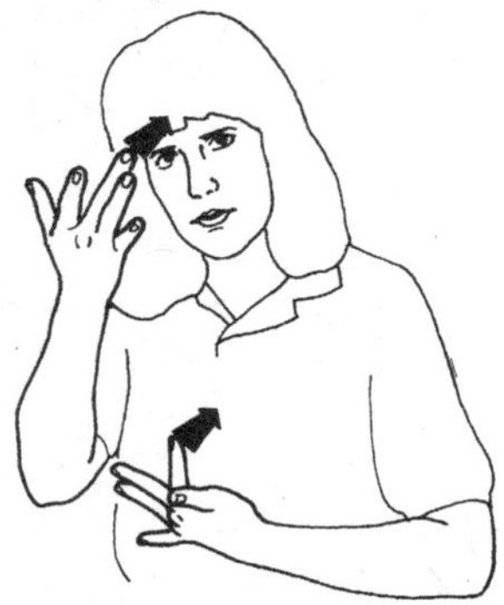

ILLNESS?

Did you have any serious illnesses?

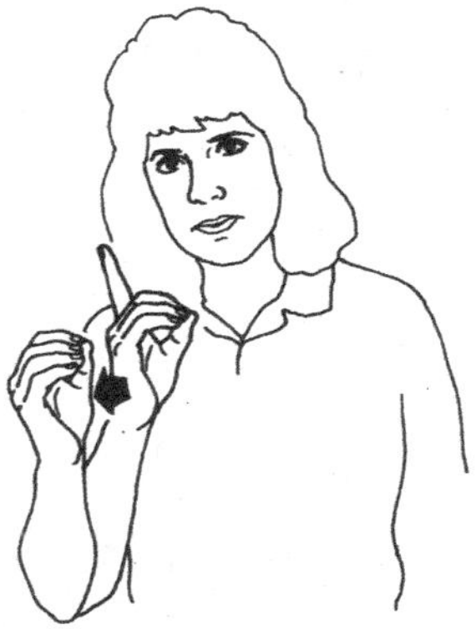

D-O

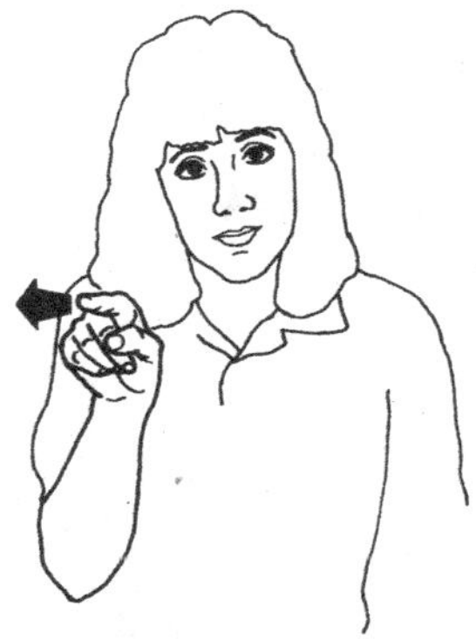

YOU

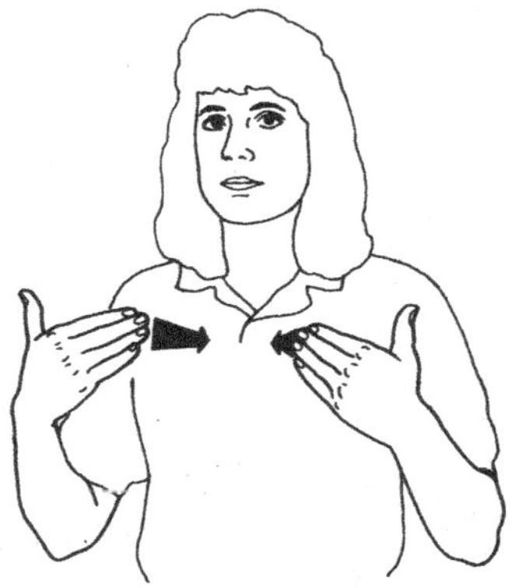

HAVE

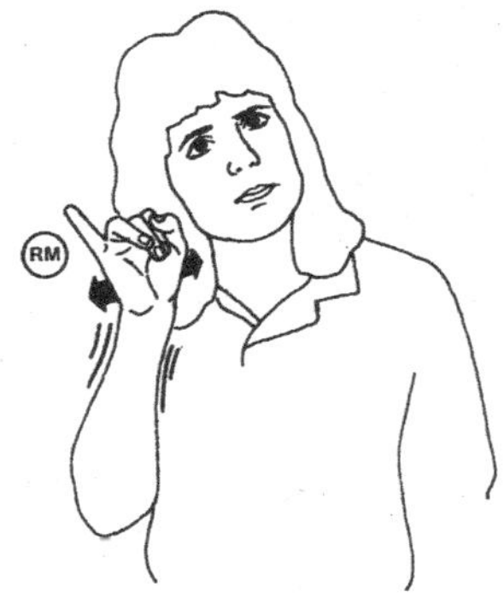

EAR-INFECTION

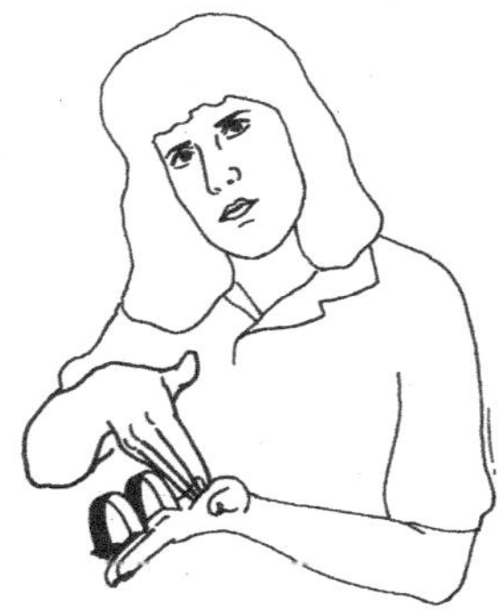

OFTEN?

Do you have ear infections often?

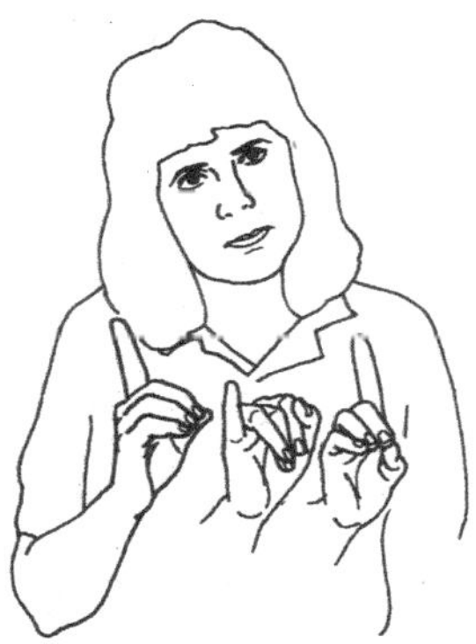

D-I-D

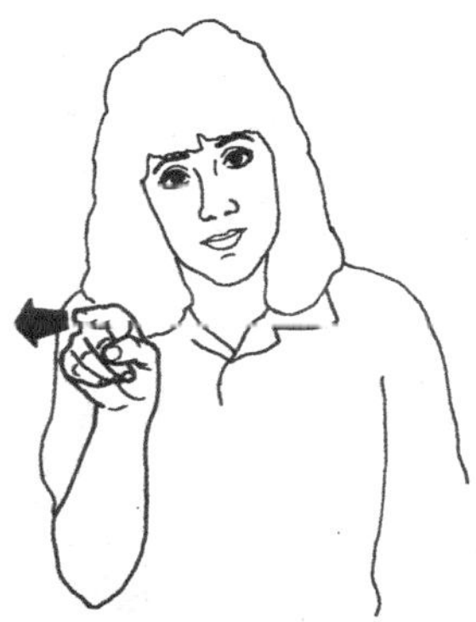

YOU

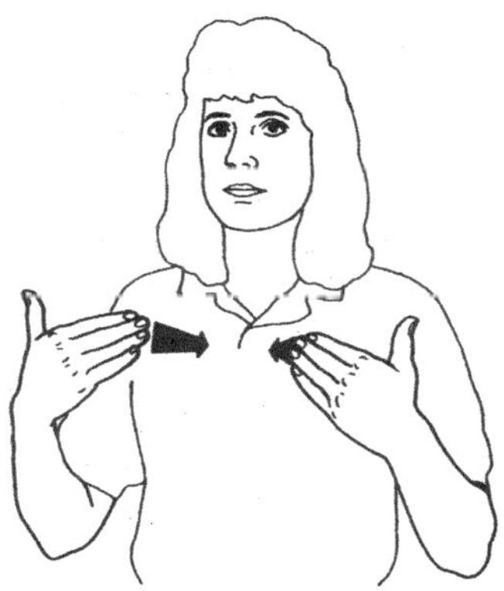

HAVE

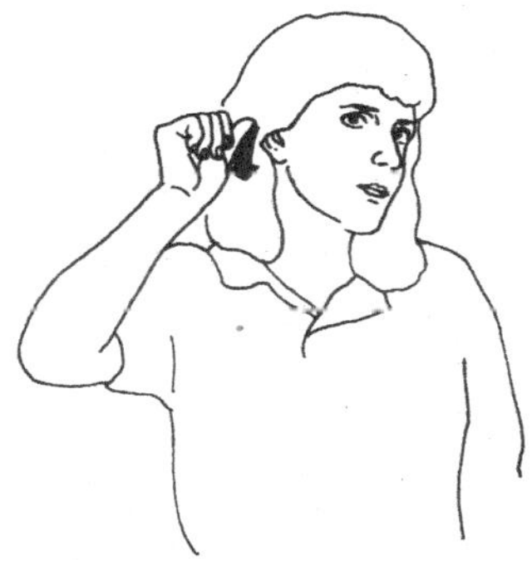

EAR-SURGERY?

Did you have ear surgery?

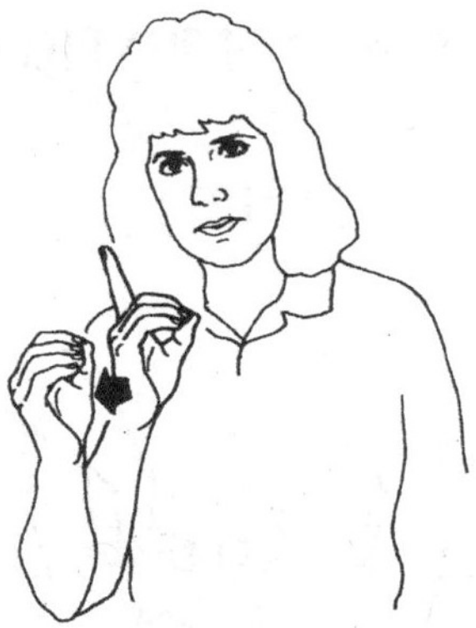

D-O

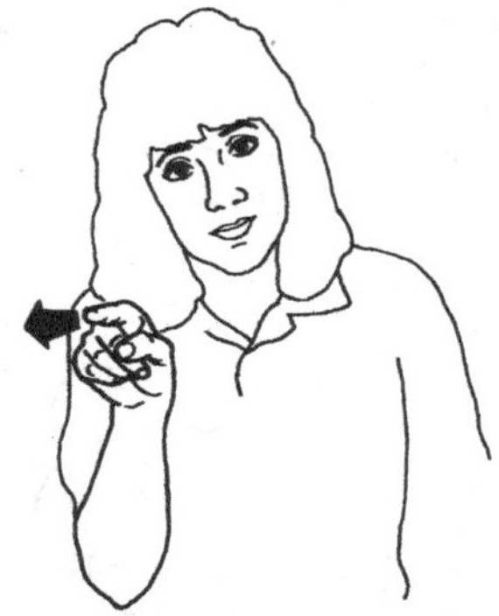

YOU

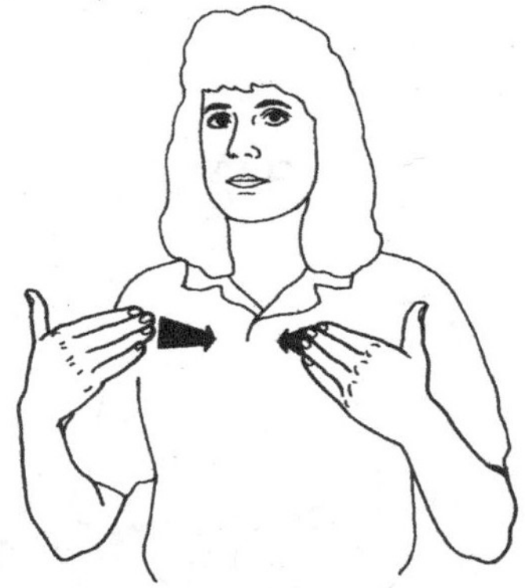

HAVE

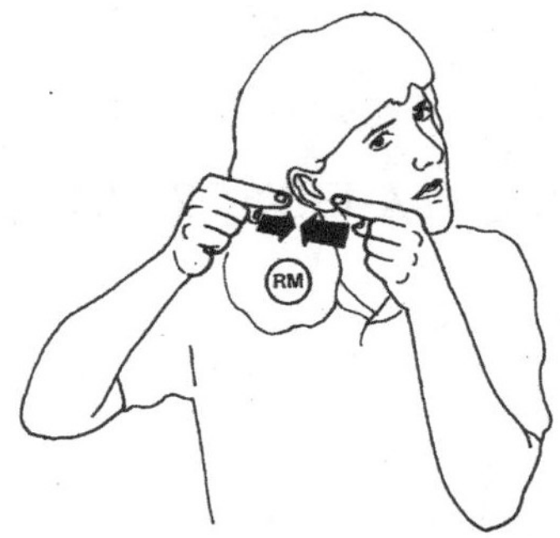

EARACHE?

Do you have earaches?

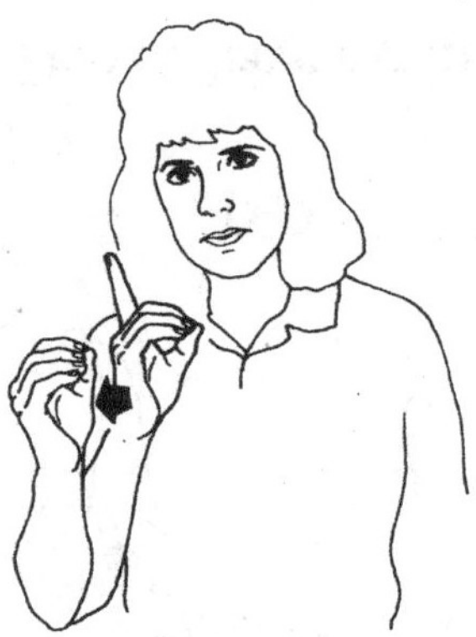

D-O

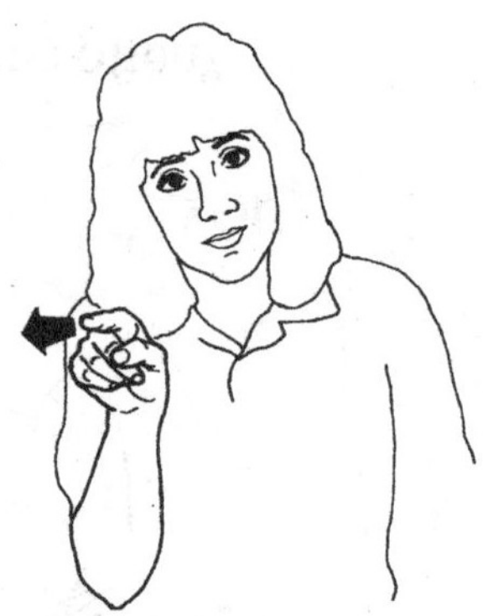

YOU

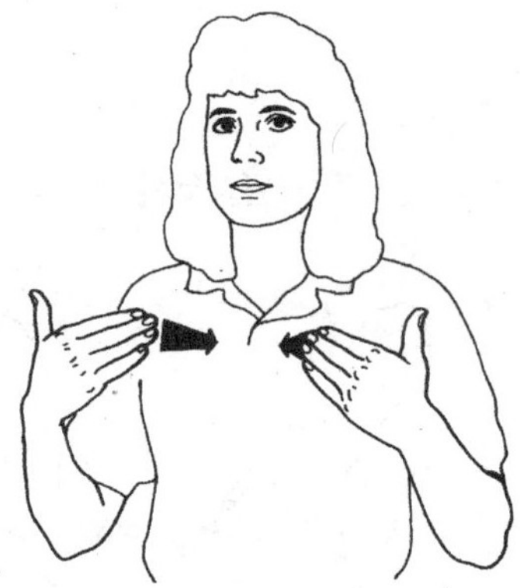

HAVE

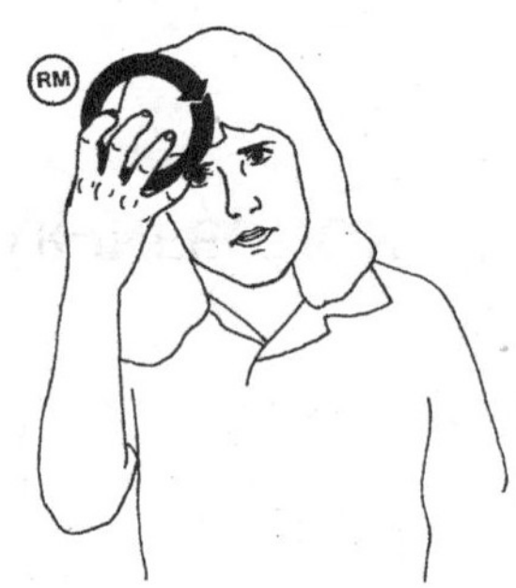

DIZZY?

Do you have dizziness?

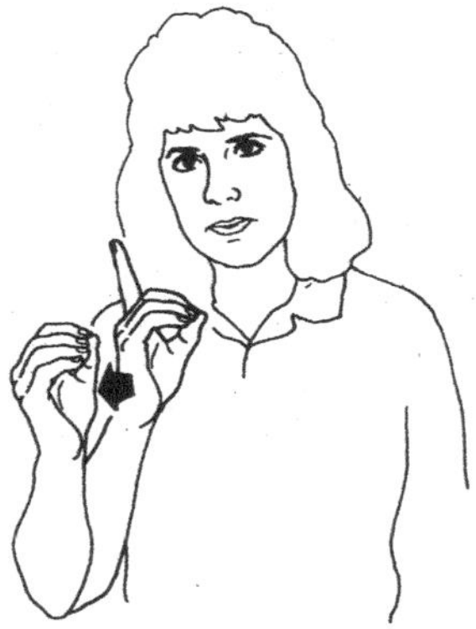

D-O

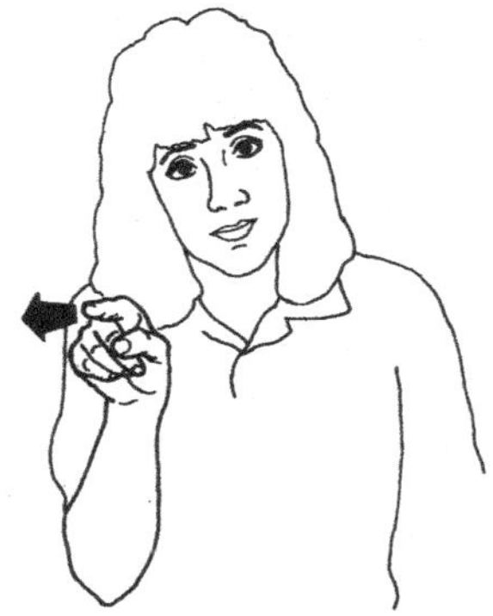

YOU

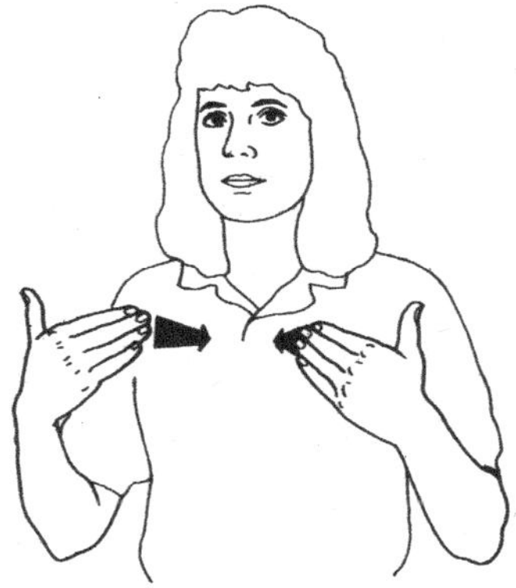

HAVE

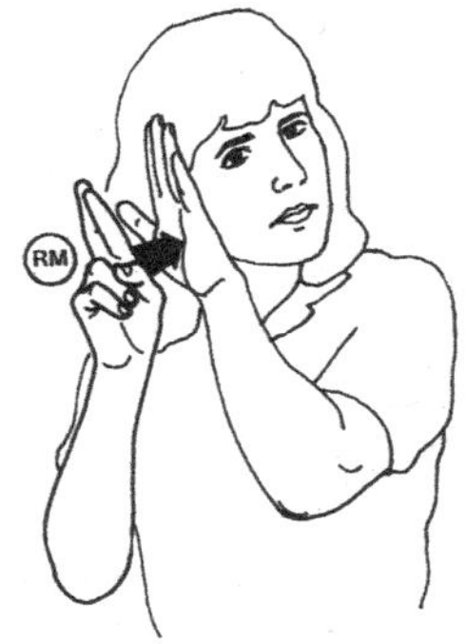

RING

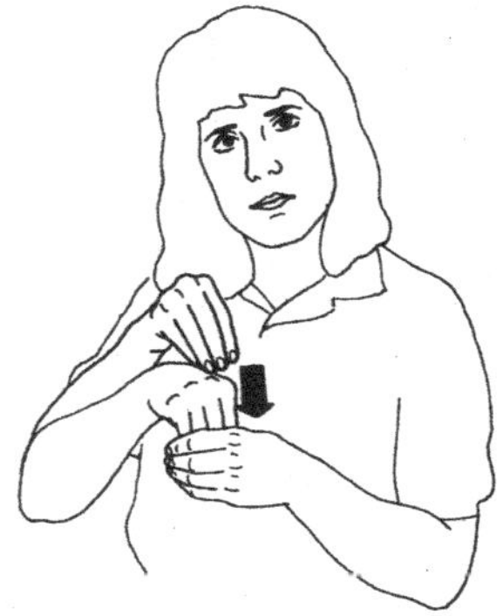

IN

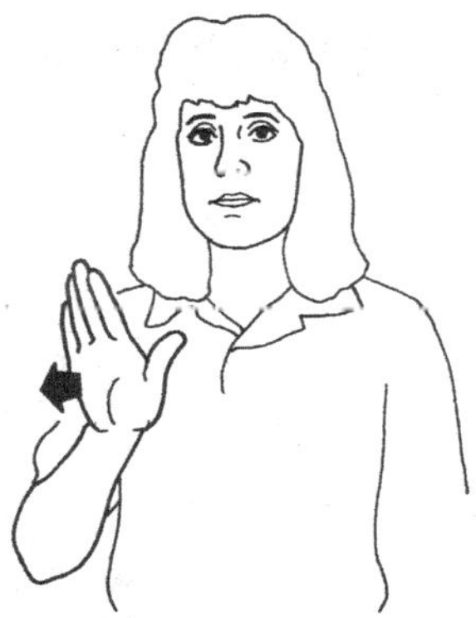

YOUR

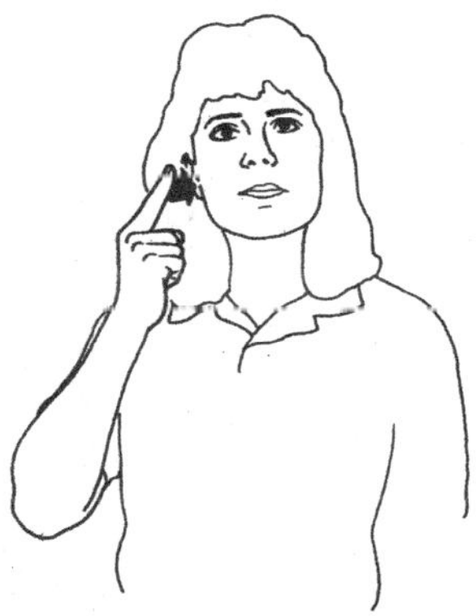

EAR?

Do you have ringing in your ears?

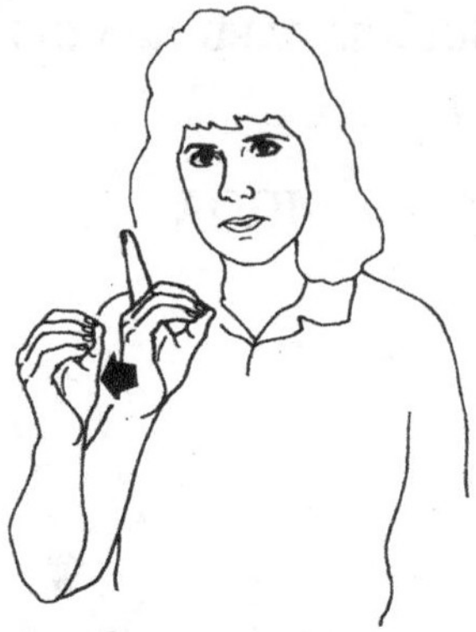

D-O

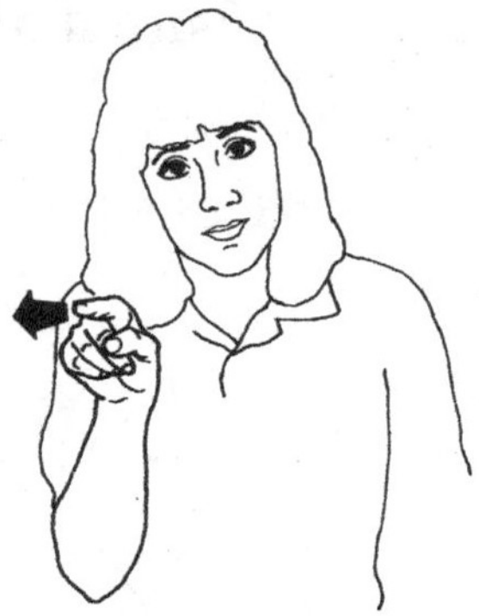

YOU

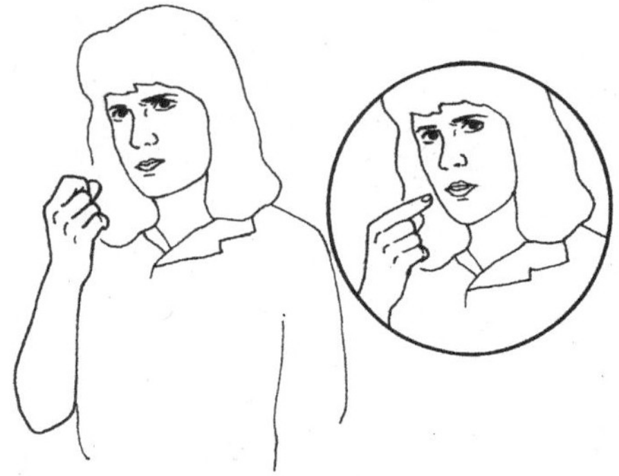

TAKE-A-PILL?

Do you take oral medication?

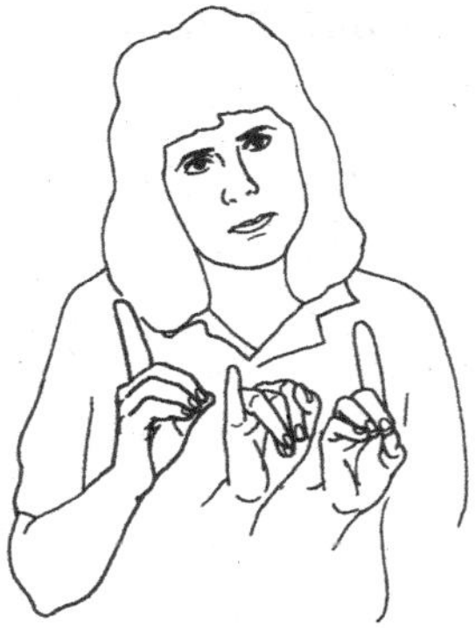

D-I-D

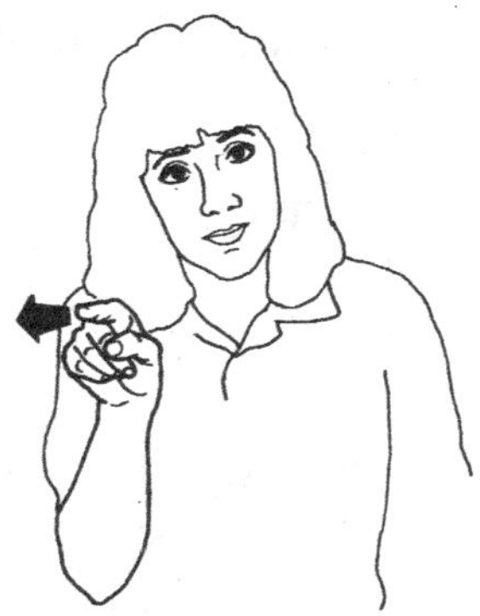

YOU

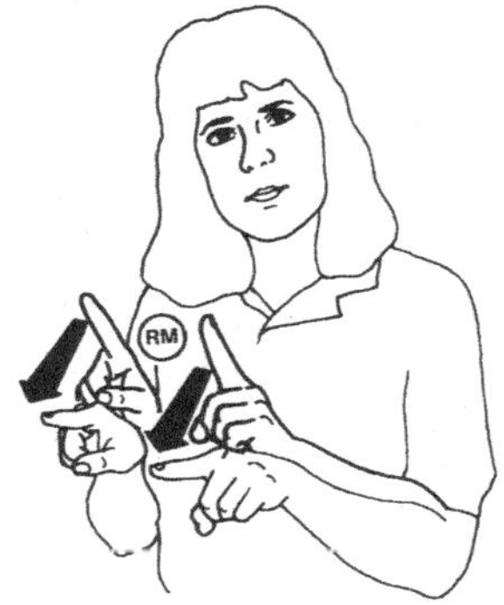

ATTEND

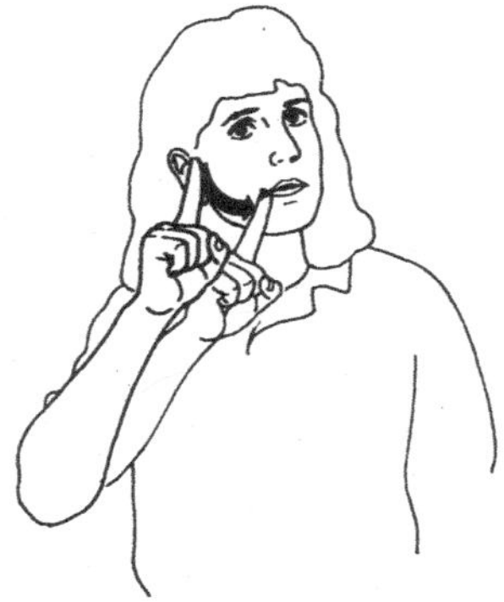

DEAF

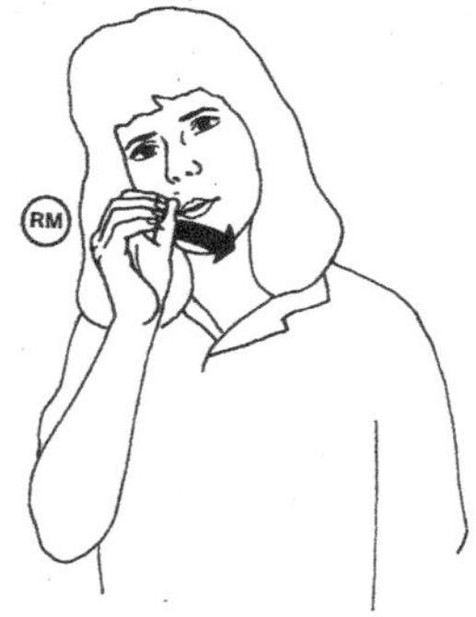

ORAL

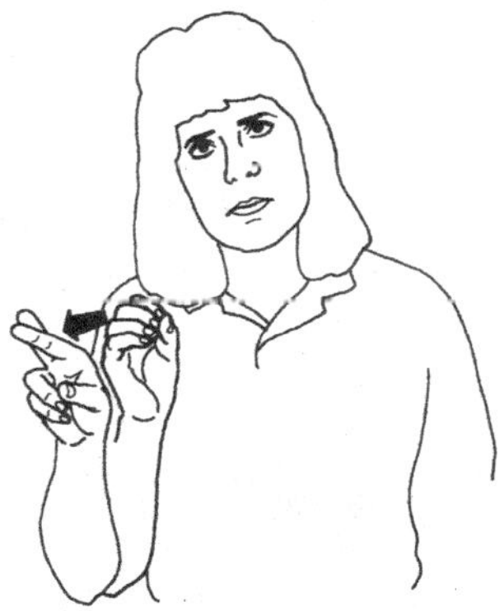

O-R

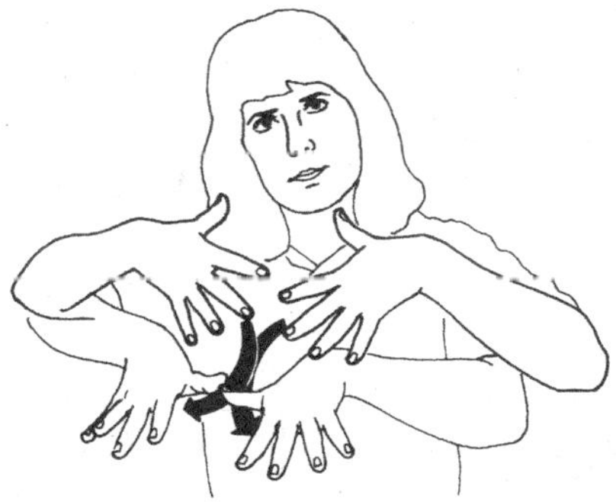

MAINSTREAM

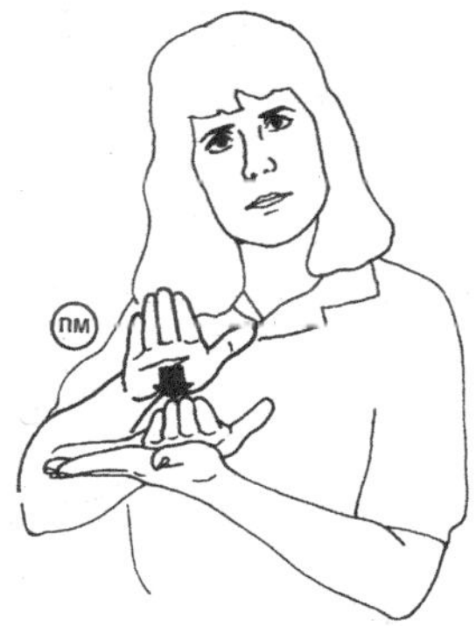

SCHOOL?

Did you attend a deaf, oral, or mainstreamed school?

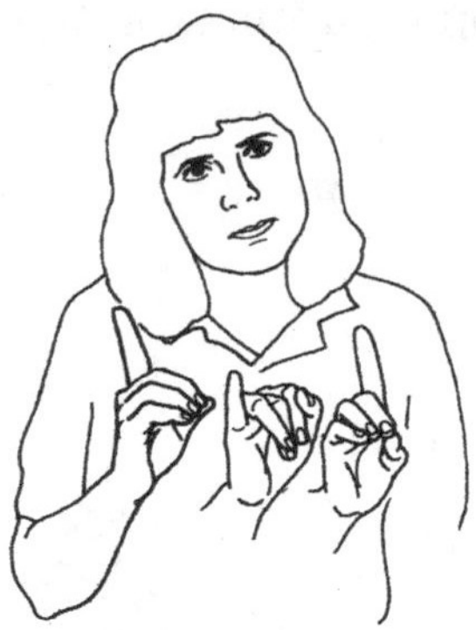

D-I-D

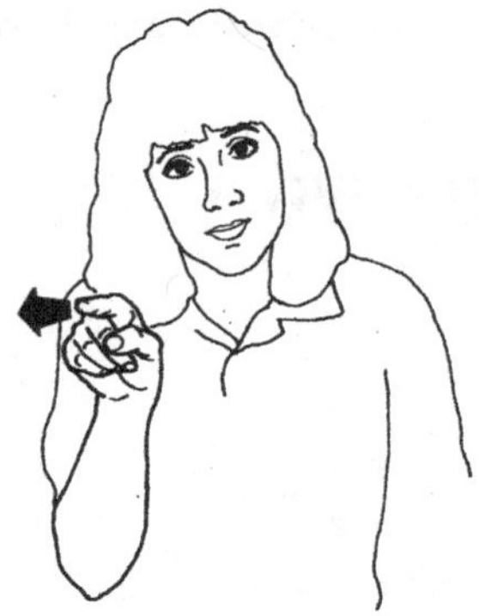

YOU

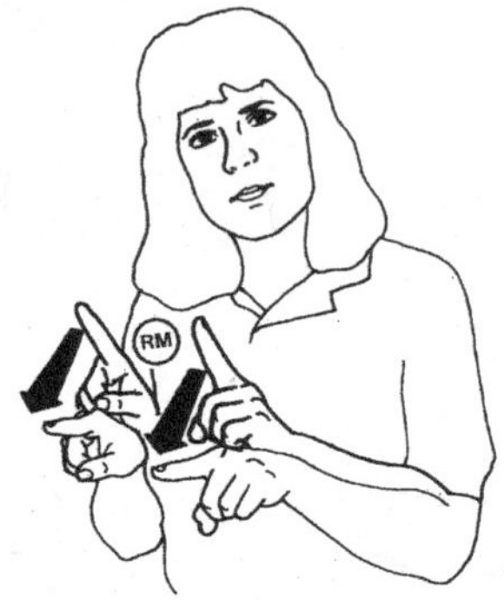

ATTEND

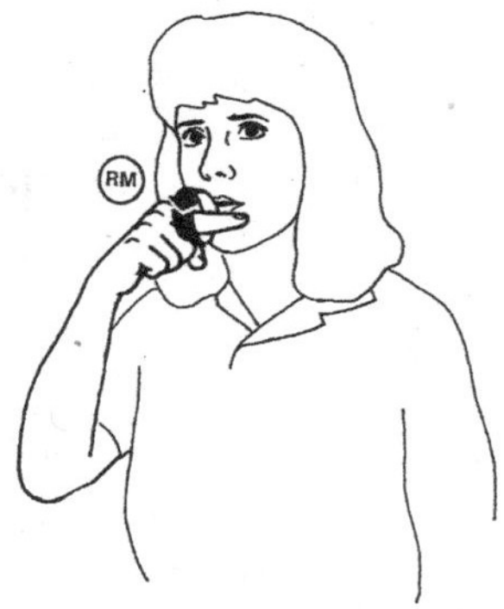

HEARING

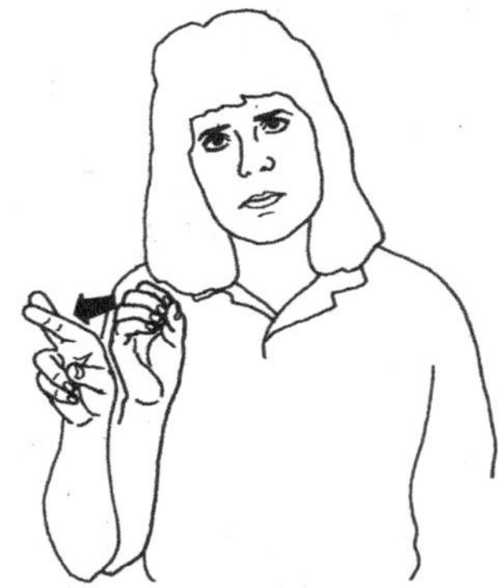

O-R

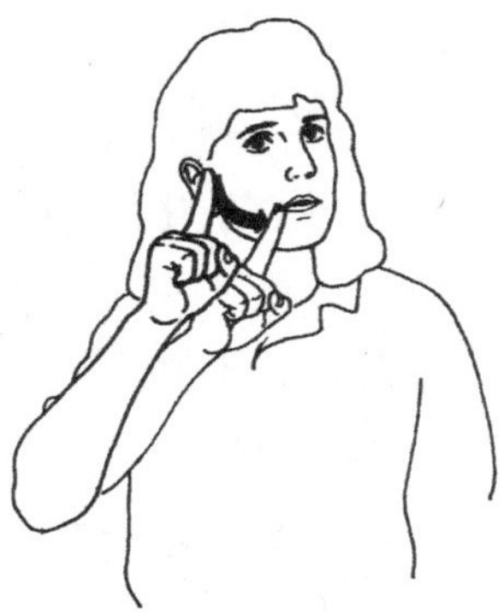

DEAF

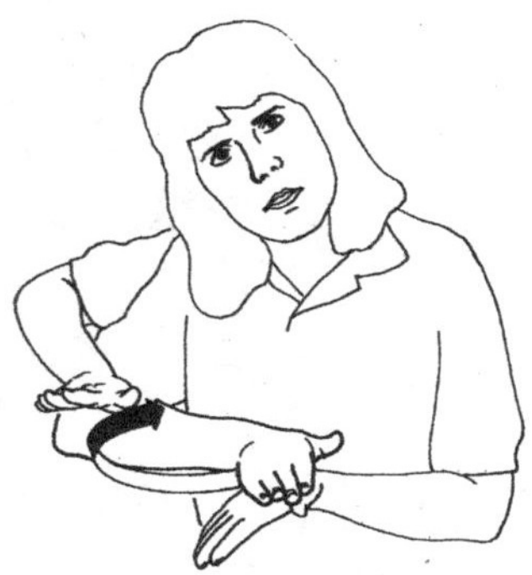

COLLEGE?

Did you attend a hearing or deaf college?

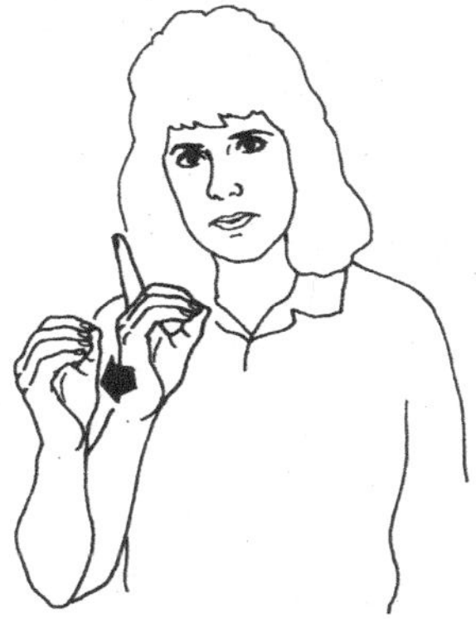

D-O

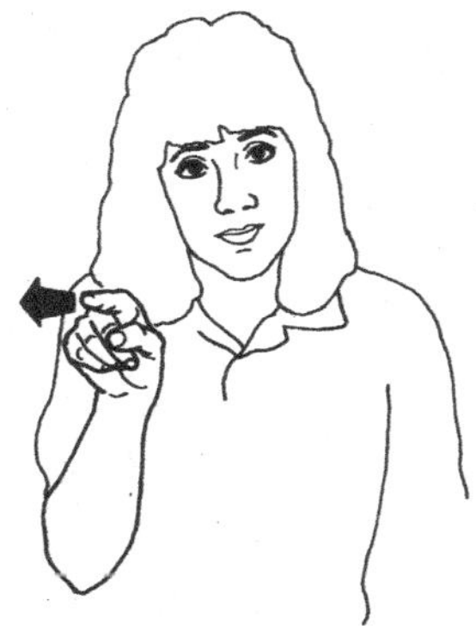

YOU

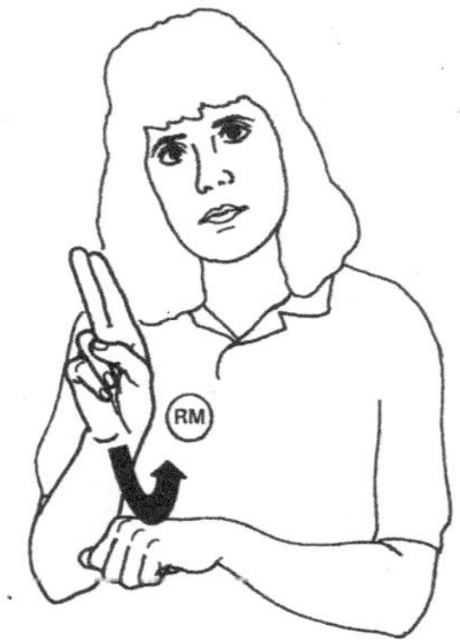

USE

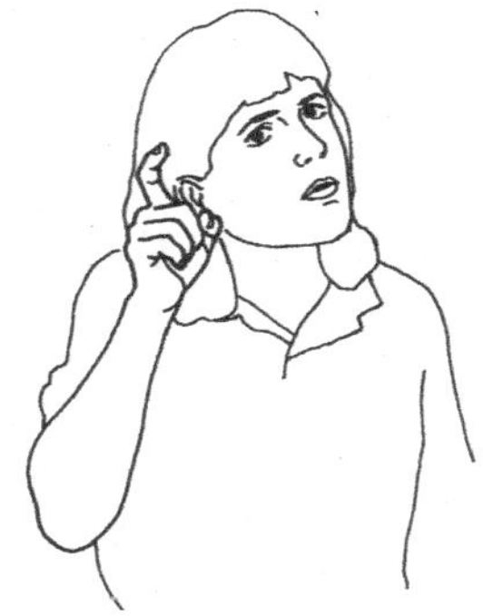

HEARING-AID?

Do you use a hearing aid?

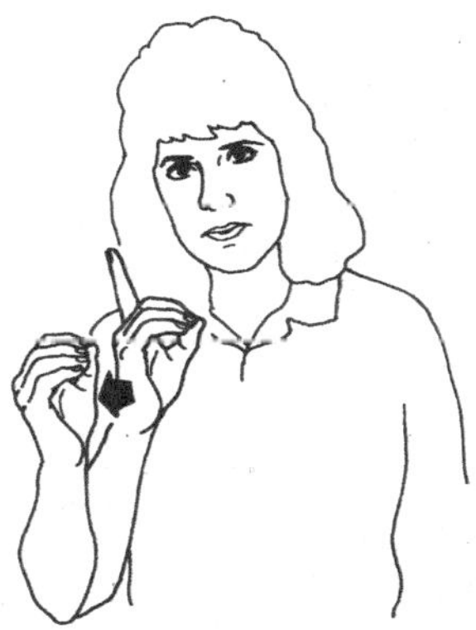

D-O

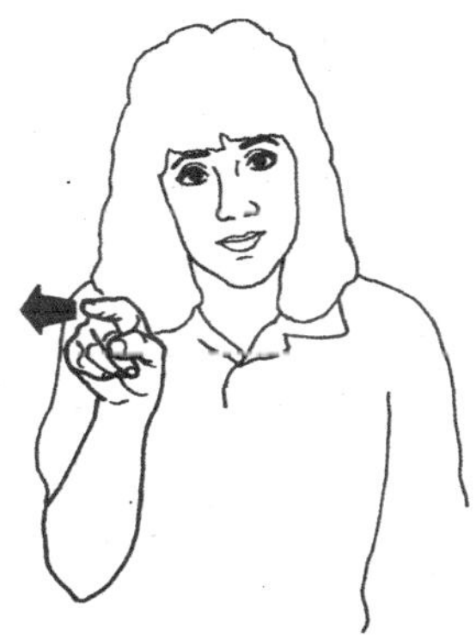

YOU

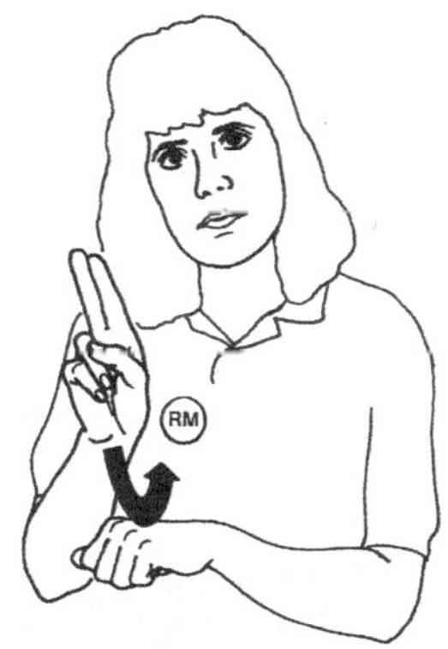

USE

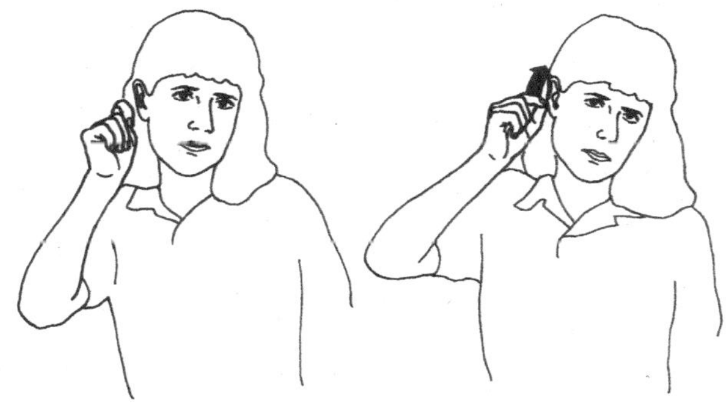

T-SWITCH?

Do you use the T-switch?

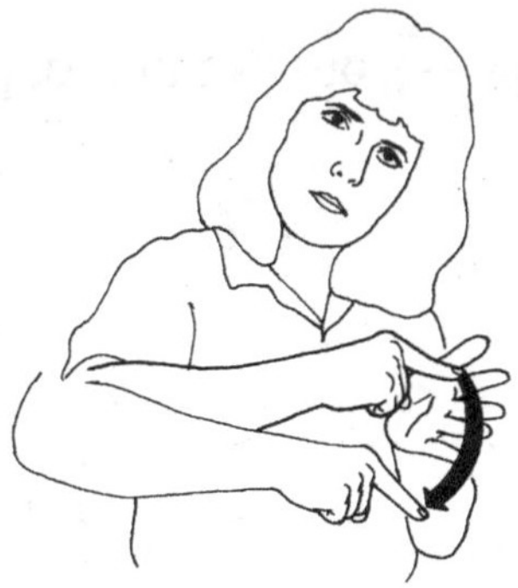

WHAT

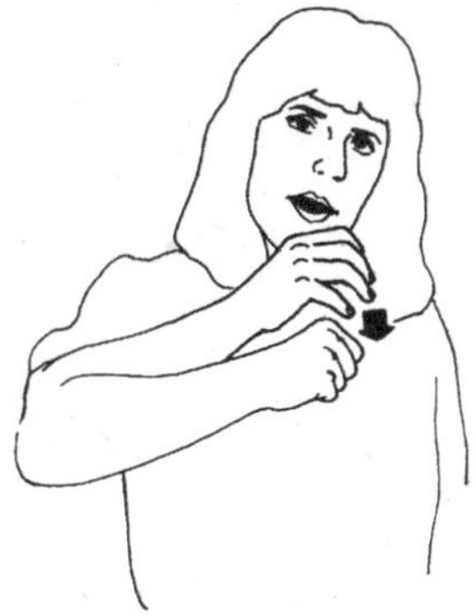

AGE

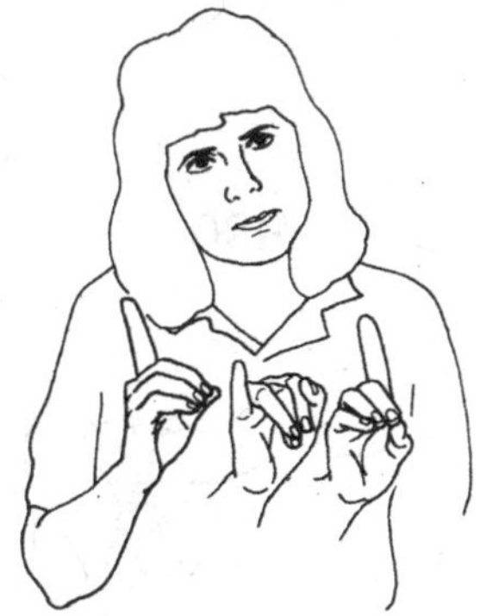

D-I-D

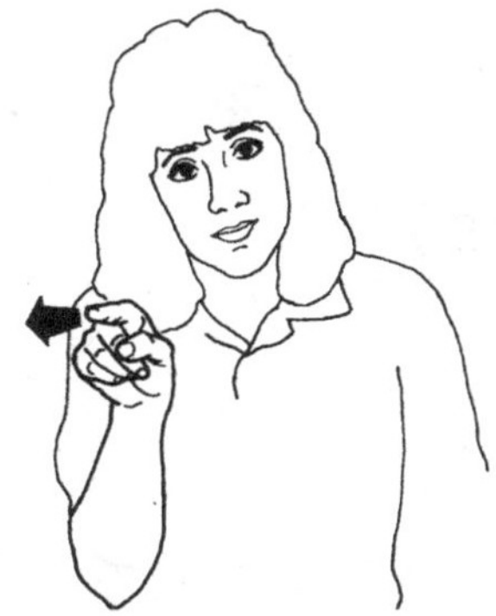

YOU

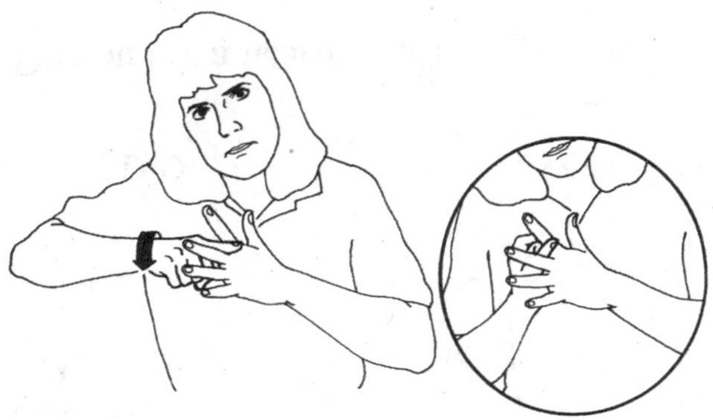

BEGIN

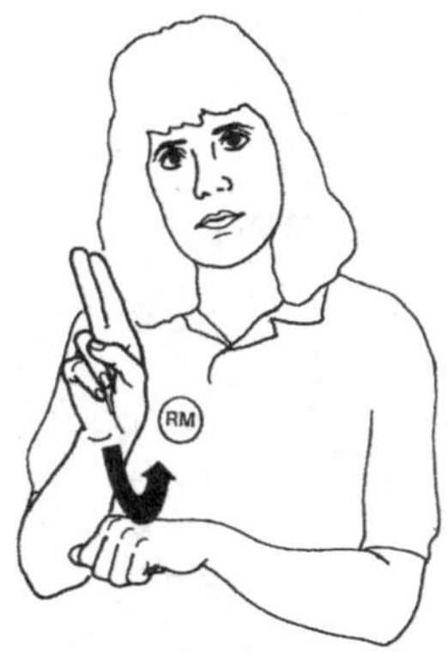

USE

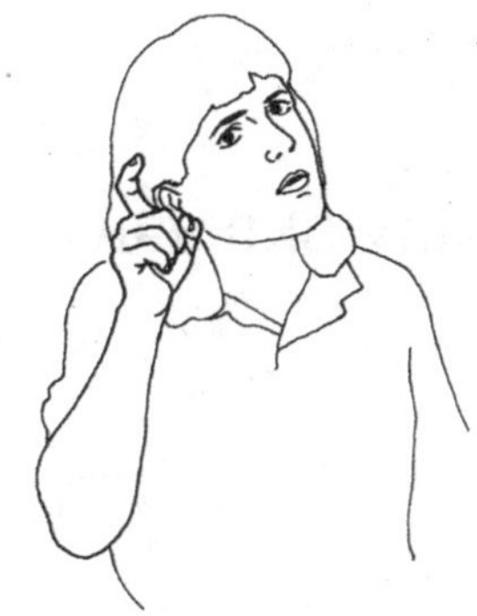

HEARING-AID?

At what age did you begin using a hearing aid?

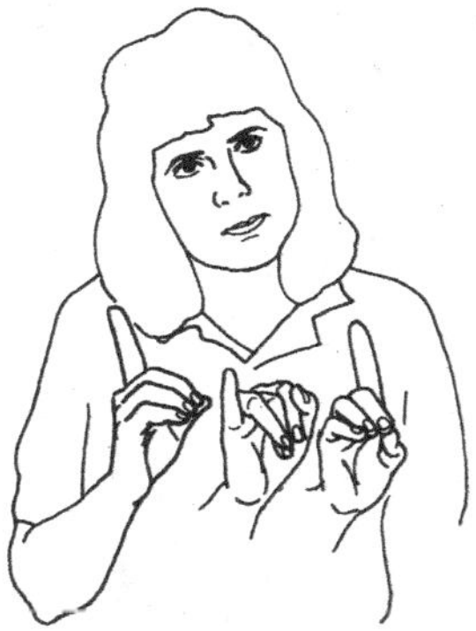

D-I-D

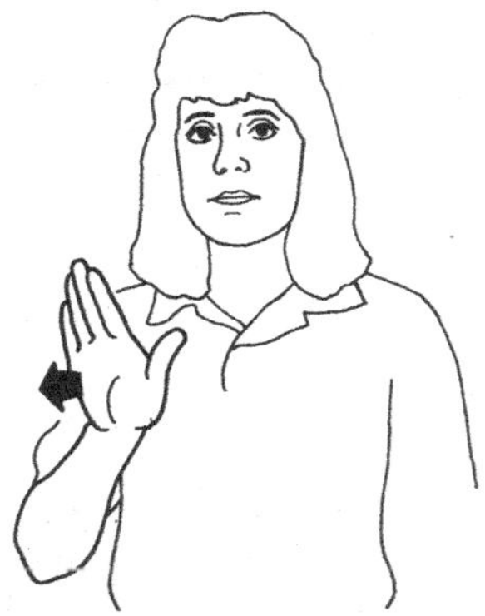

YOUR

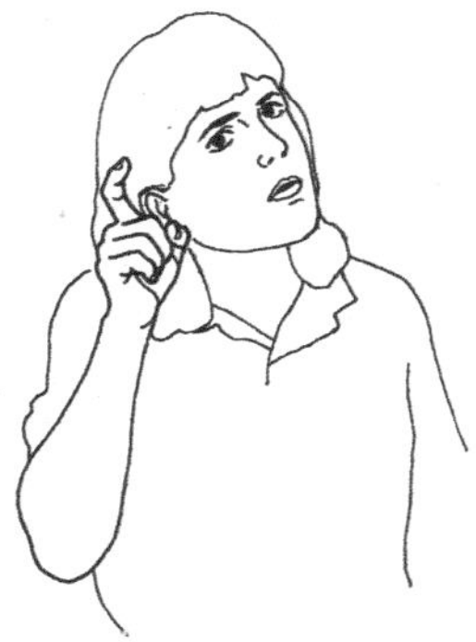

HEARING-AID

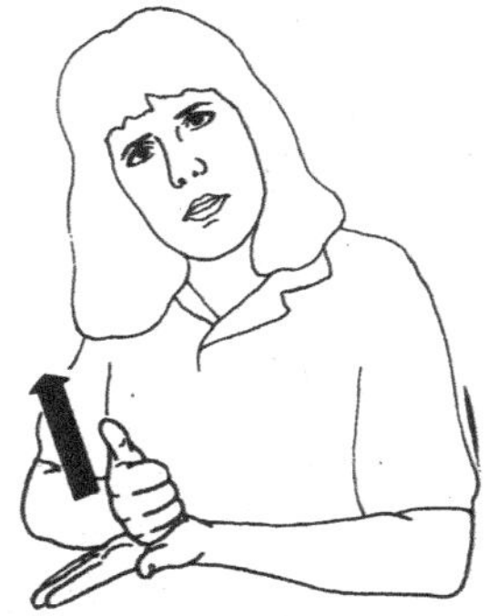

HELP

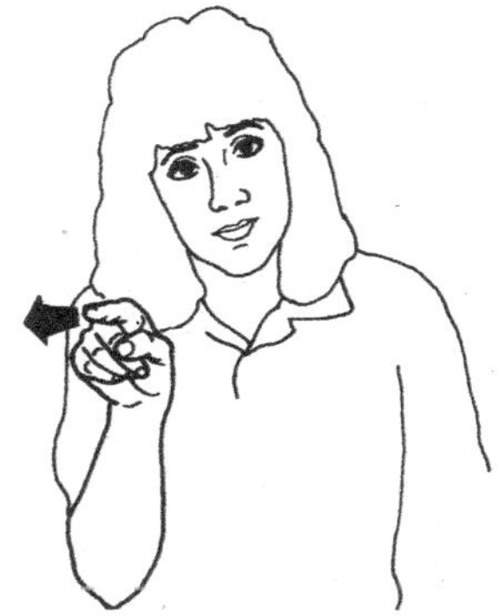

YOU?

Did your hearing aid help you?

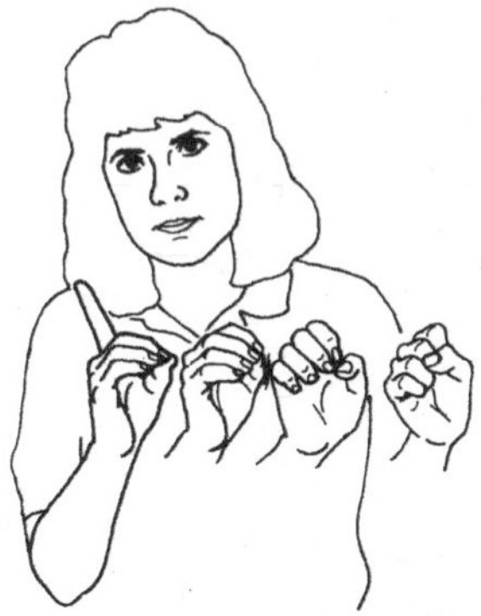

D-O-E-S

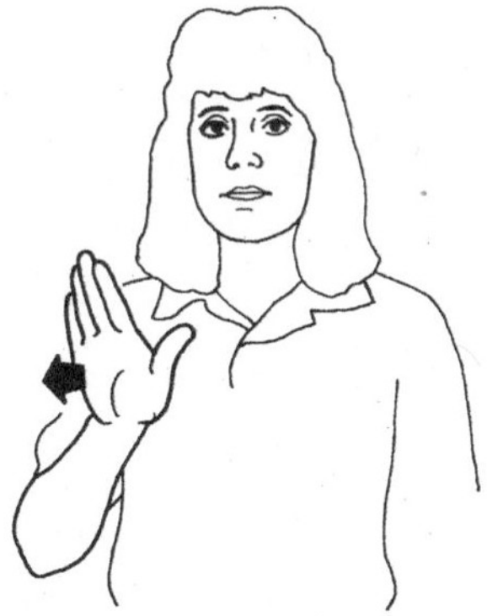

YOUR

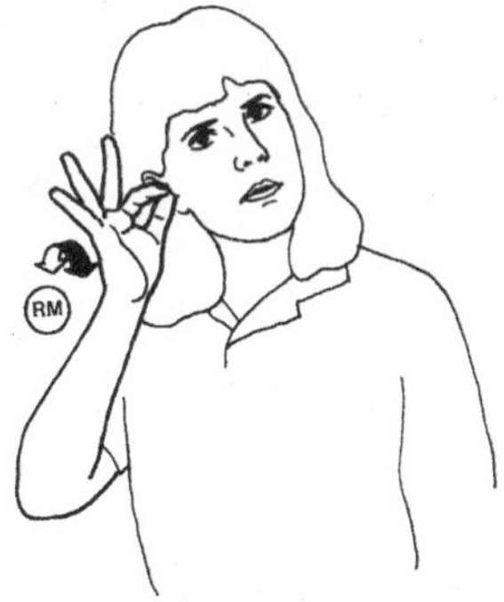

EARMOLD

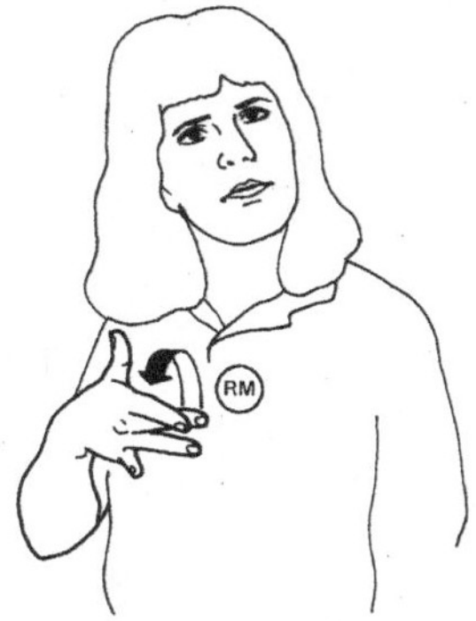

FEEL

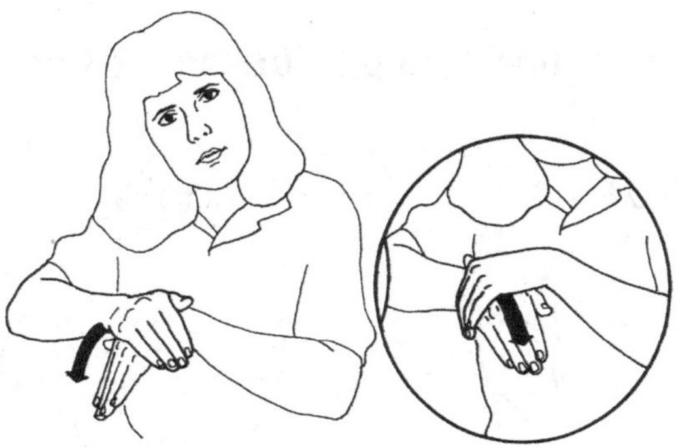

COMFORTABLE?

Does your earmold feel comfortable?

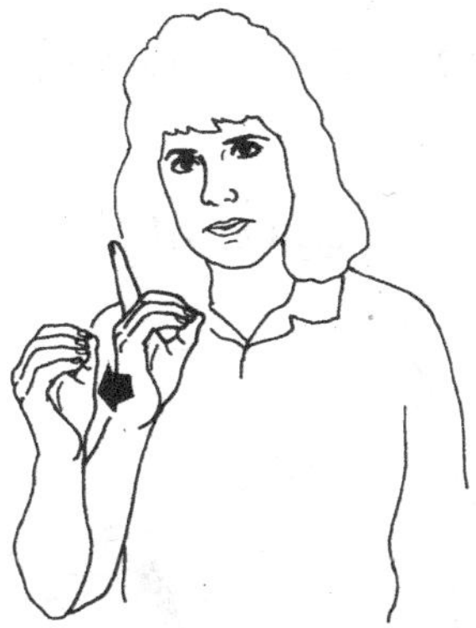

D-O

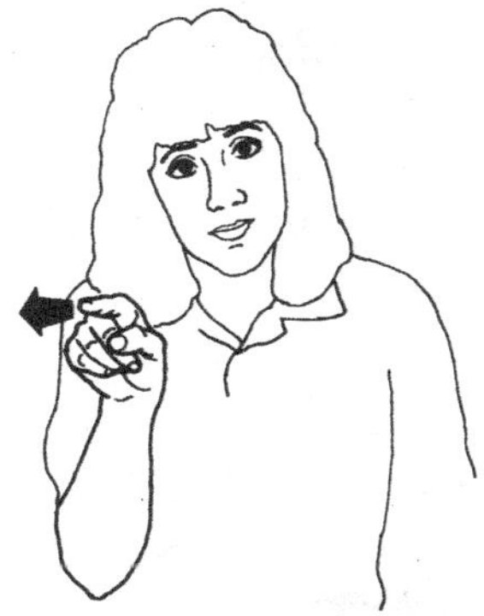

YOU

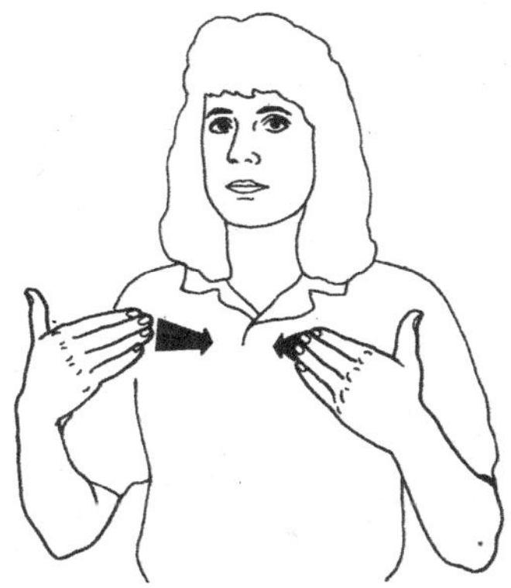

HAVE

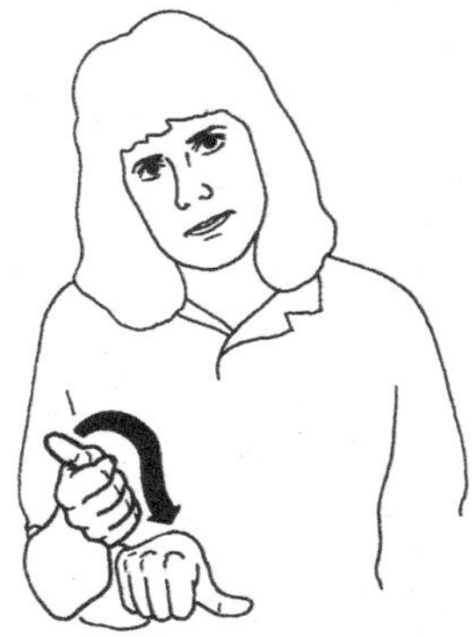

ANY

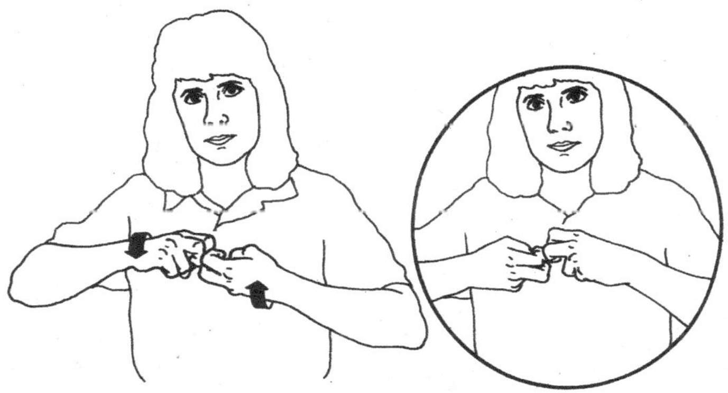

PROBLEM

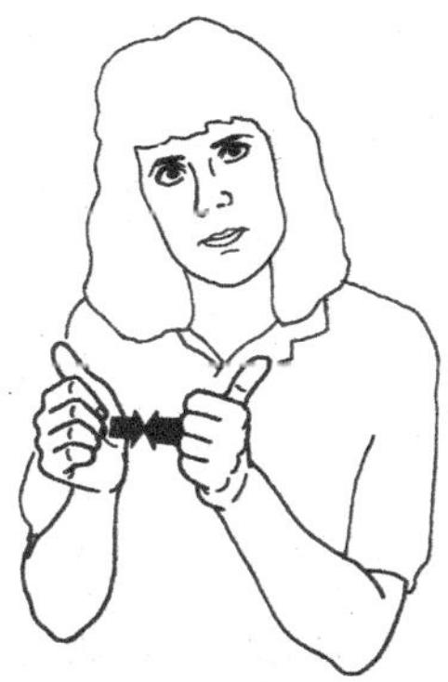

WITH

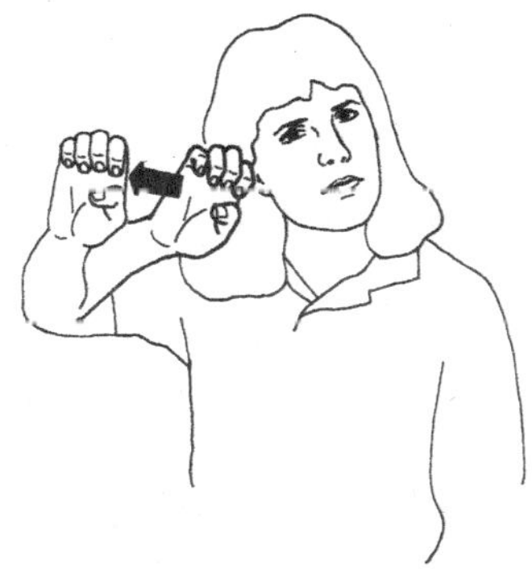

FEEDBACK?

Do you have any problem with feedback?

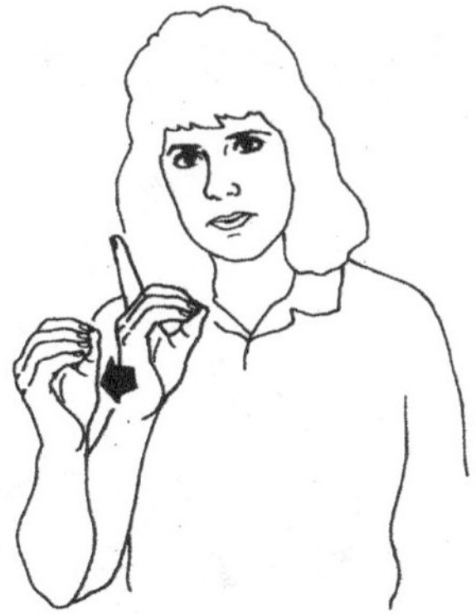

D-O

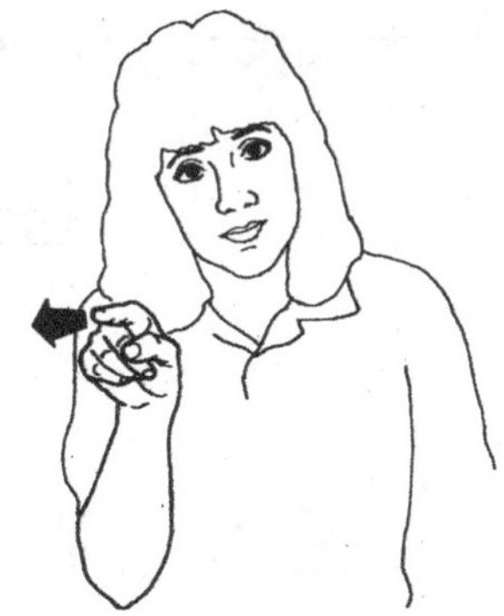

YOU

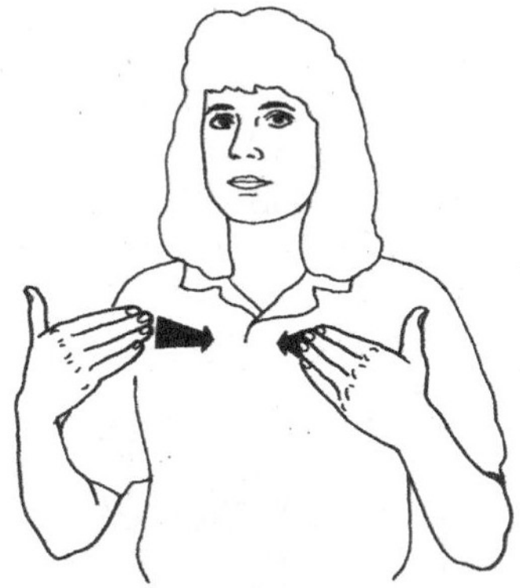

HAVE

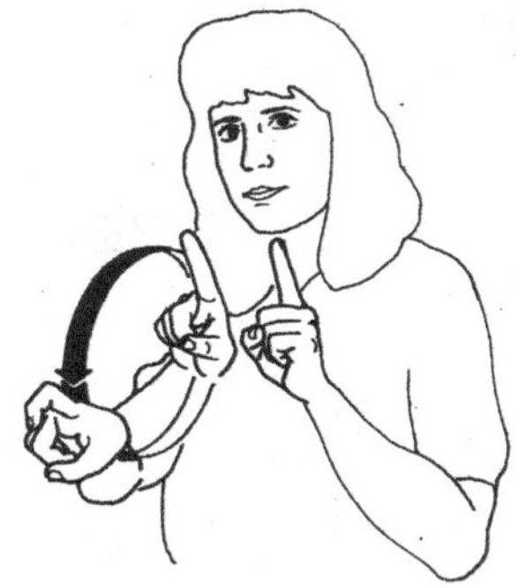

QUESTION

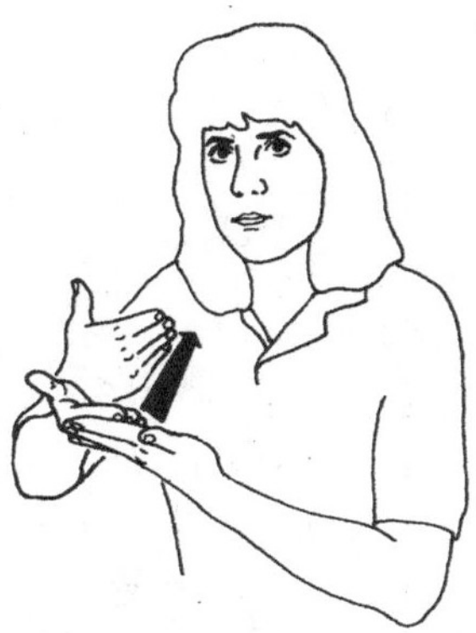

BEFORE

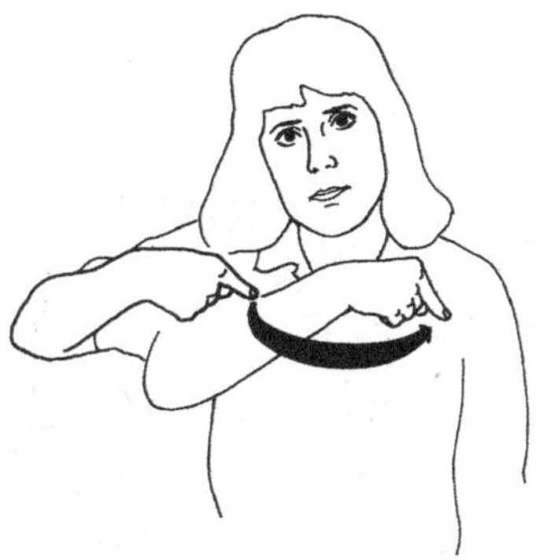

WE

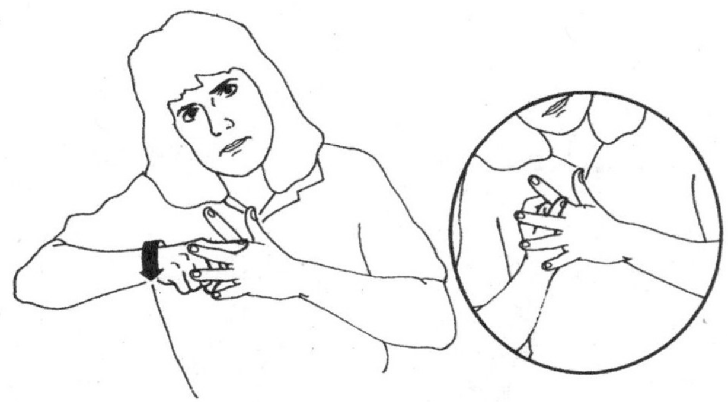

BEGIN

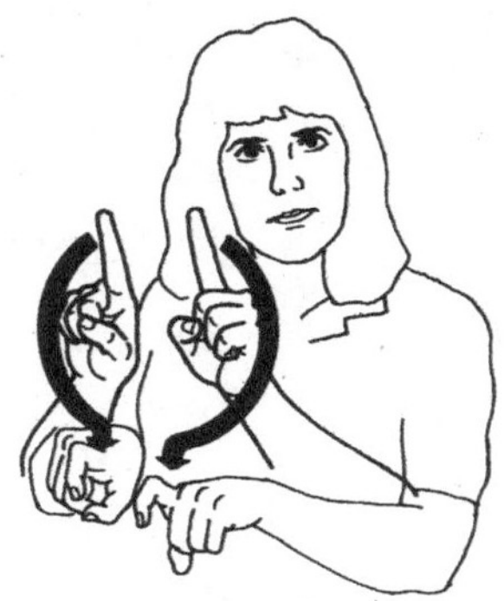

TEST?

Do you have questions before we begin the testing?

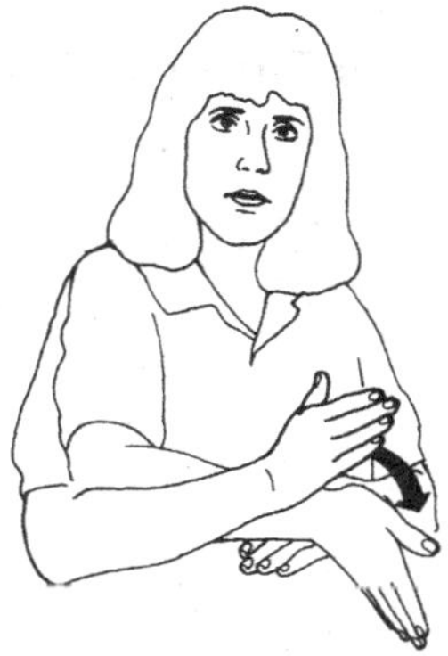

AFTER

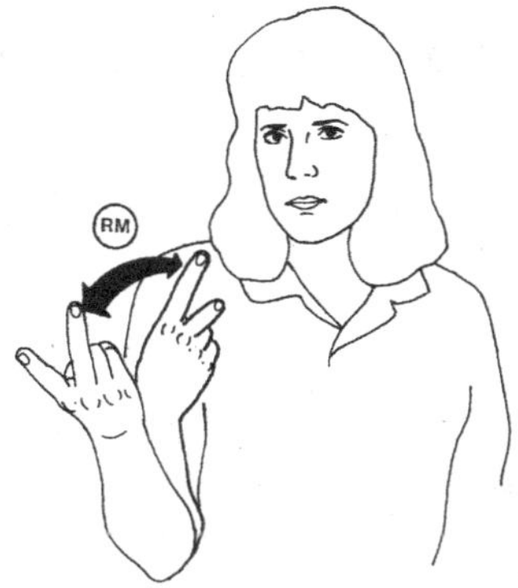

TWO-OF-US

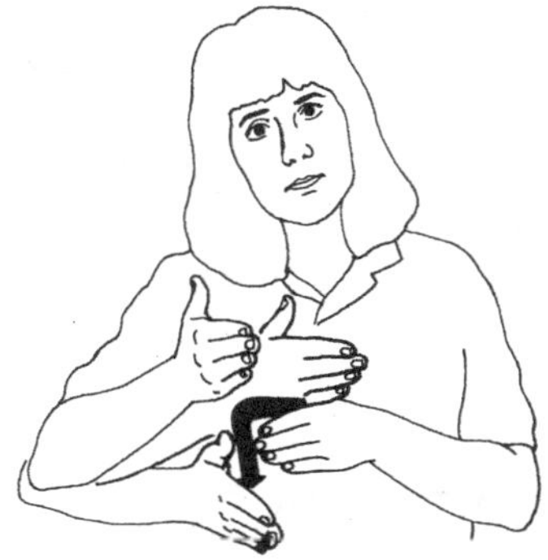

COMPLETE

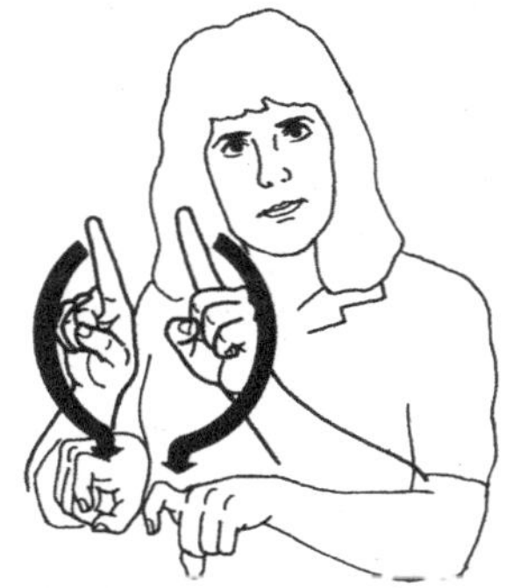

TEST

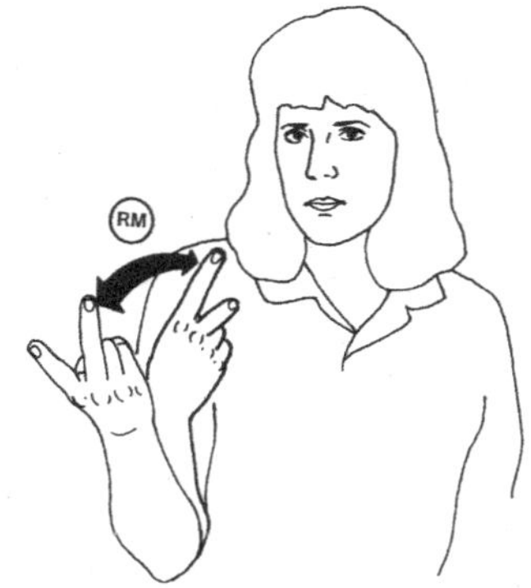

TWO-OF-US

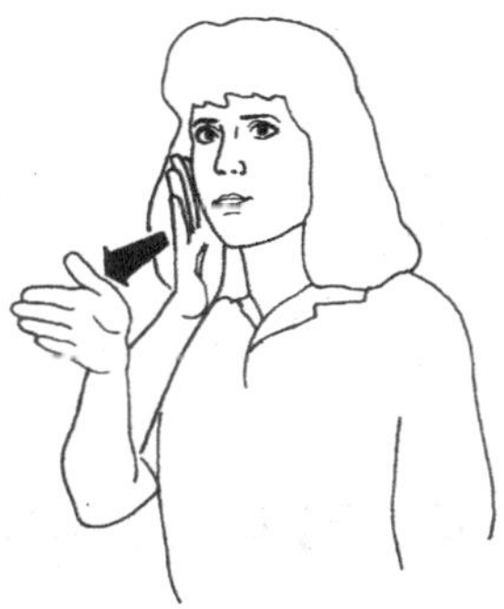

WILL

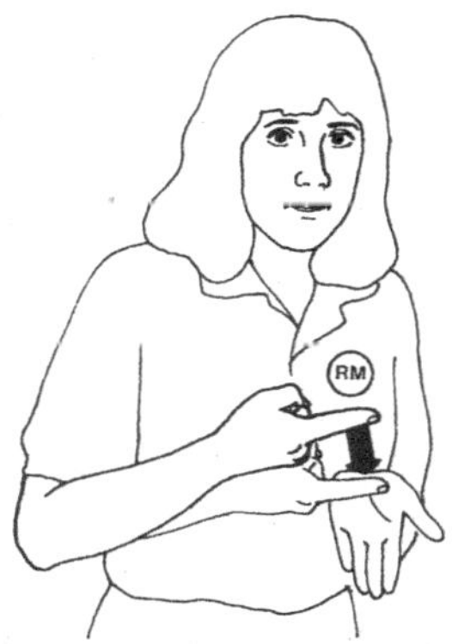

DISCUSS

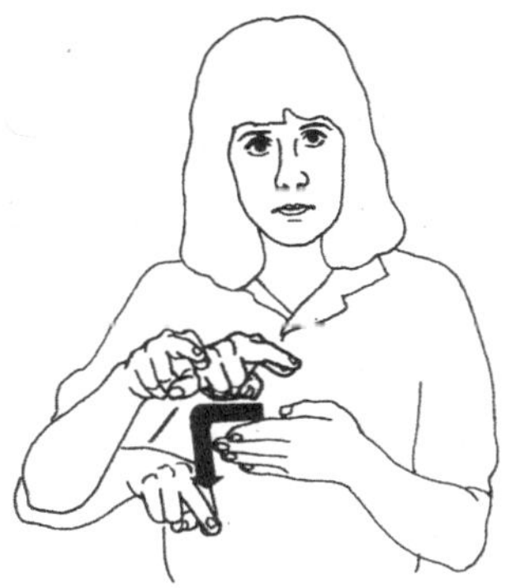

RESULTS.

After we complete the testing, we will discuss the results.

Chapter 3

Audiologic Testing of a Young Deaf Child

Pure-tone Testing

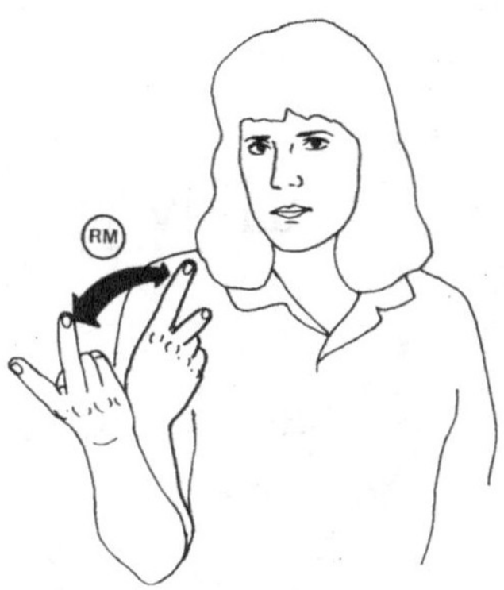

TWO-OF-US

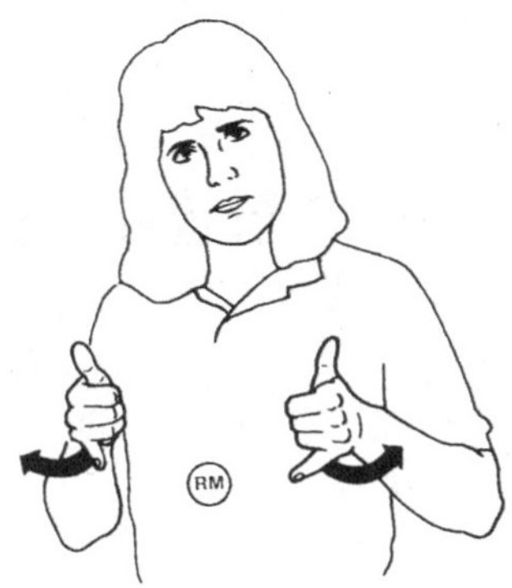

PLAY

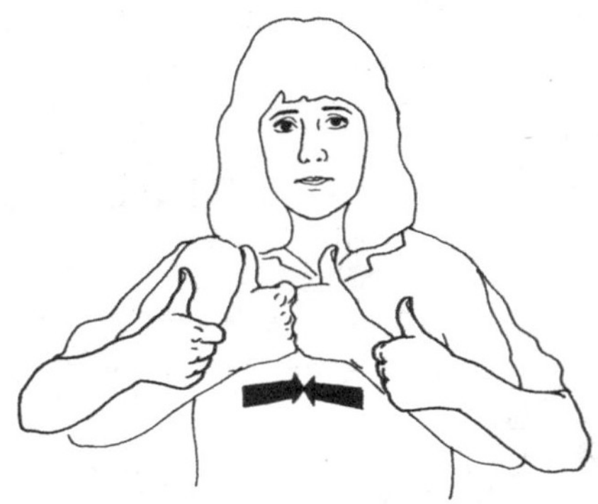

GAME

We are going to play a game called "airplane pilot."

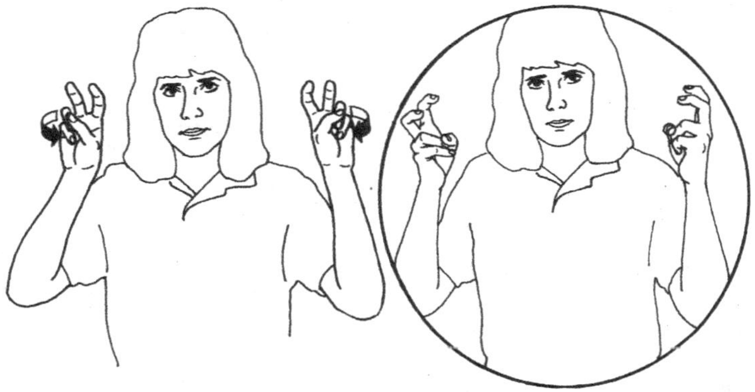

TOPIC

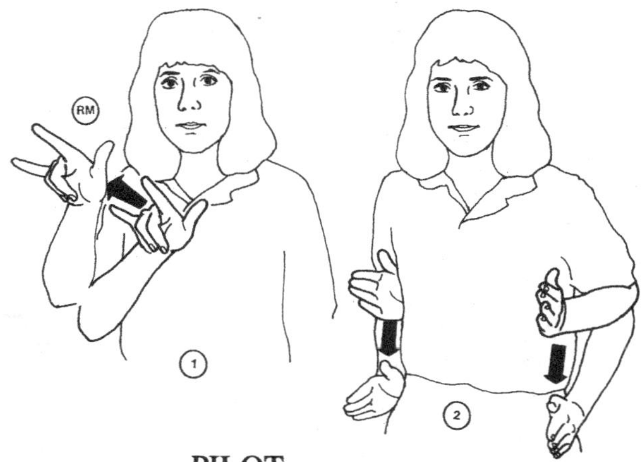

PILOT.

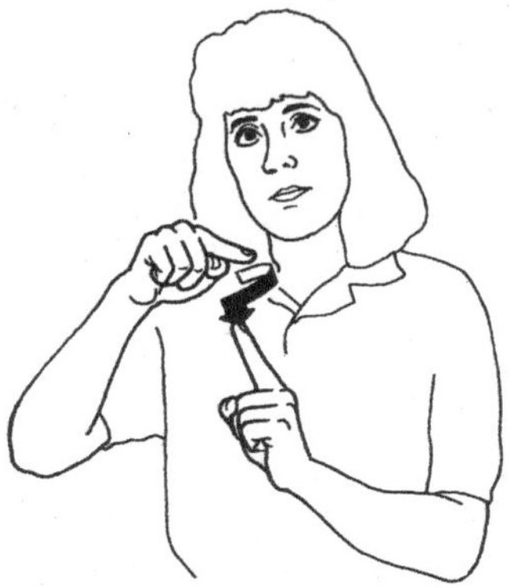

WHEN

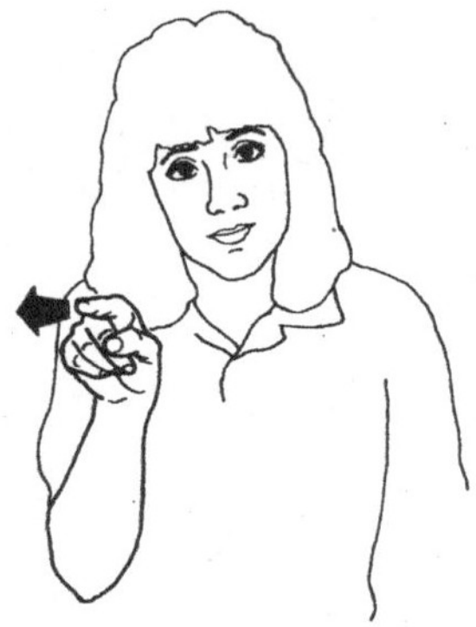

YOU

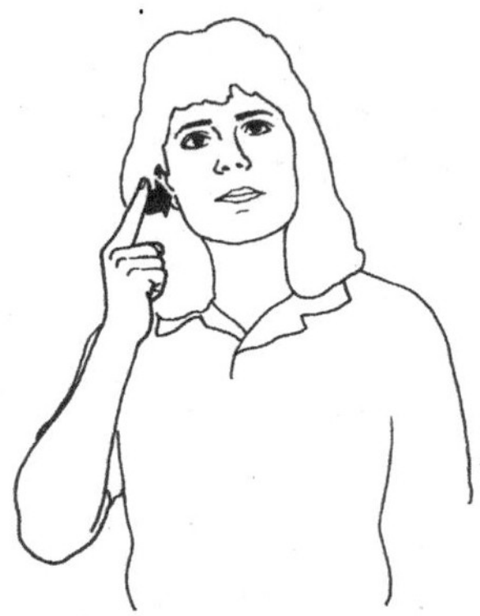

HEAR

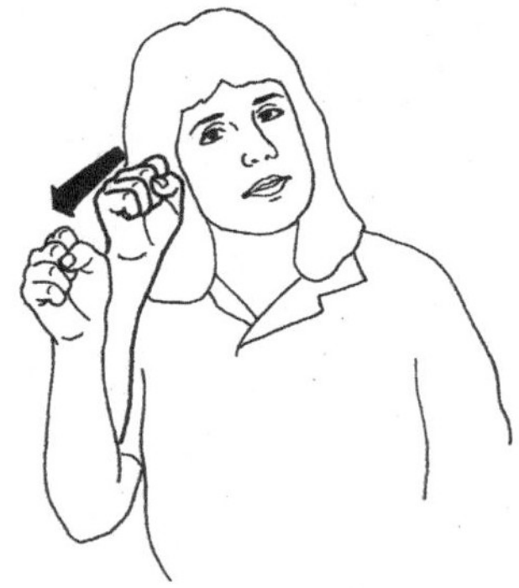

SOUND

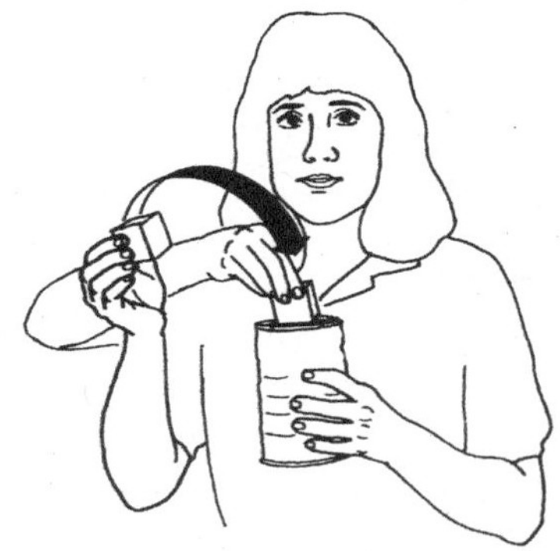

PUT-BLOCK-IN-CAN.

When you hear a sound, put this block in the can.

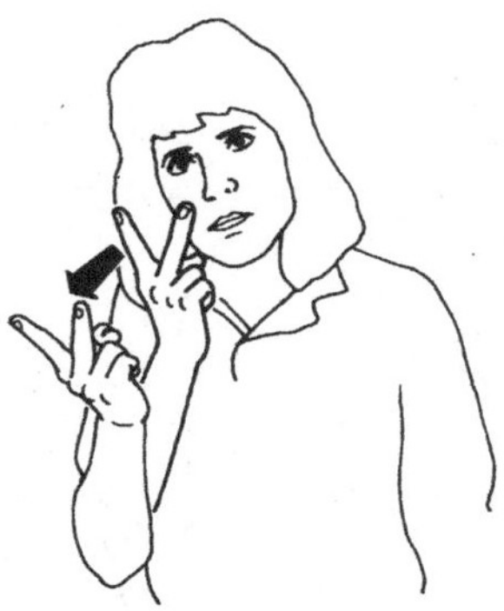

WILL-SEE

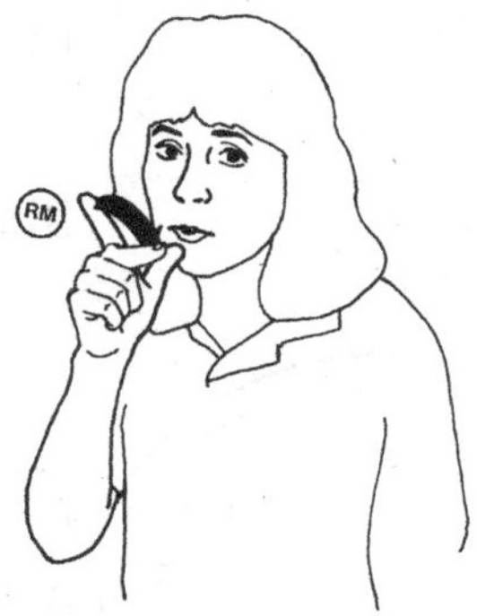

WHO

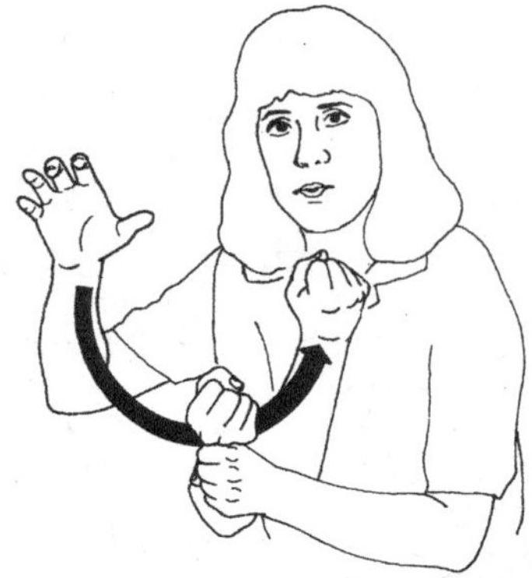

WIN.

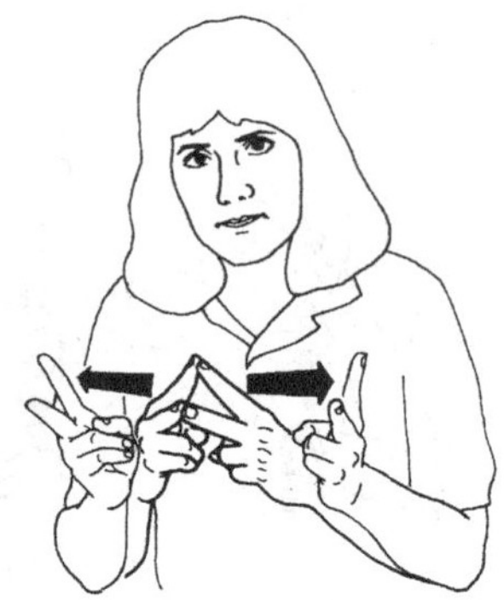

VERY

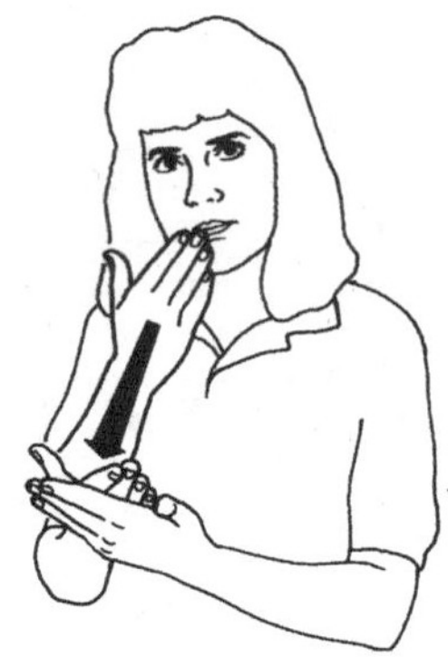

GOOD.

Let's see who wins!

Very good!

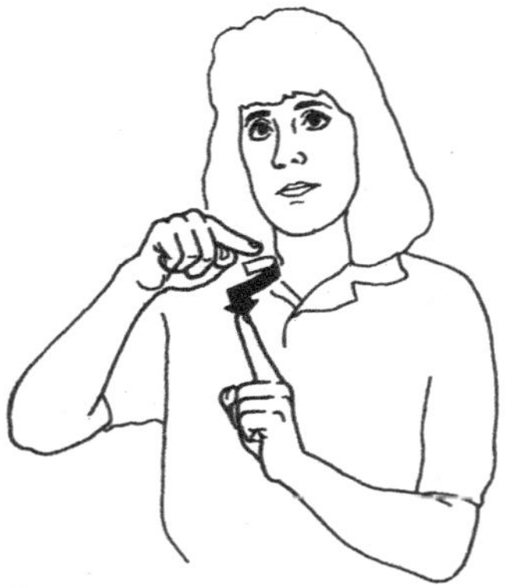

WHEN

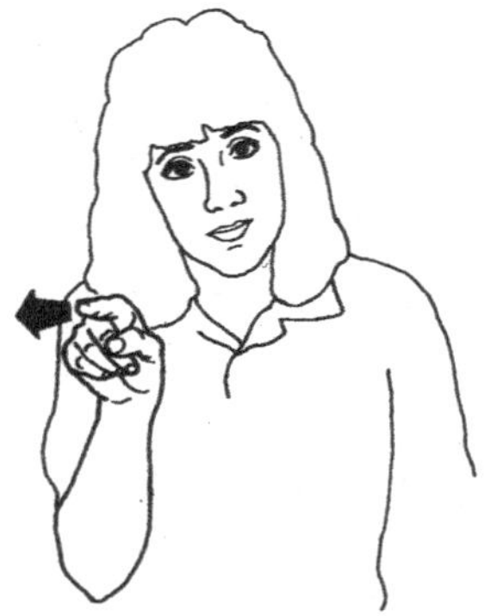

YOU

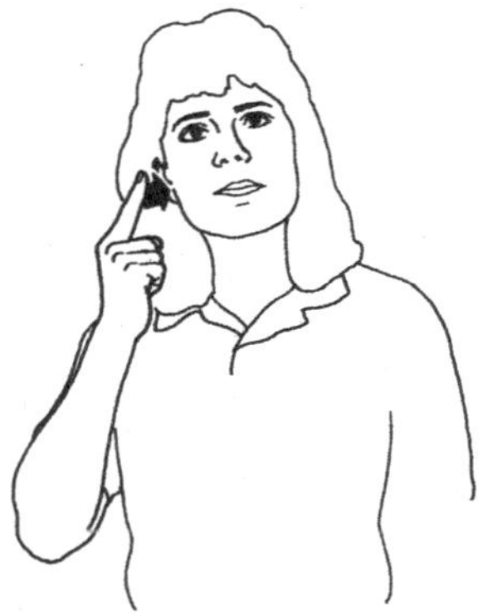

HEAR

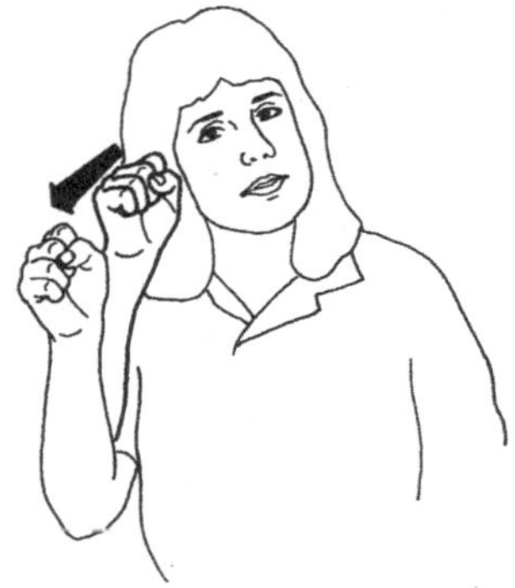

SOUND

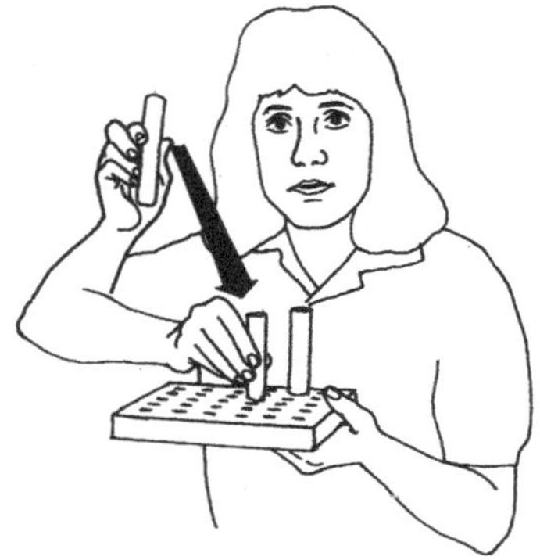

PUT-PEG-IN-BOARD.

When you hear the sound, put the peg in the board.

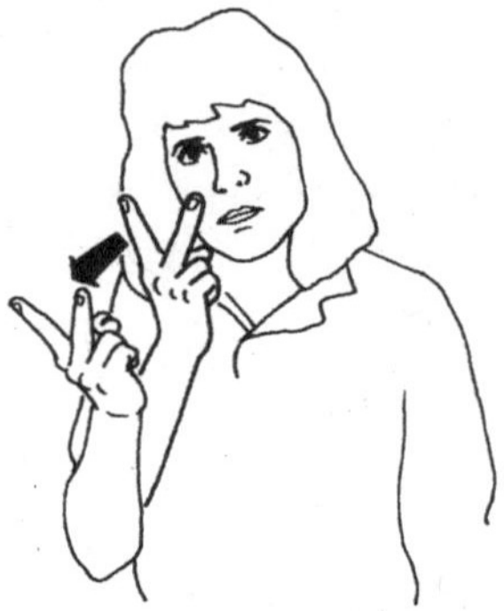

SEE

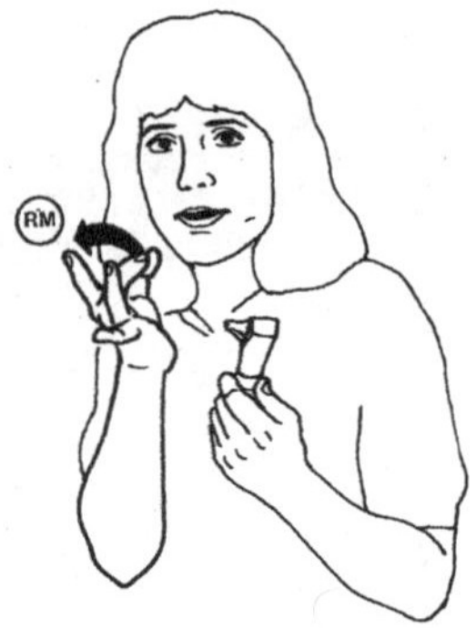

LIGHT?

See this light?

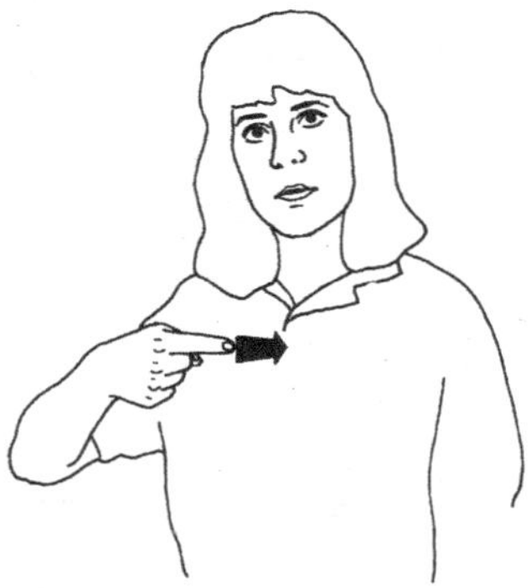

I

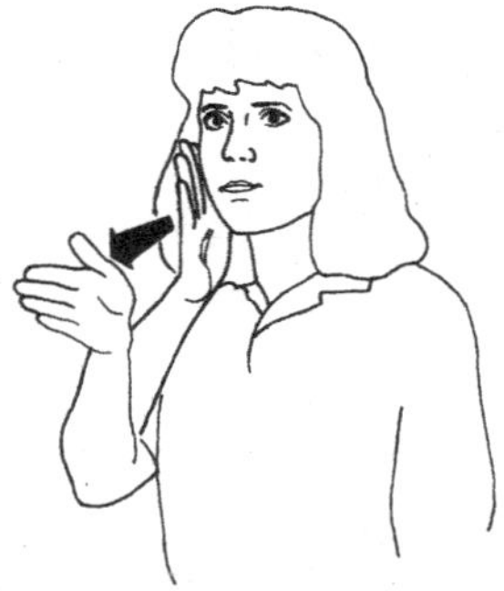

WILL

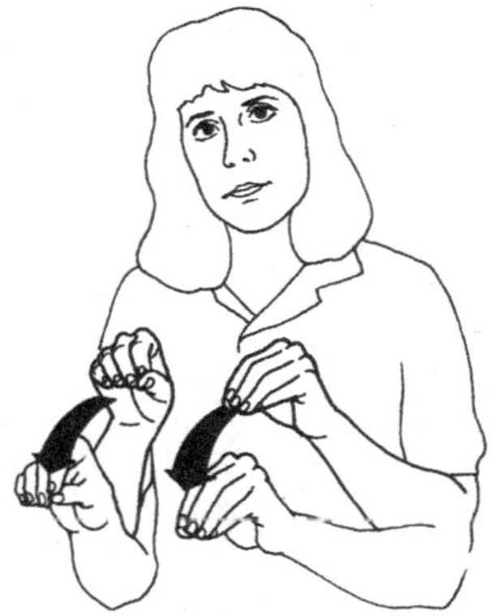

PUT

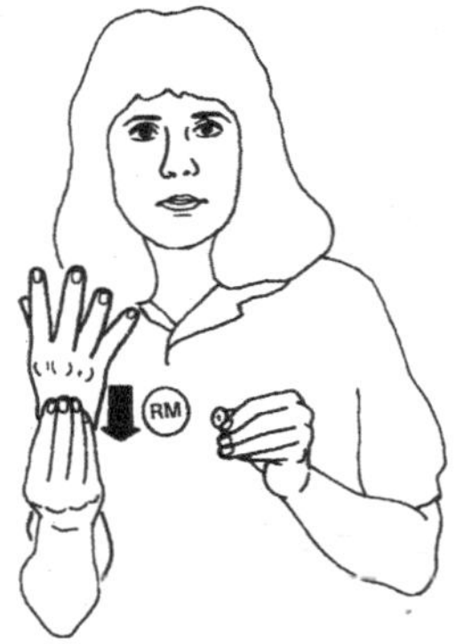

SOFT

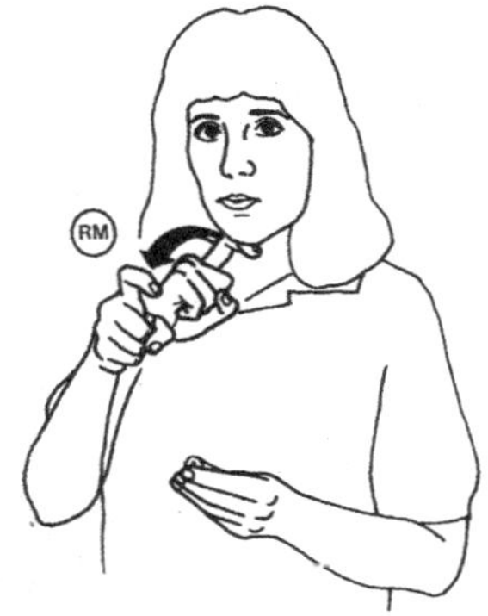

RUBBER

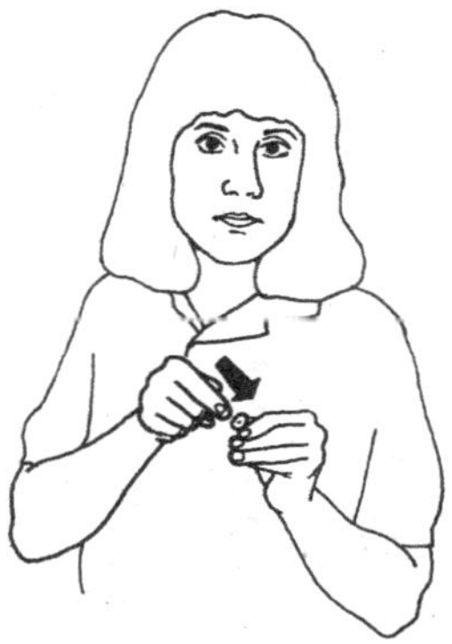

TIP

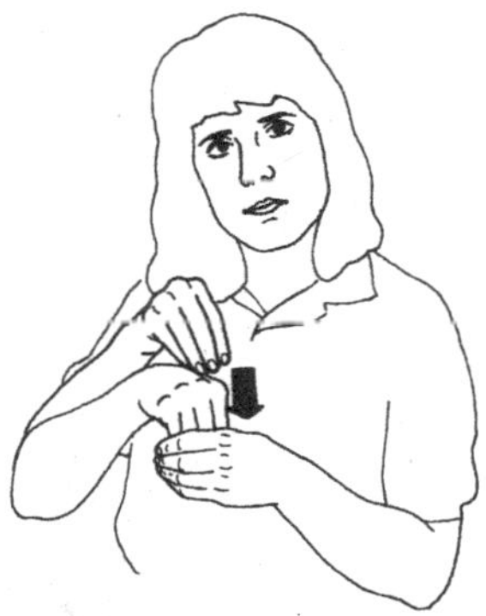

IN

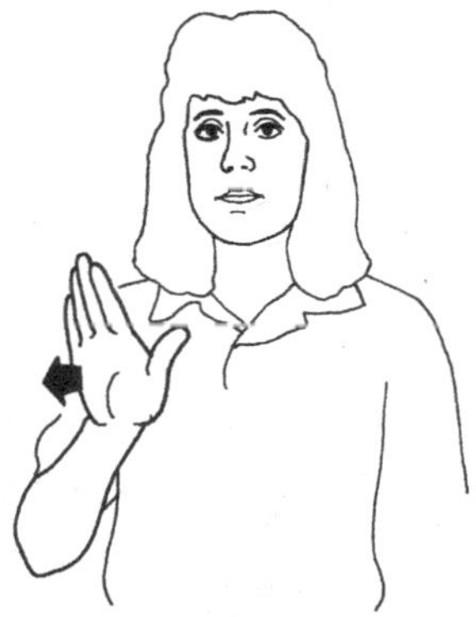

YOUR

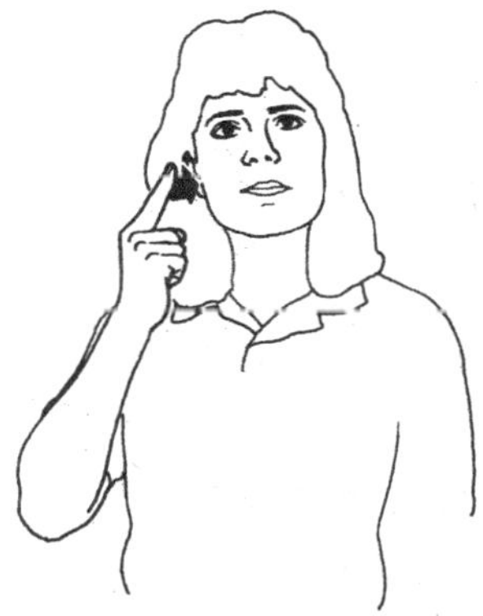

EAR.

I will put this soft rubber tip in your ear.

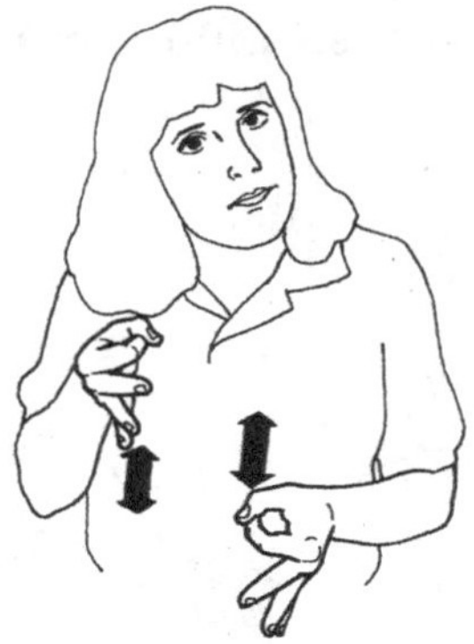

IF

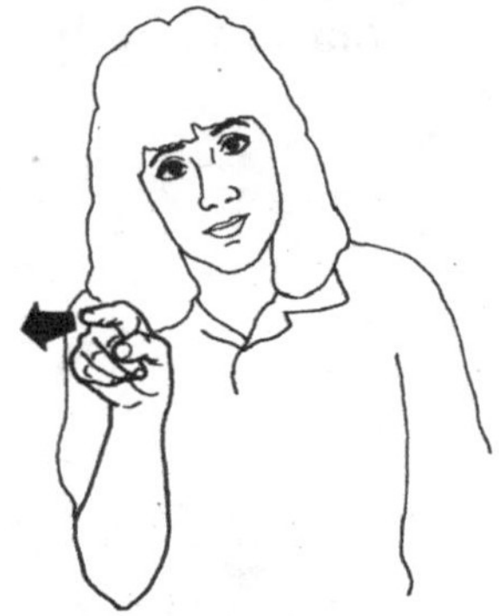

YOU

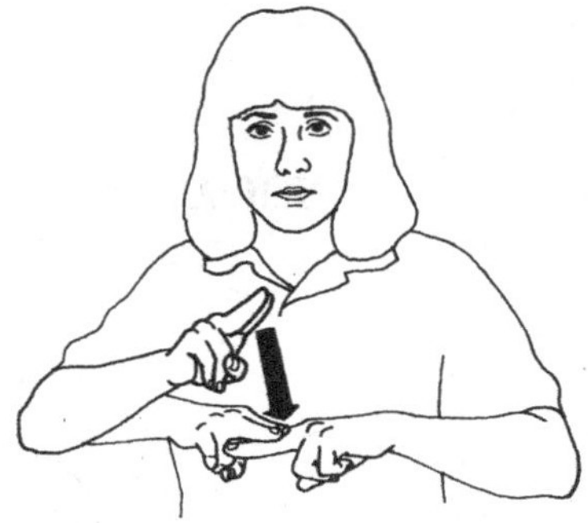

SIT

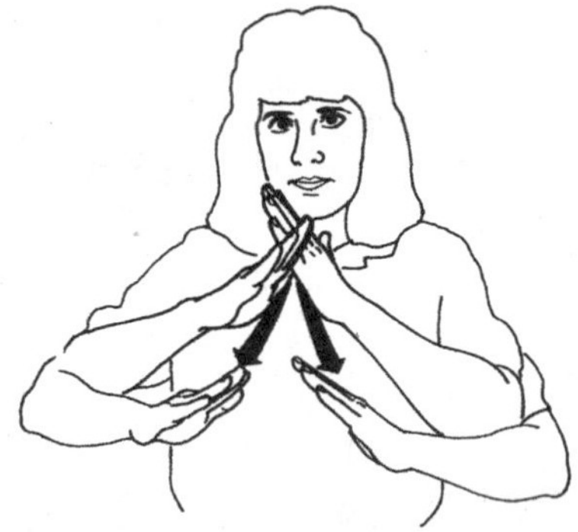

QUIET

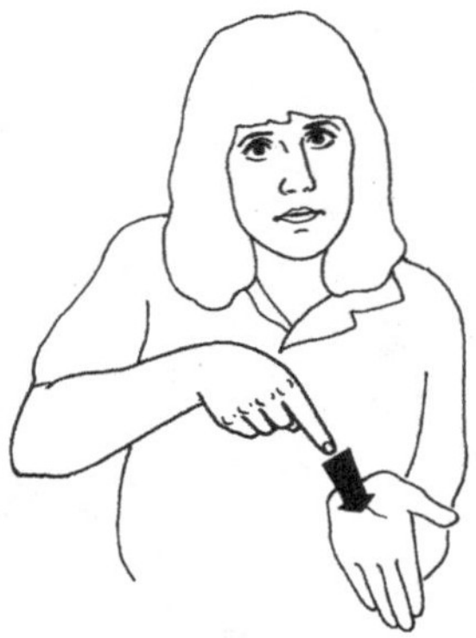

THIS

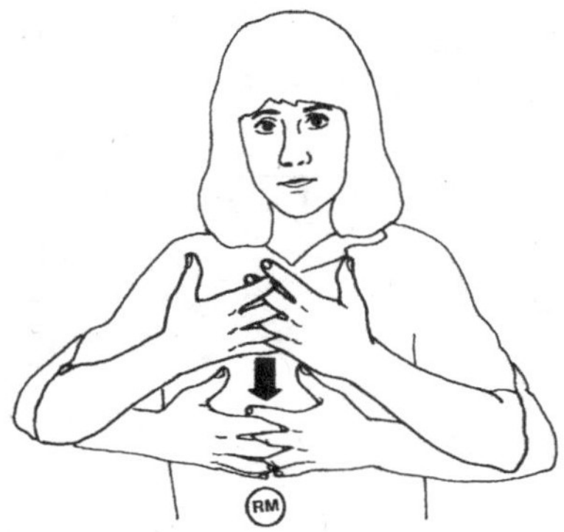

MACHINE

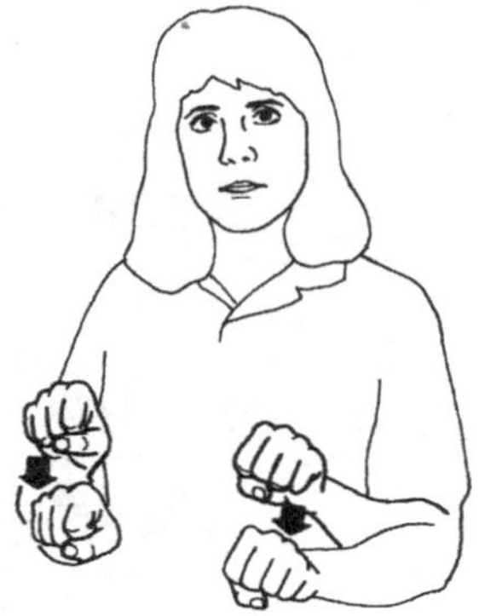

CAN

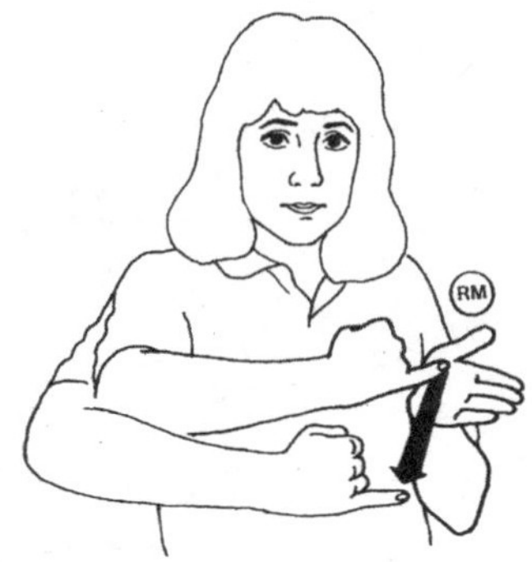

DRAW

If you sit quietly, this machine can draw a picture of a mountain.

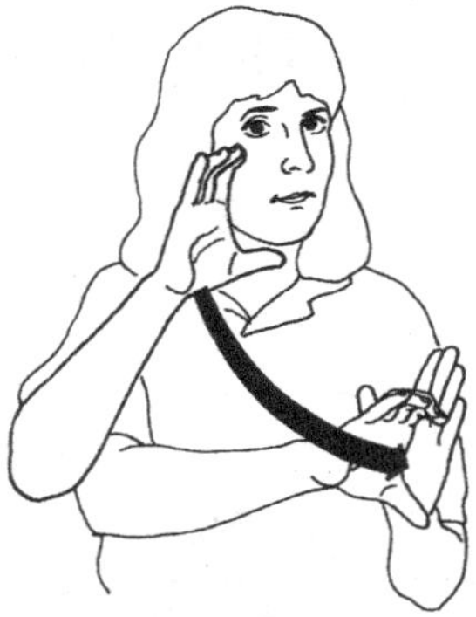

PICTURE

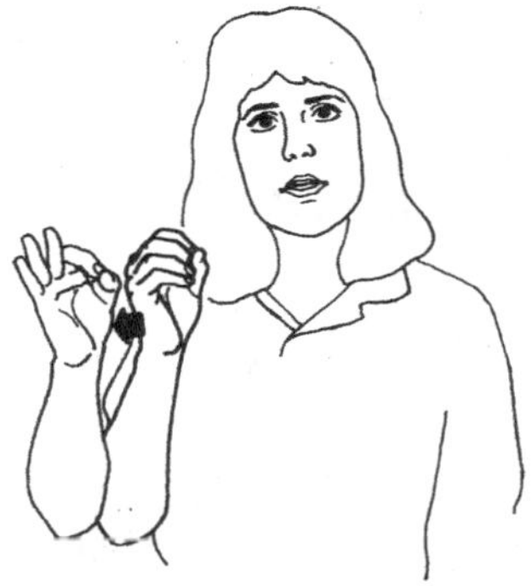

O-F

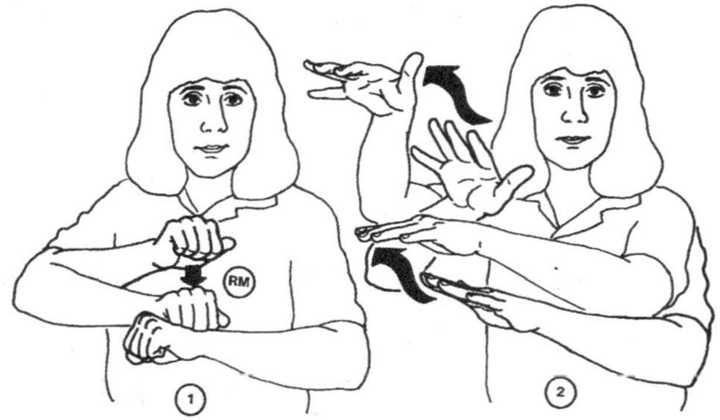

MOUNTAIN.

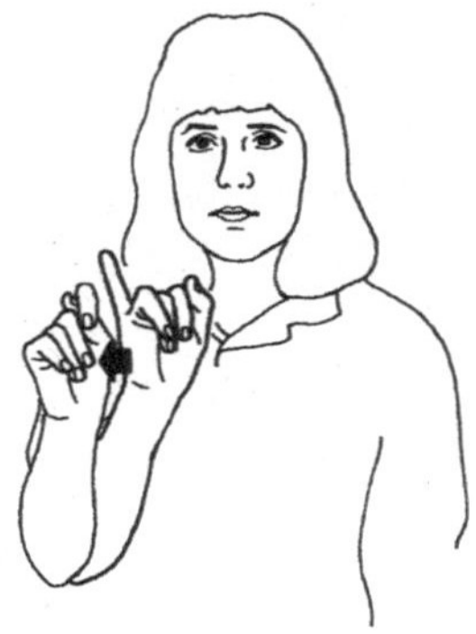

I-T

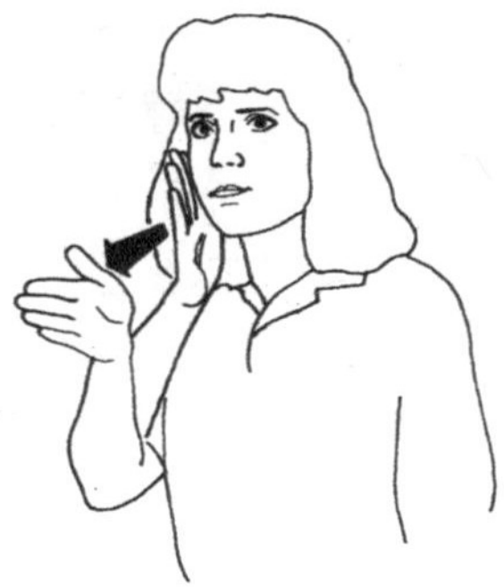

WILL

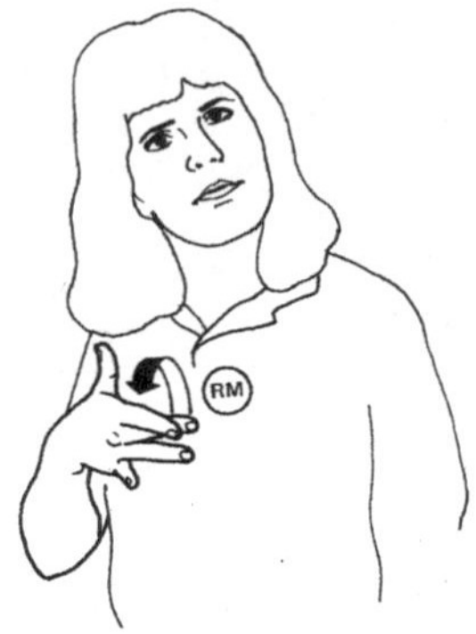

FEEL

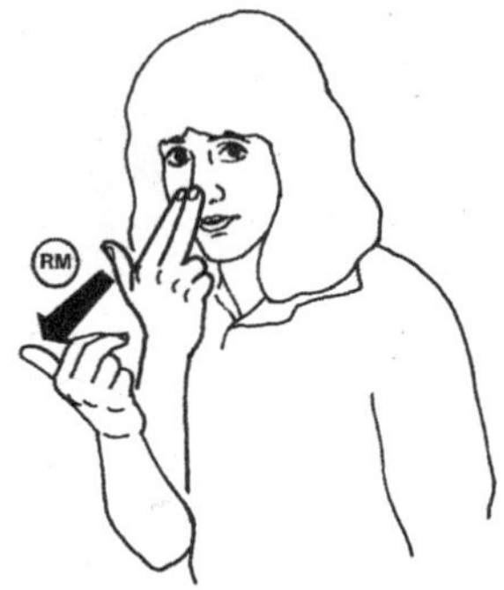

FUNNY

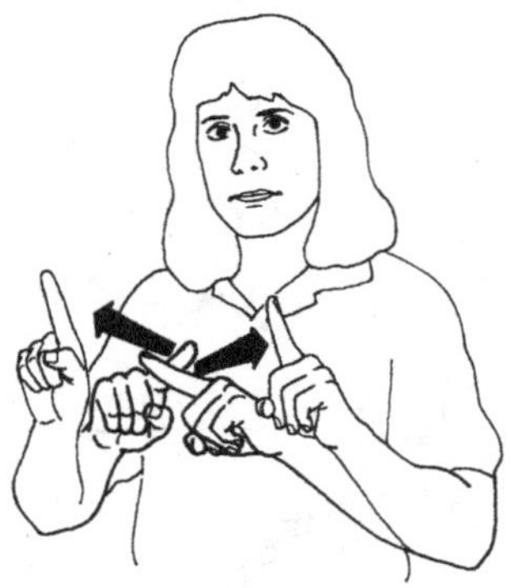

BUT

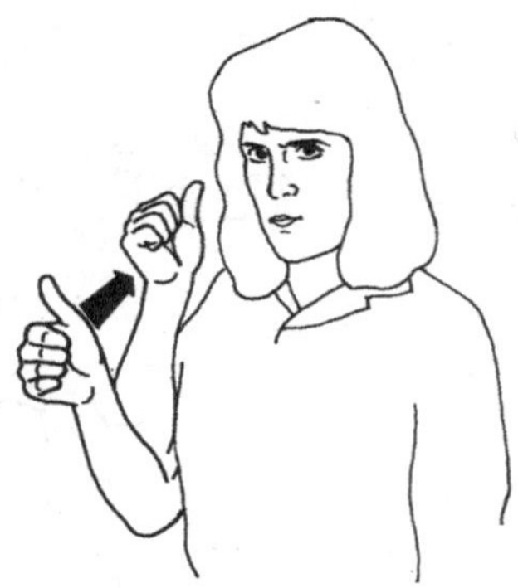

WON'T

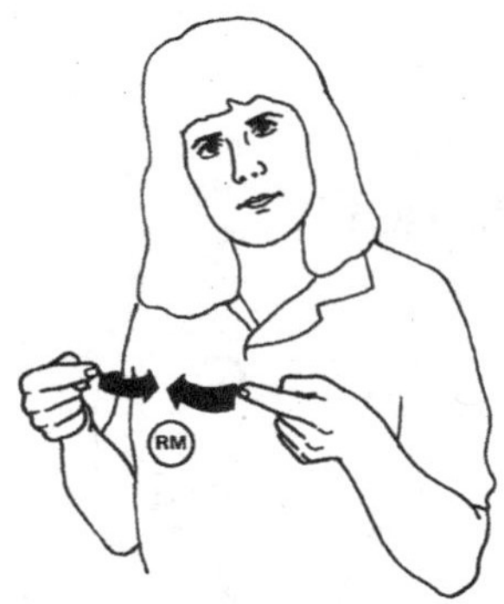

HURT.

It will feel funny, but it won't hurt.

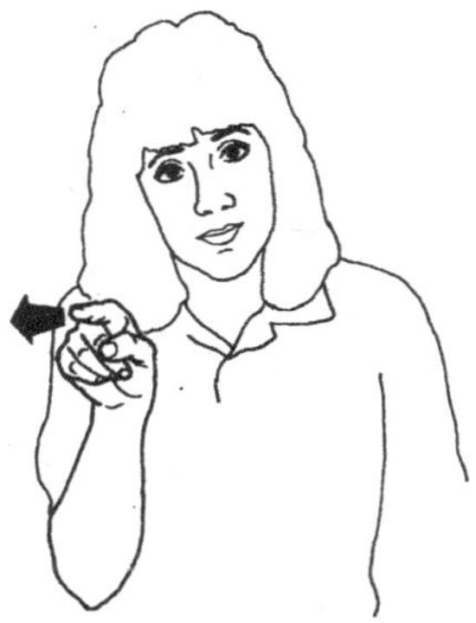

YOU

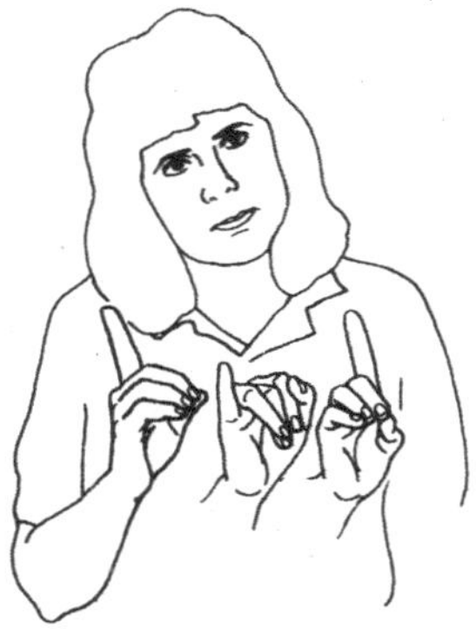

D-I-D

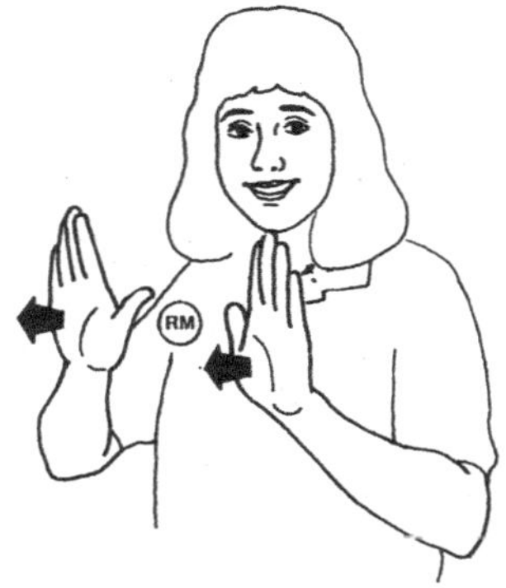

FANTASTIC

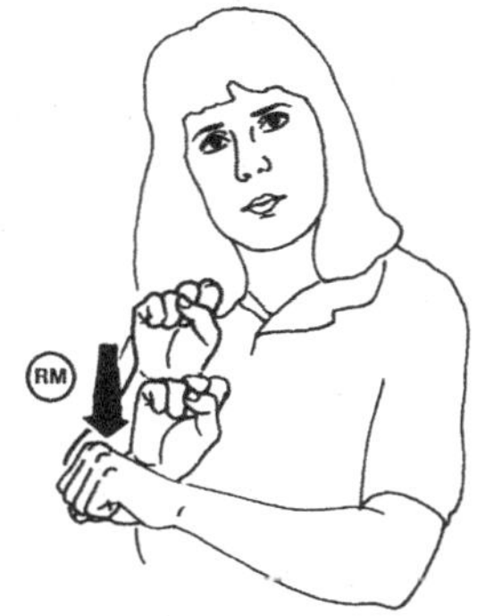

JOB.

You did a fantastic job.

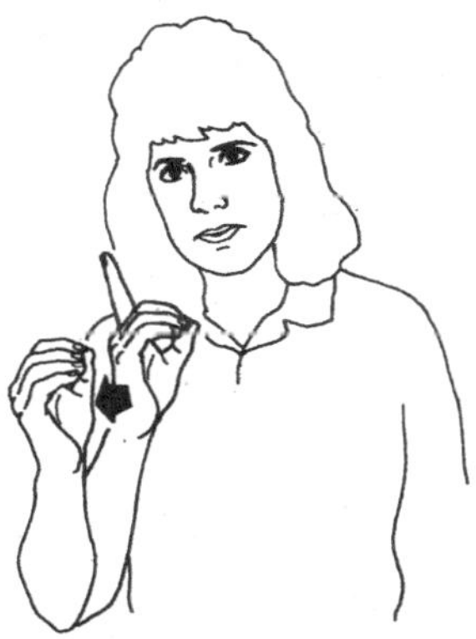

D-O

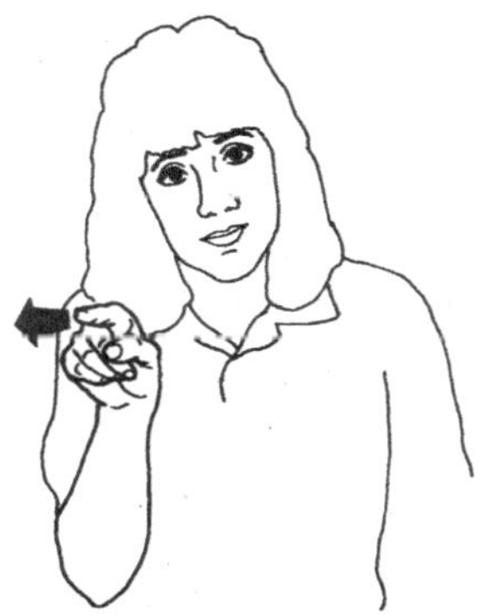

YOU

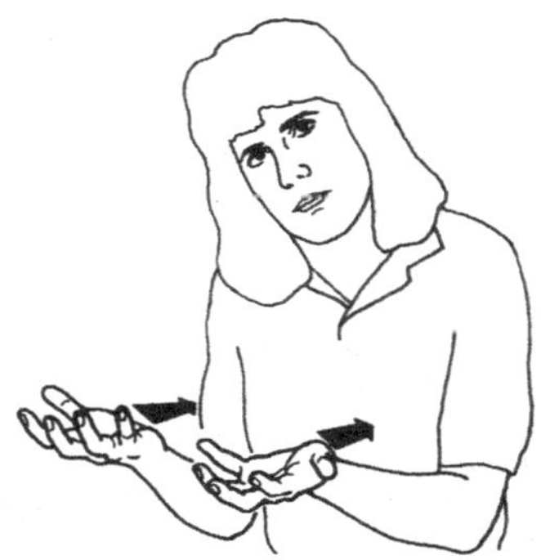

WANT

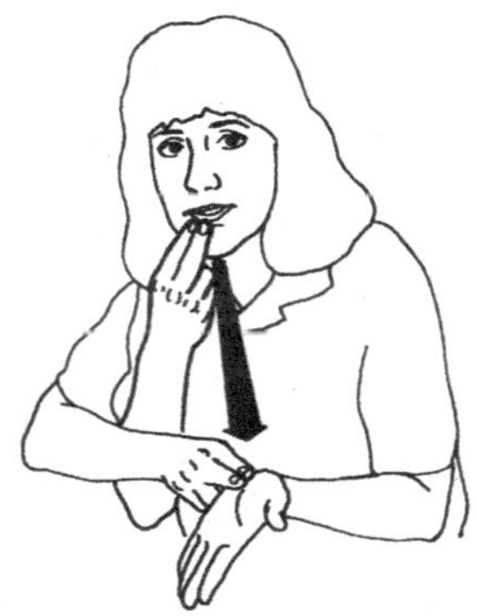

STICKER?

Do you want a sticker?

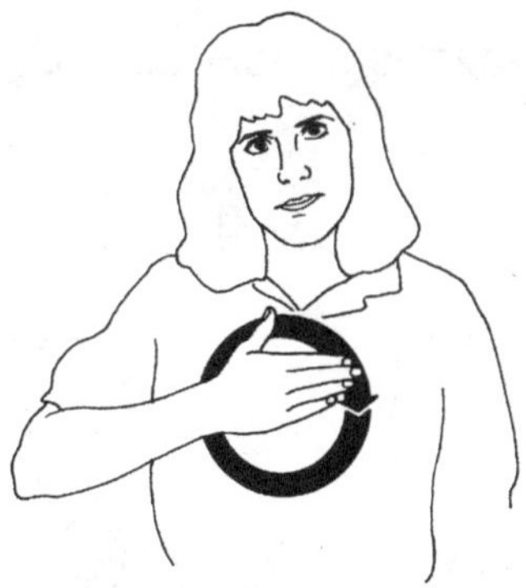

PLEASE

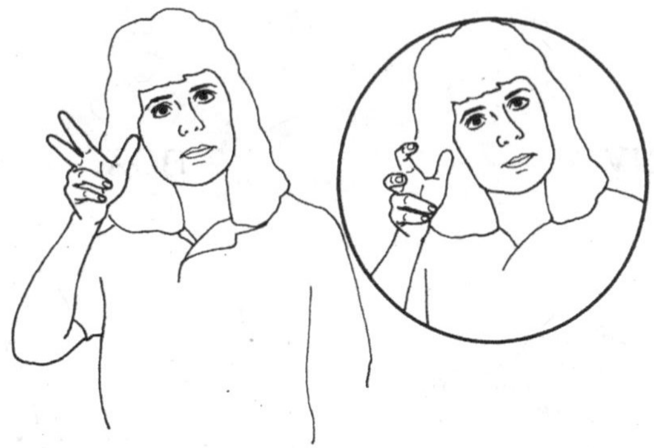

LISTEN

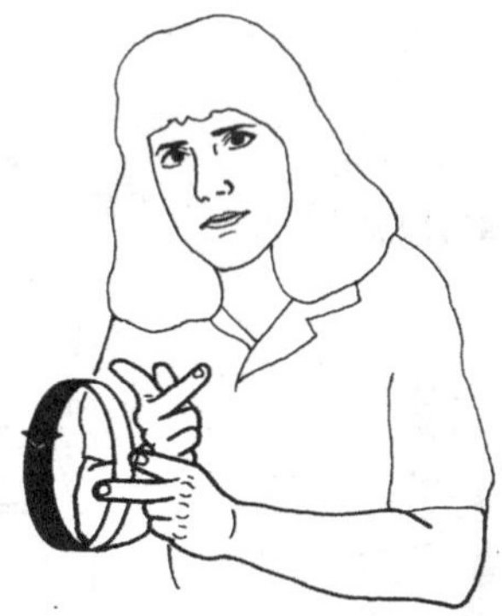

CAREFUL.

Please listen carefully.

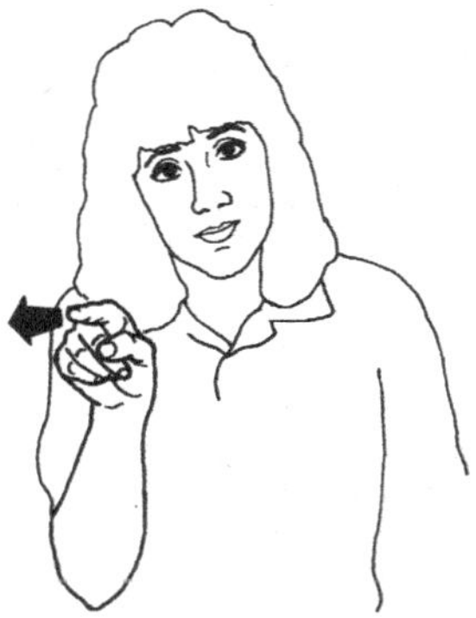

YOU

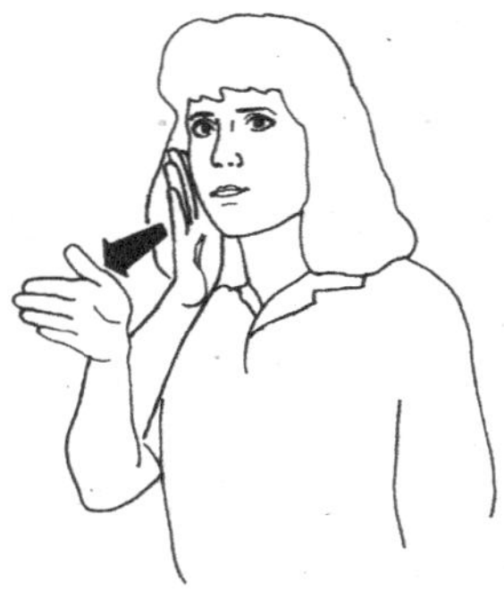

WILL

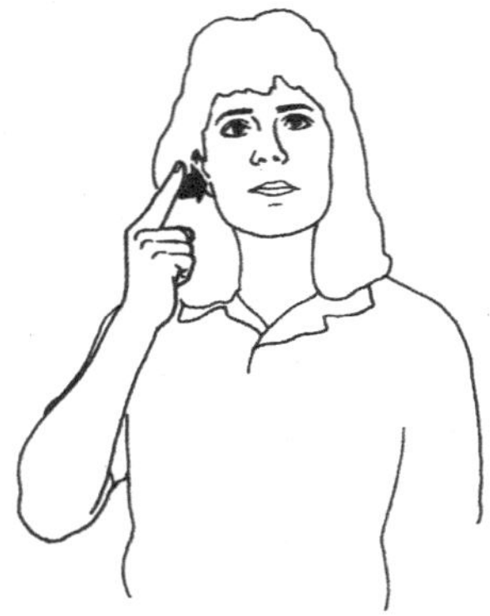

HEAR

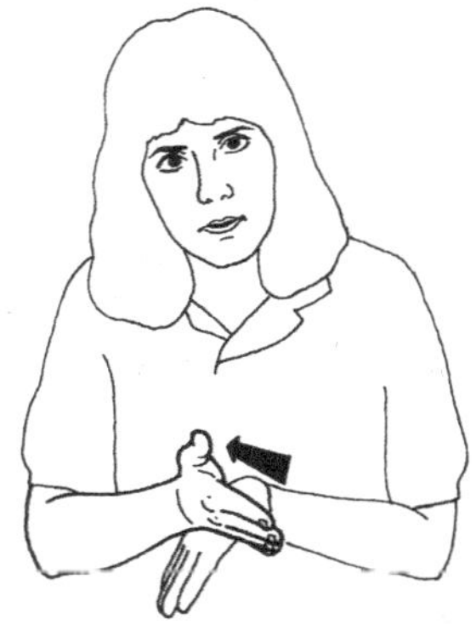

SOME

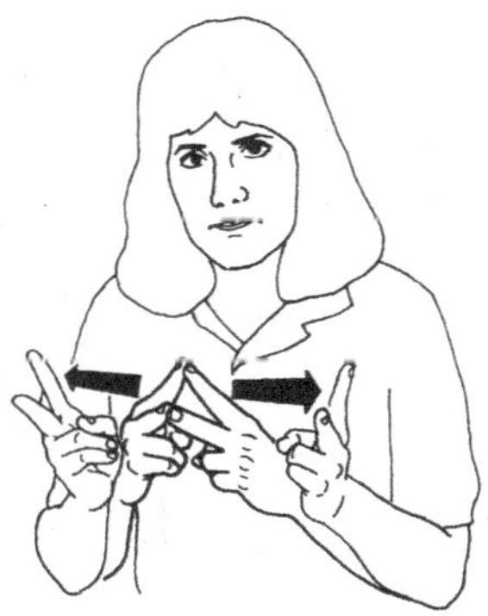

VERY

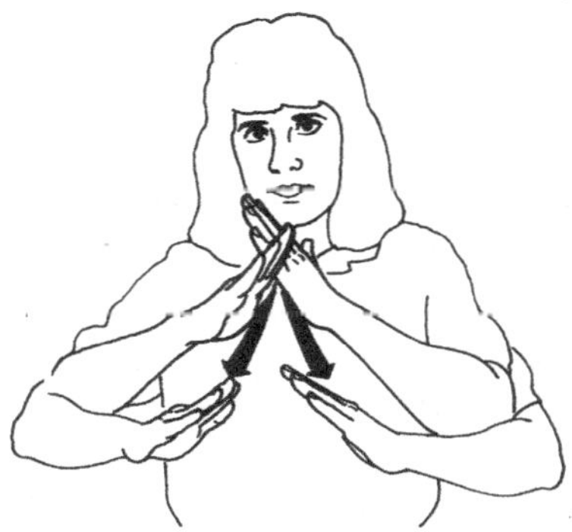

QUIET

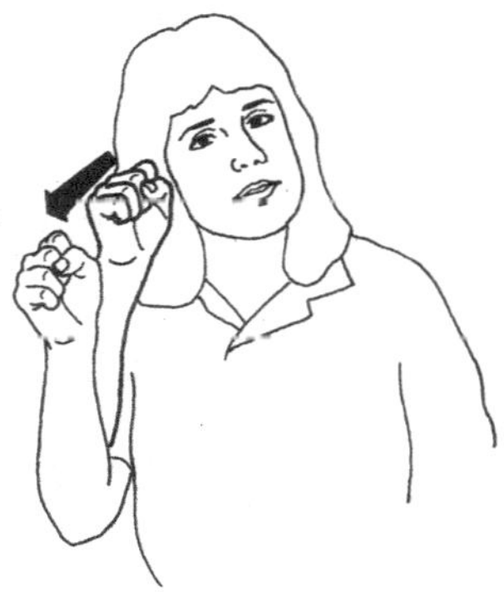

SOUND.

You will hear some very quiet sounds.

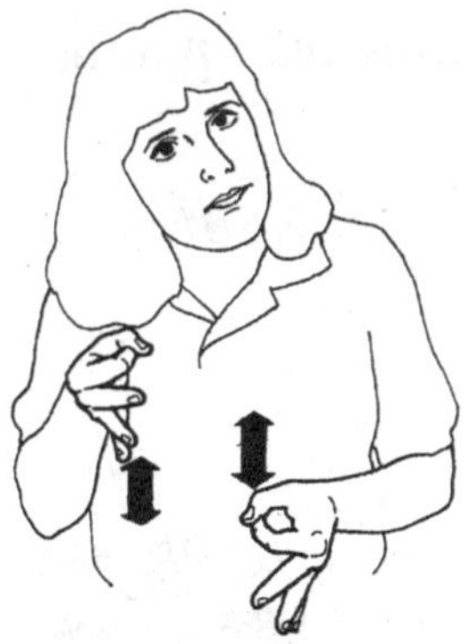

IF

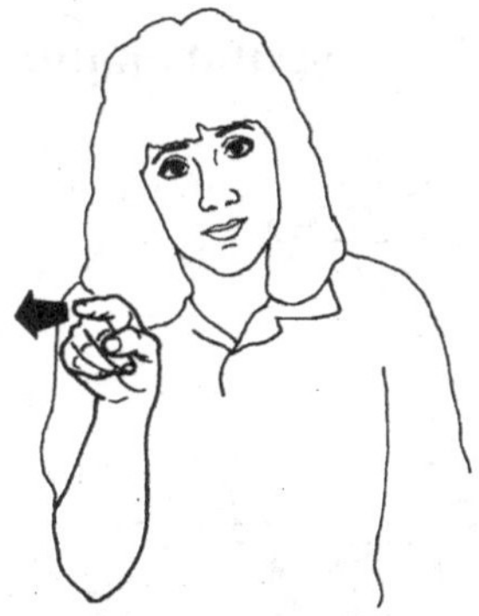

YOU

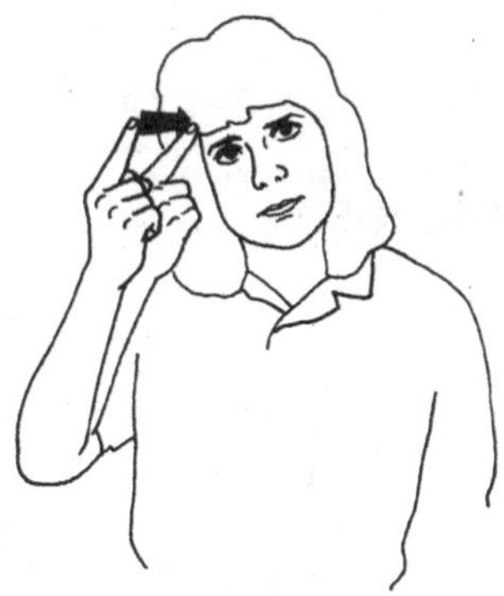

THINK

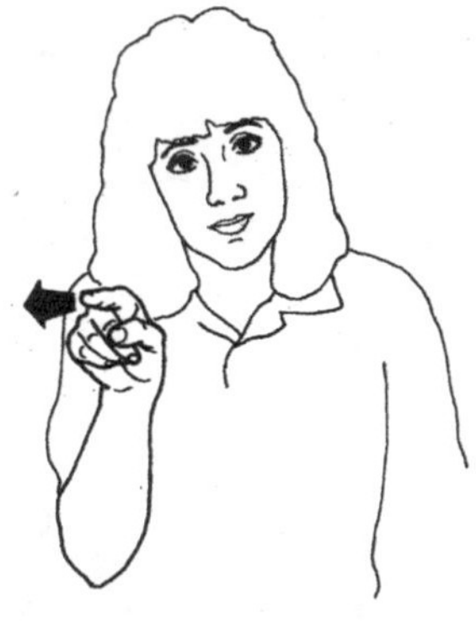

YOU

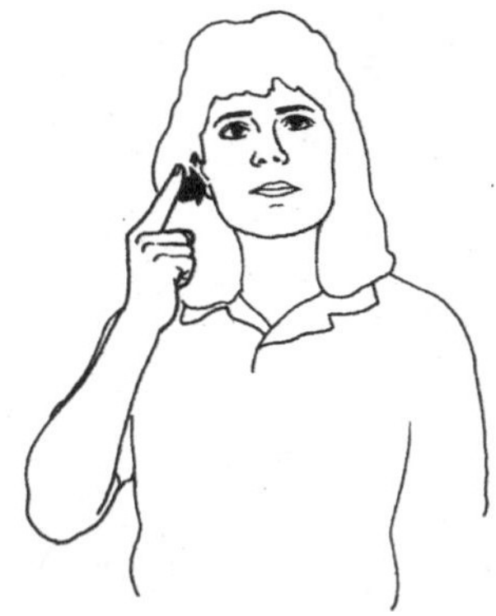

HEAR

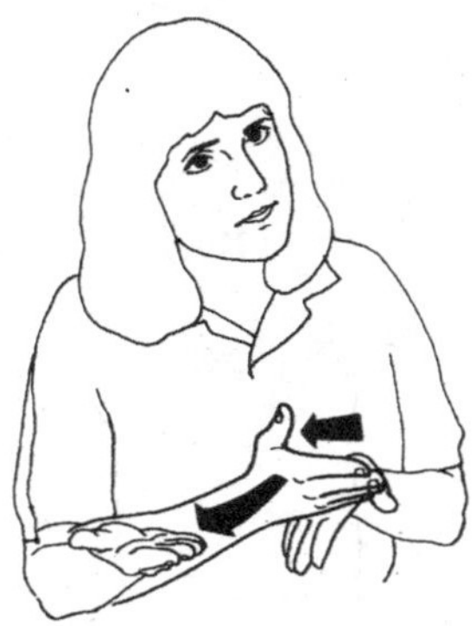

SOMETHING

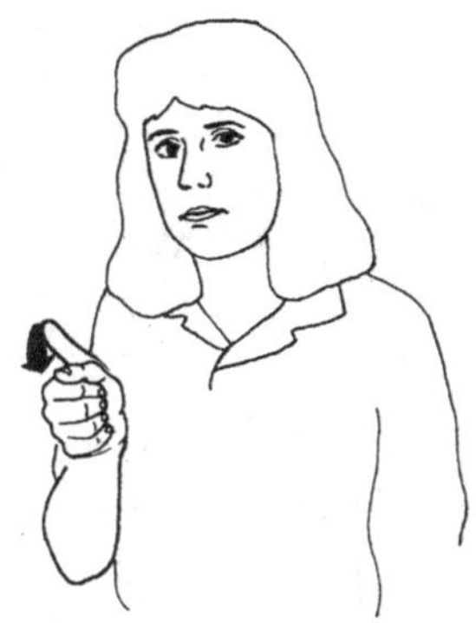

PRESS-BUTTON.

If you think you hear something, press the button.

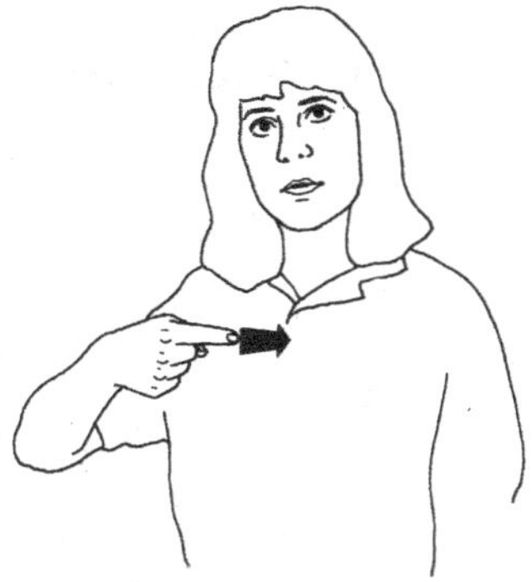

I

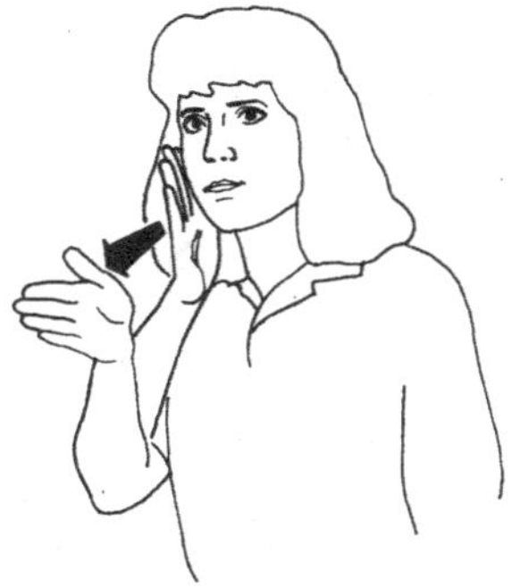

WILL

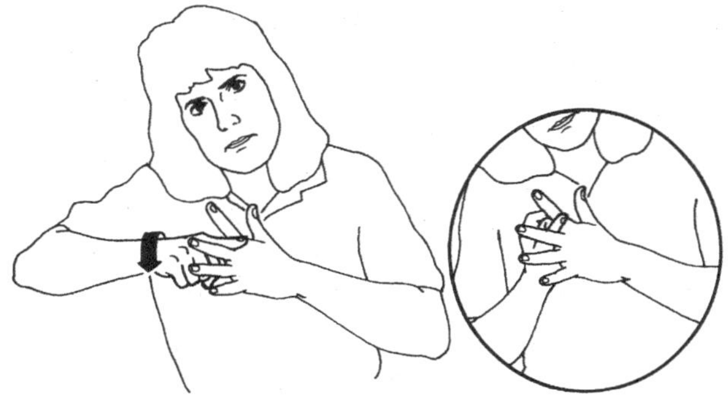

START

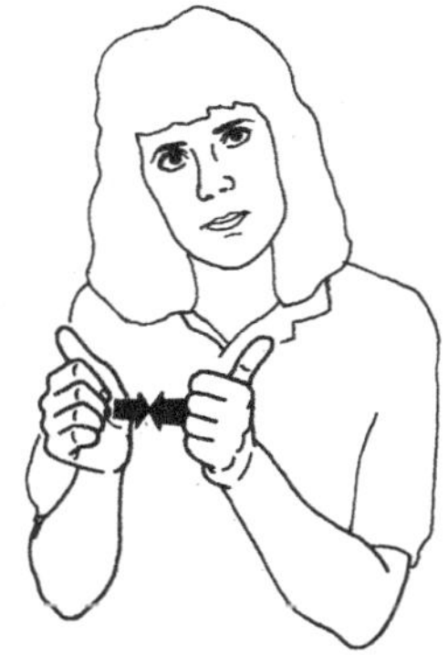

WITH

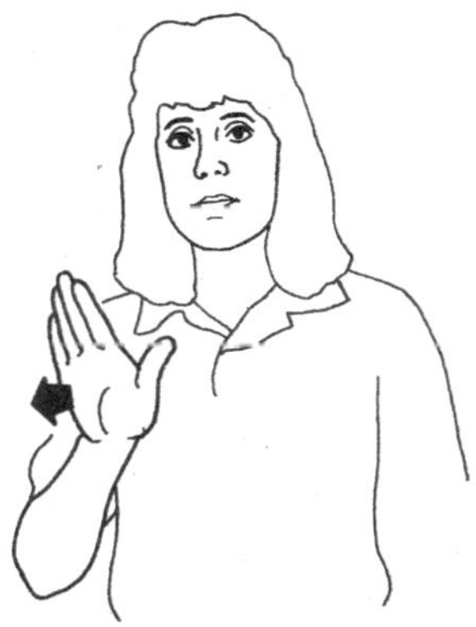

YOUR

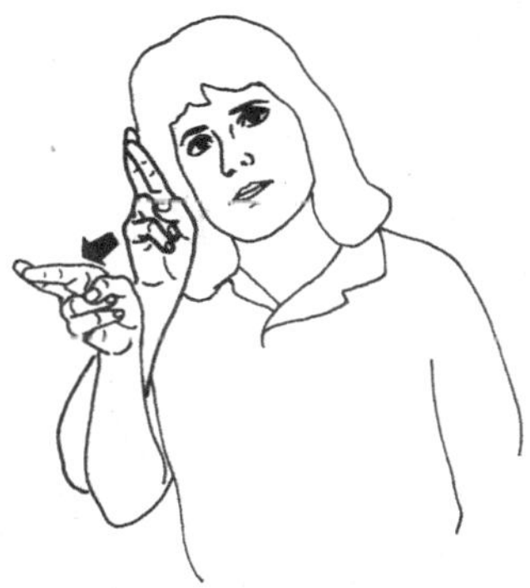

RIGHT

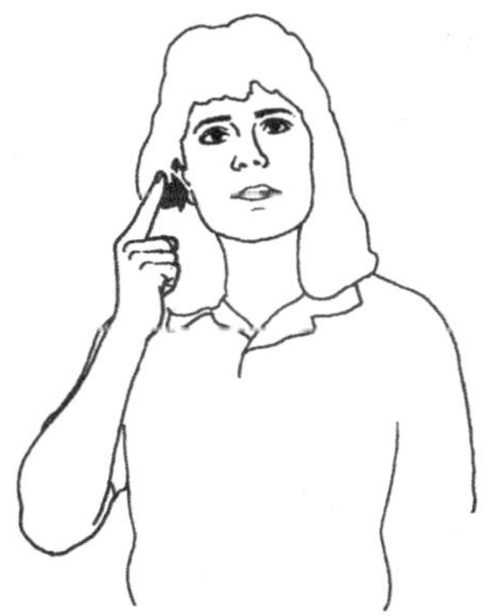

EAR.

I will start with your right ear.

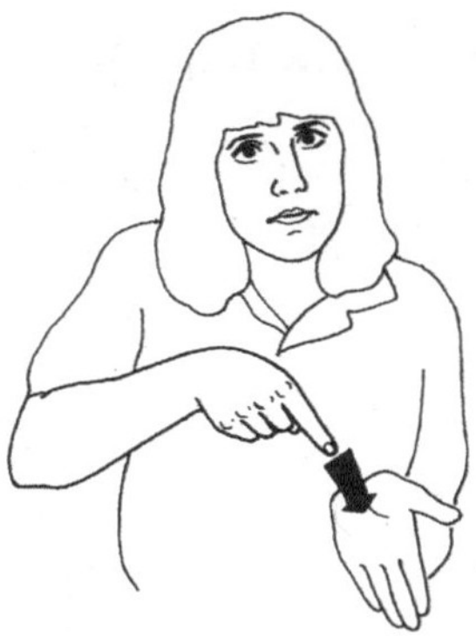

THIS

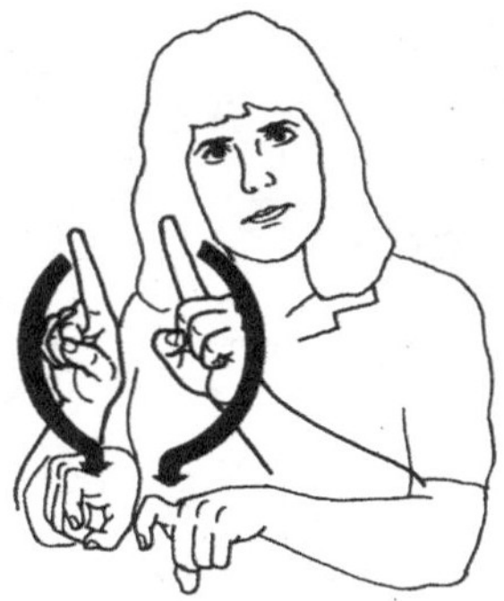

TEST

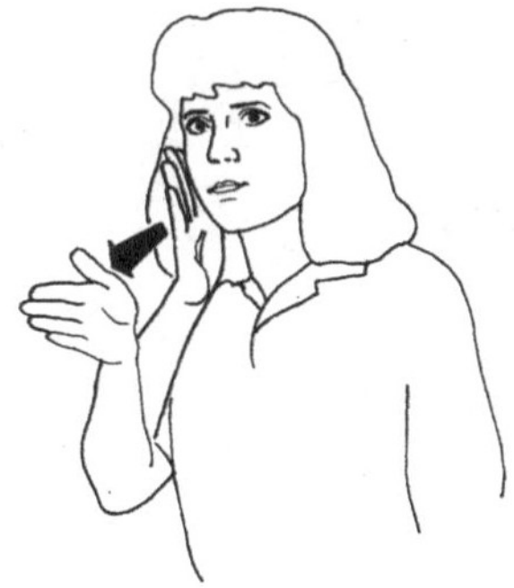

WILL

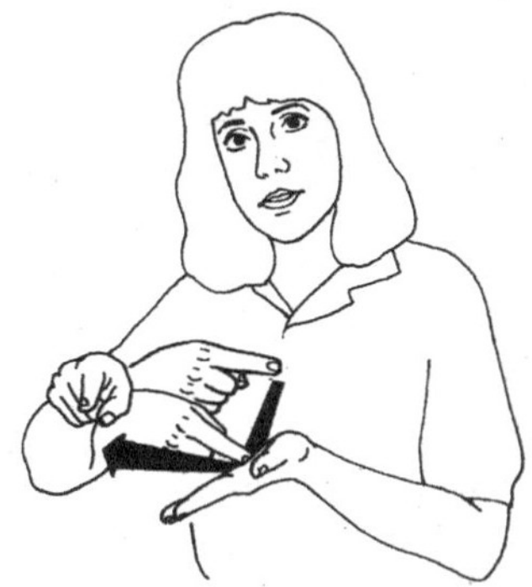

CHECK

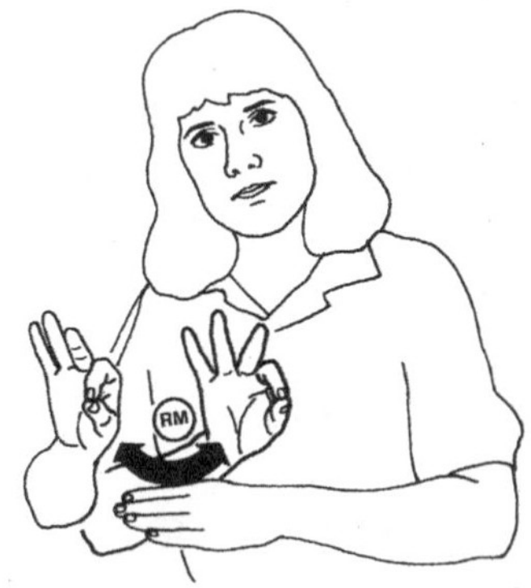

FUNCTION

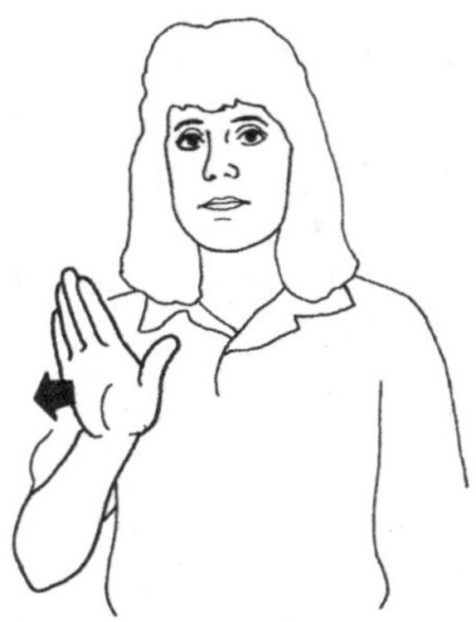

YOUR

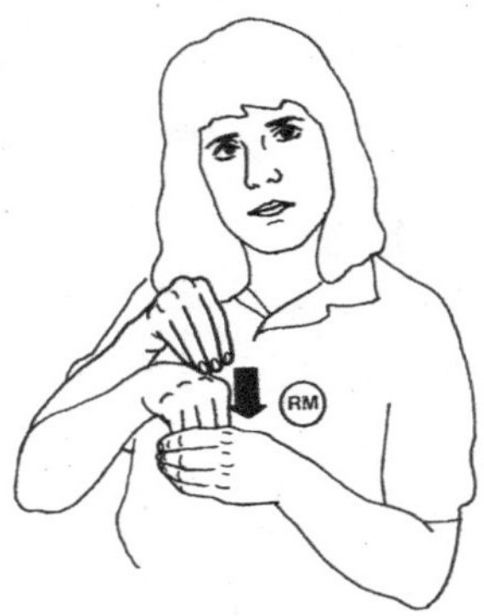

IN

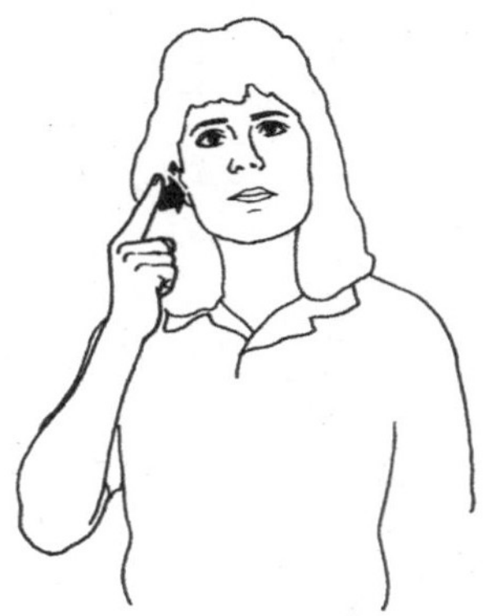

EAR.

This test will check the functioning of your inner ear.

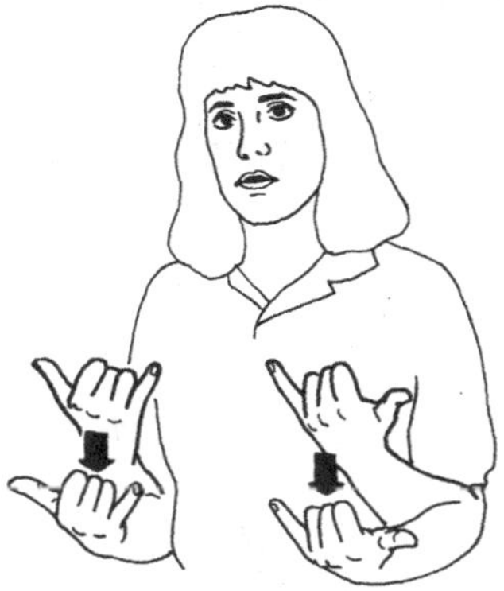

NOW

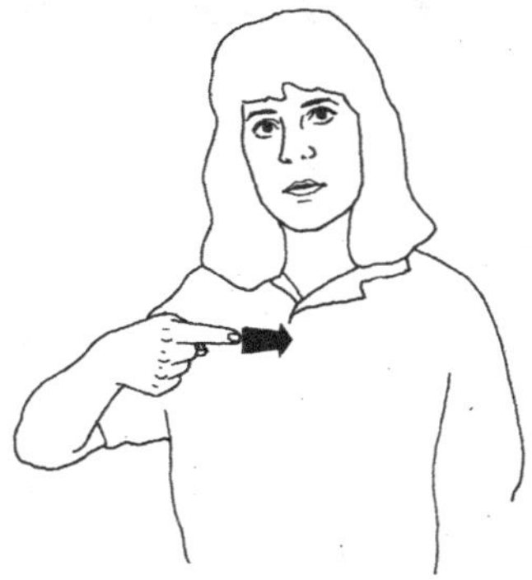

I

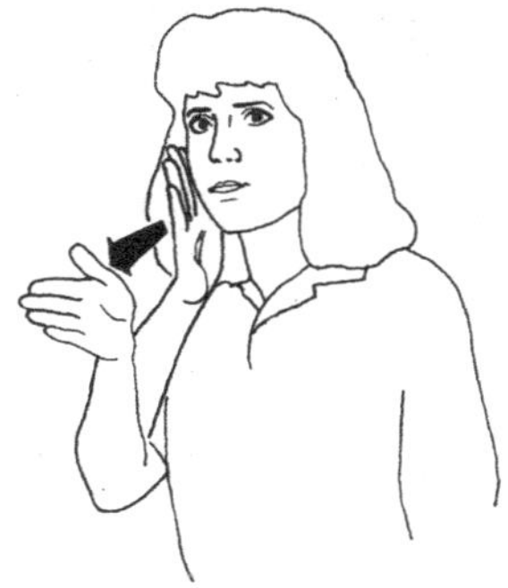

WILL

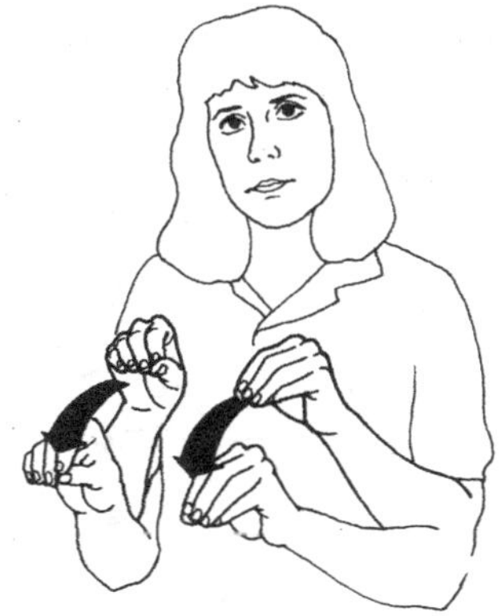

PUT

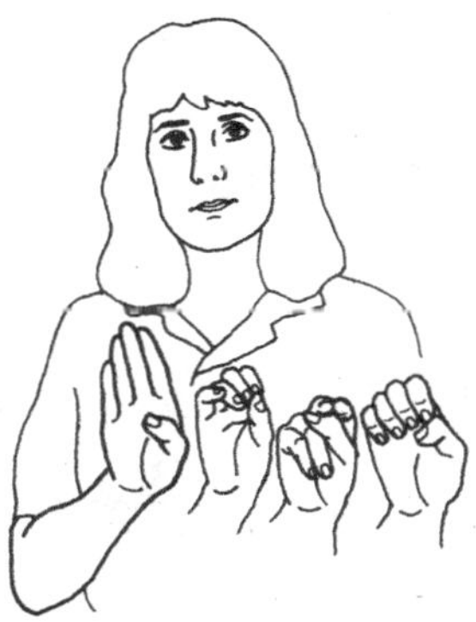

B-O-N-E

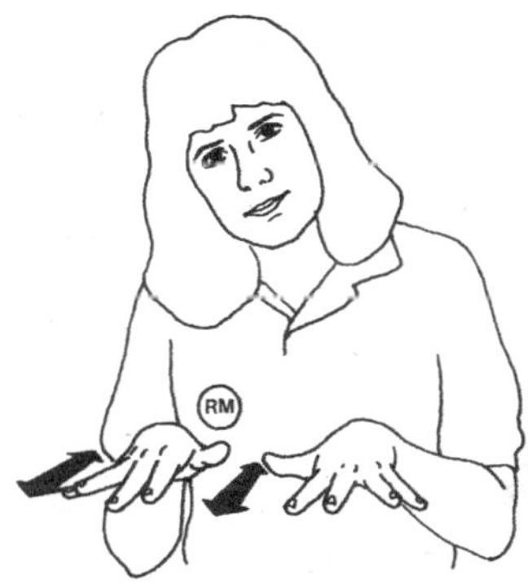

VIBRATOR

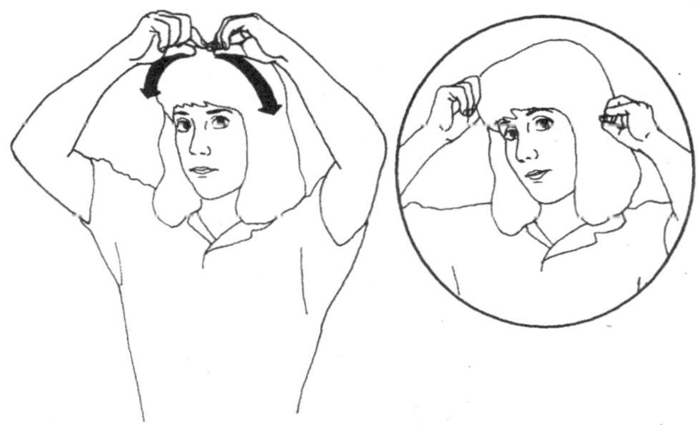

HEADBAND.

Now I will put the bone vibrator behind your ear.

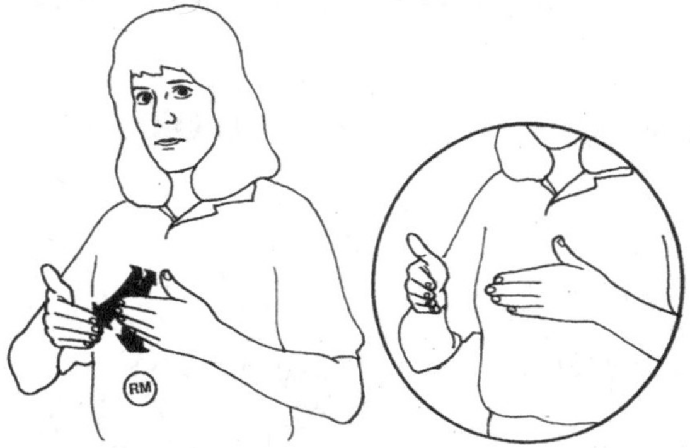

DOESN'T-MATTER

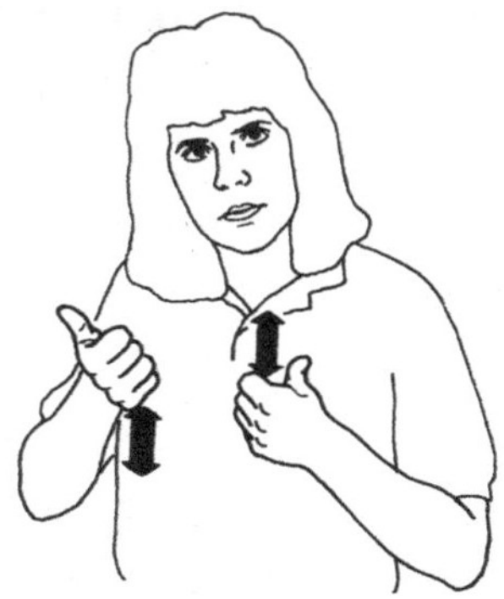

WHICH

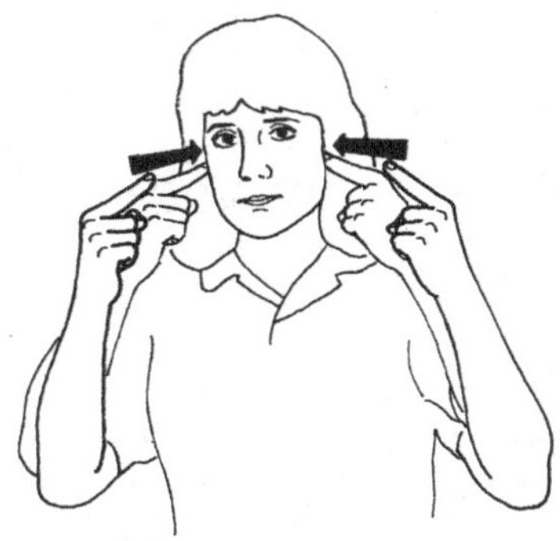

POINT-TO-EARS

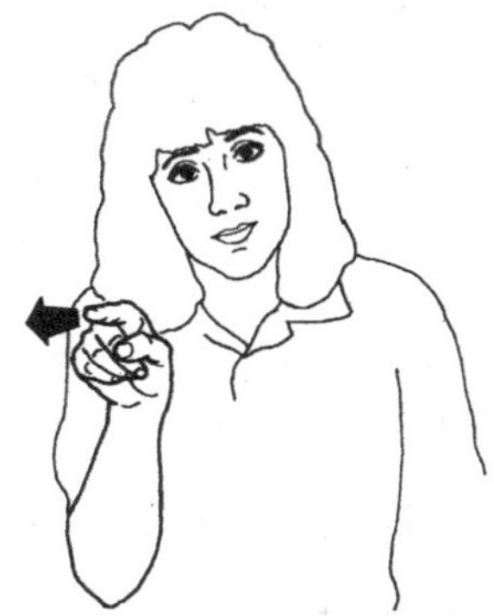

YOU

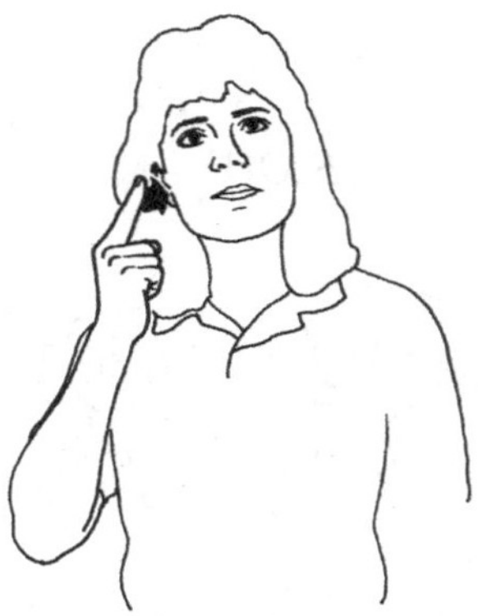

HEAR

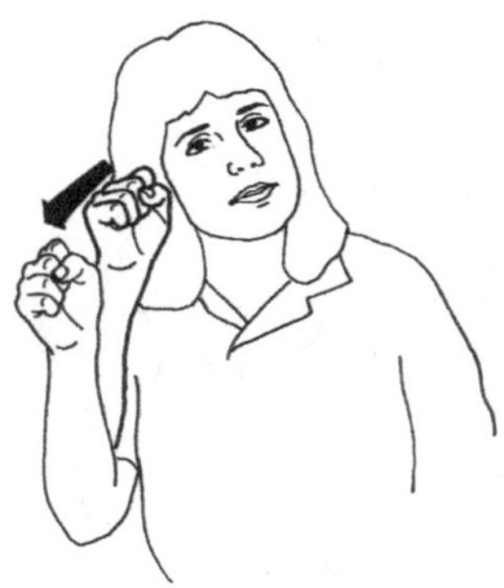

SOUND.

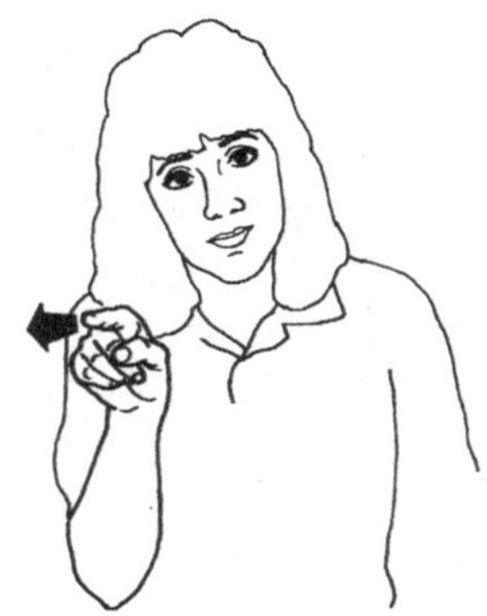

YOU

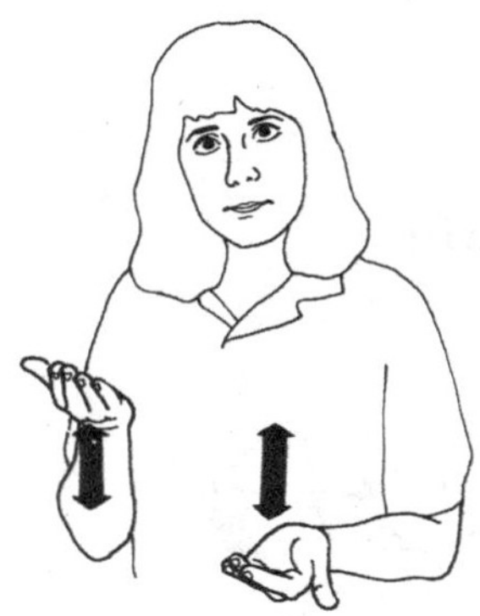

MAYBE

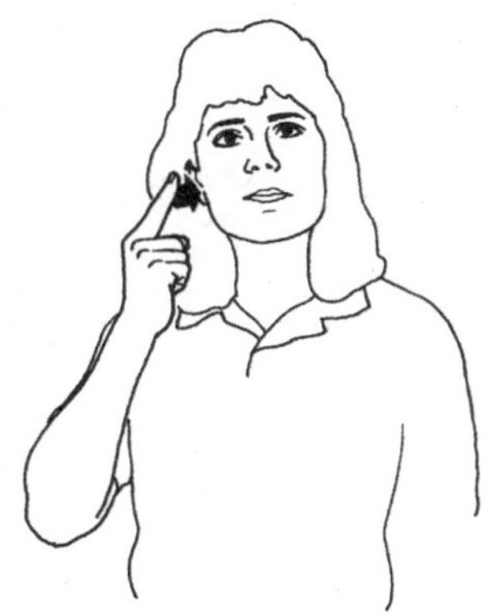

HEAR

It doesn't matter in which ear you hear the sound. You might hear something in the middle of your head.

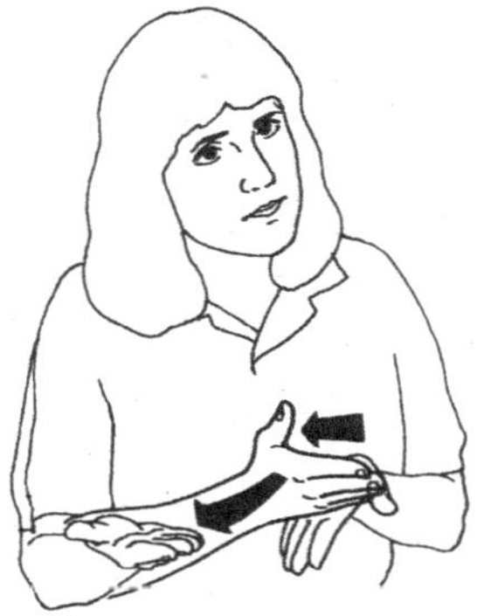

SOMETHING

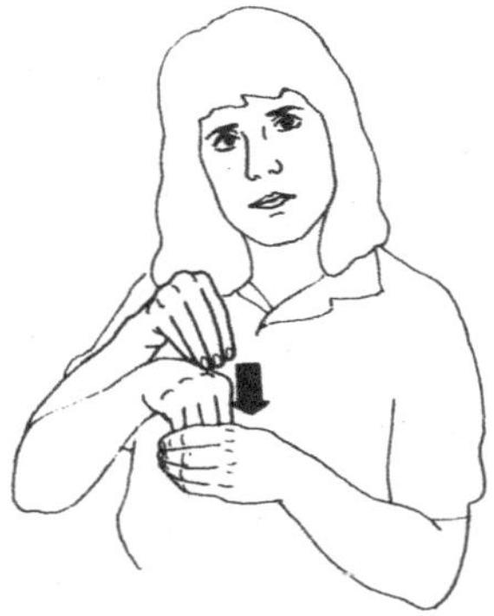

IN

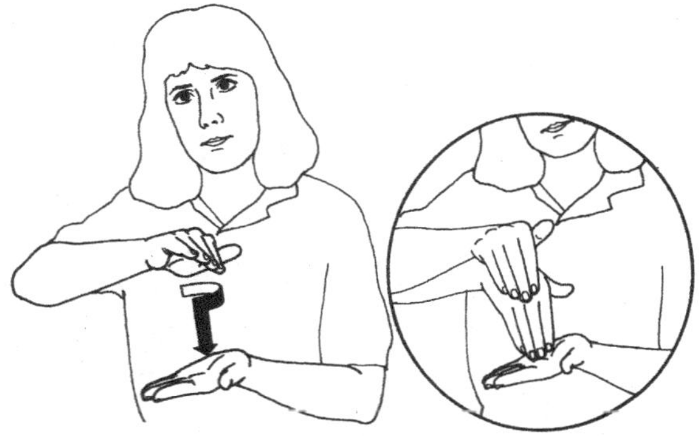

MIDDLE

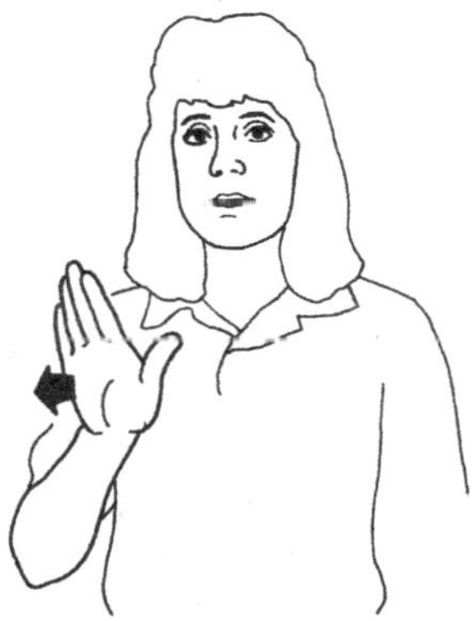

YOUR

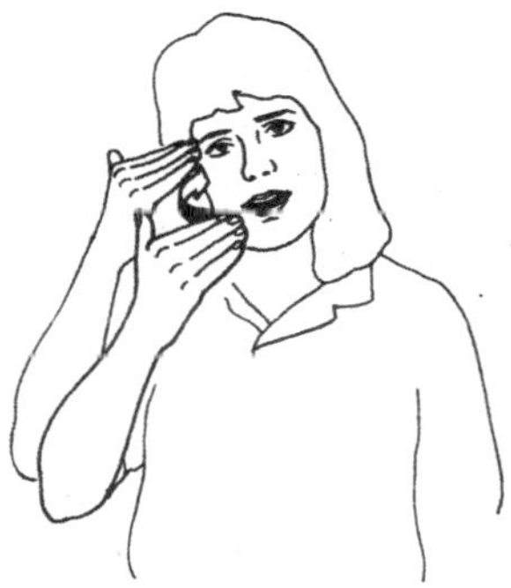

HEAD.

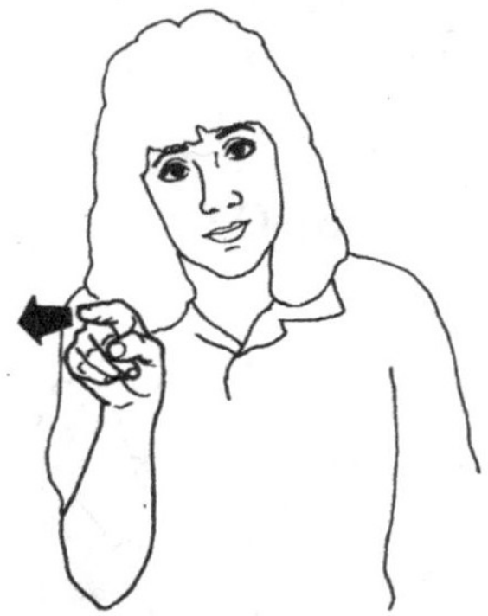

YOU

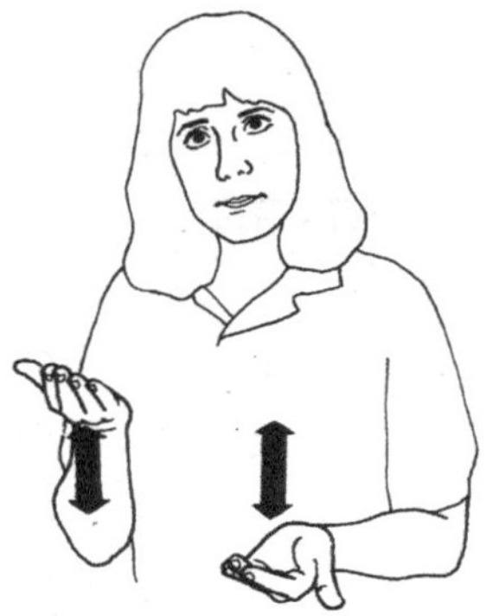

MAYBE

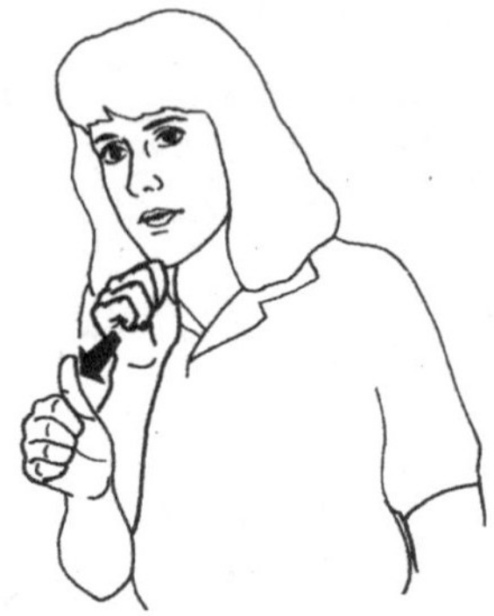

NOT

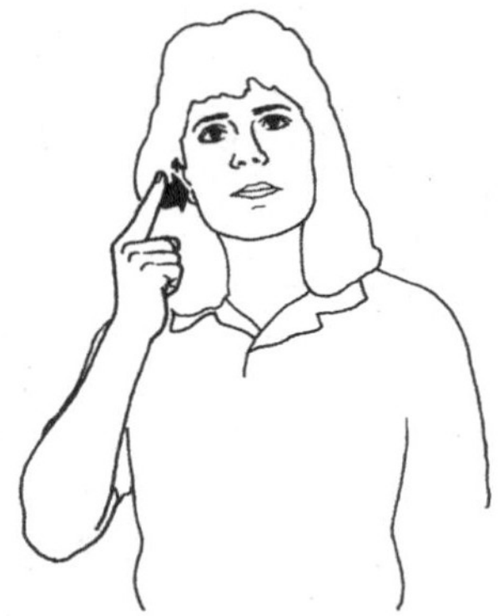

HEAR

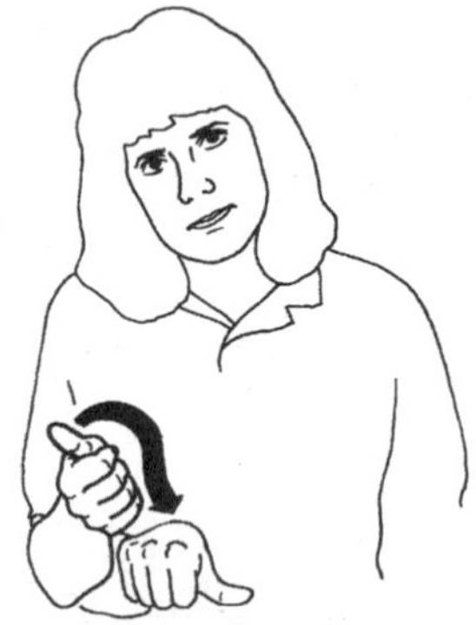

ANY

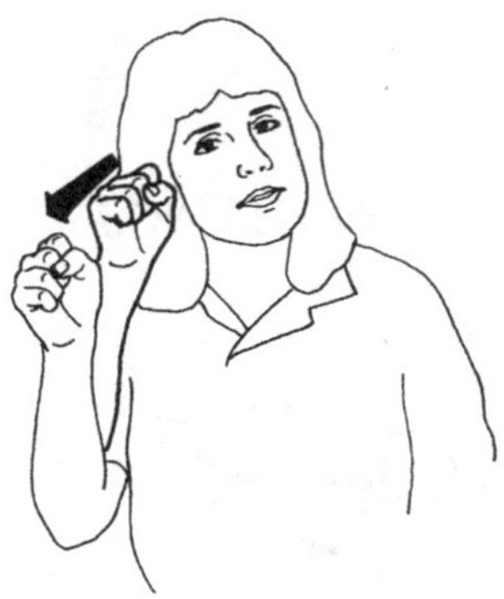

SOUND

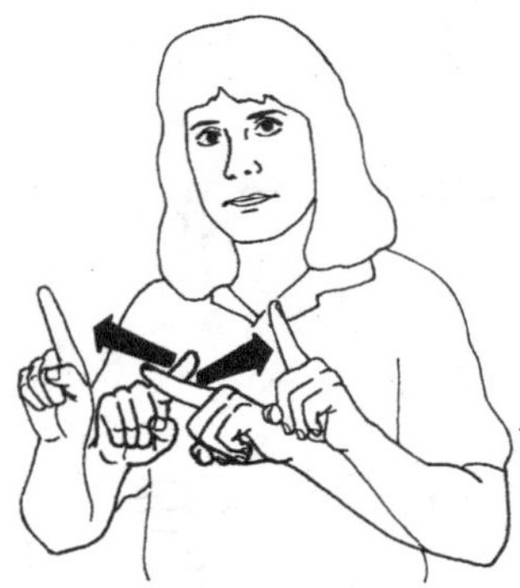

BUT

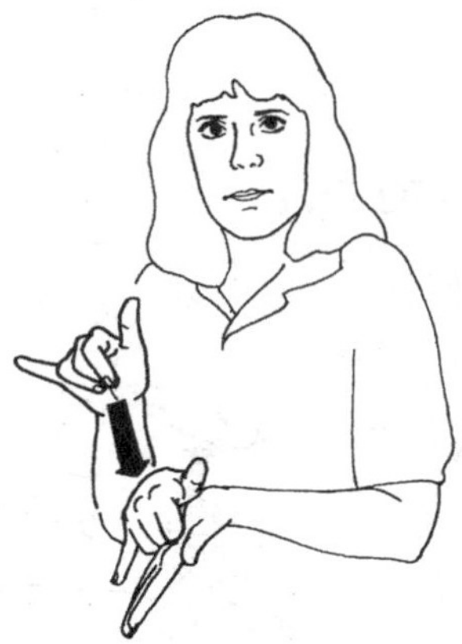

THAT

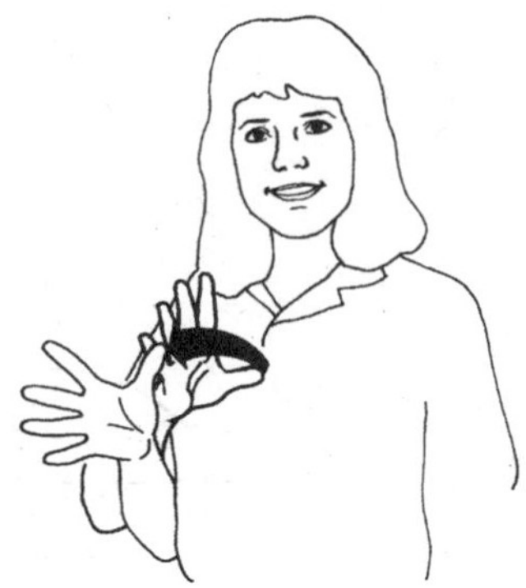

FINE.

You might not hear any of the sounds, but that's fine.

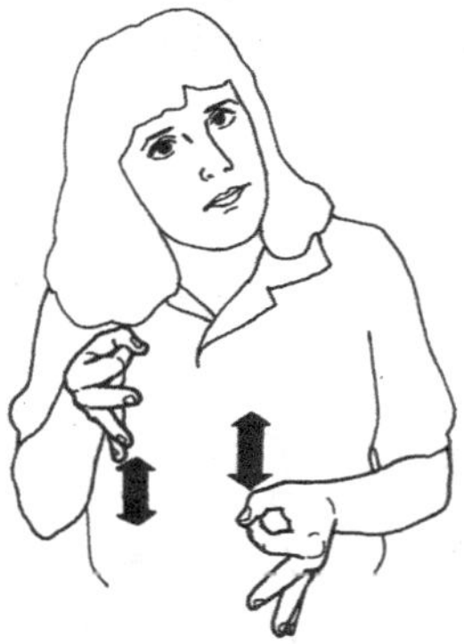

IF

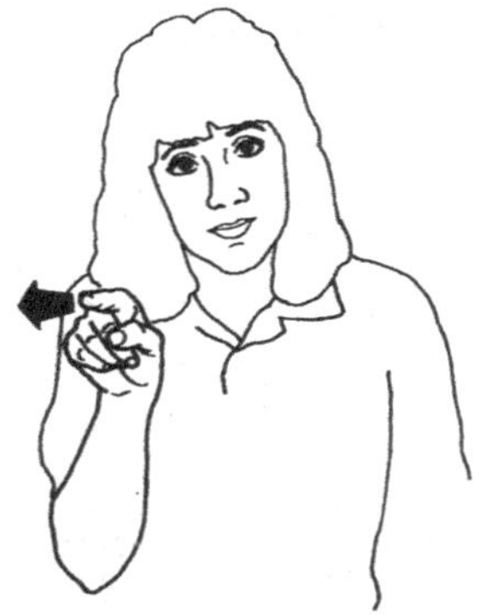

YOU

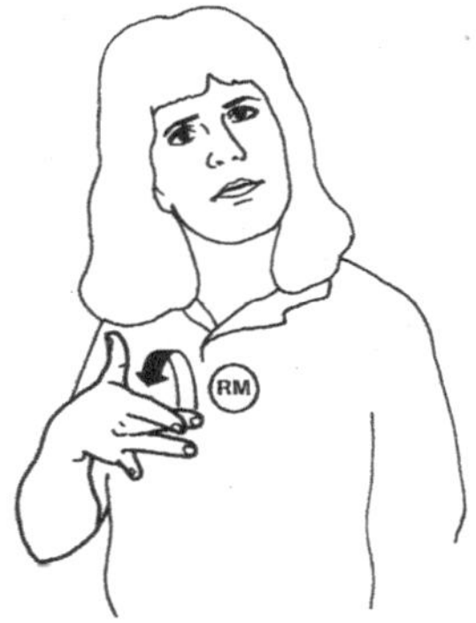

FEEL

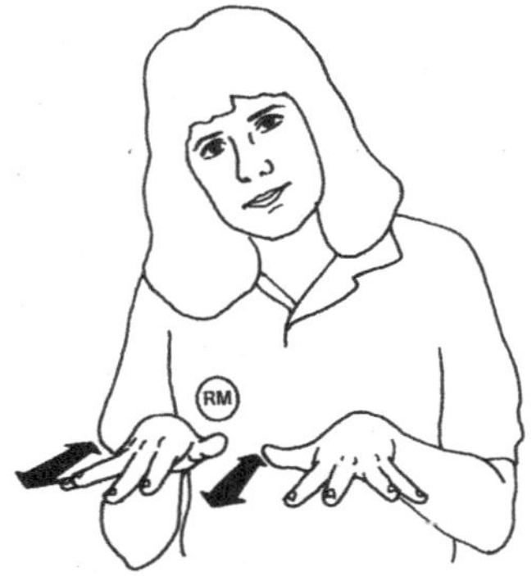

VIBRATION

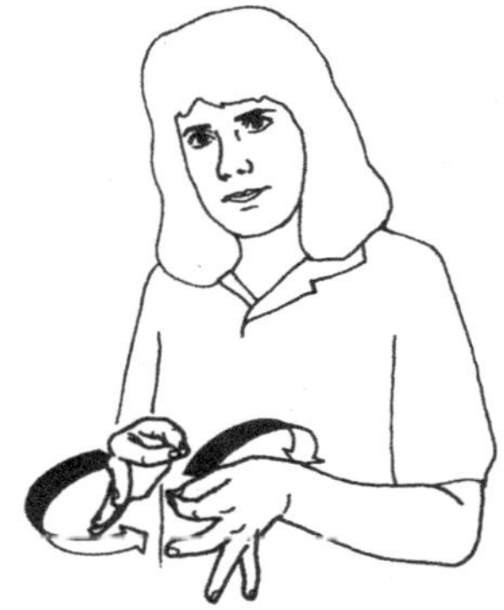

INSTEAD

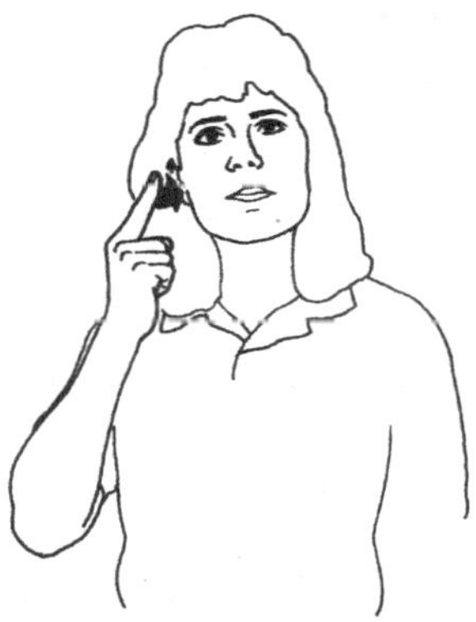

HEAR

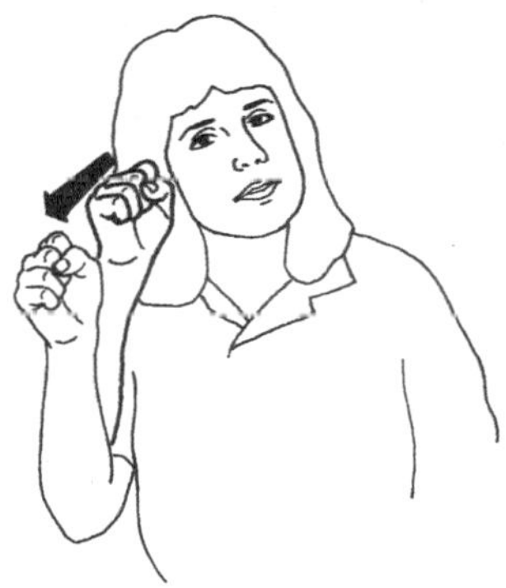

SOUND

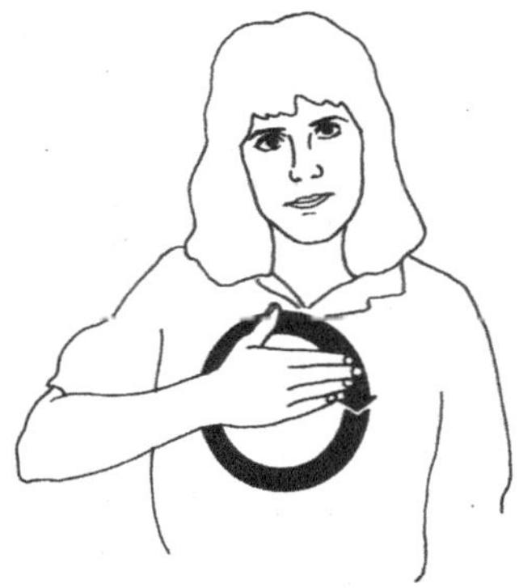

PLEASE

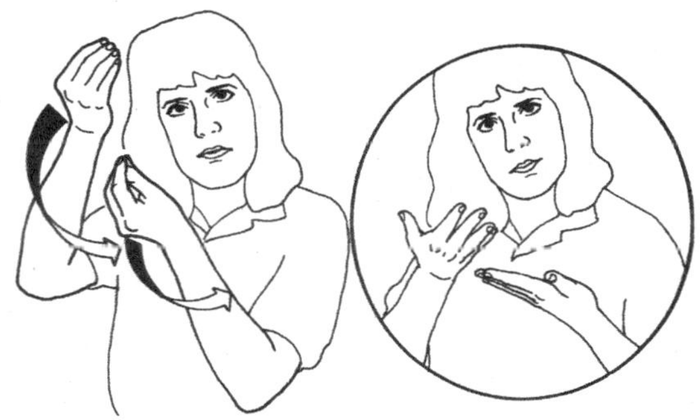

LET-ME-KNOW.

If you feel vibration instead of hearing sound, please let me know.

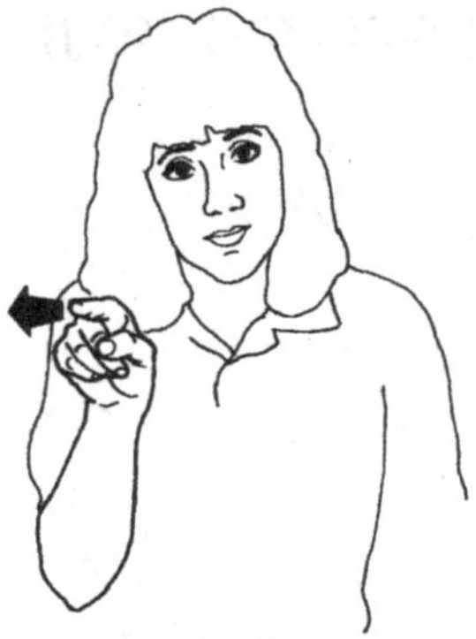

YOU

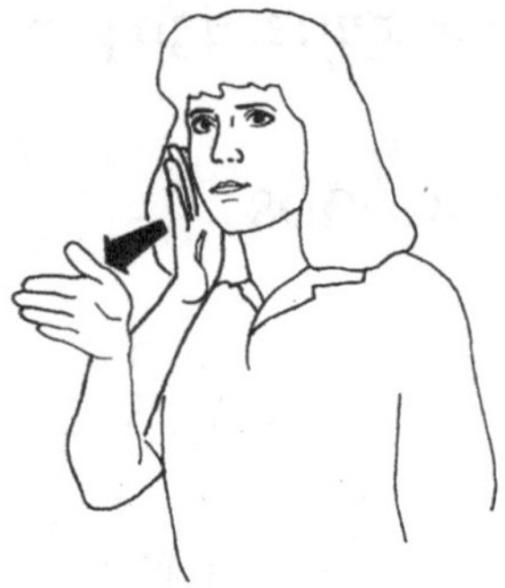

WILL

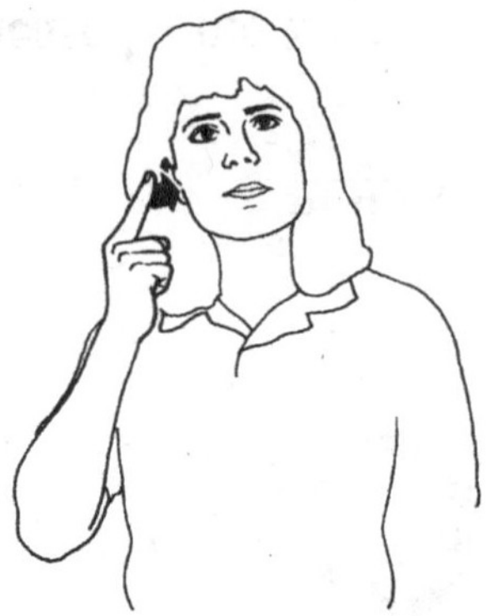

HEAR

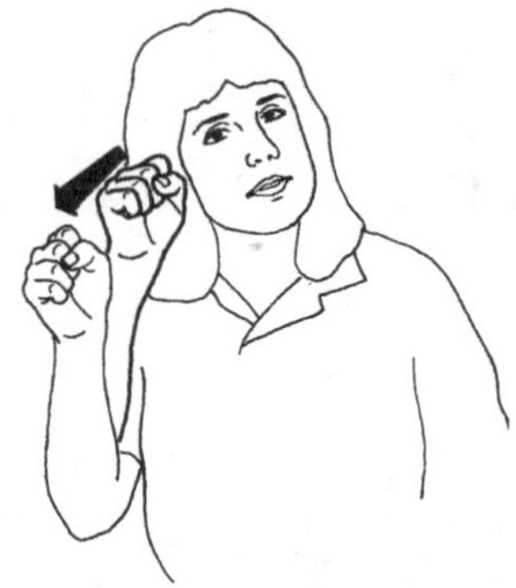

SOUND

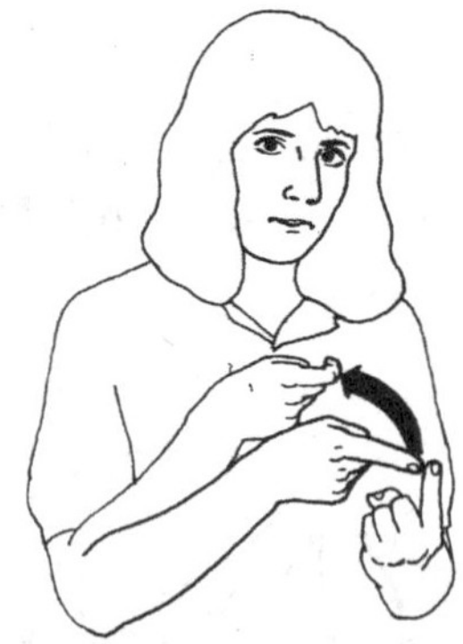

FROM

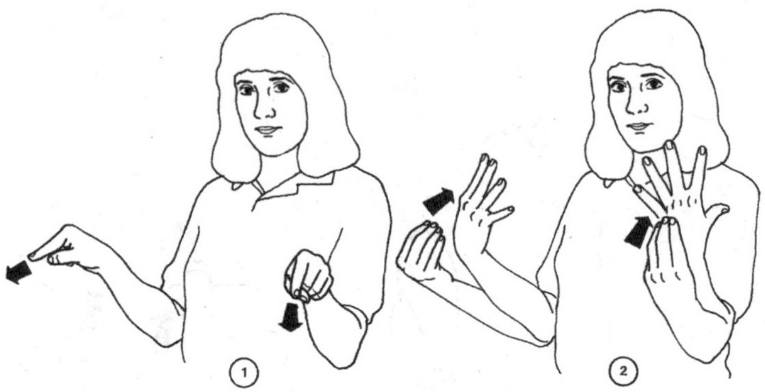

SPEAKER.

You will hear sounds from the speakers.

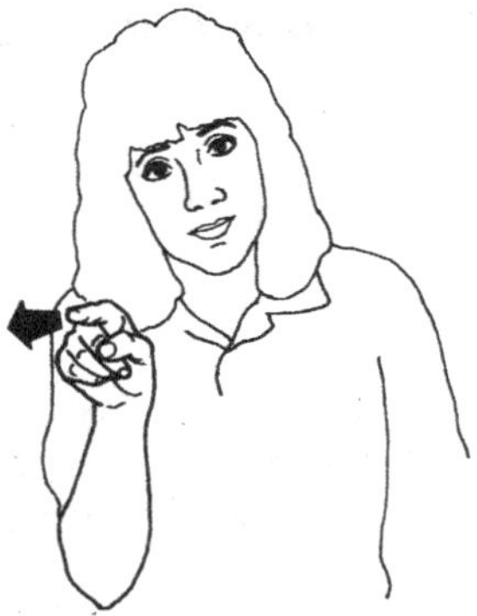

YOU

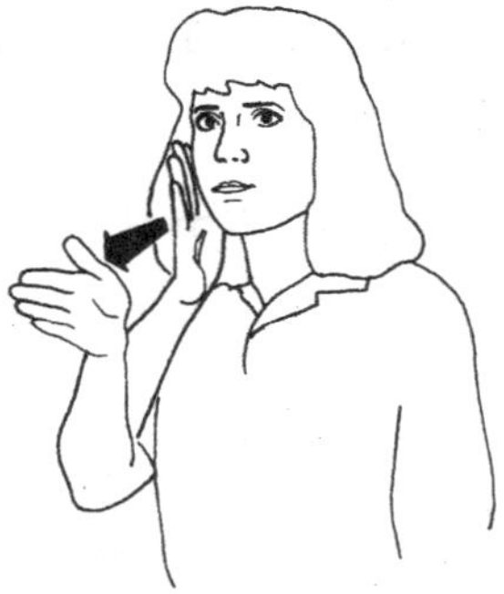

WILL

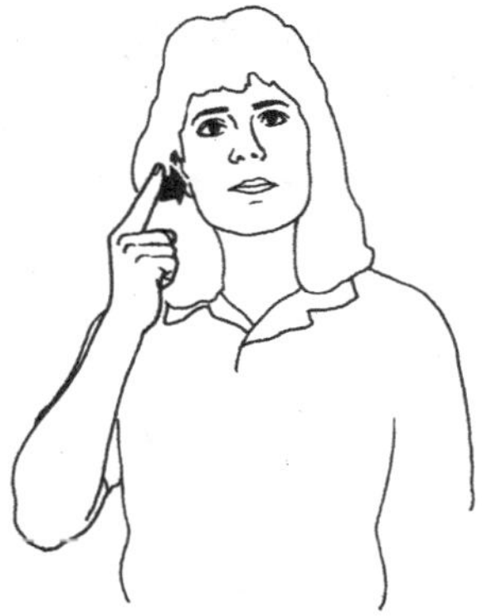

HEAR

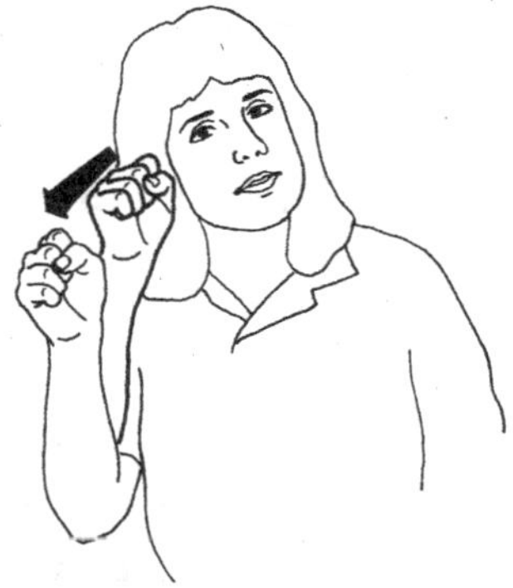

SOUNDS

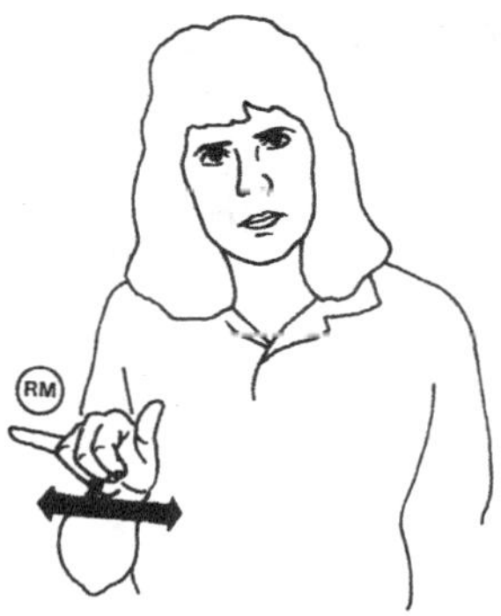

LIKE

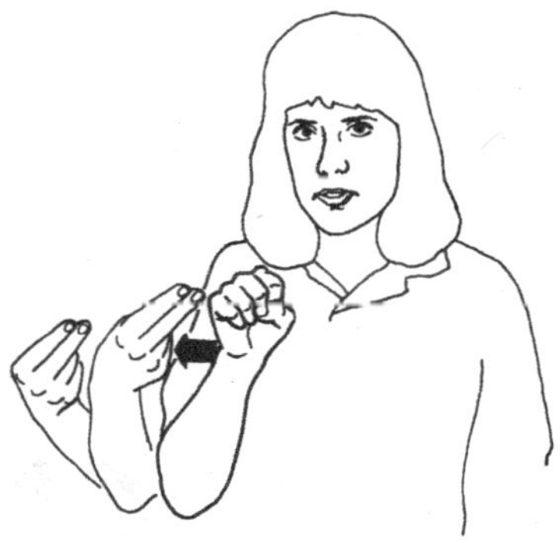

S-H-H.

You will hear sounds like "shhhh."

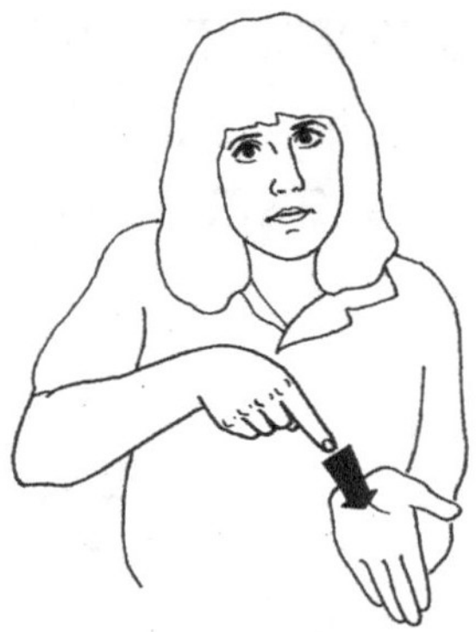

THIS

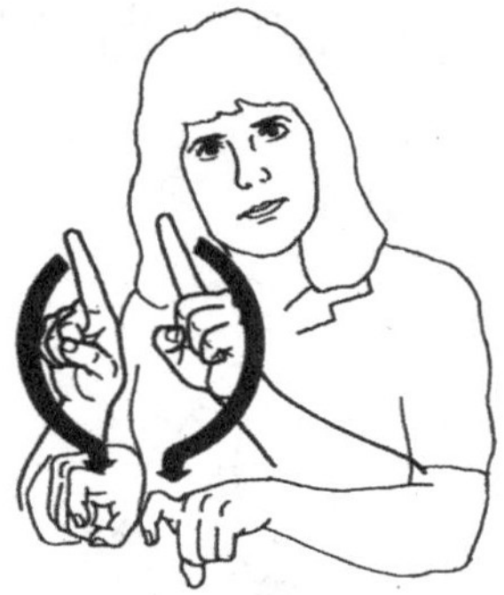

TEST

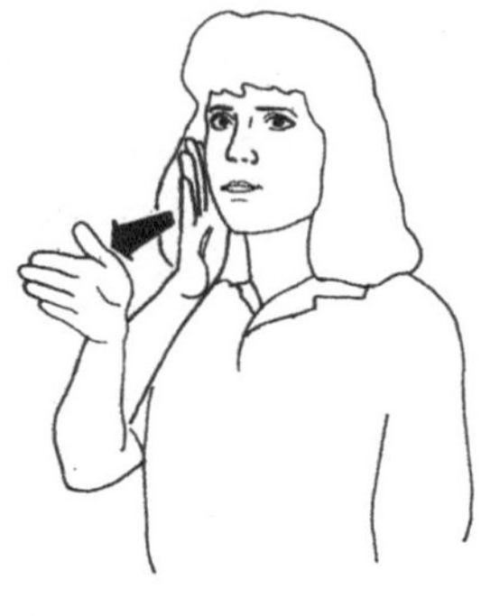

WILL

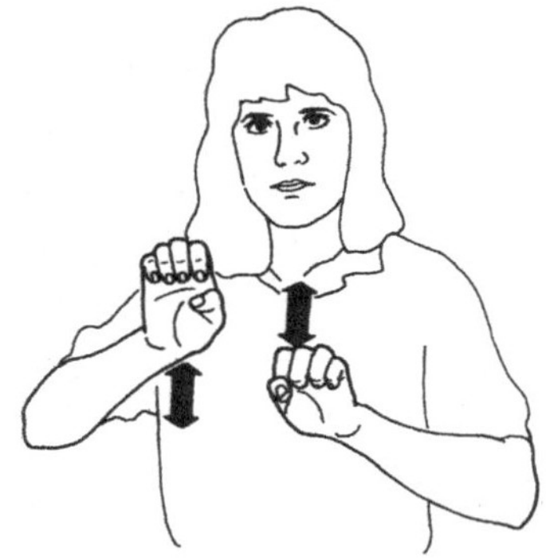

EVALUATE

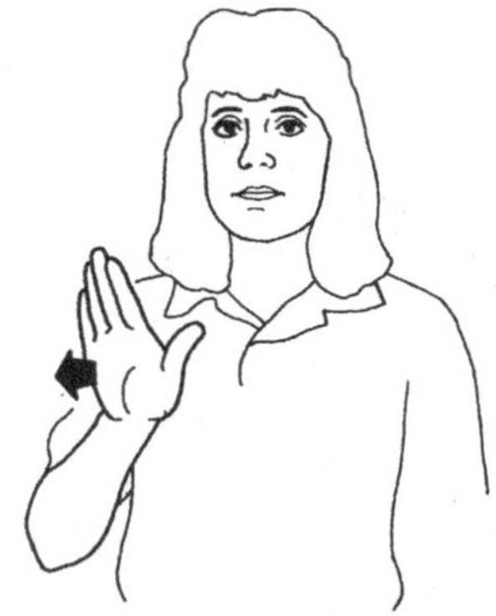

YOUR

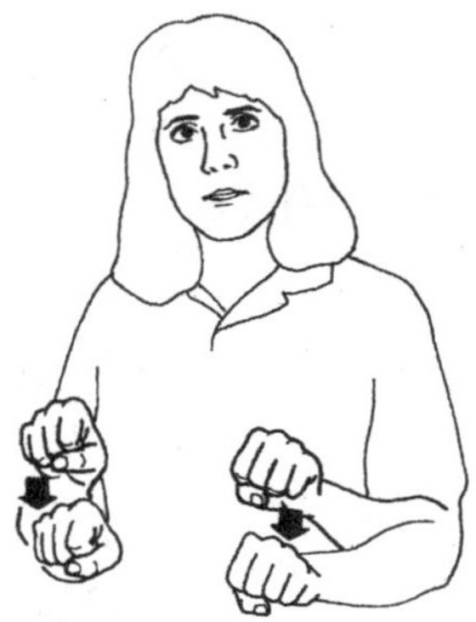

ABILITY

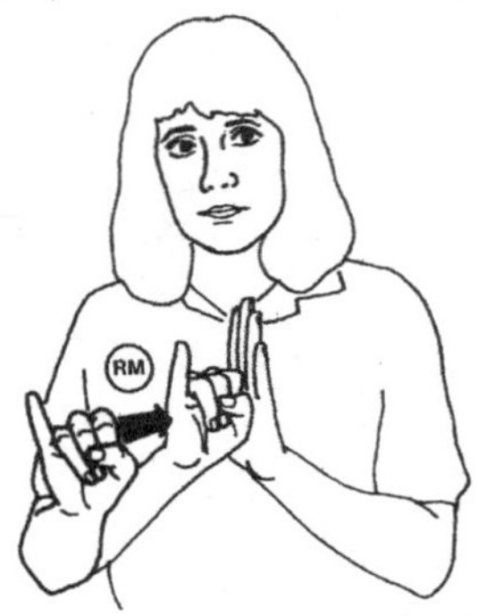

IDENTIFY

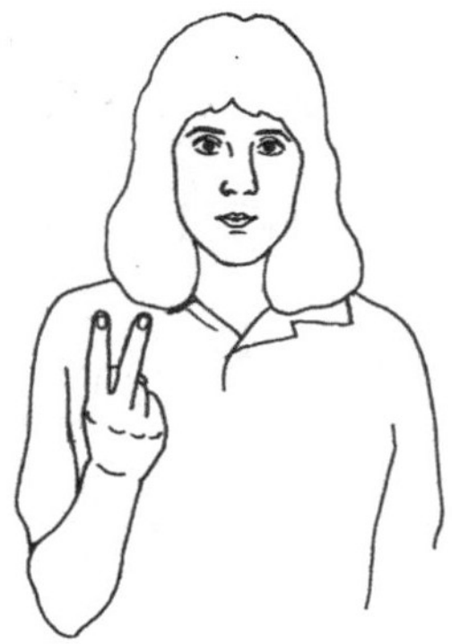

TWO

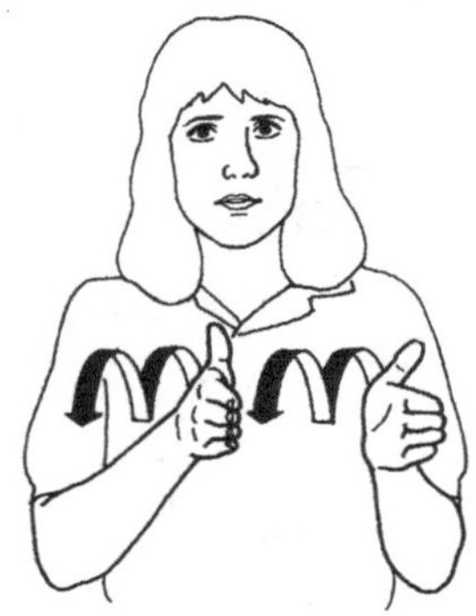

SYLLABLE

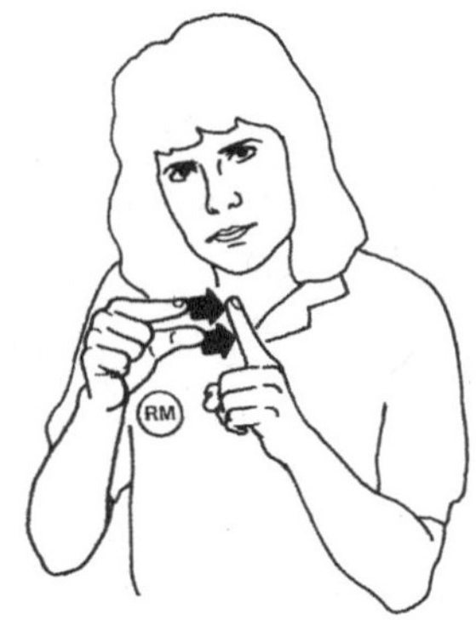

WORD.

This test will evaluate your ability to identify two-syllable words.

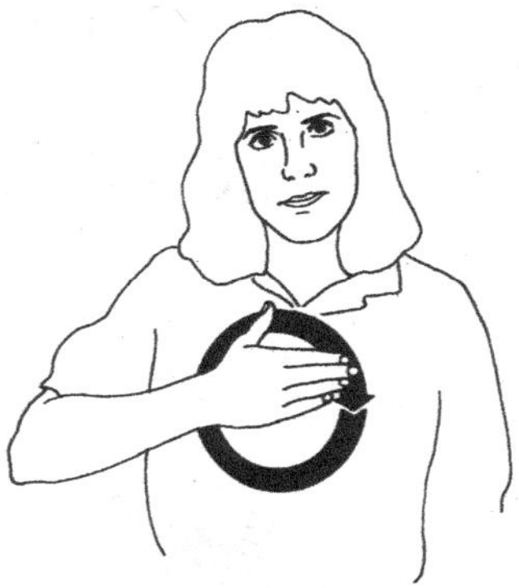

PLEASE

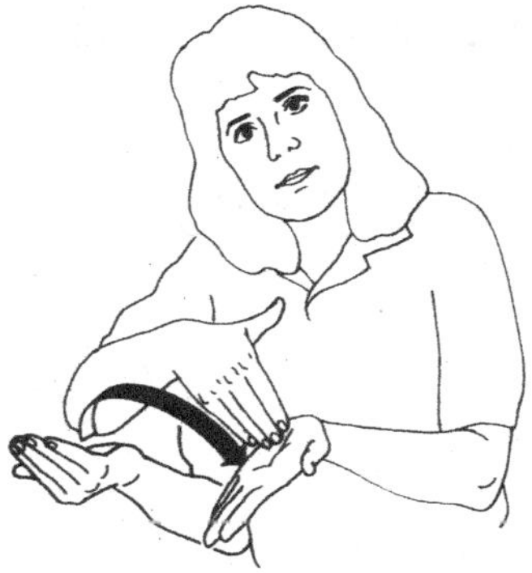

REPEAT

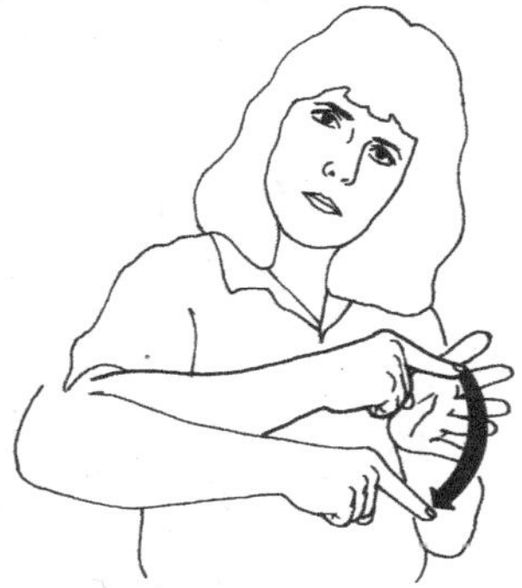

WHAT

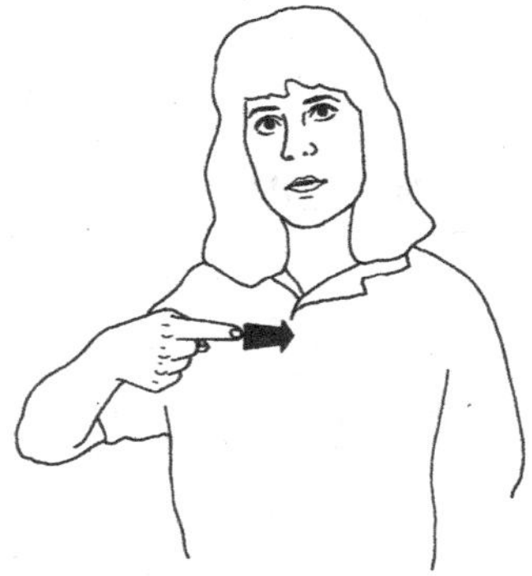

I

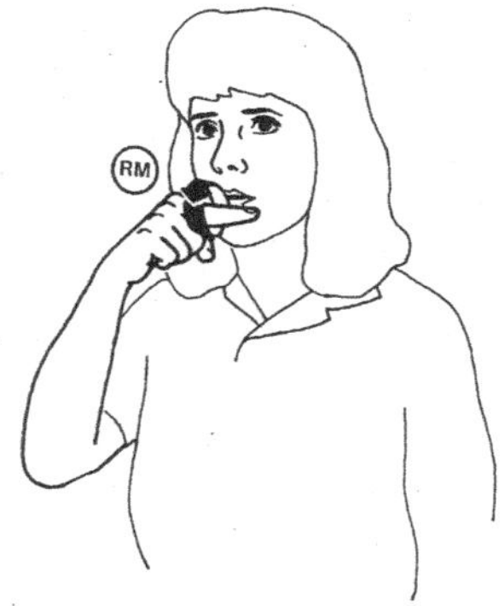

SAY.

Please repeat what I say.

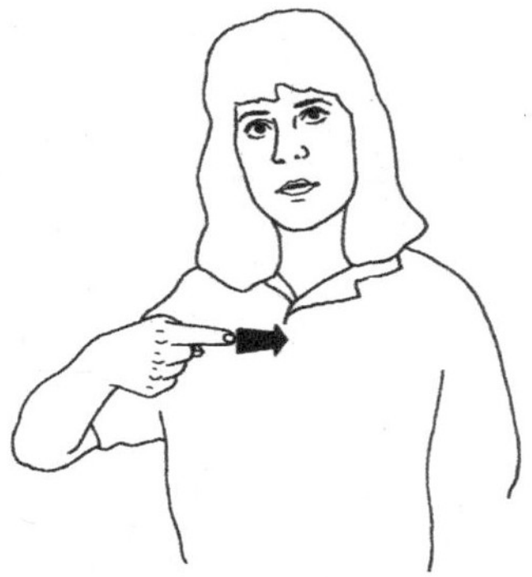

I

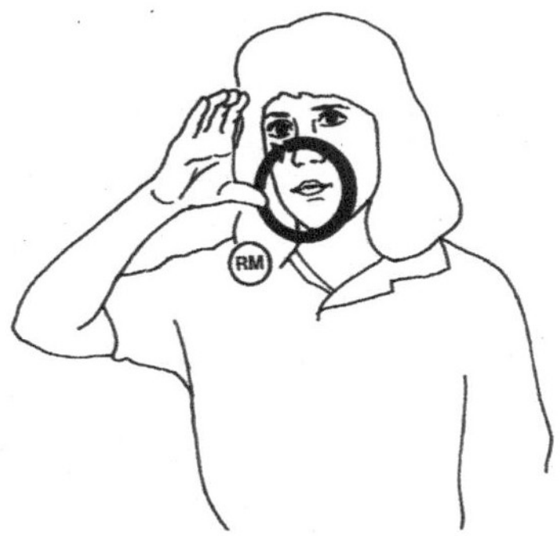

LOOK-FOR

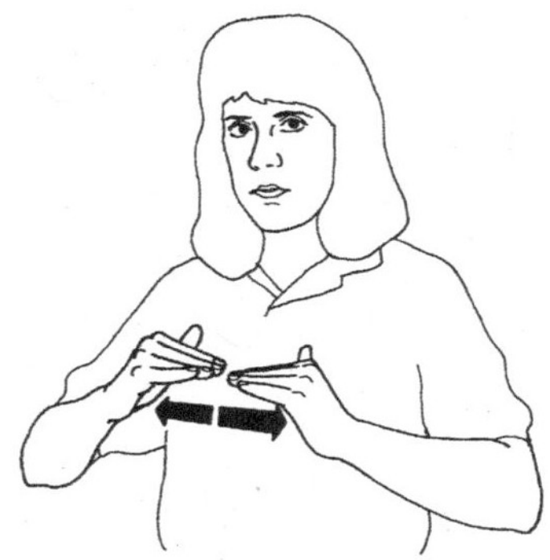

LEVEL

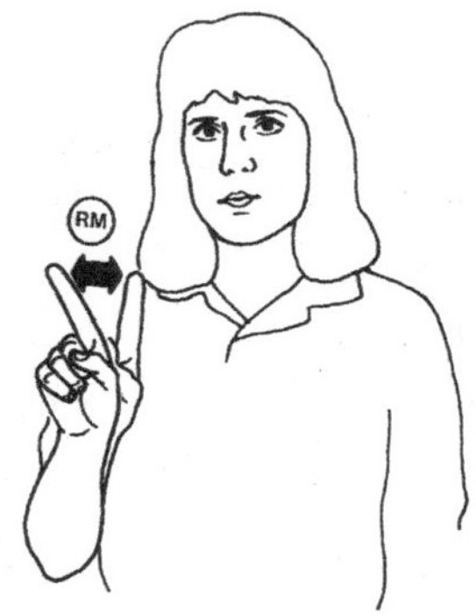

WHERE

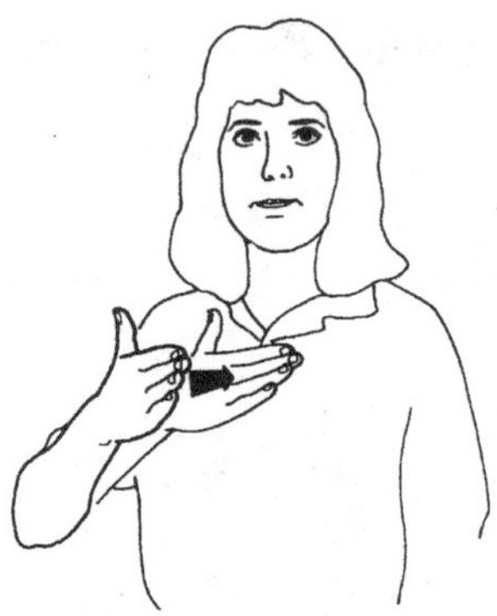

MY

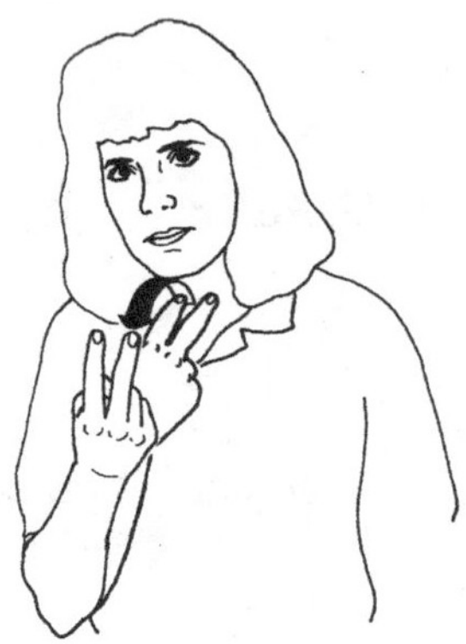

VOICE

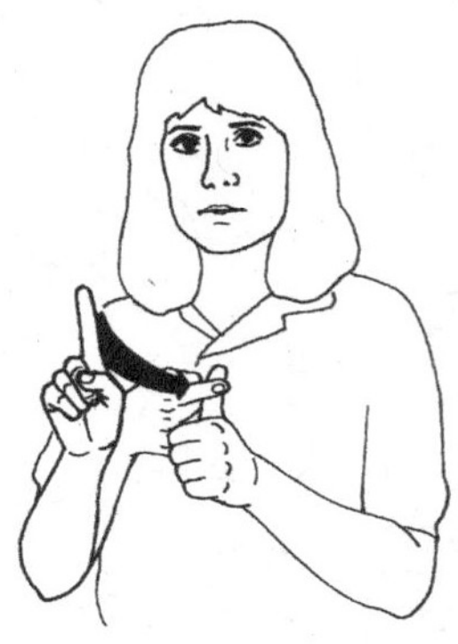

FIRST

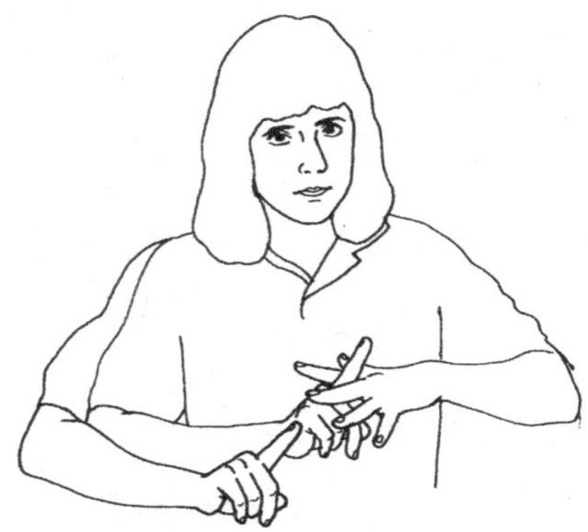

APPEARS.

I am looking for the level where my voice first appears.

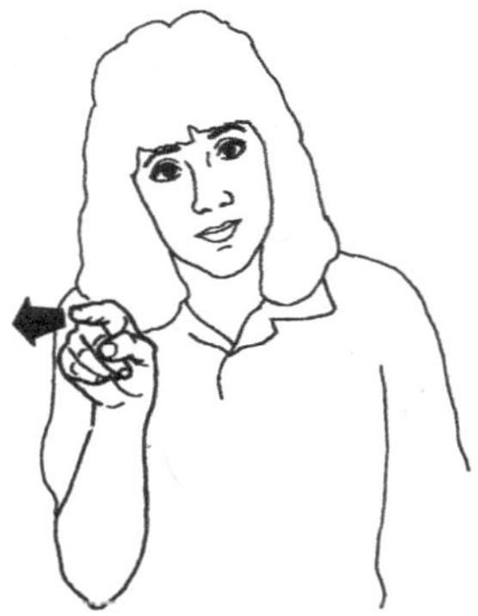

YOU

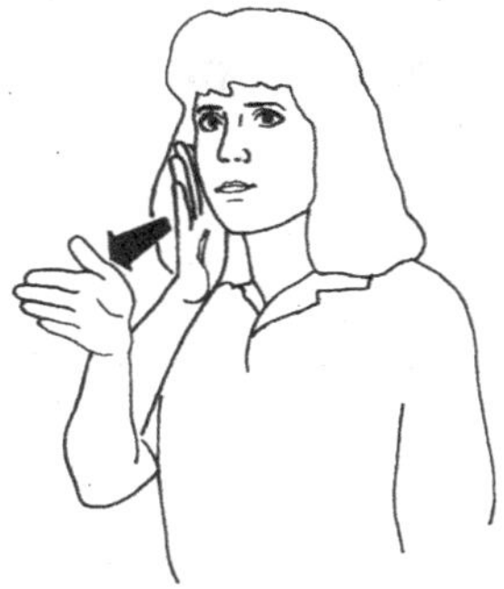

WILL

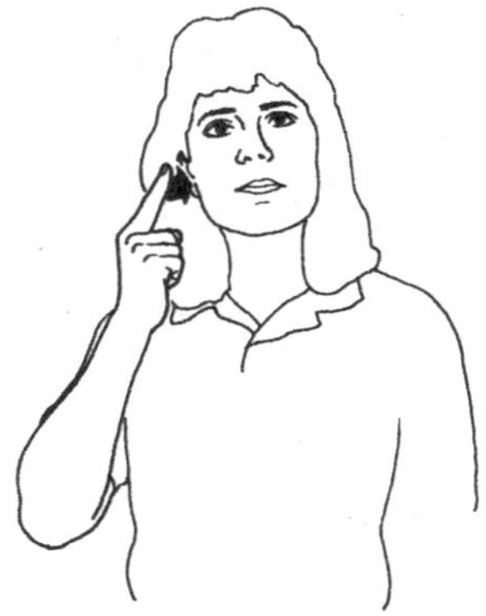

HEAR

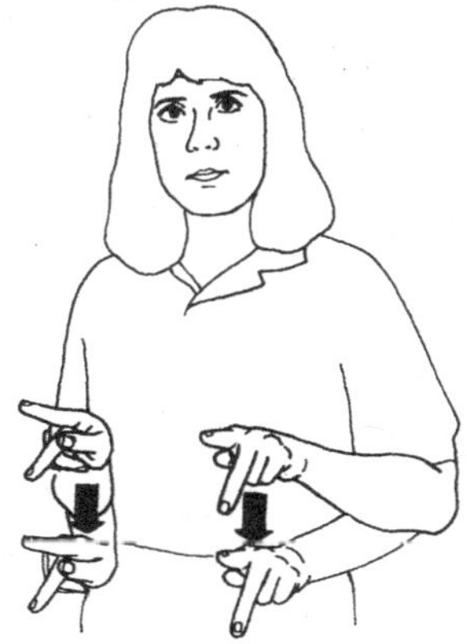

PERSON

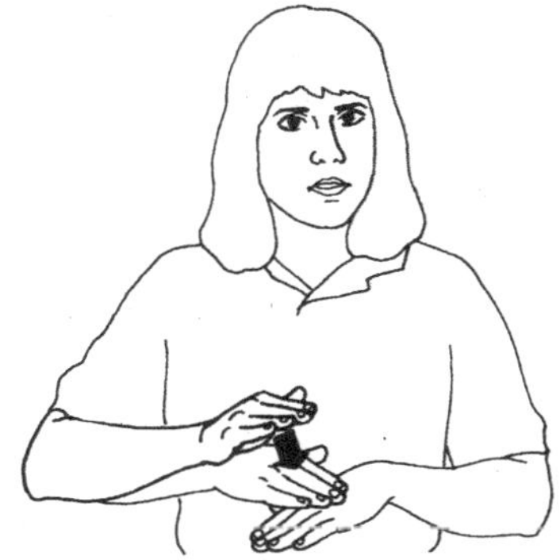

ON

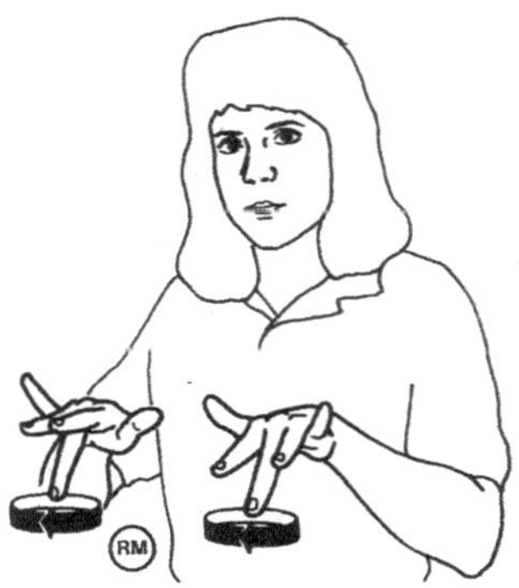

TAPE

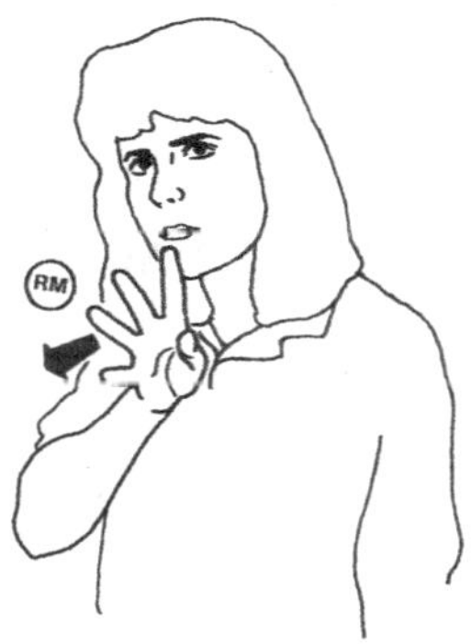

TALK.

You will hear a person on the tape talking.

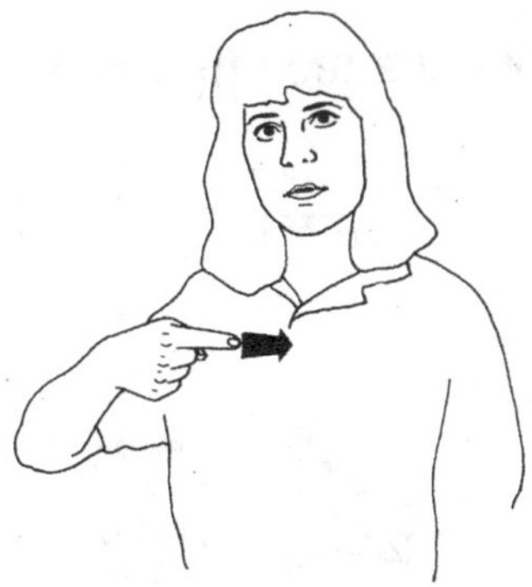

I

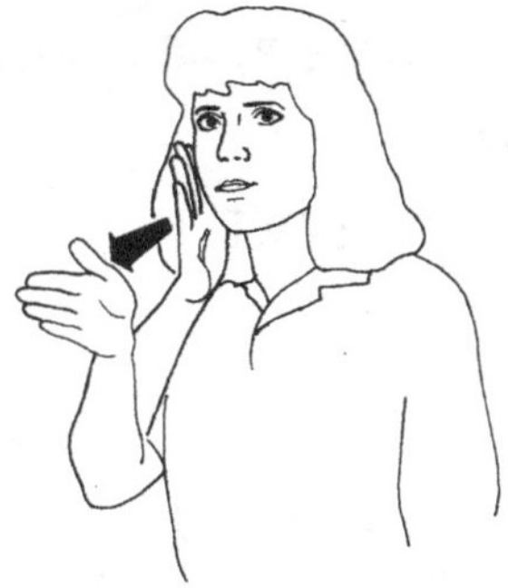

WILL

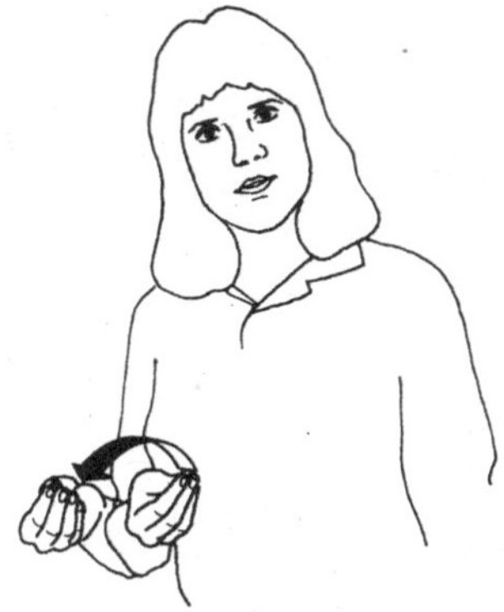

GIVE

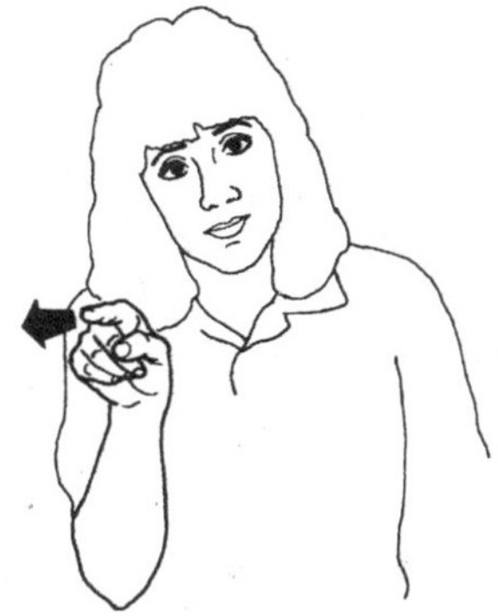

YOU

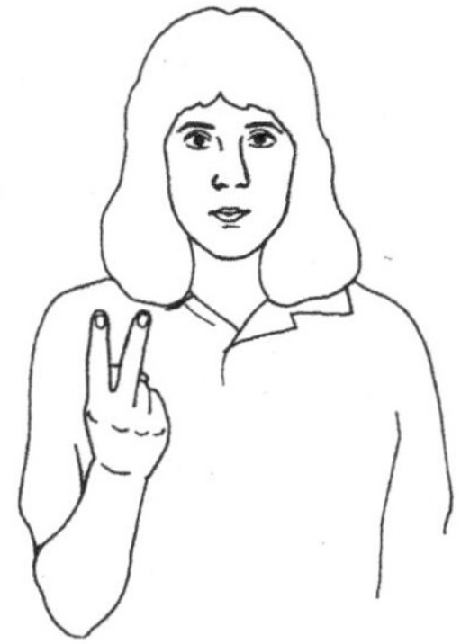

TWO

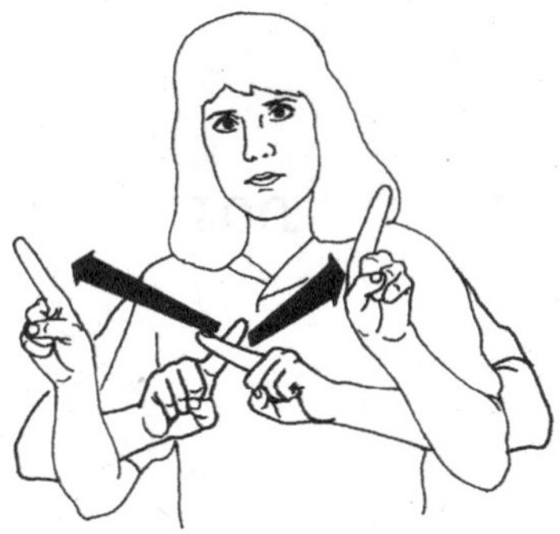

DIFFERENT

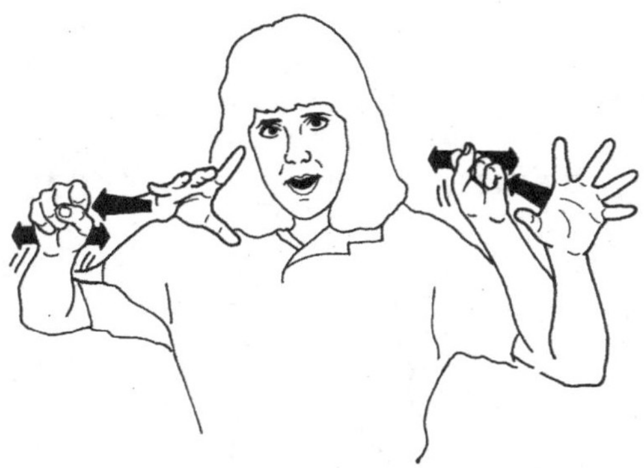

LOUD

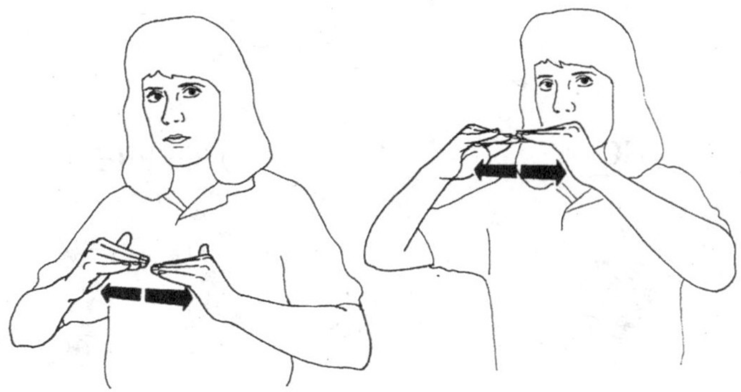

LEVEL-LEVEL

I will give you two different loudness levels, level one and level two.

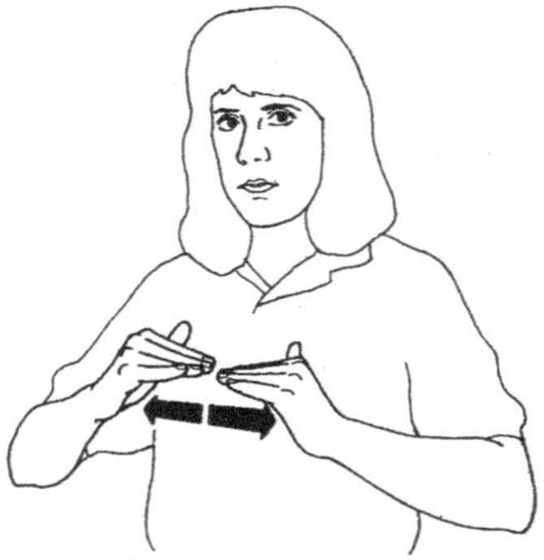

LEVEL

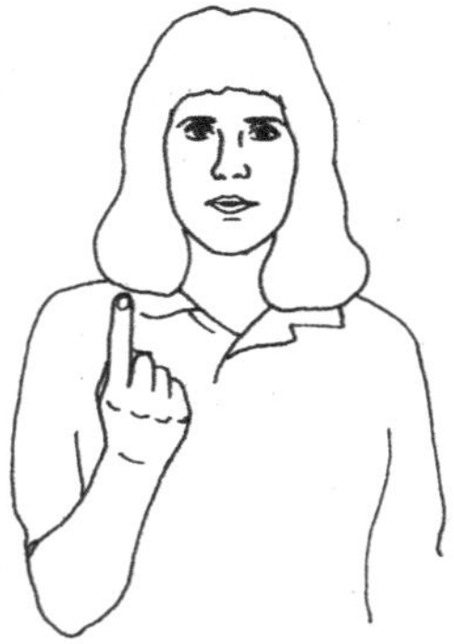

ONE

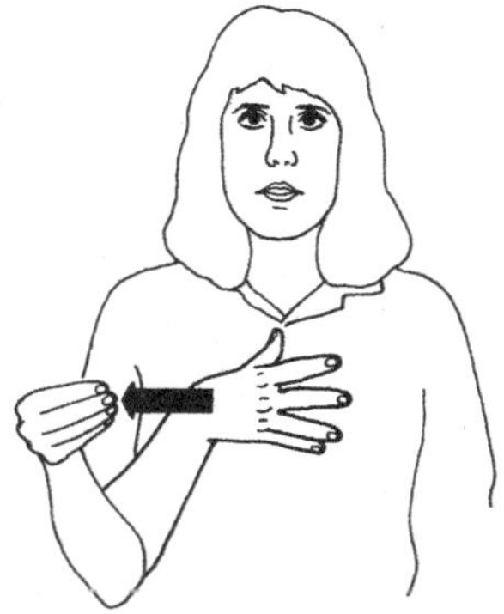

AND

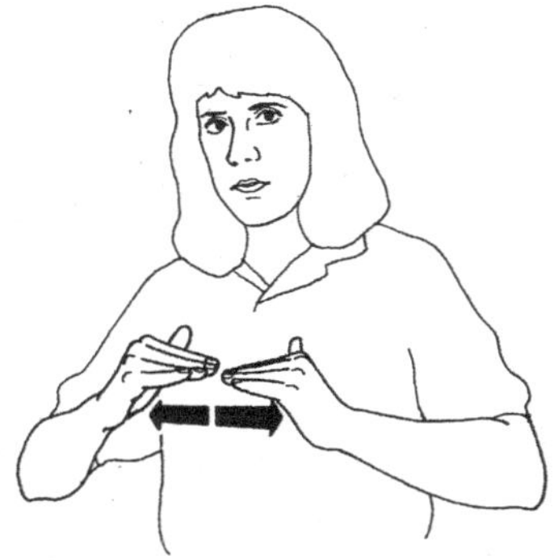

LEVEL

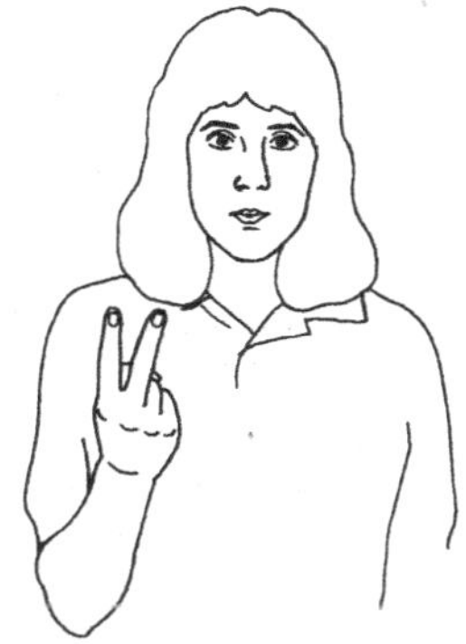

TWO.

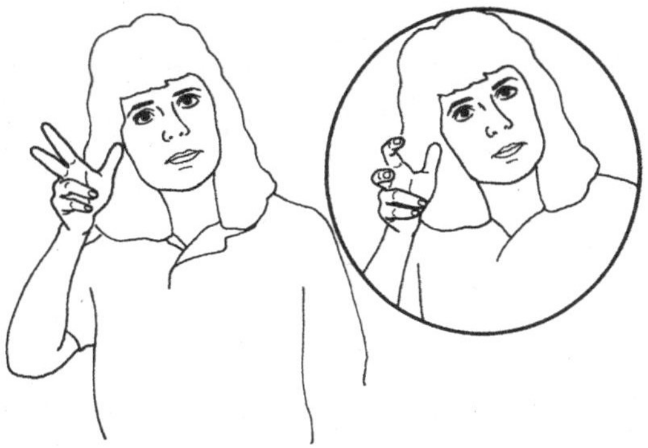

LISTEN

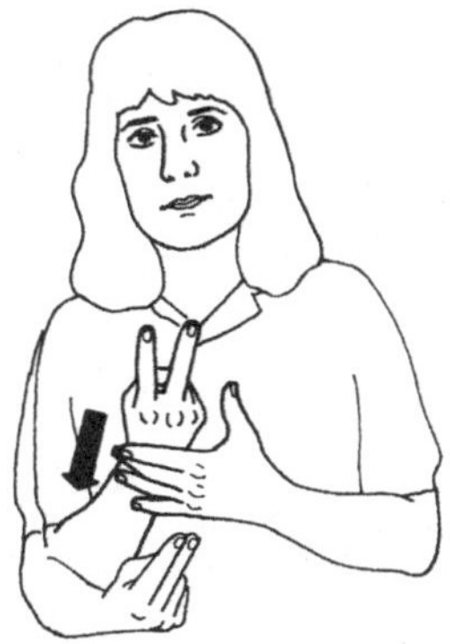

BOTH

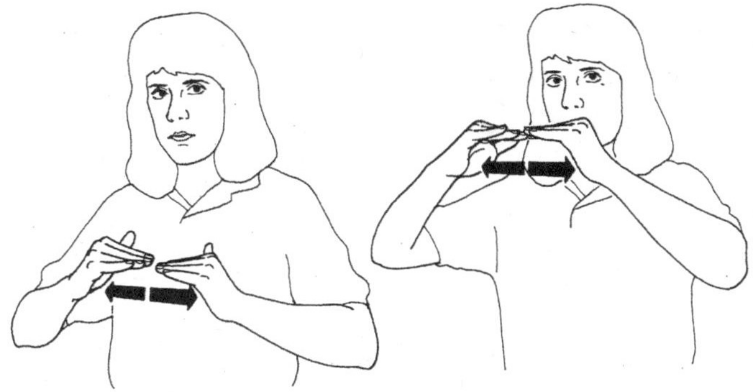

LEVEL-LEVEL

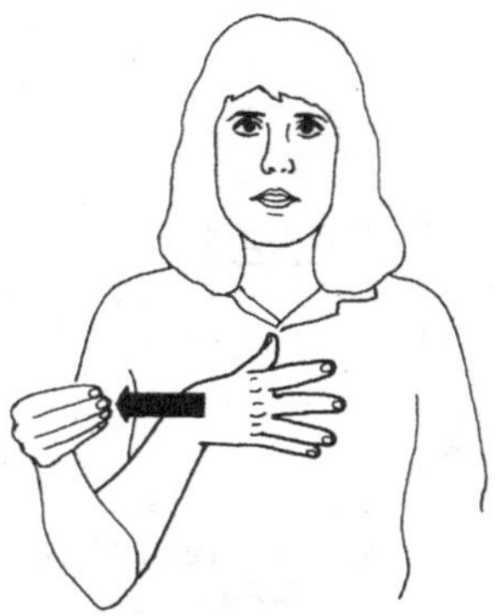

AND

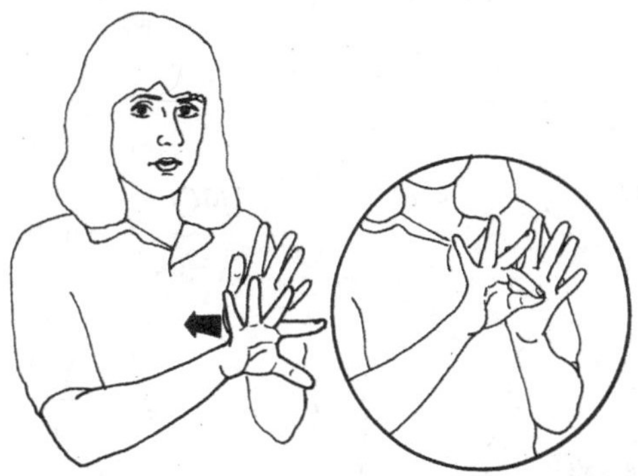

CHOOSE

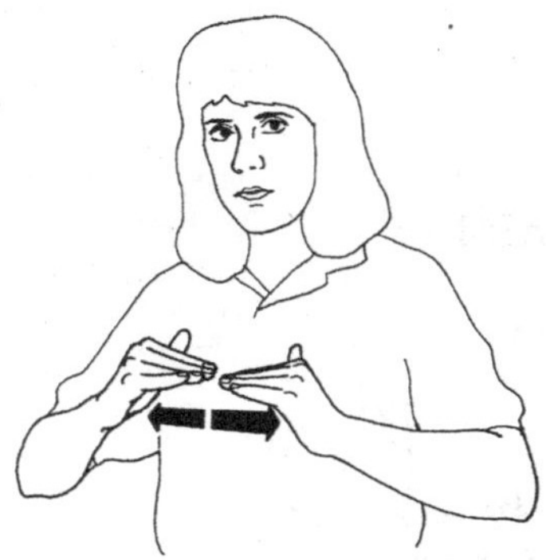

LEVEL

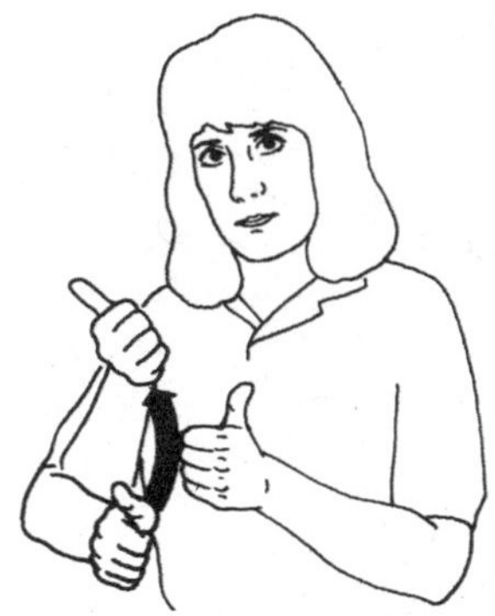

MOST

Listen to both levels and choose the level that is most comfortable for you.

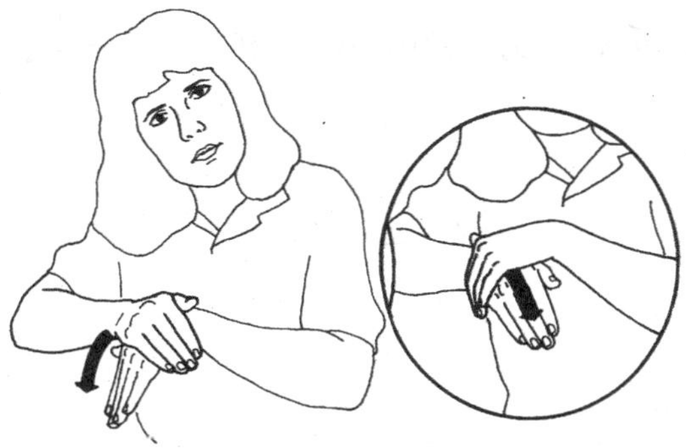

COMFORTABLE

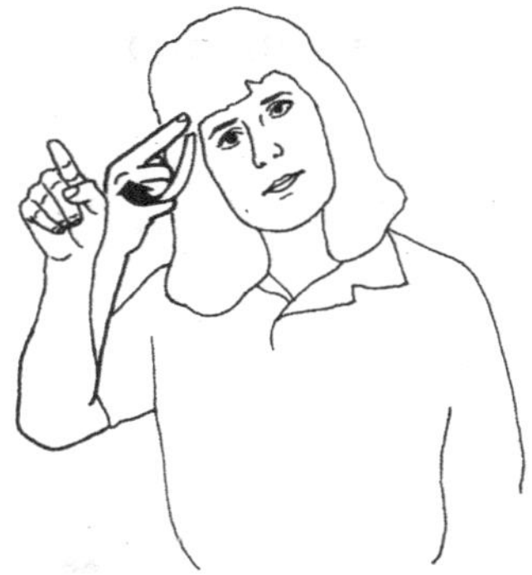

FOR

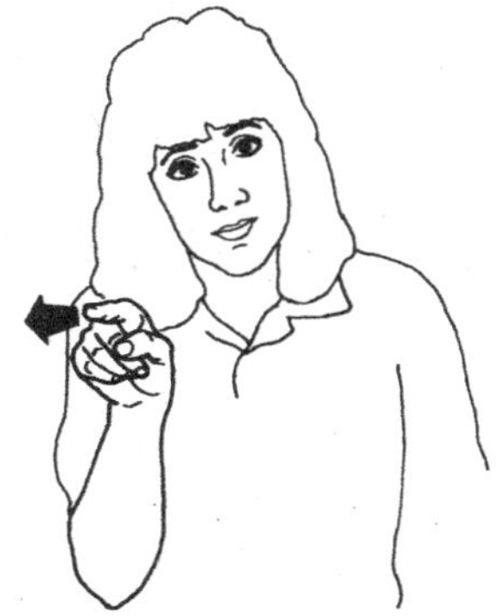

YOU.

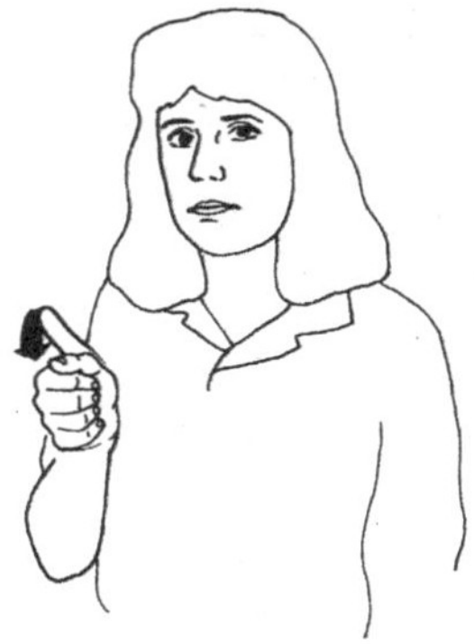

PRESS-BUTTON

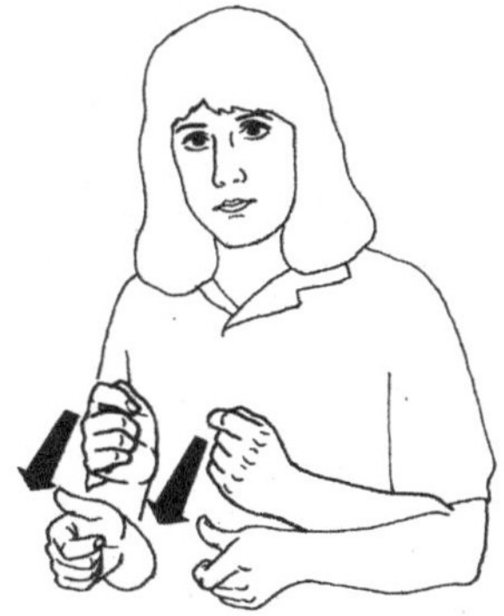

IMMEDIATELY

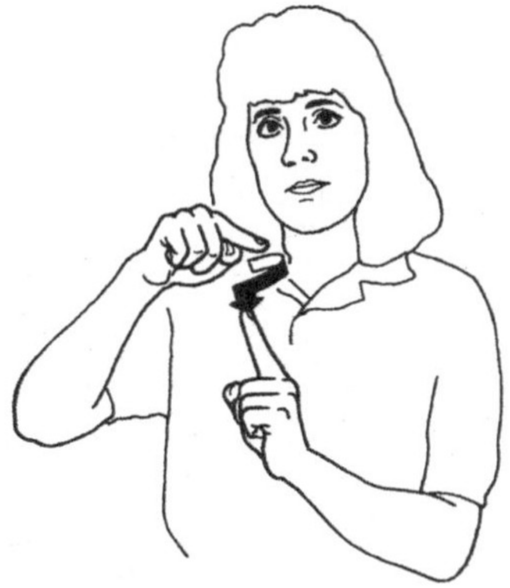

WHEN

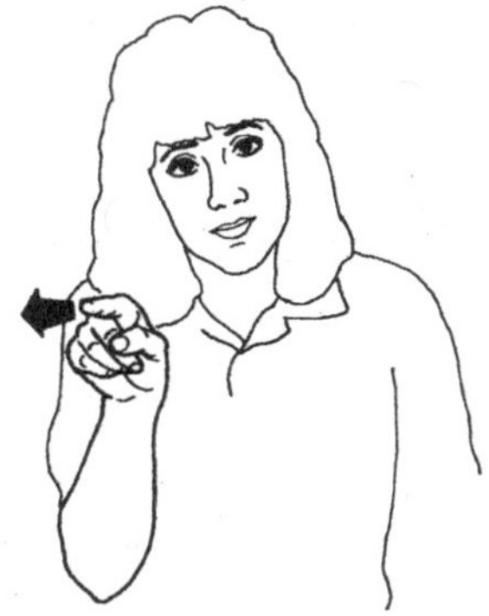

YOU

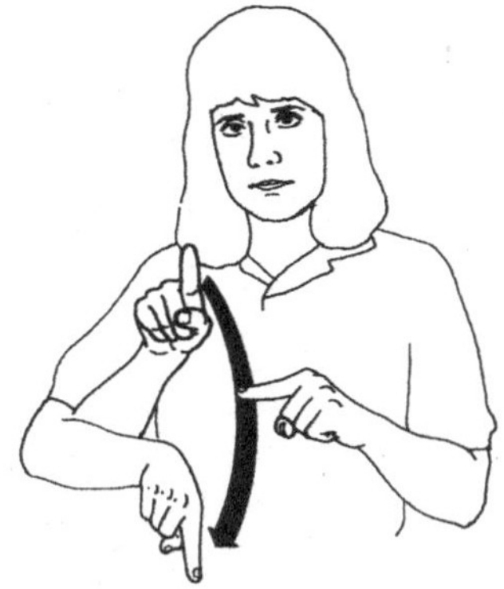

CAN'T

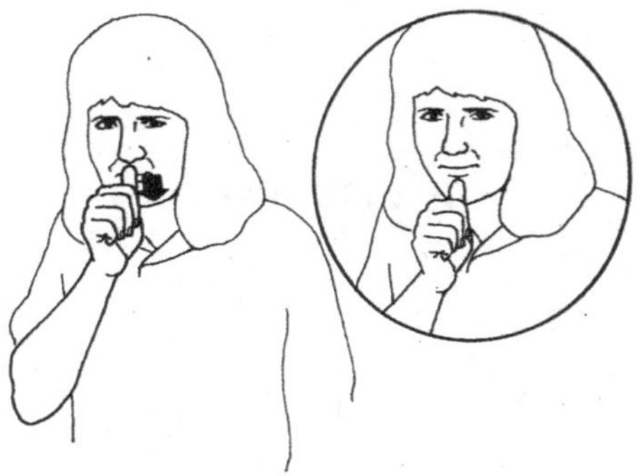

TOLERATE

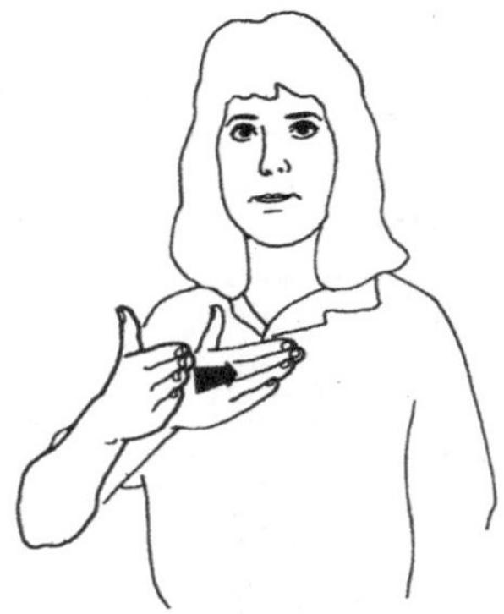

MY

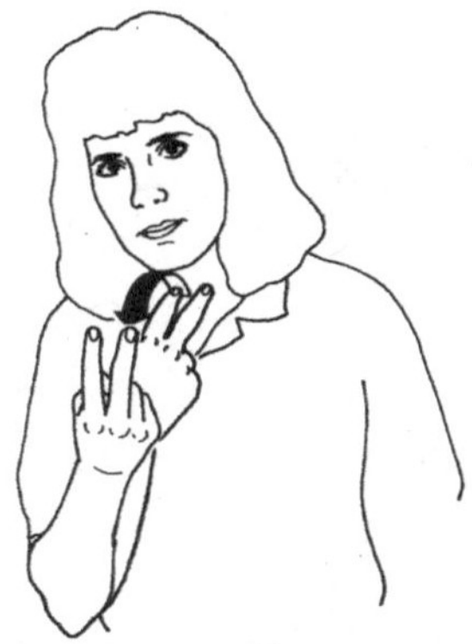

VOICE.

Press the button immediately when you can't tolerate my voice.

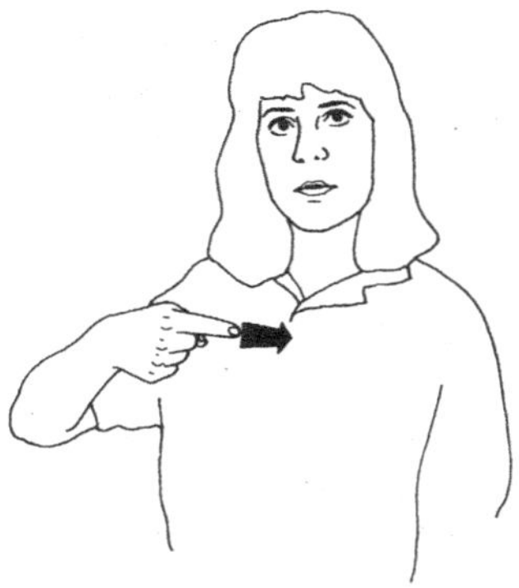

I

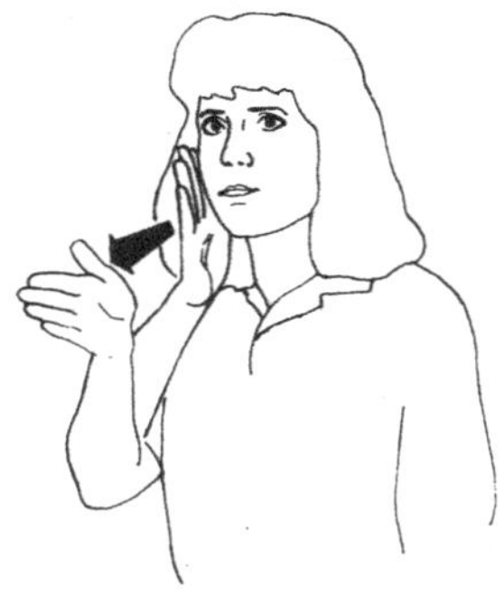

WILL

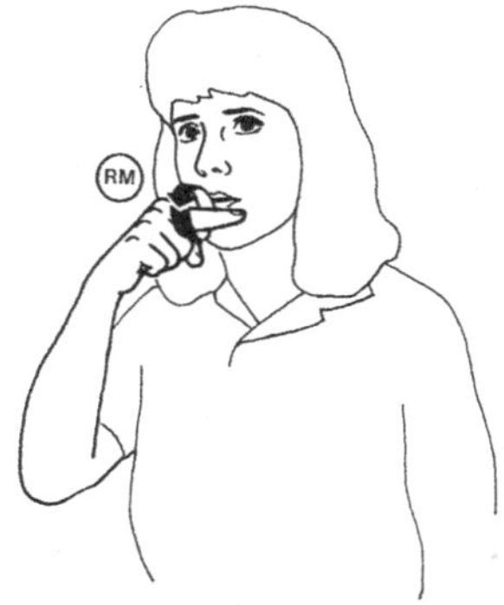

SAY

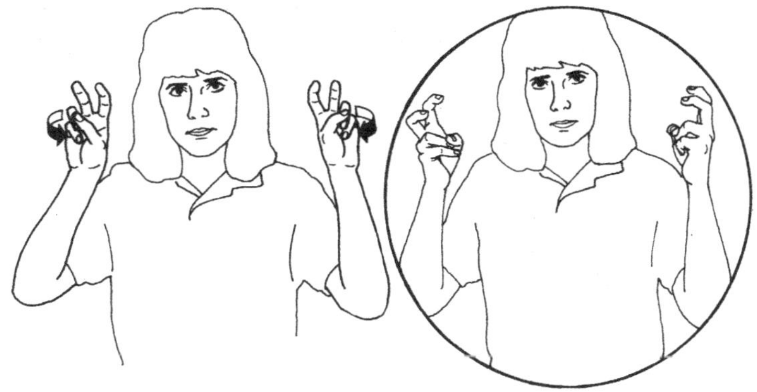

QUOTE

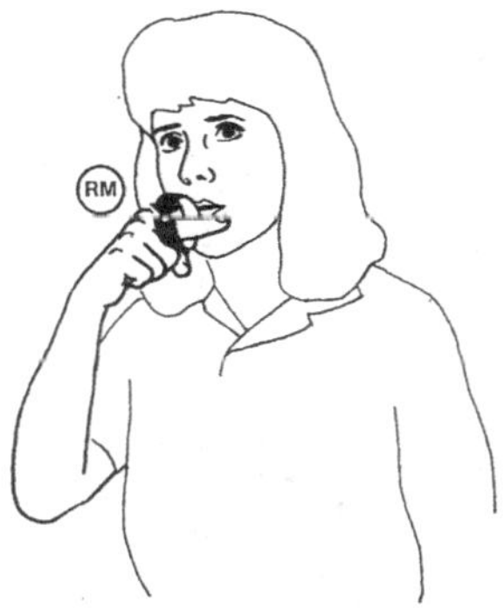

SAY

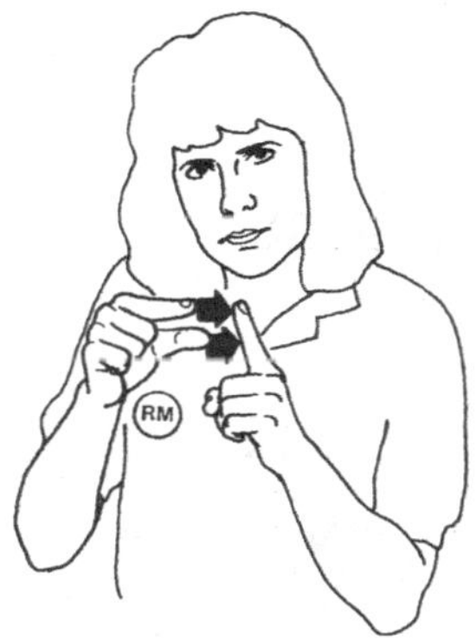

WORD ________________.

I will say, "Say the word ________________."

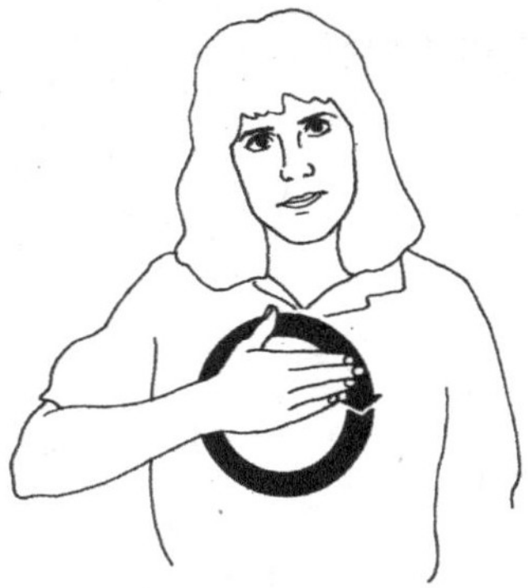

PLEASE

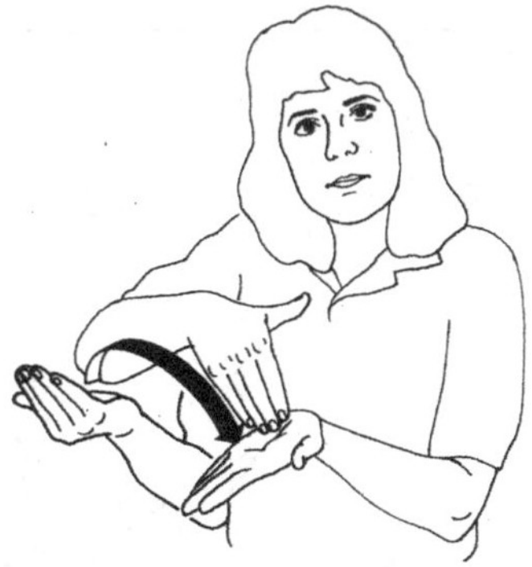

REPEAT

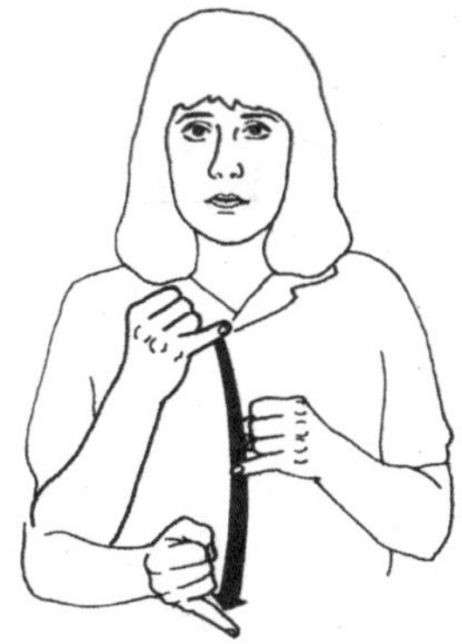

LAST

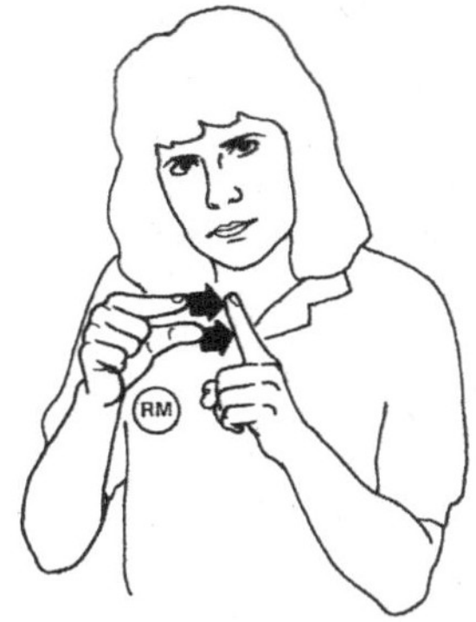

WORD.

Please repeat the last word.

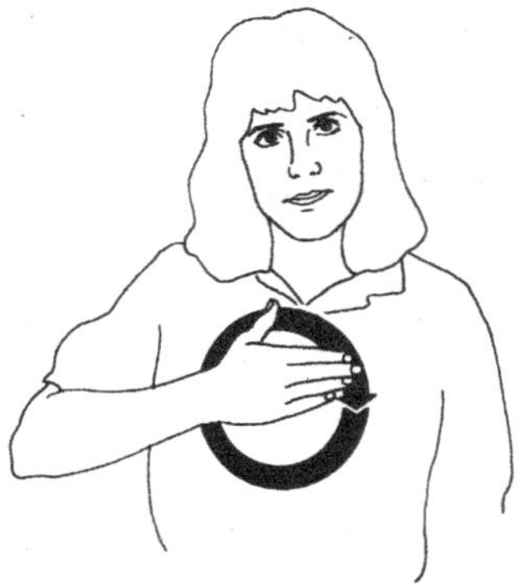

PLEASE

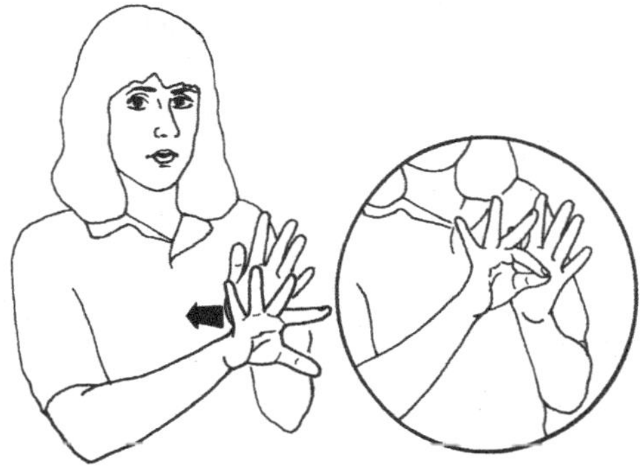

CHOOSE

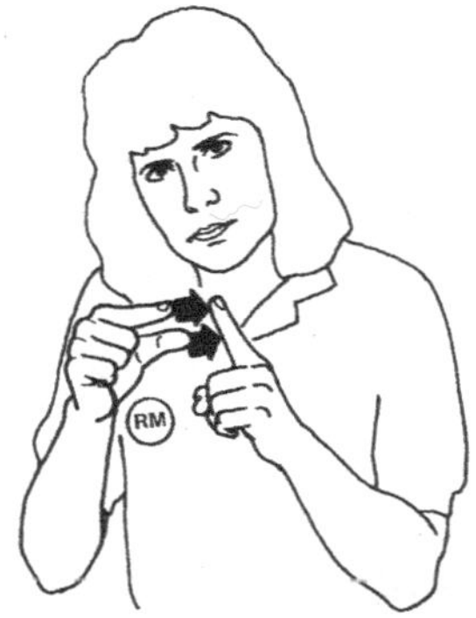

WORD

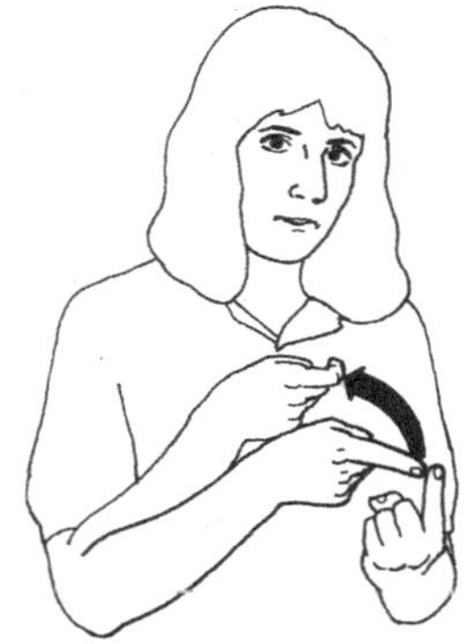

FROM

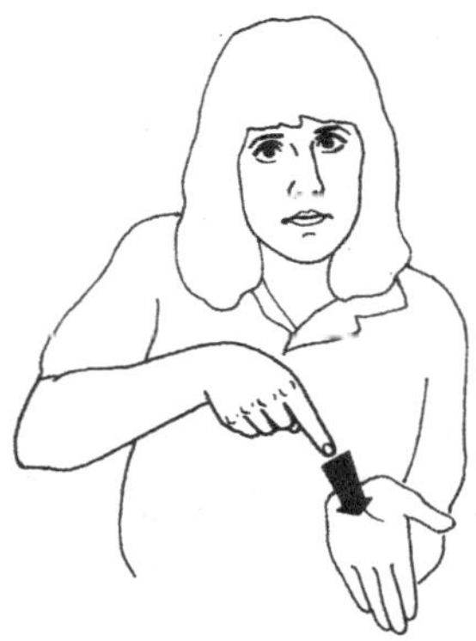

THIS

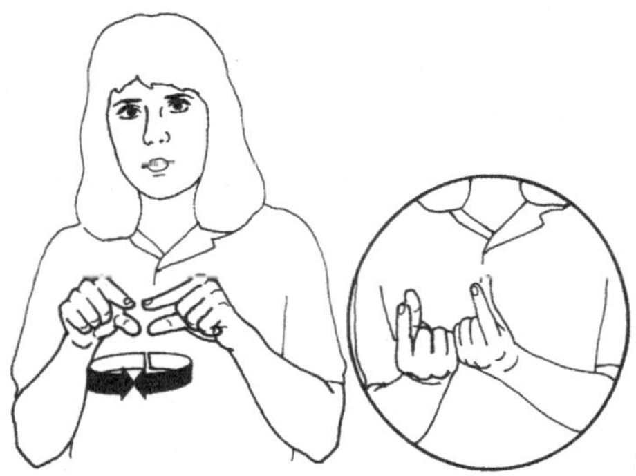

GROUP.

Please choose the word from this group.

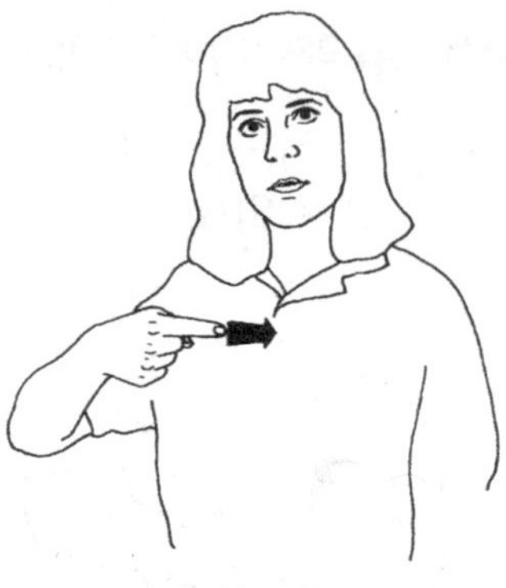

I

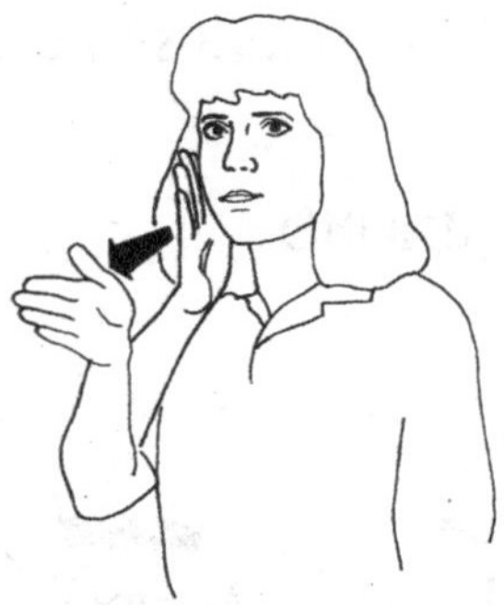

WILL

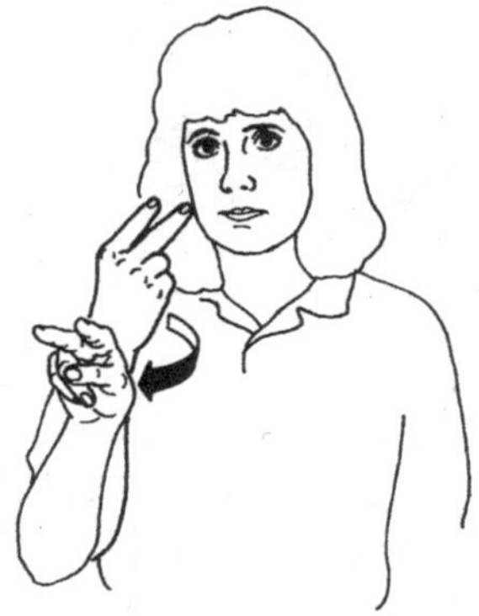

LOOK

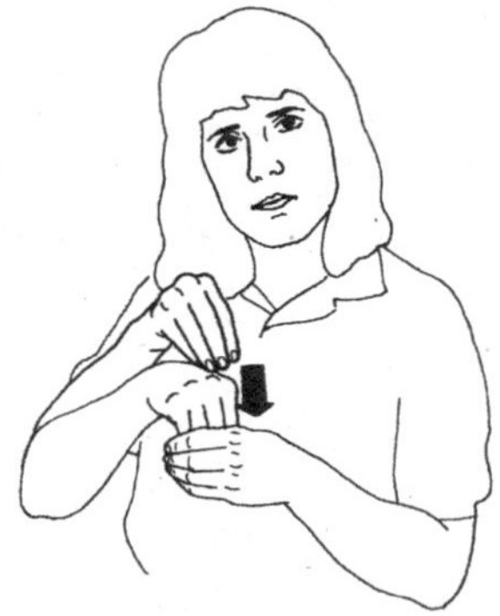

IN

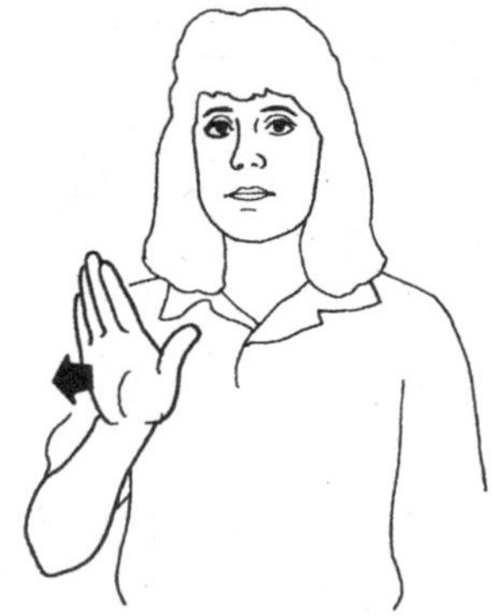

YOUR

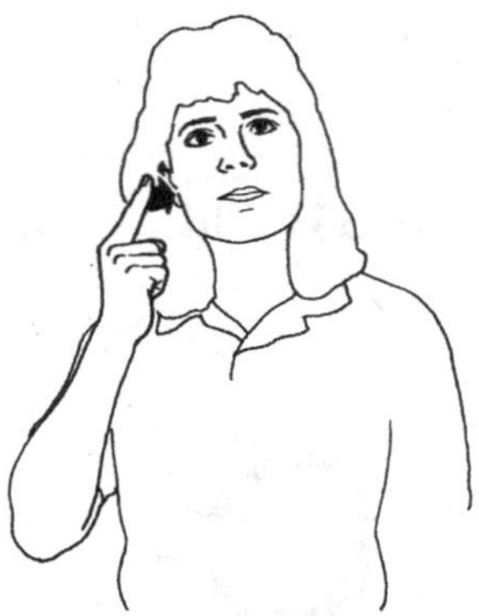

EAR.

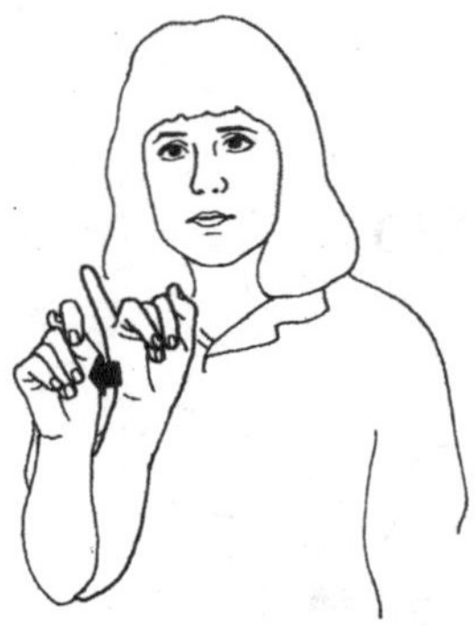

I-T

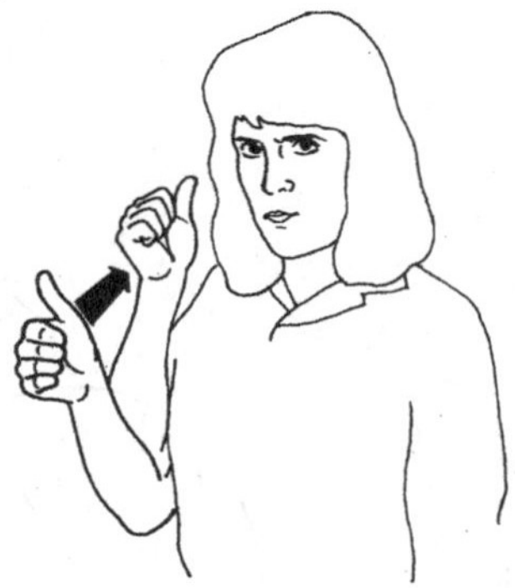

WON'T

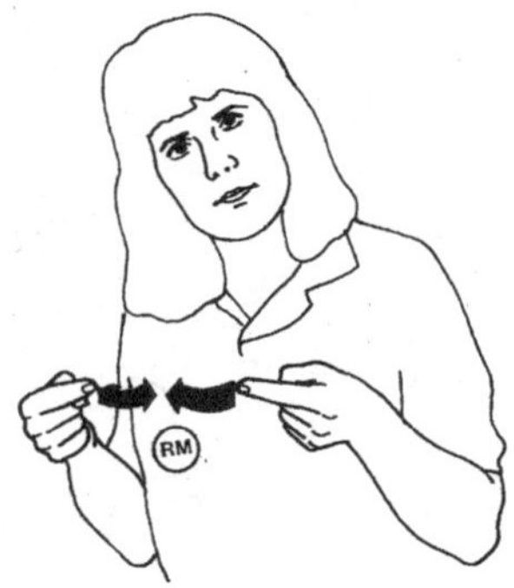

HURT.

I will look into your ears. It won't hurt.

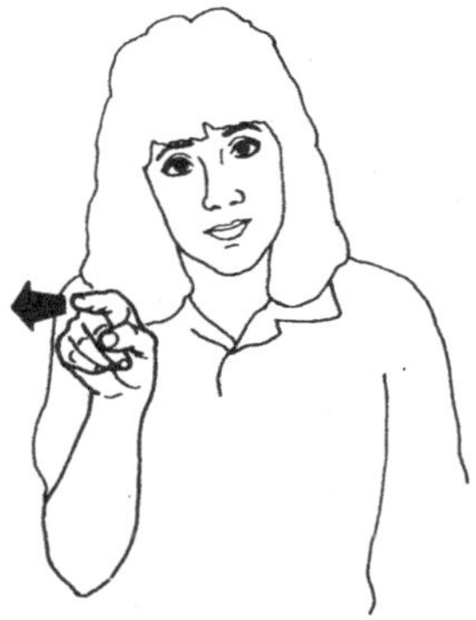

YOU

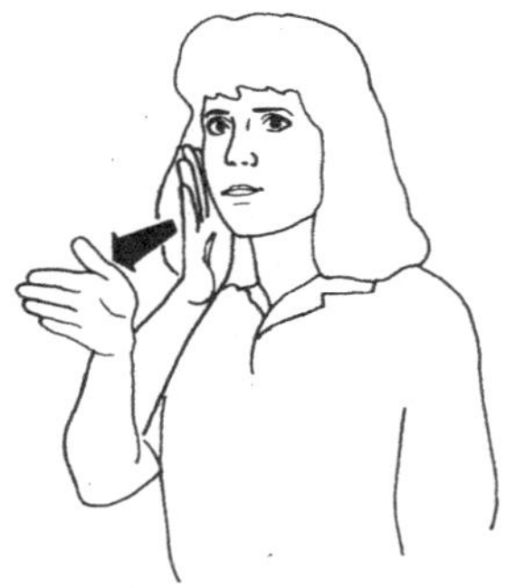

WILL

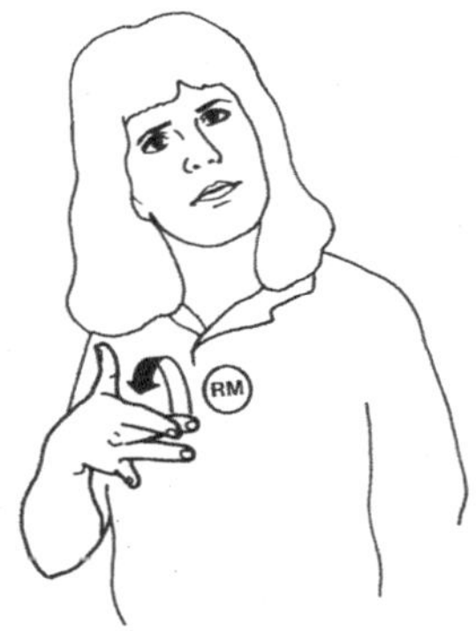

FEEL

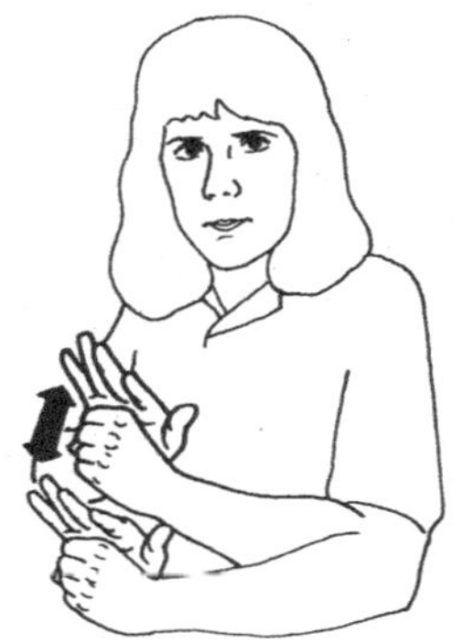

PRESSURE

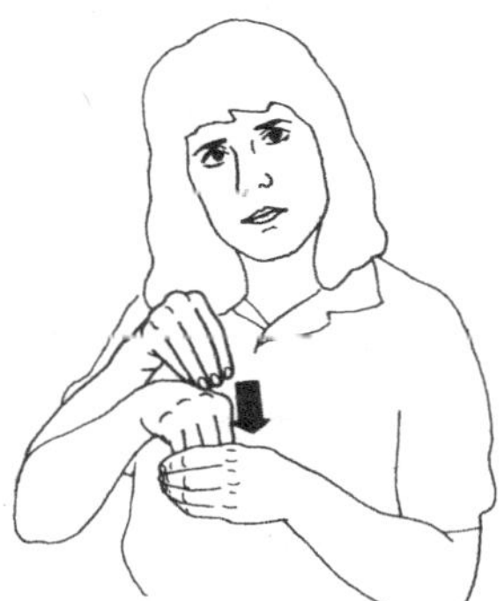

IN

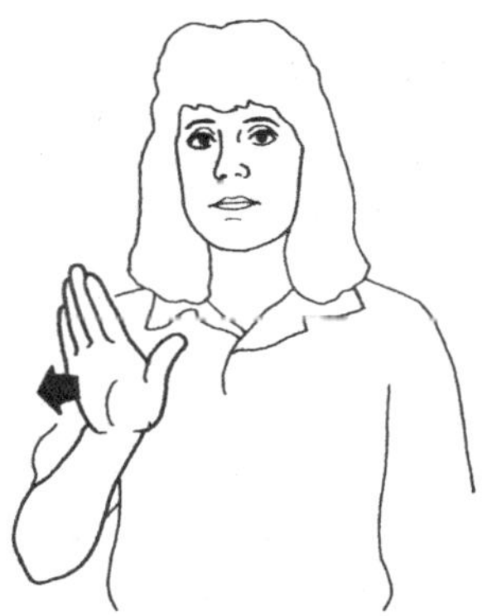

YOUR

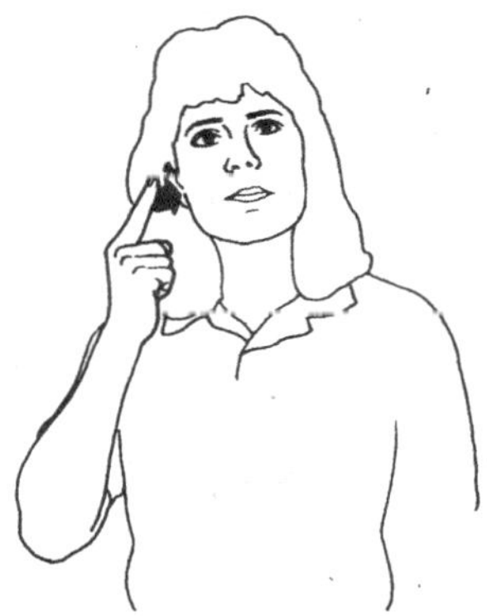

EAR

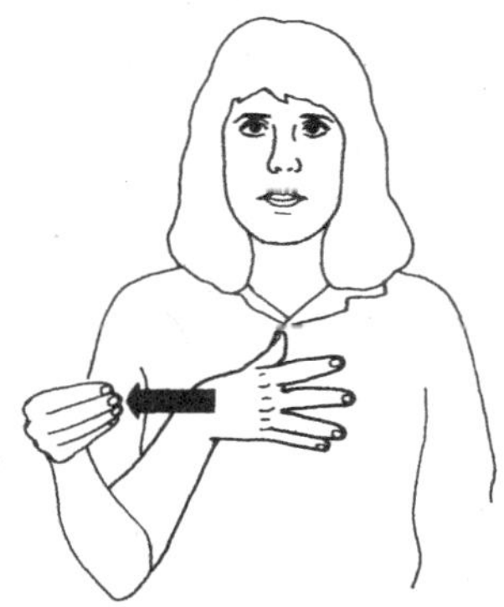

AND

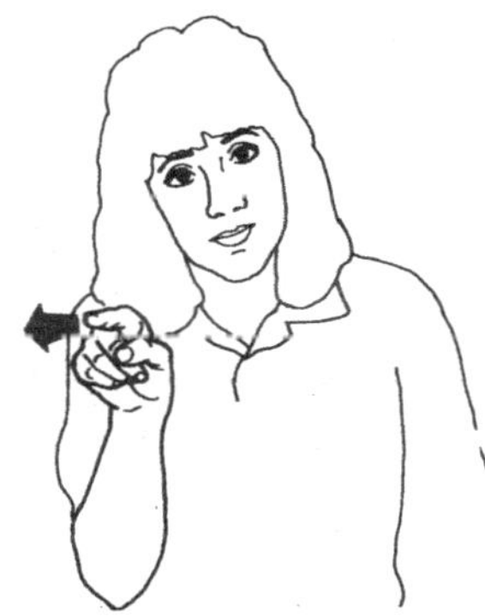

YOU

You will feel pressure in your ears, and you might hear some sounds.

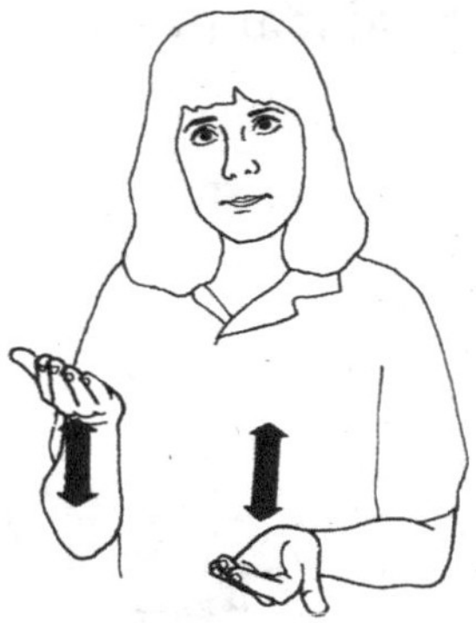

MAYBE

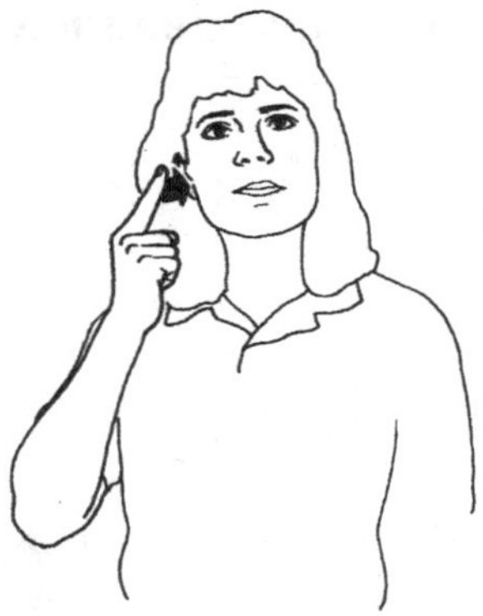

HEAR

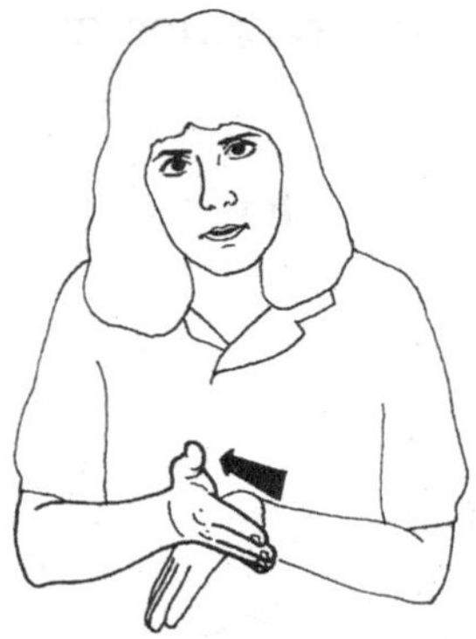

SOME

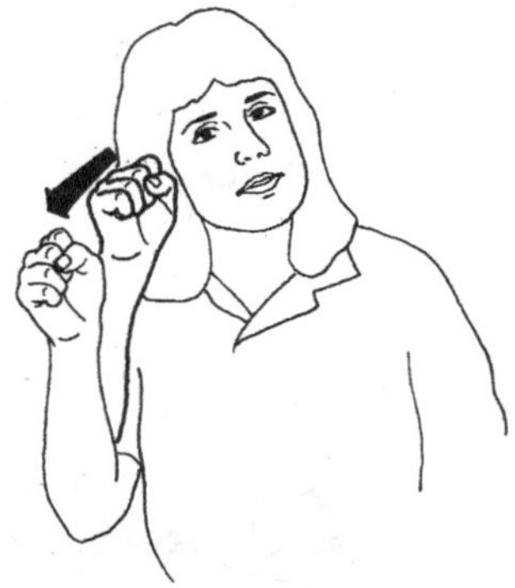

SOUND.

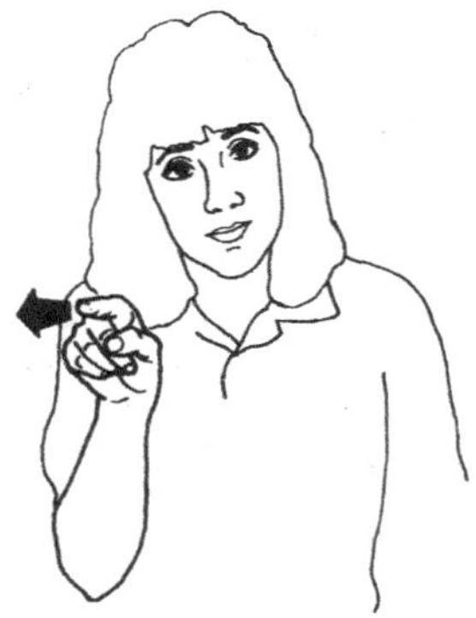

YOU

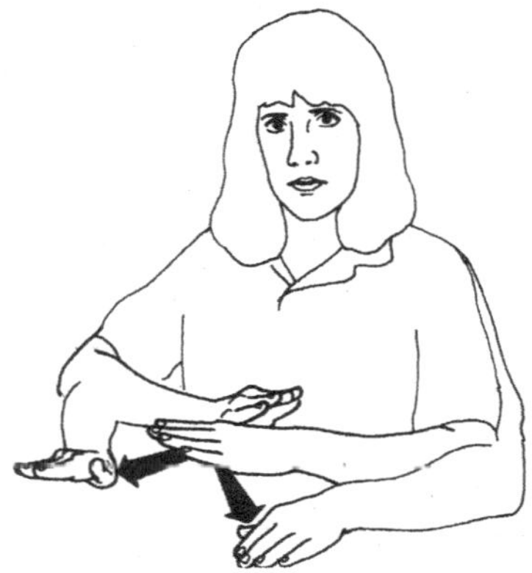

DON'T

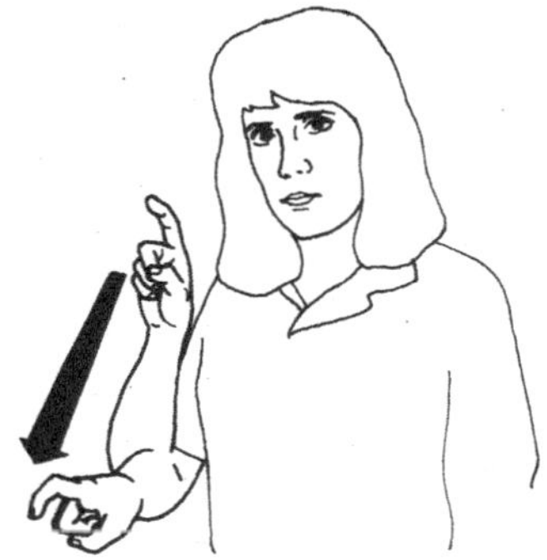

HAVE-TO

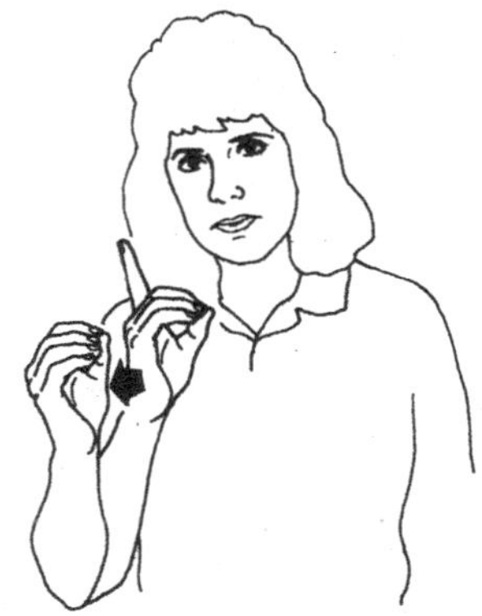

D-O

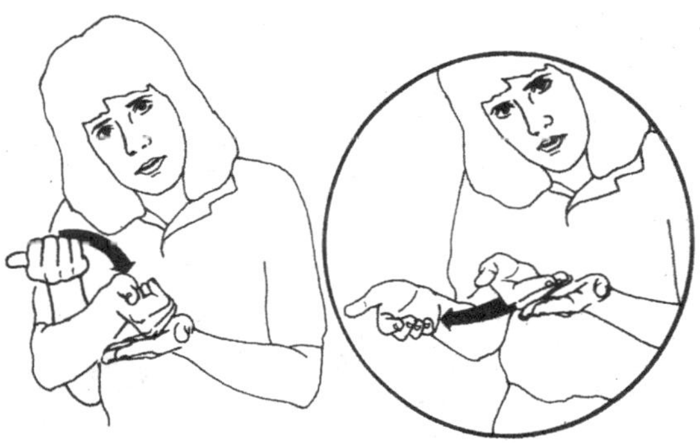

ANYTHING.

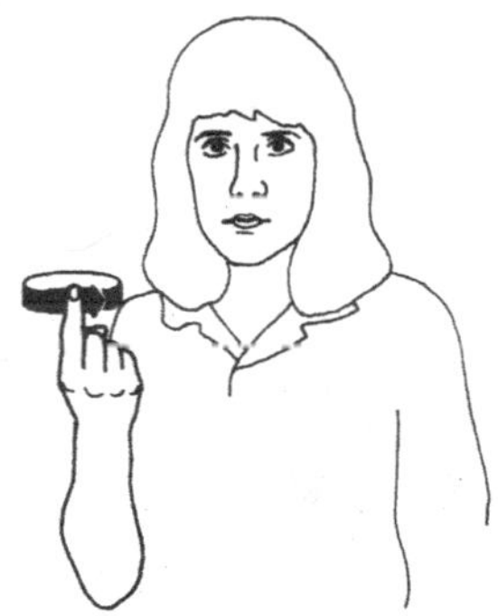

ONLY

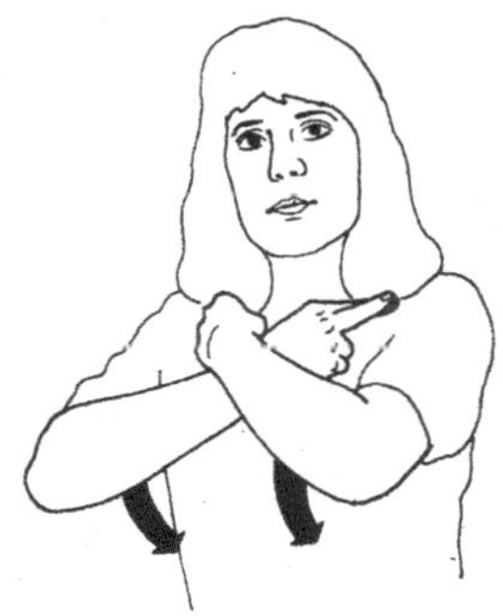

RELAX

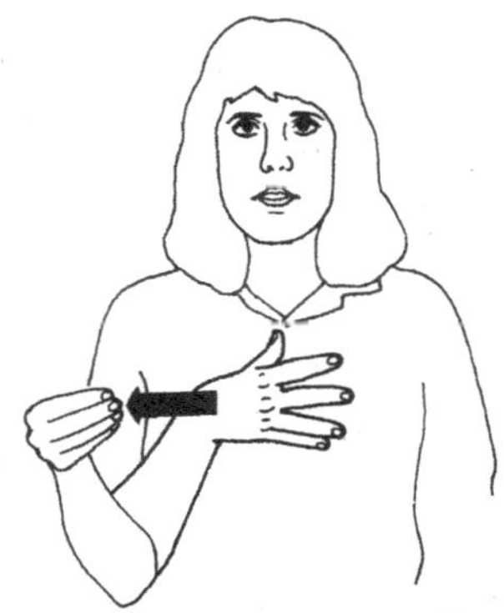

AND

You don't have to do anything; just relax and try not to move or talk.

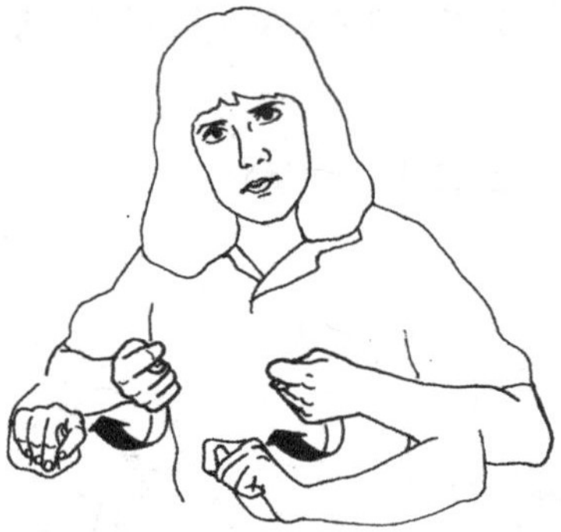

TRY

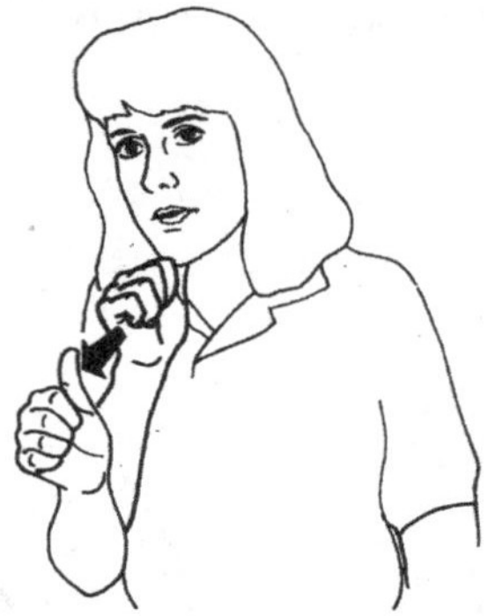

NOT

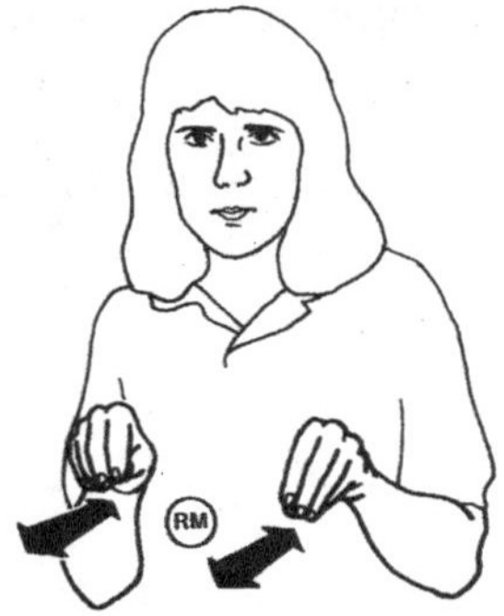

MOVE

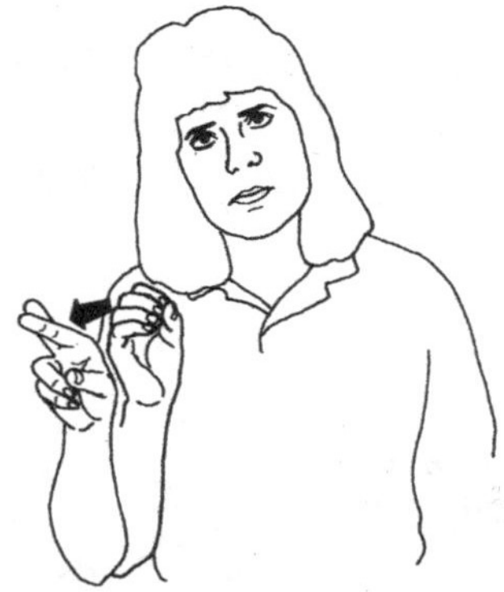

O-R

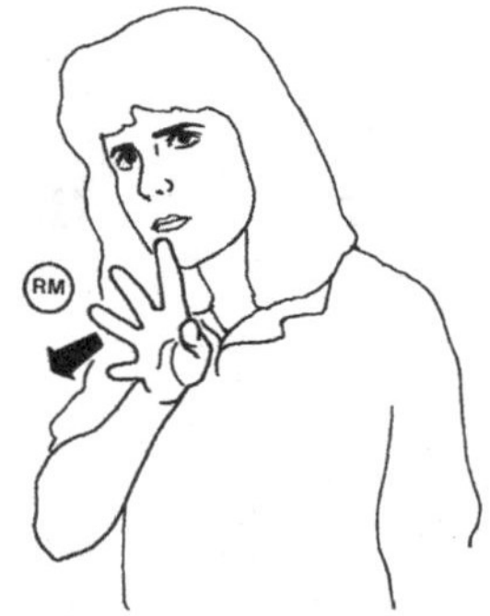

TALK.

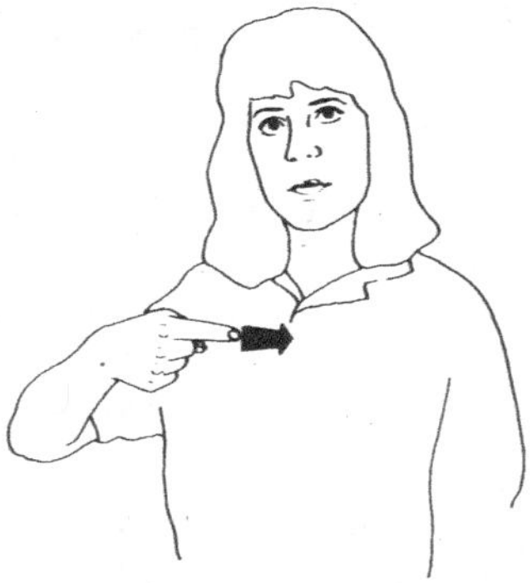

I

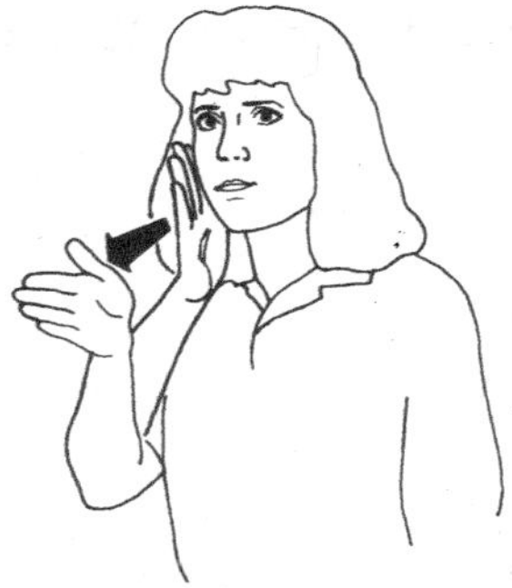

WILL

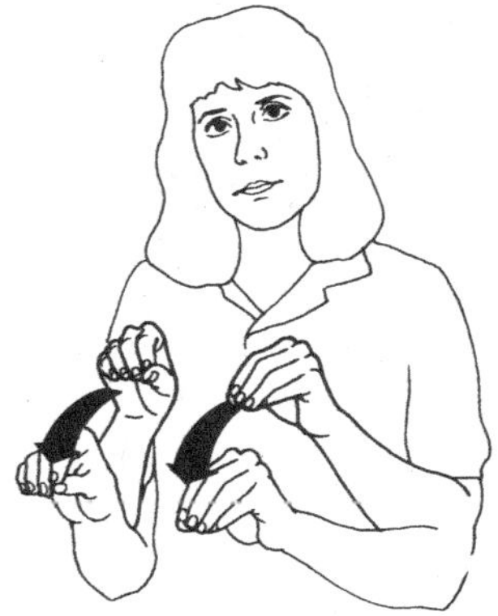

PUT

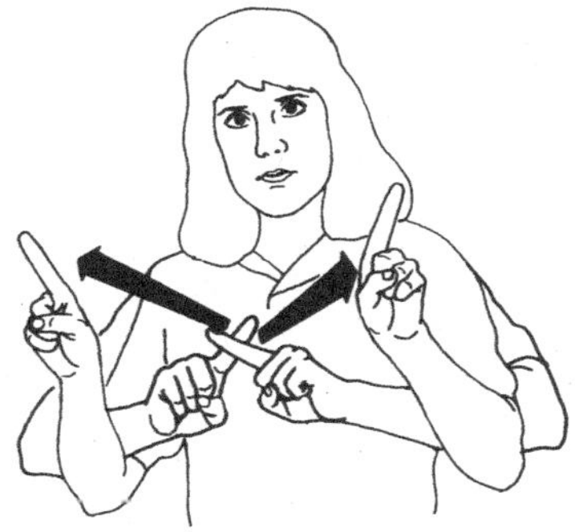

DIFFERENT

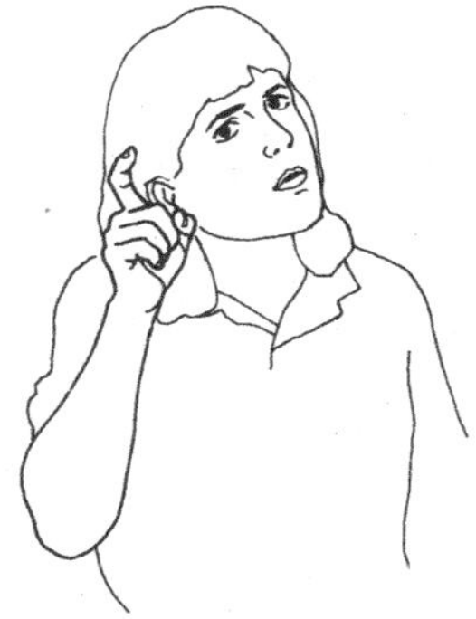

HEARING-AID

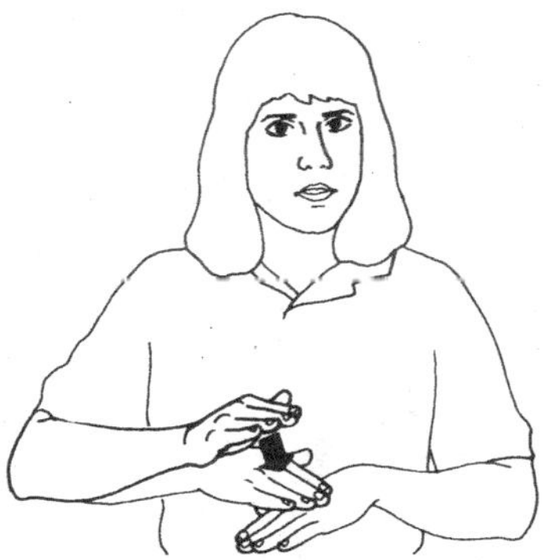

ON

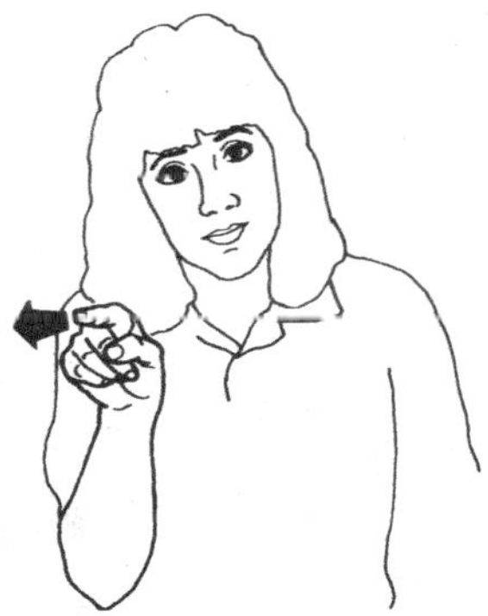

YOU

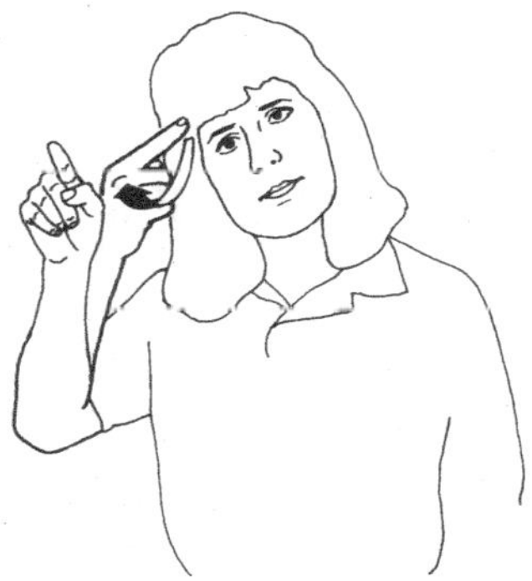

FOR

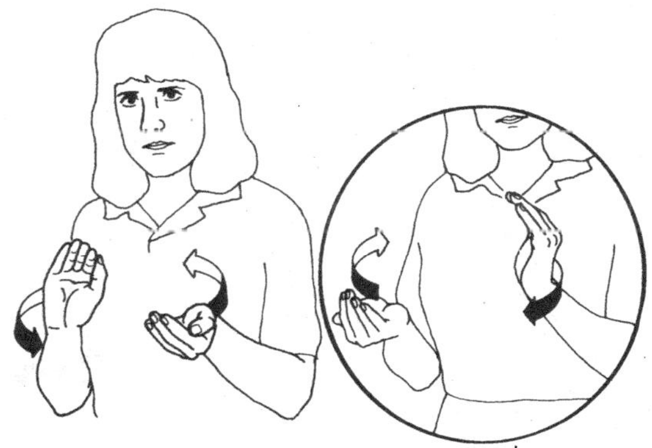

COMPARISON.

I will put different hearing aids on you for comparison.

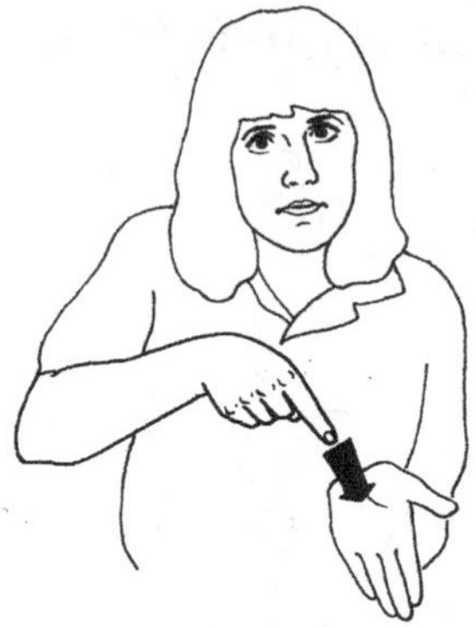
THIS

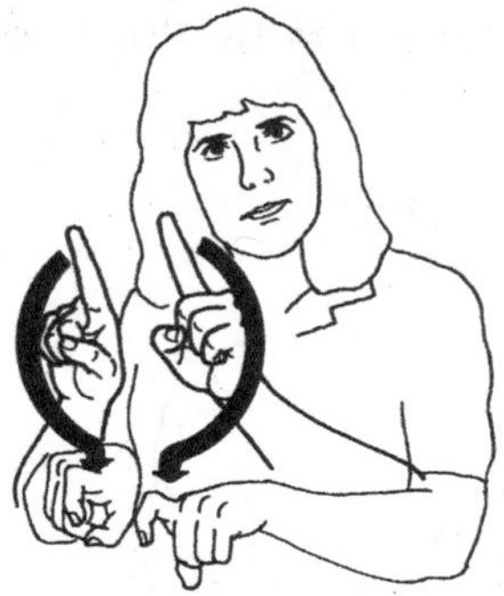
TEST

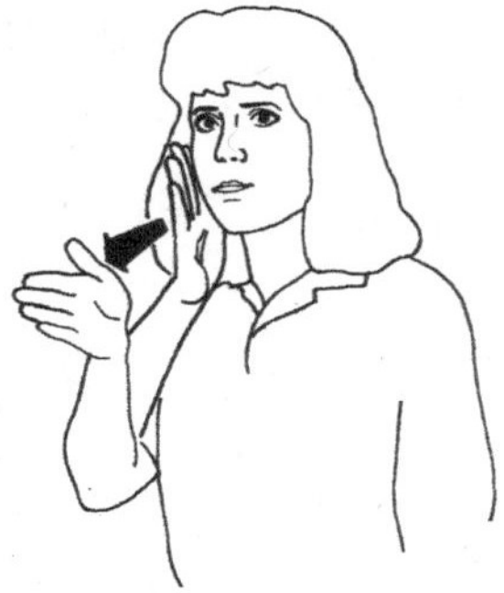
WILL

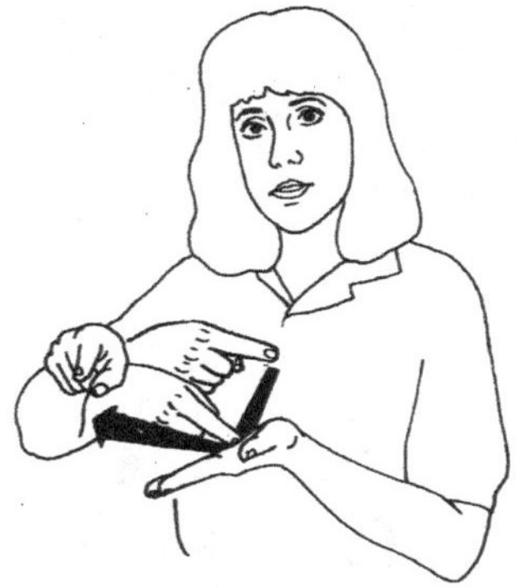
CHECK

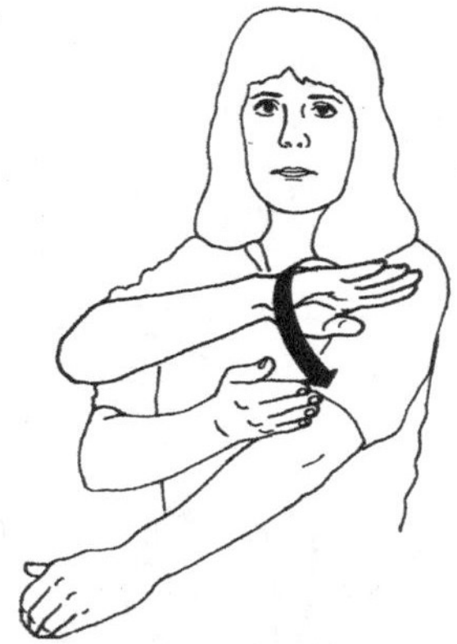
POWER

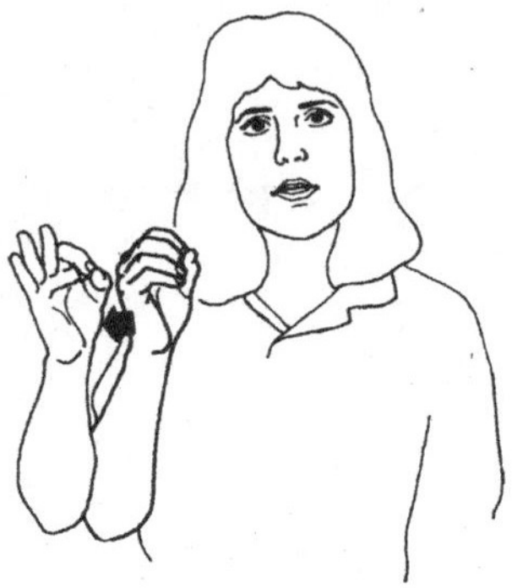
O-F

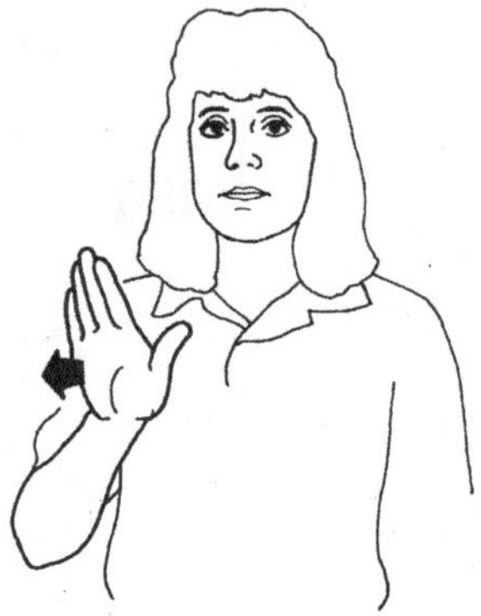
YOUR

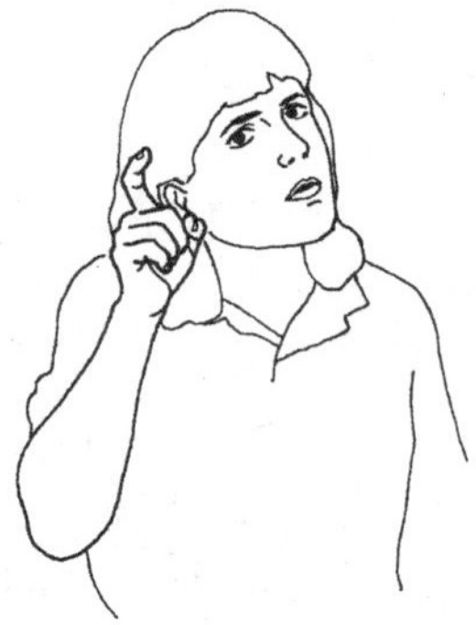
HEARING-AID.

This test will check the power of your hearing aid.

Chapter 4

Aural Rehabilitation Evaluation of a Deaf Child

Introduction

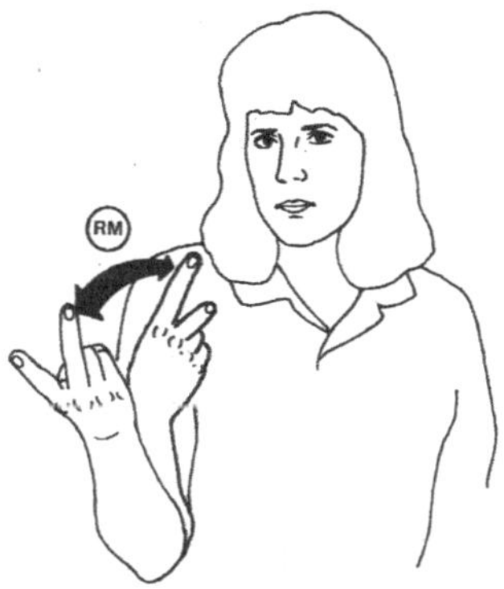

TWO-OF-US

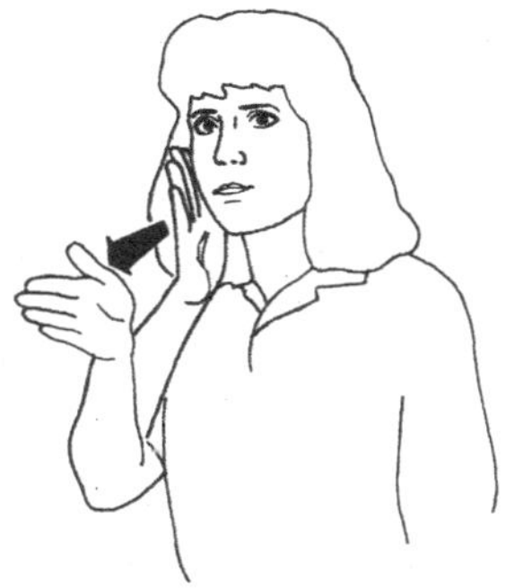

WILL

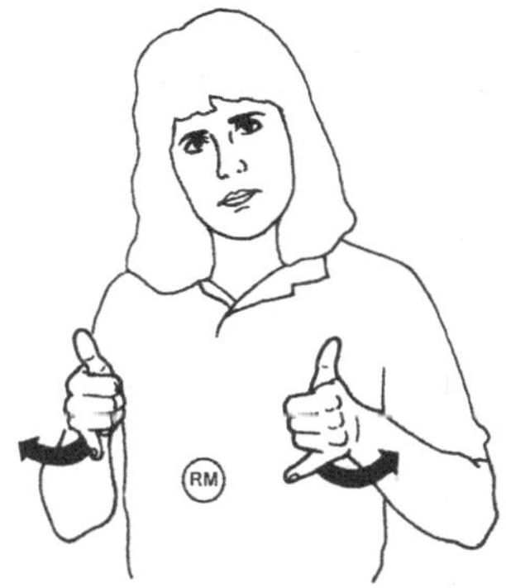

PLAY

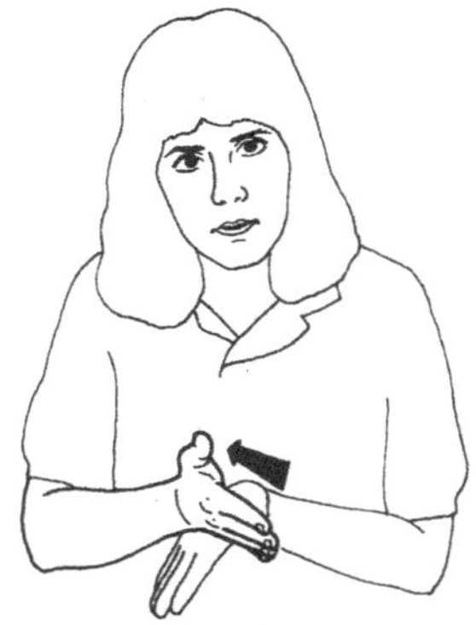

SOME

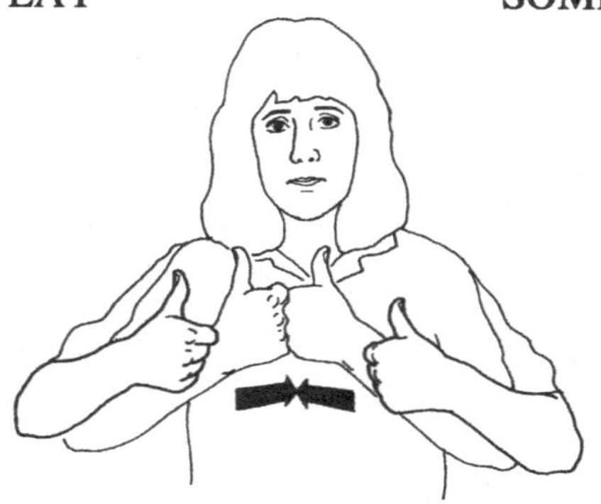

GAME

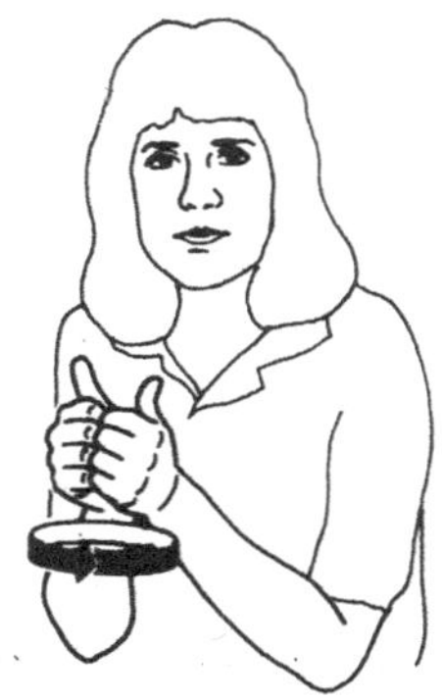

TOGETHER.

We will play some games together.

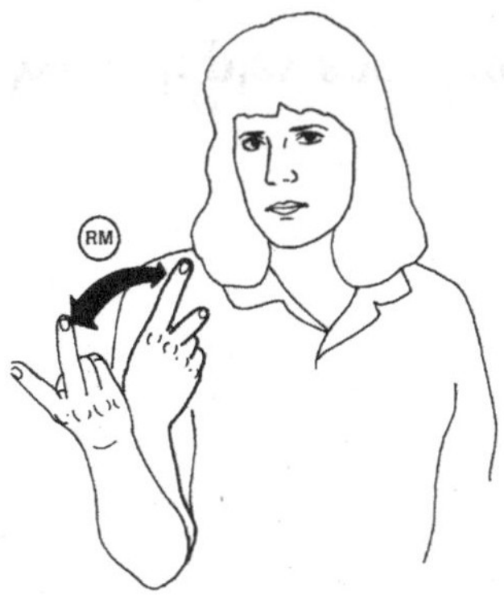

TWO-OF-US

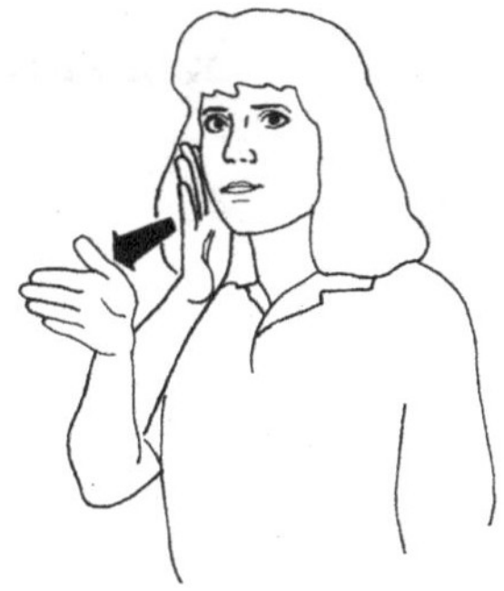

WILL

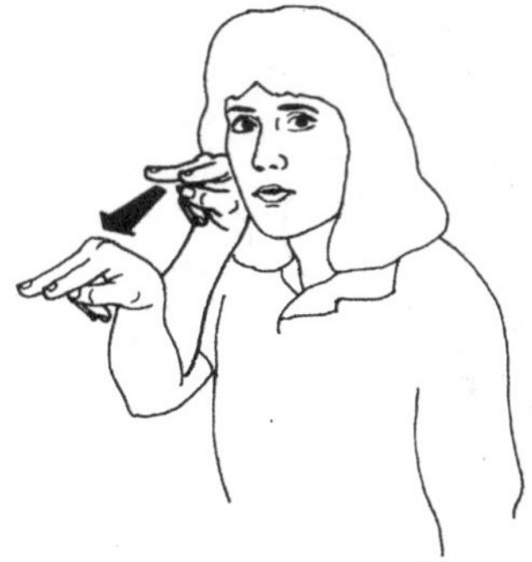

LOOK-AT

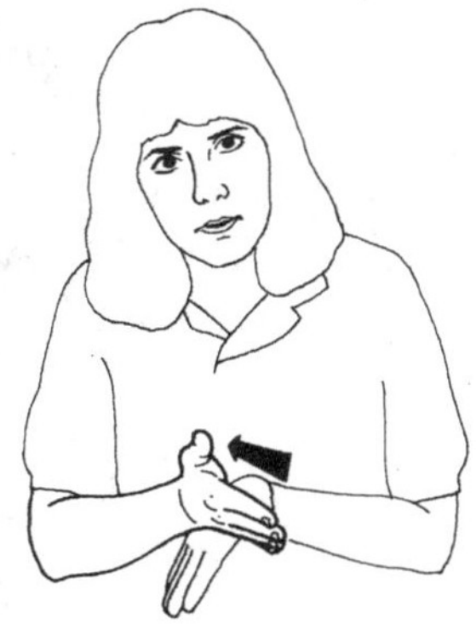

SOME

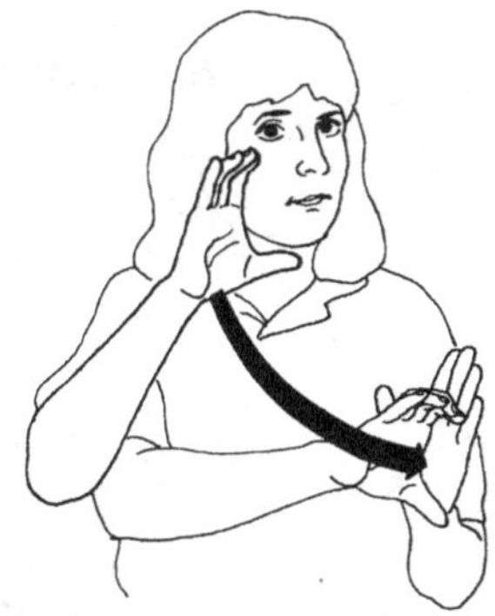

PICTURE.

We will look at some pictures.

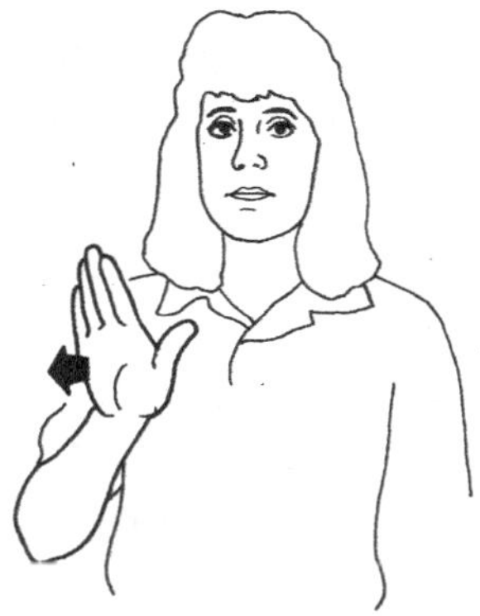

YOUR

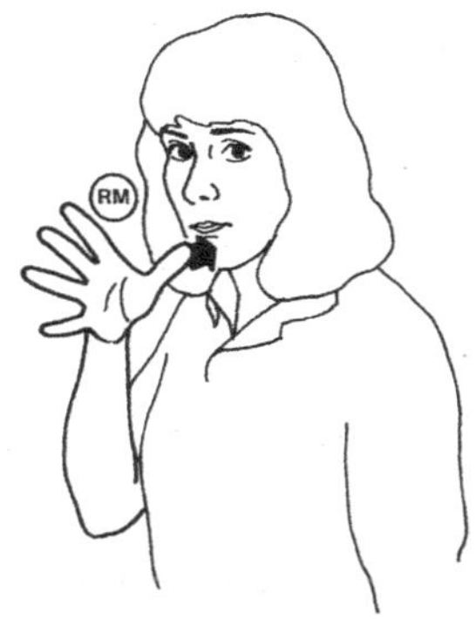

MOTHER

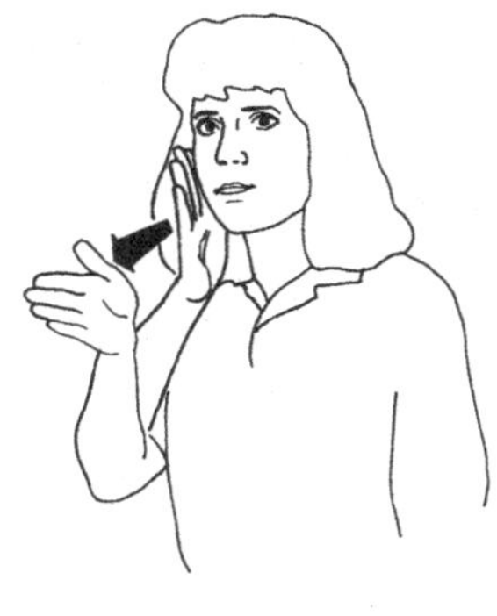

WILL

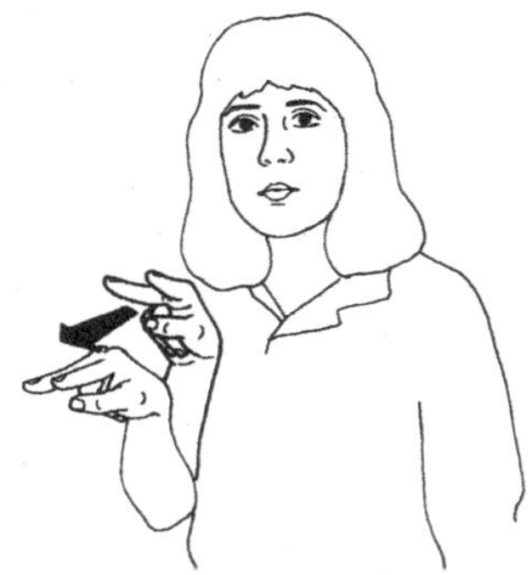

WATCH

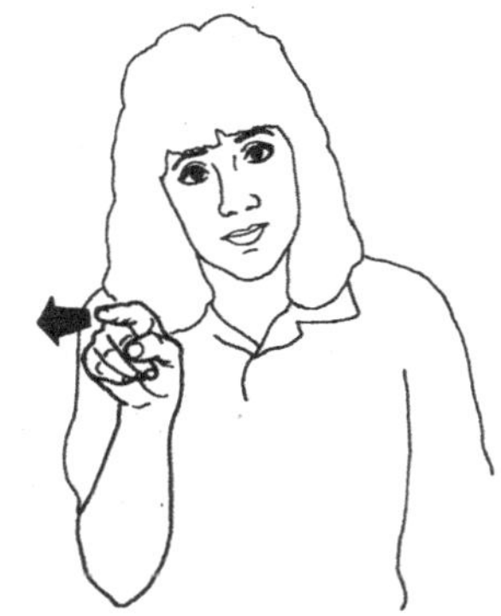

YOU

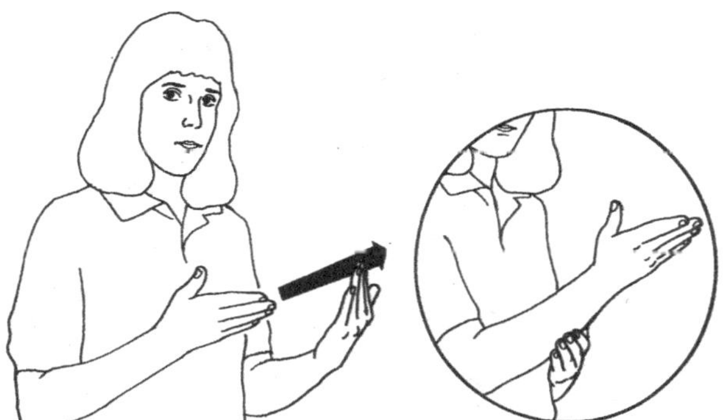

THROUGH

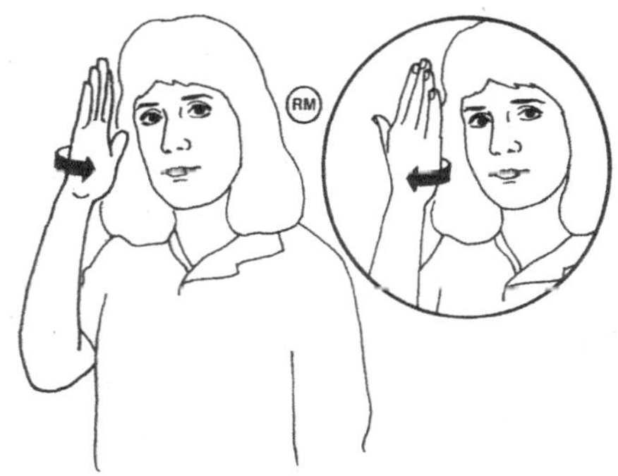

MIRROR.

Your mom will watch you through the mirror.

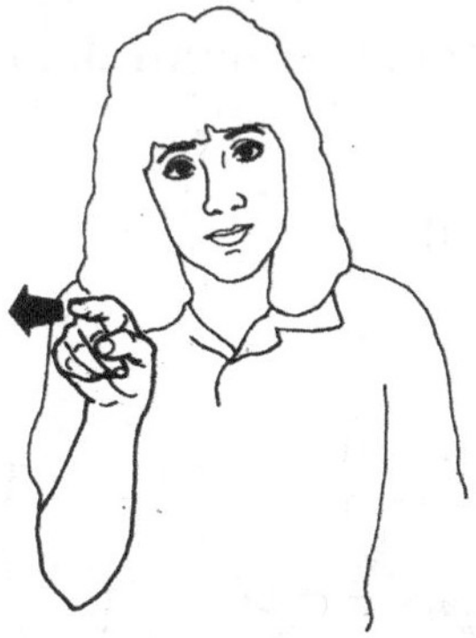

YOU

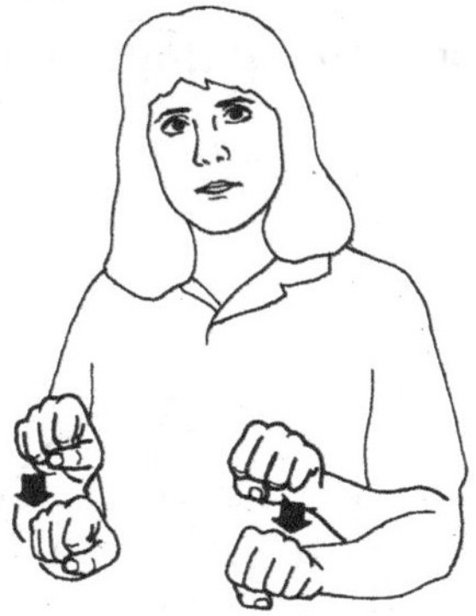

CAN

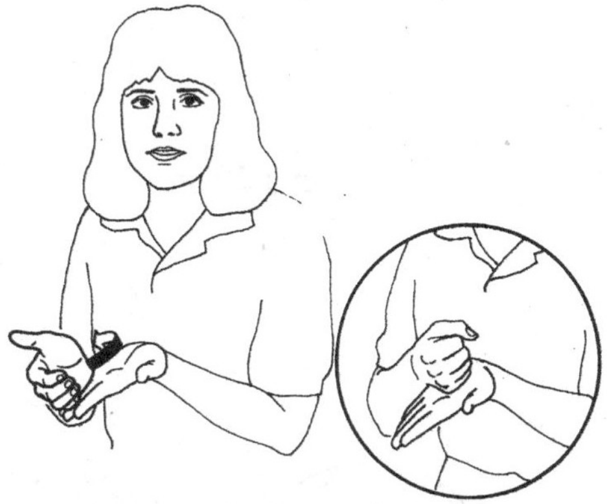

EARN

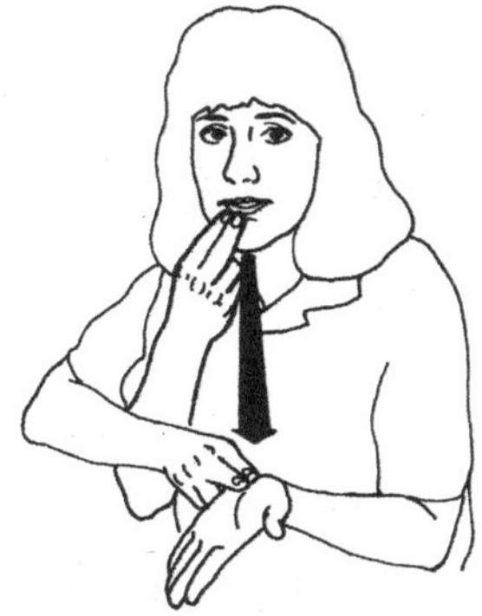

STICKER.

You can earn a sticker.

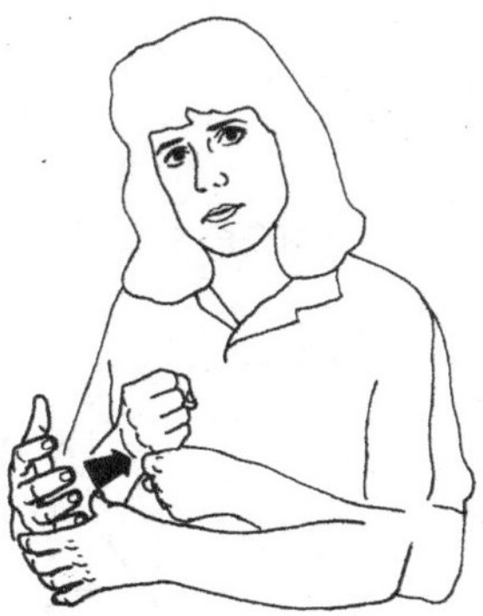

GET

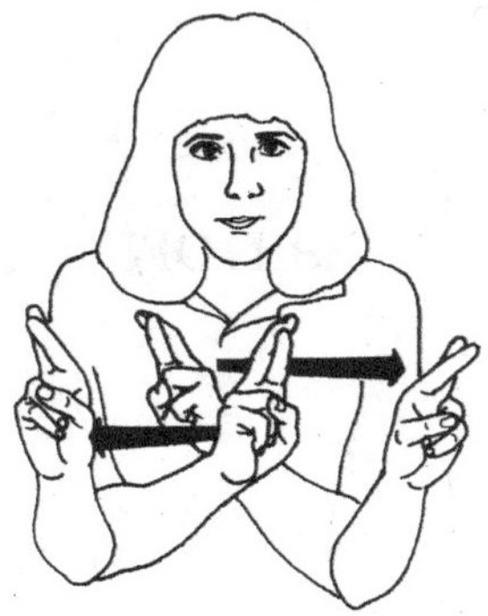

READY.

Get ready.

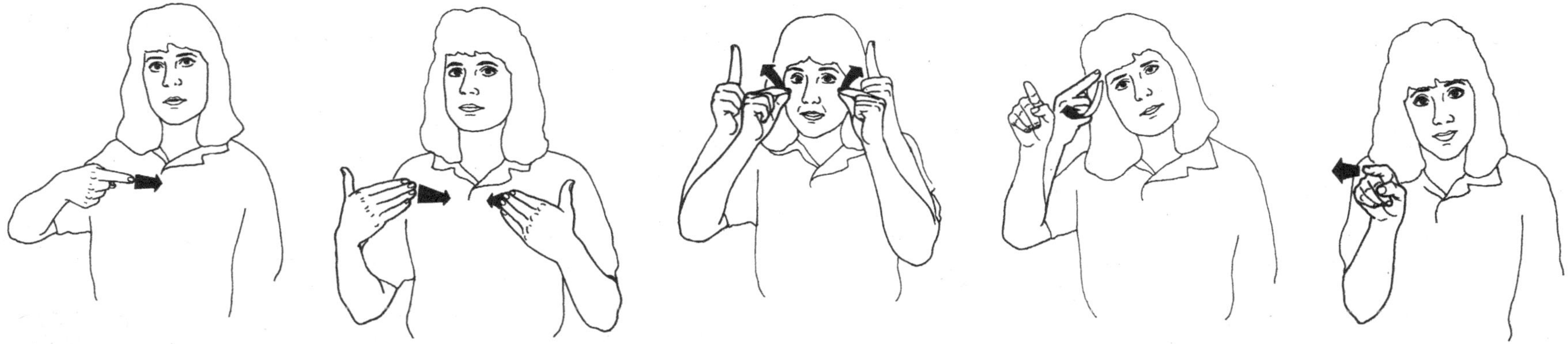

I HAVE SURPRISE FOR YOU.

I have a surprise for you.

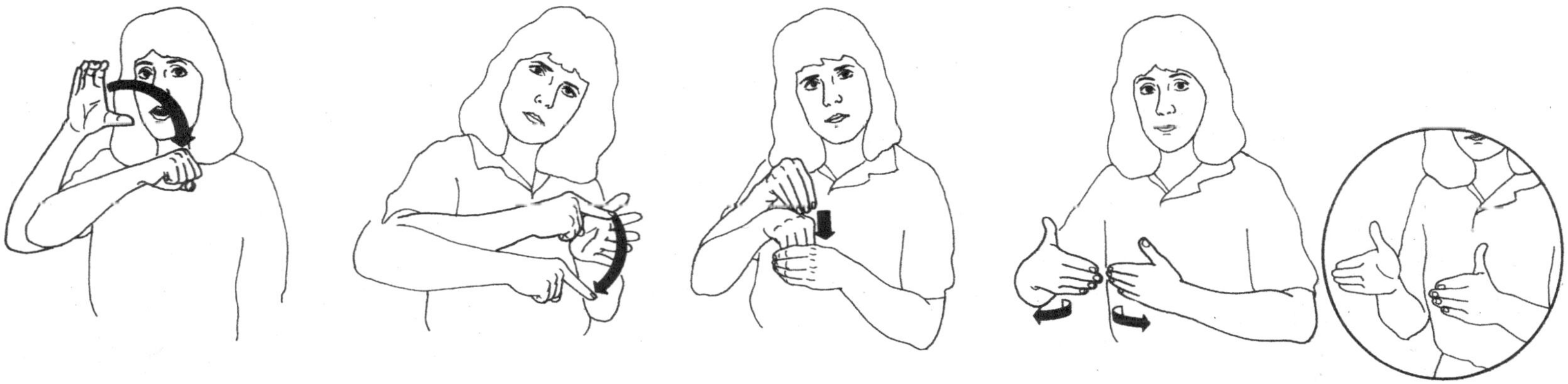

GUESS WHAT IN BOX.

Guess what's in the box.

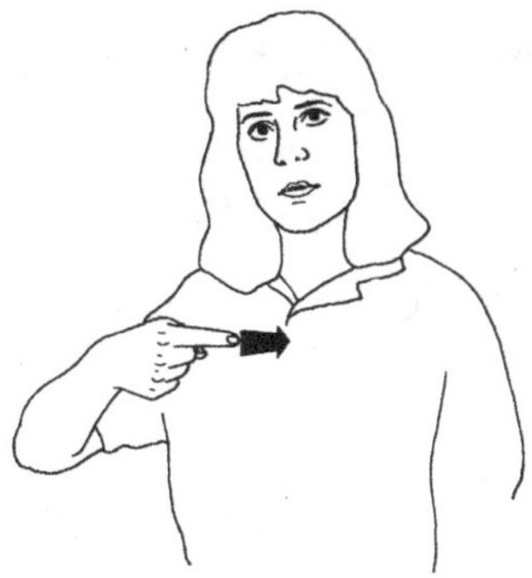

I

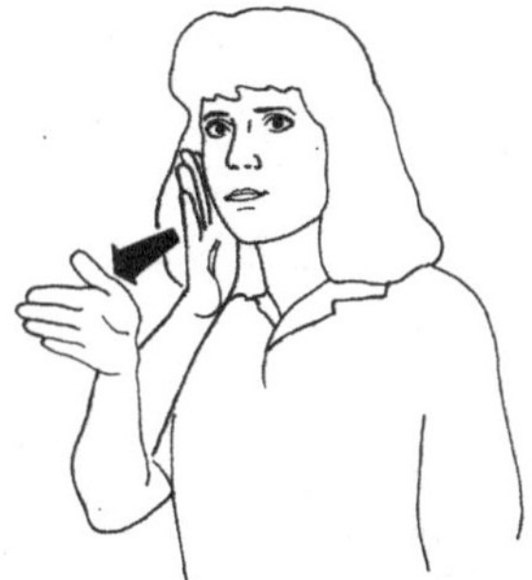

WILL

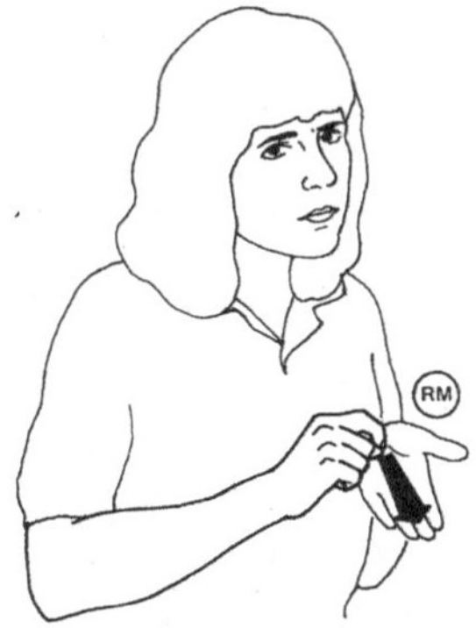

WRITE

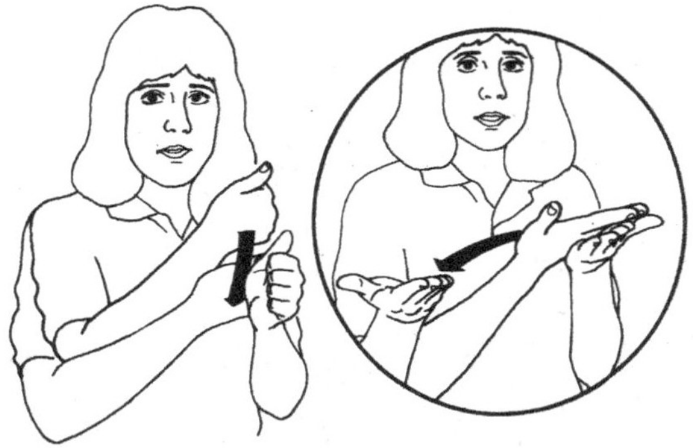

EVERYTHING

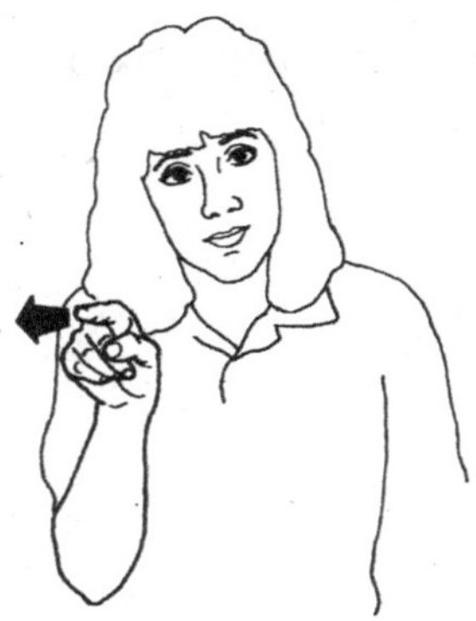

YOU

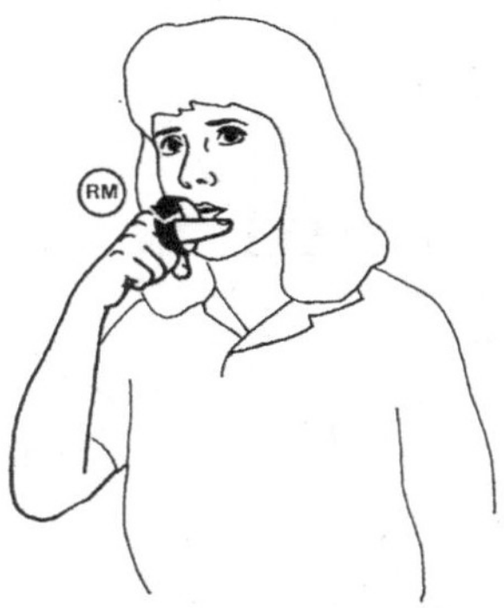

SAY.

I will write everything you say.

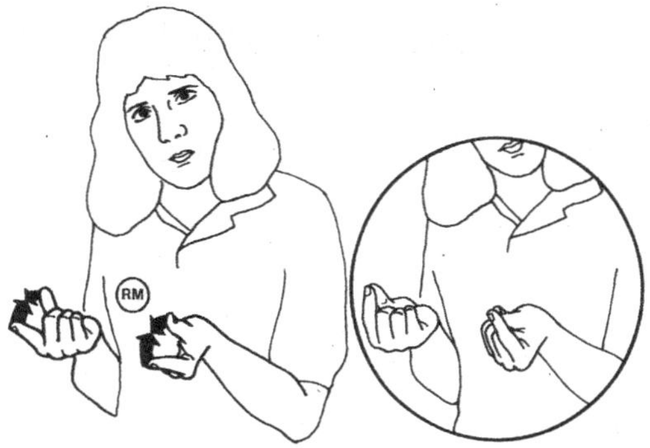

WHAT-DO

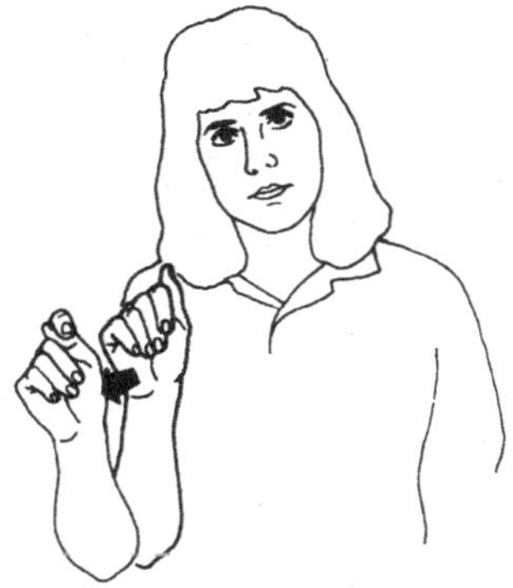

A-T

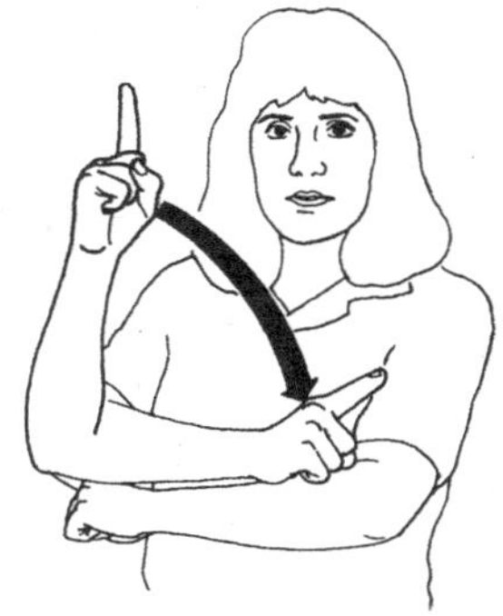

DAY

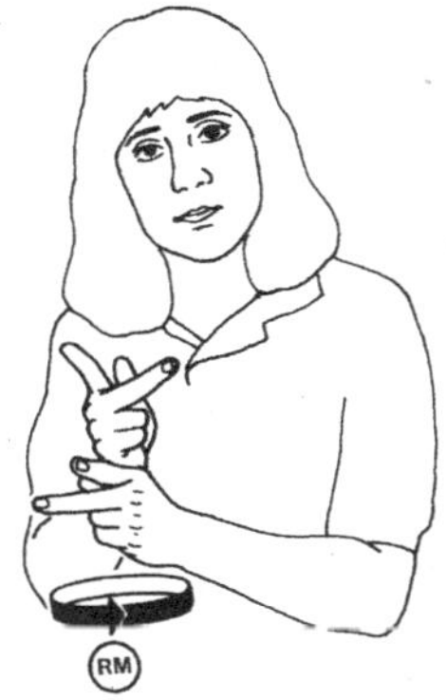

CARE

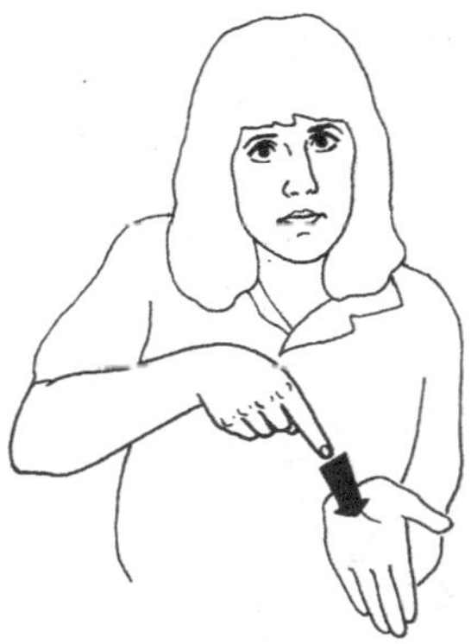

THIS

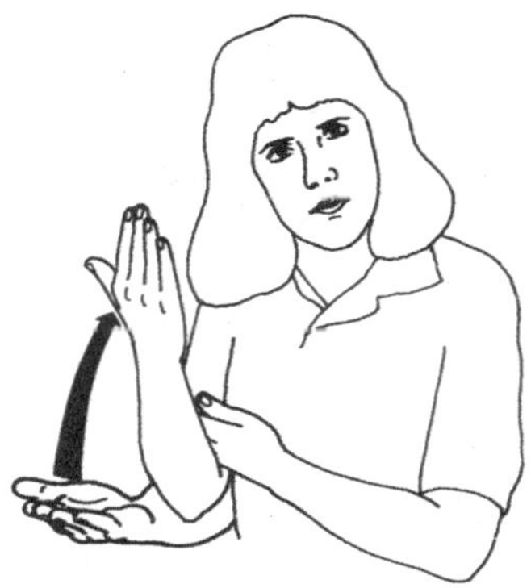

MORNING?

What did you do at day care this morning?

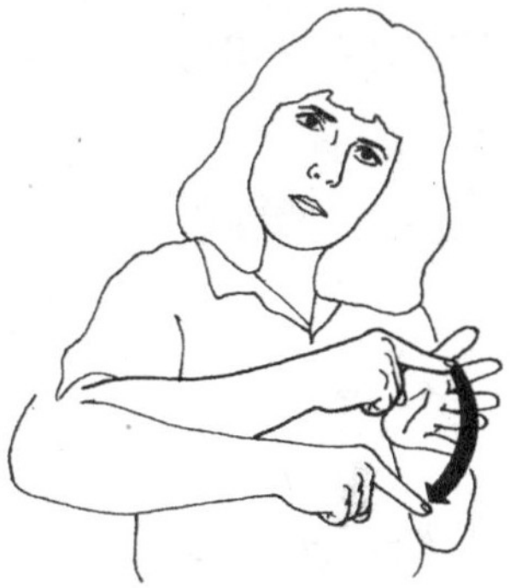

WHAT

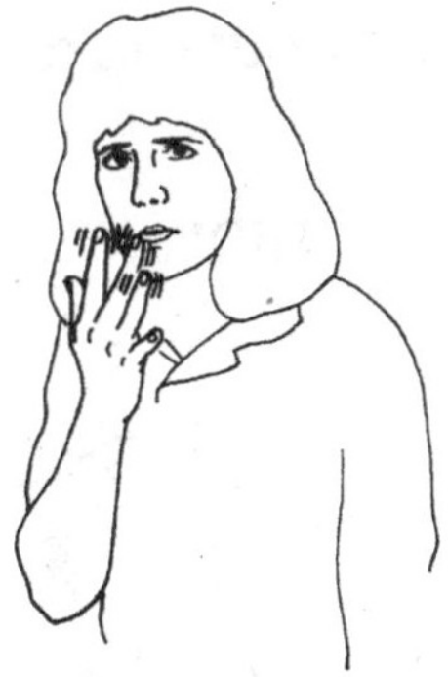

COLOR

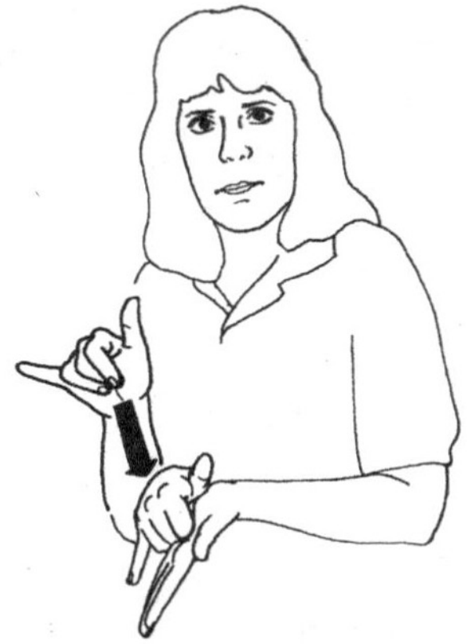

THAT?

What color is that?

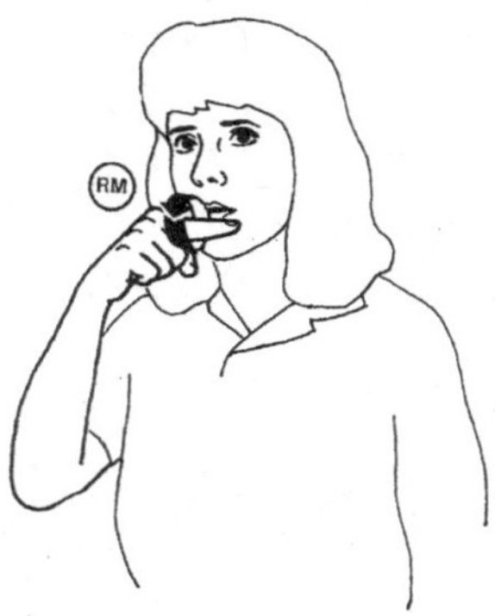

SAY

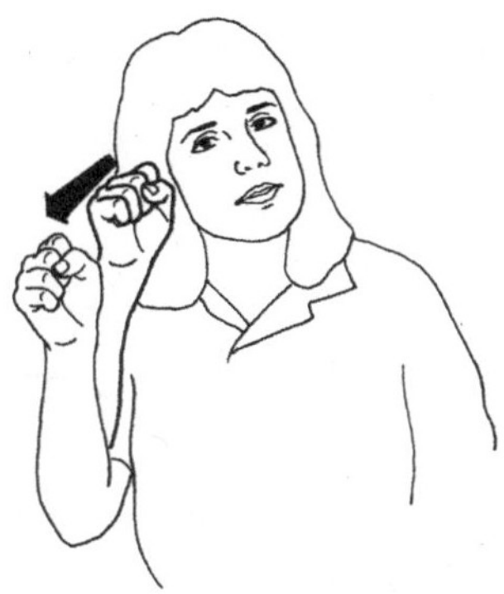

SOUND

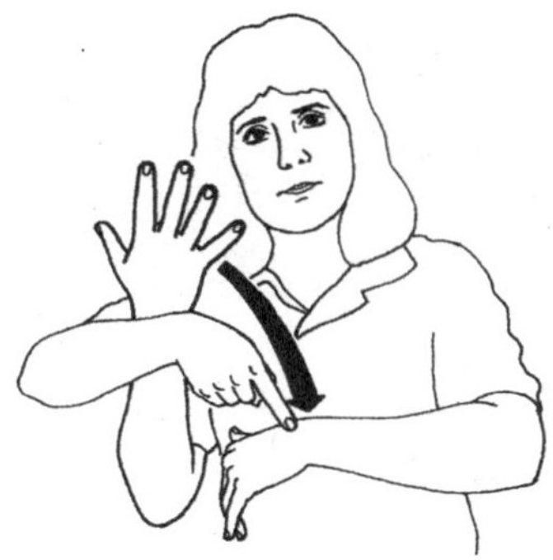

FIVE-TIME.

Say the sound five times.

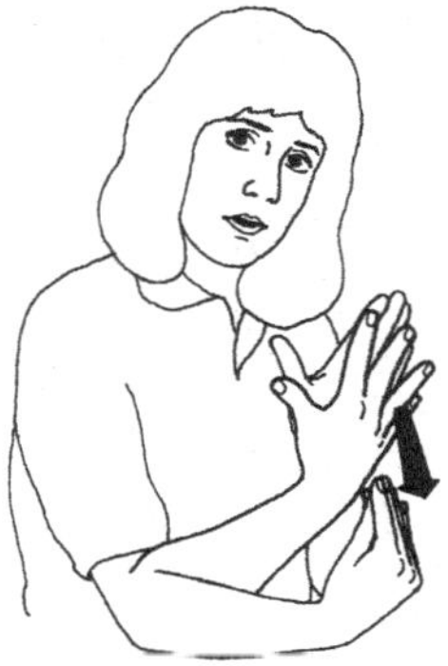

COPY

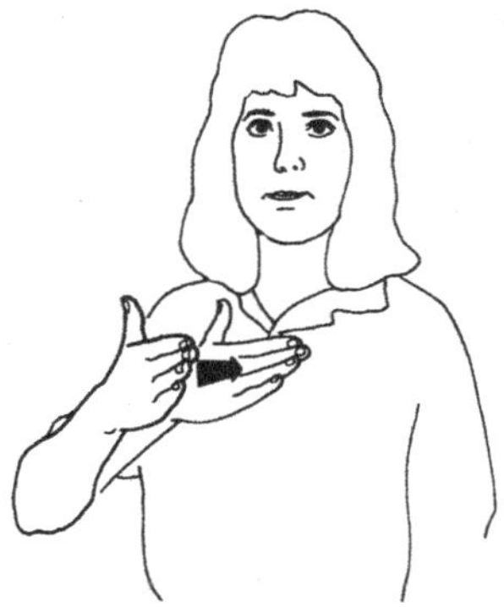

MY

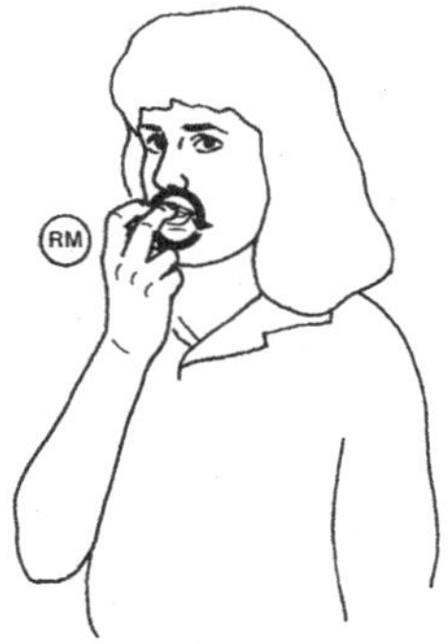

SPEECH.

Copy my speech.

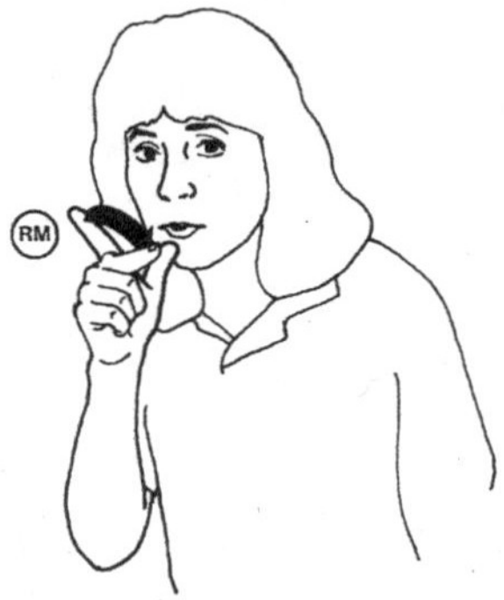

WHO

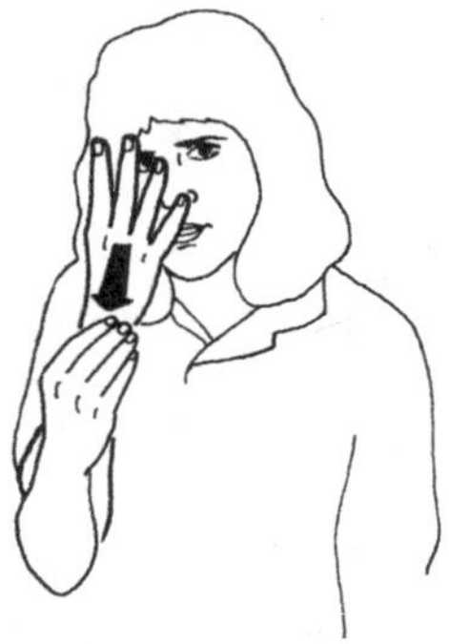

SLEEP?

Who is sleeping?

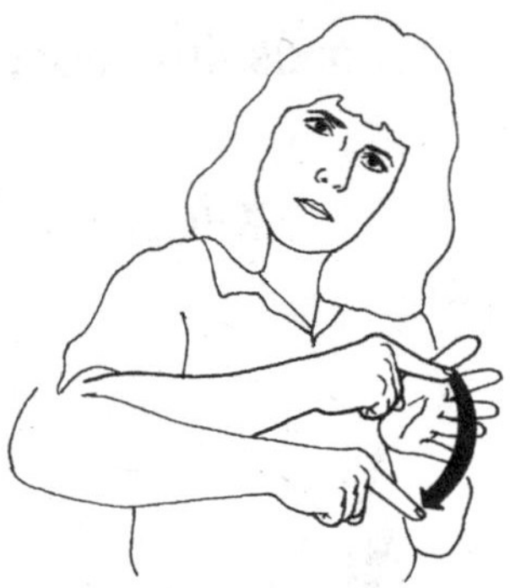

WHAT

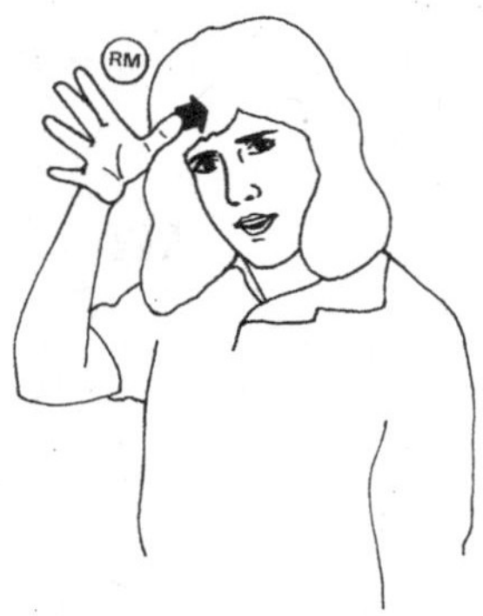

FATHER

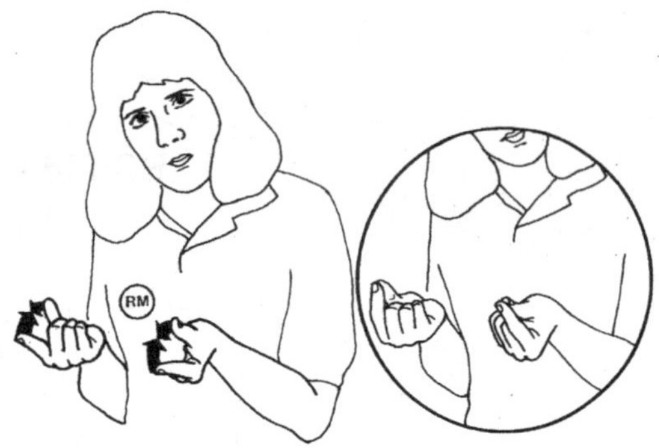

DO?

What is daddy doing?

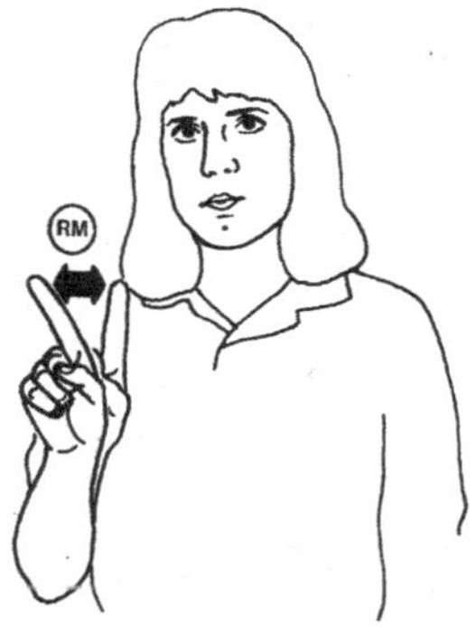

WHERE

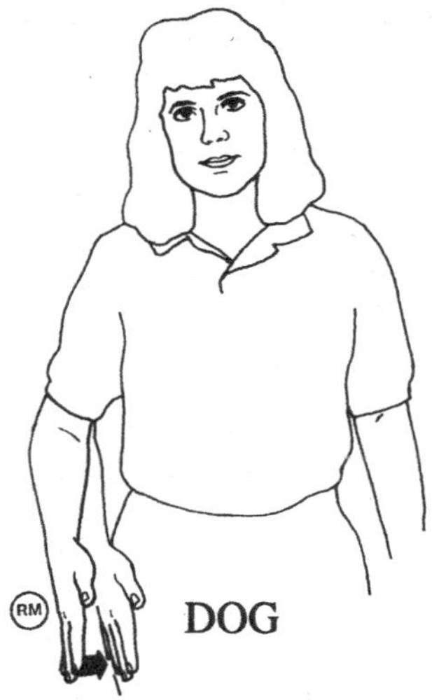

DOG

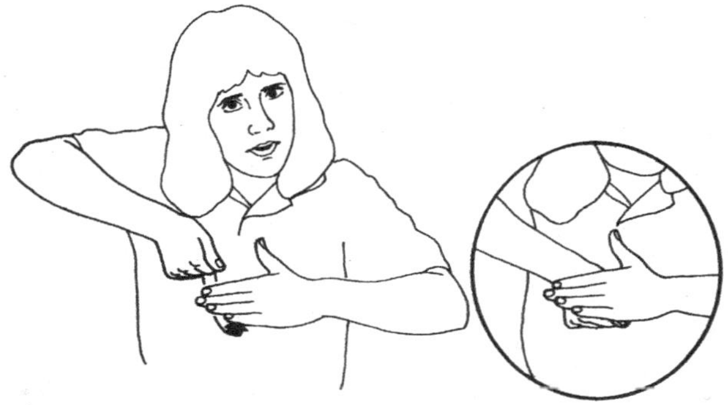

HIDE?

Where is the dog hiding?

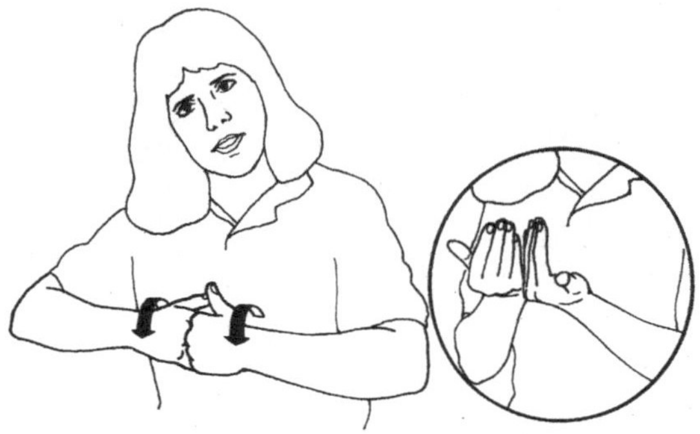

HOW

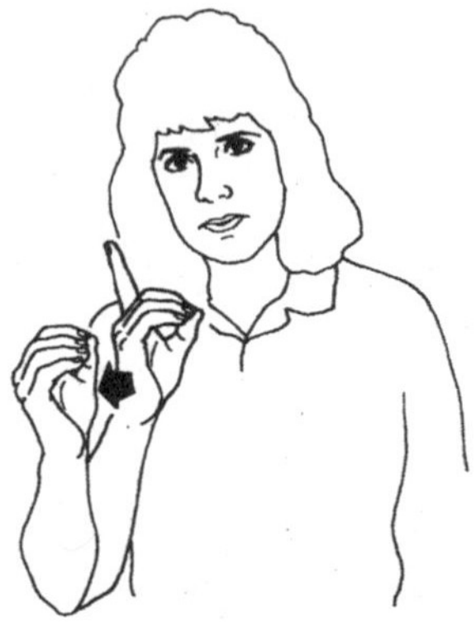

D-O

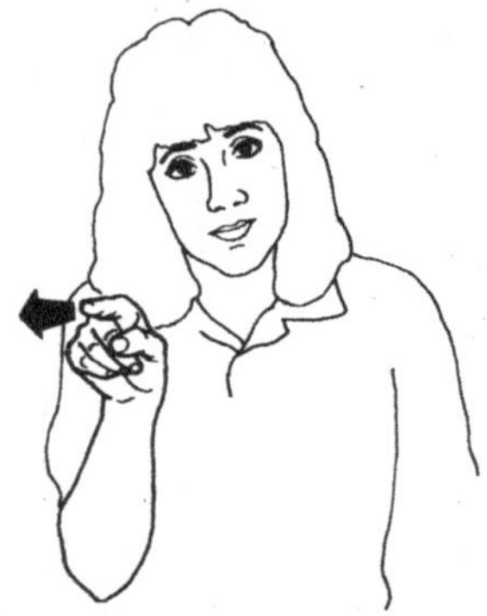

YOU

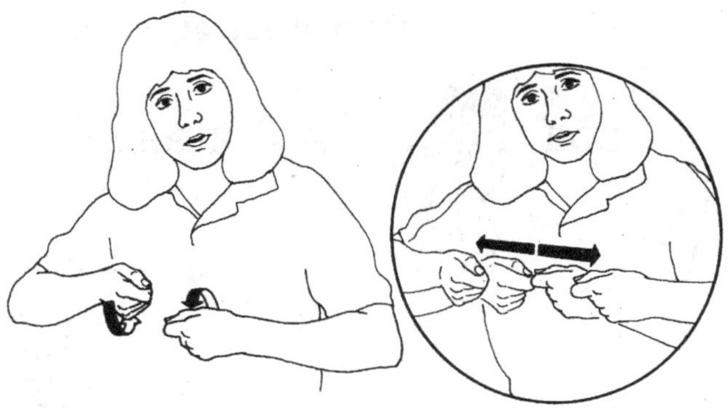

TIE

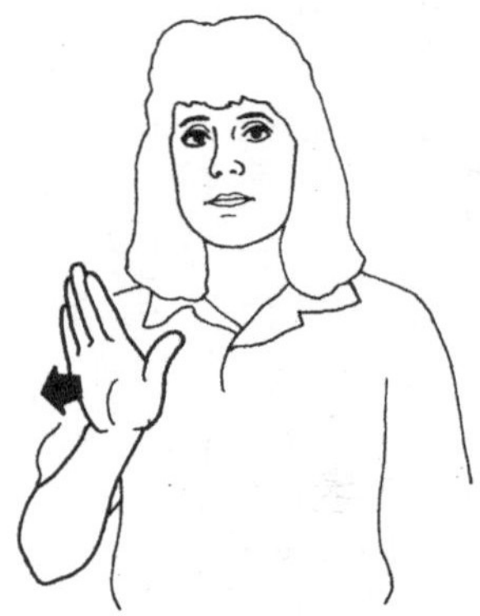

YOUR

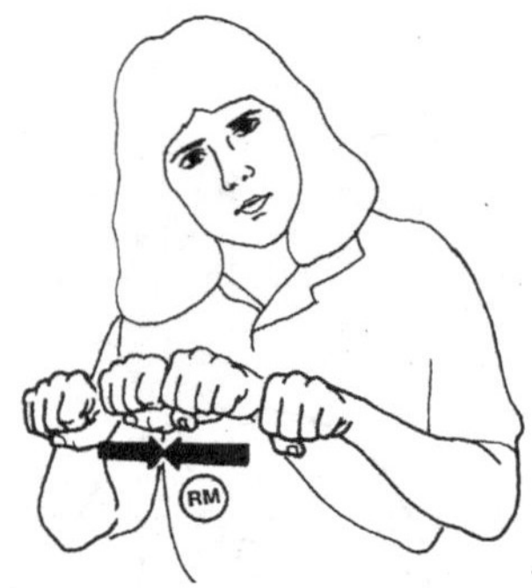

SHOE?

How do you tie your shoes?

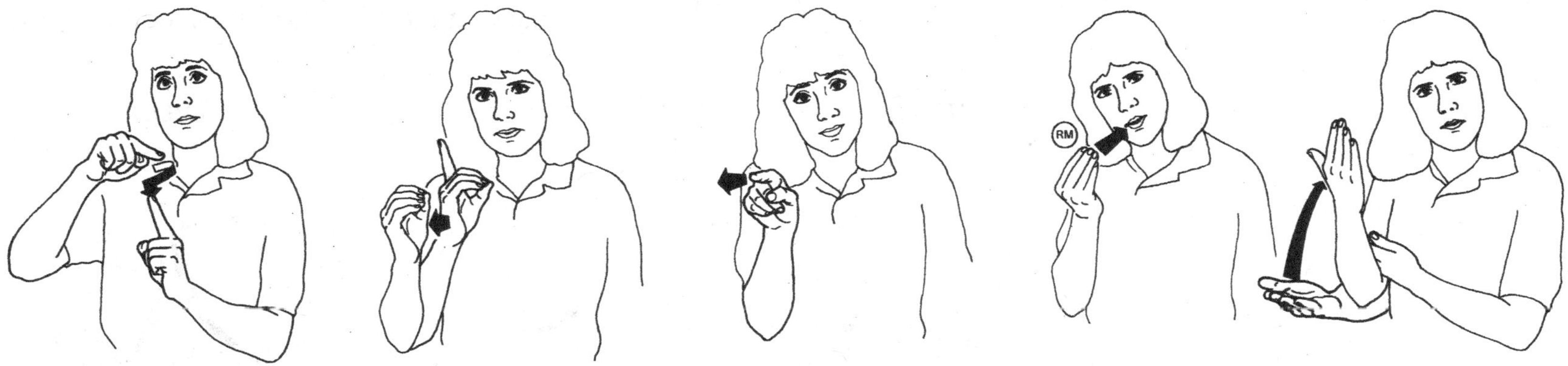

WHEN D-O YOU EAT-BREAKFAST?

When do you eat breakfast?

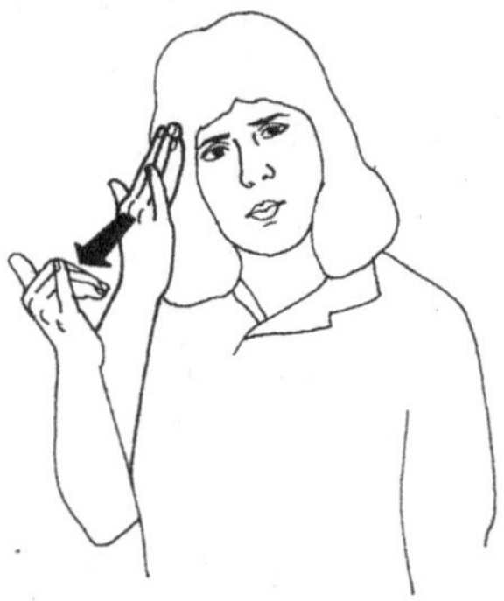

WHY

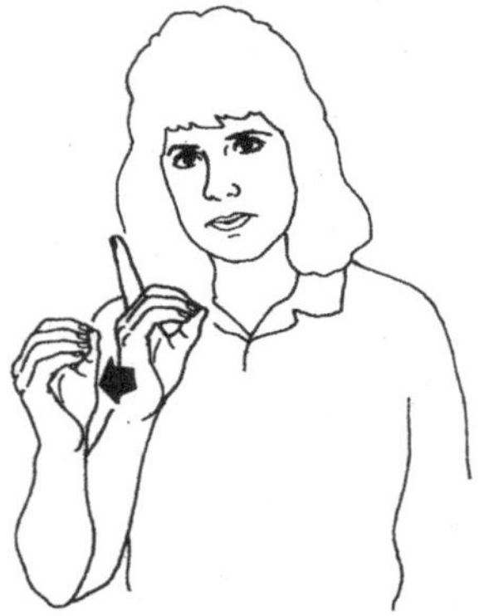

D-O

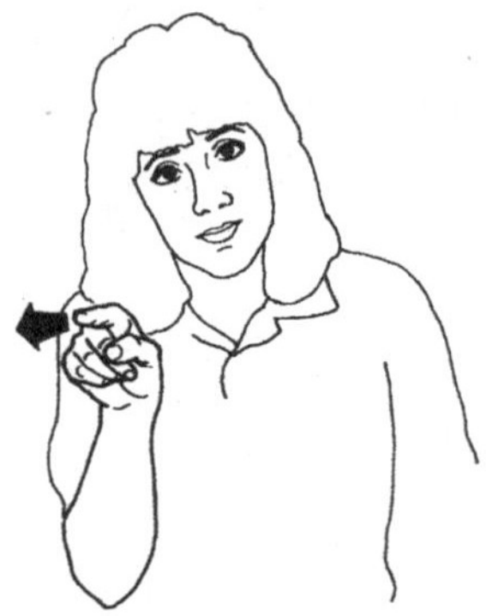

YOU

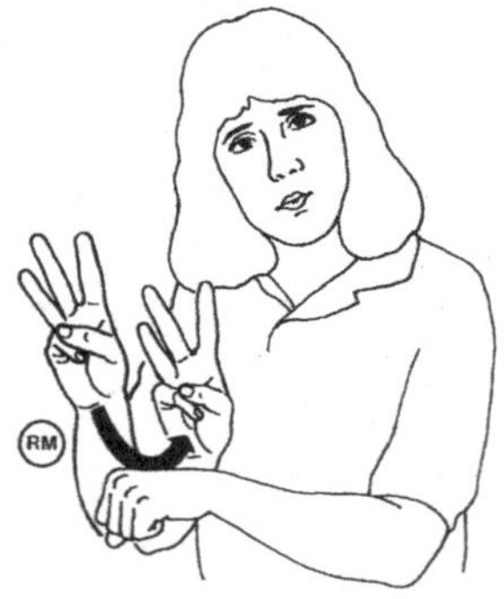

WEAR

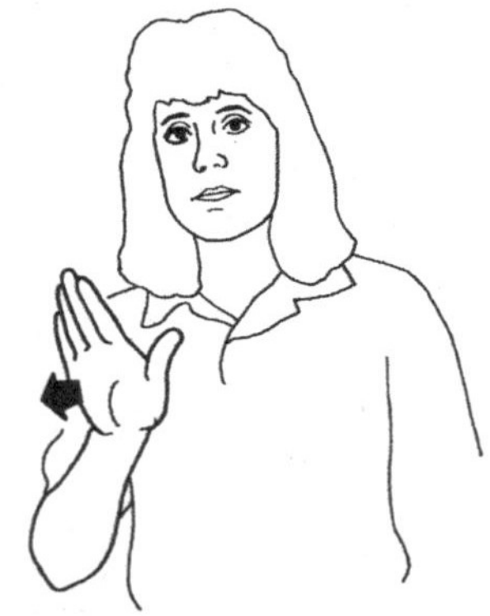

YOUR

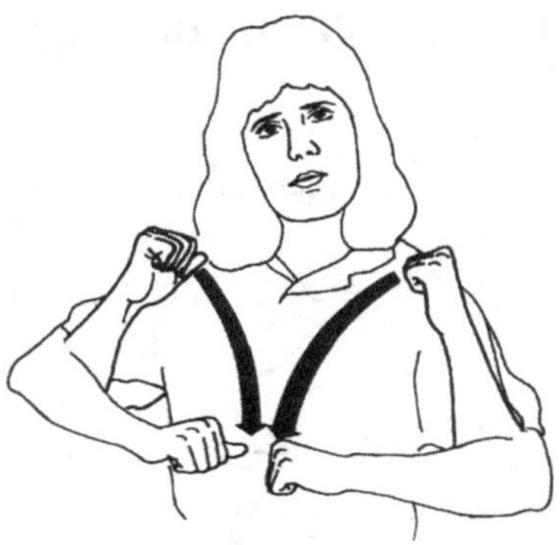

COAT

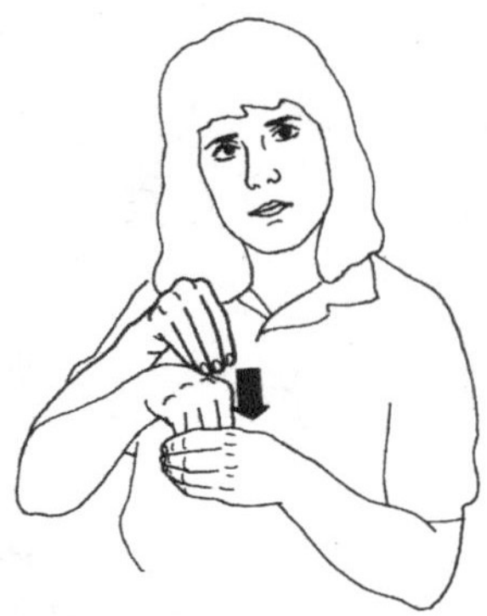

IN

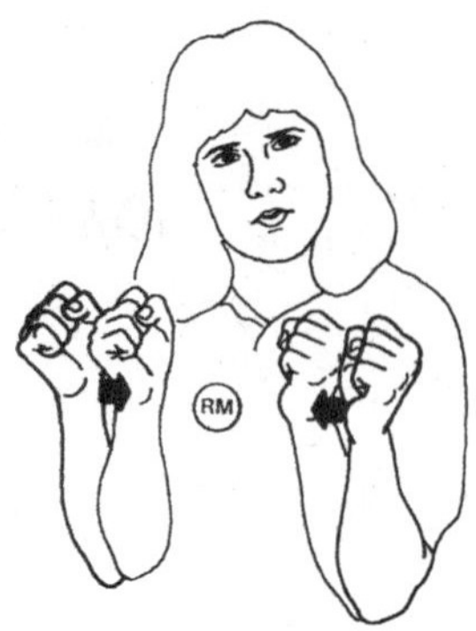

WINTER?

Why do you wear your coat in the winter?

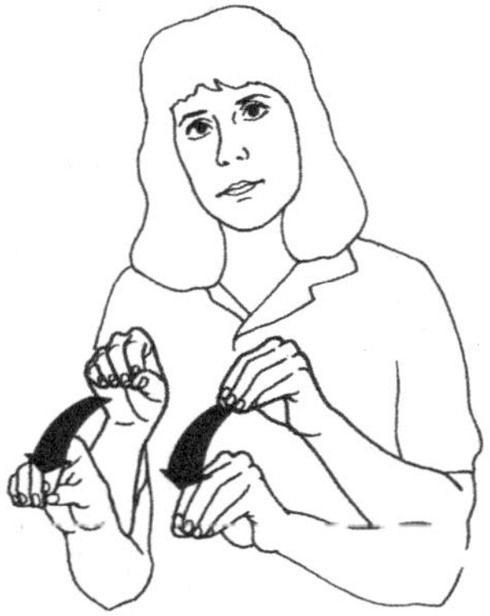

PUT

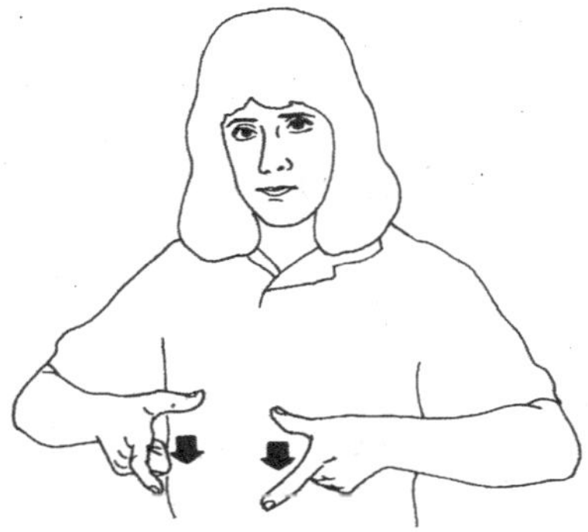

PLATE

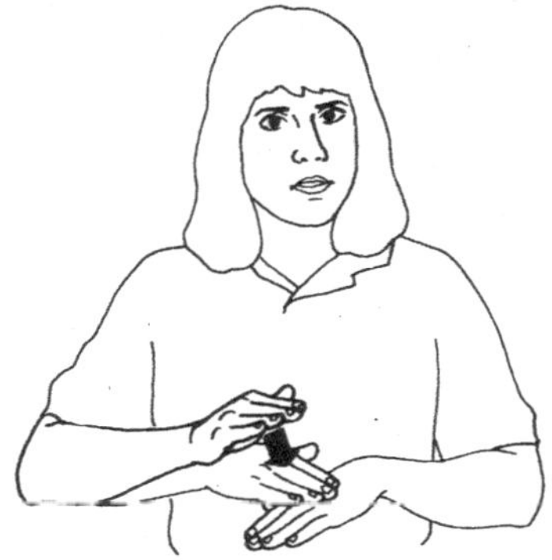

ON

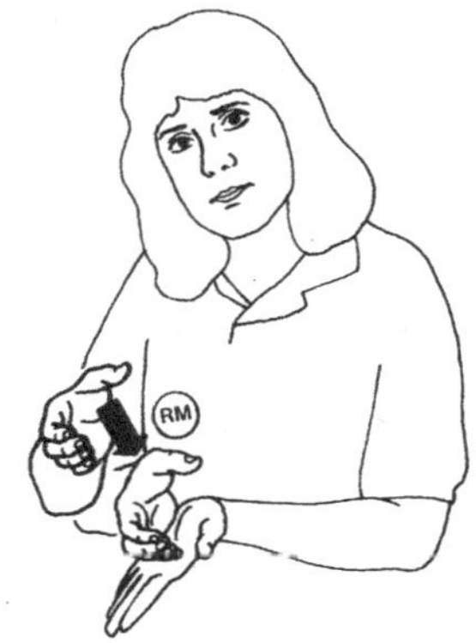

CUP.

Put the plate on the cup.

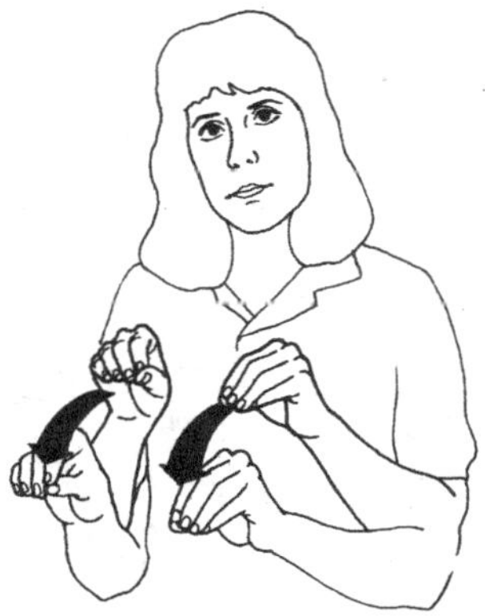

PUT

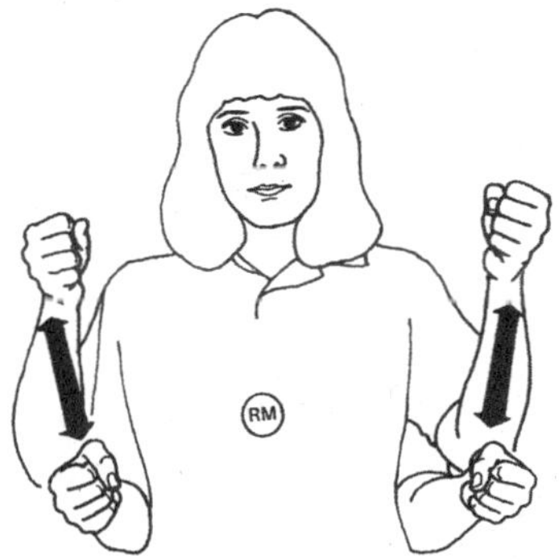

TRUCK

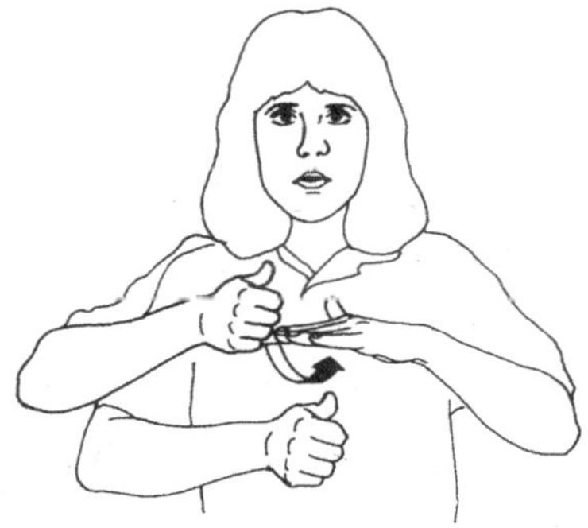

UNDER

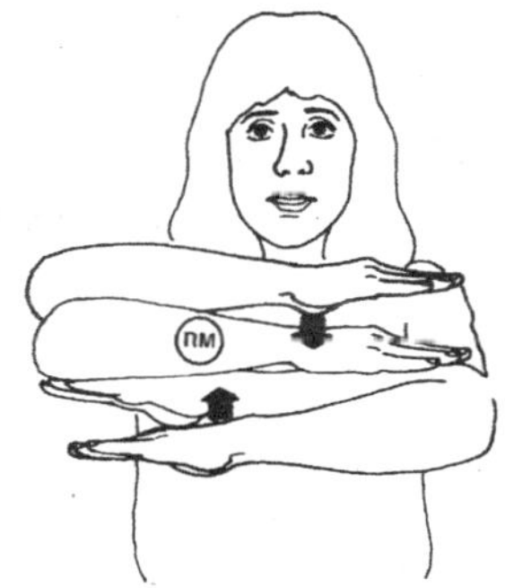

TABLE.

Put the truck under the table.

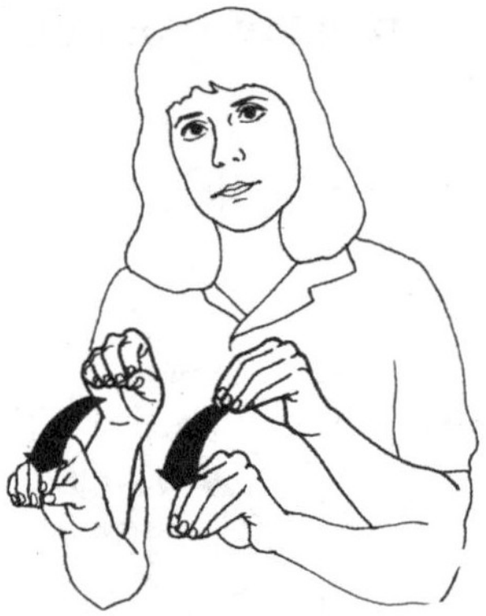

PUT

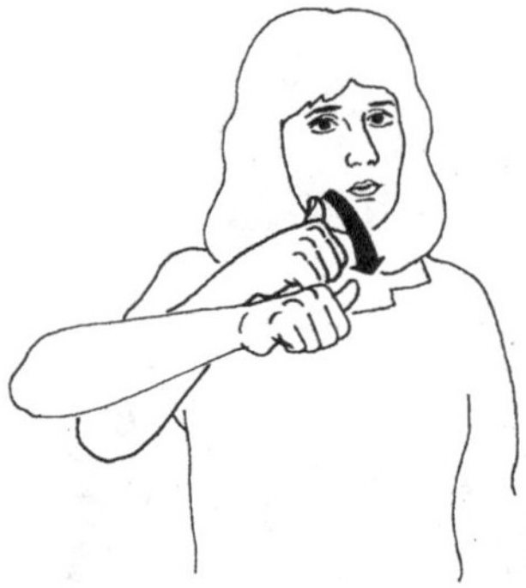

GIRL

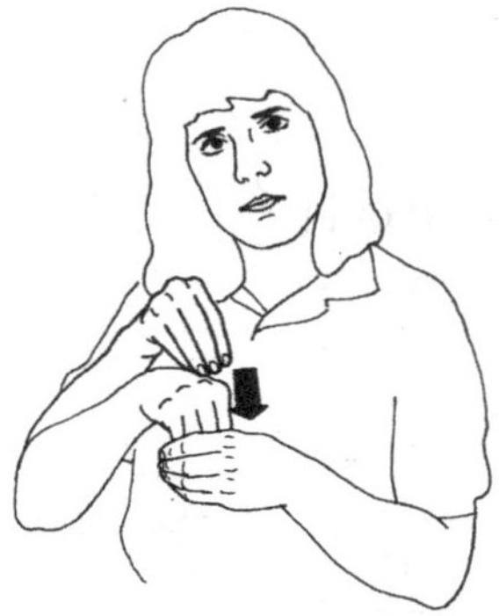

IN

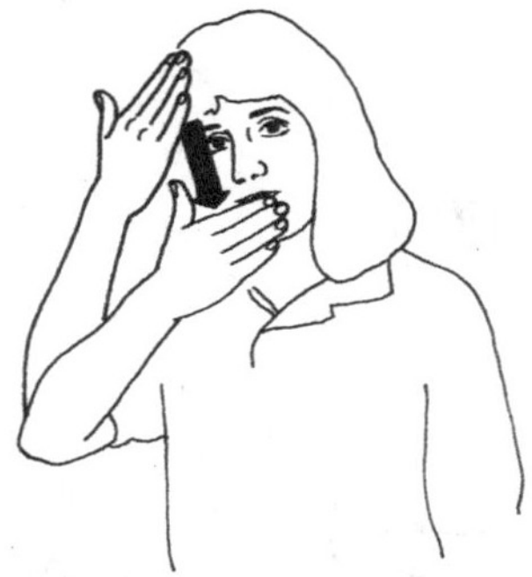

FRONT

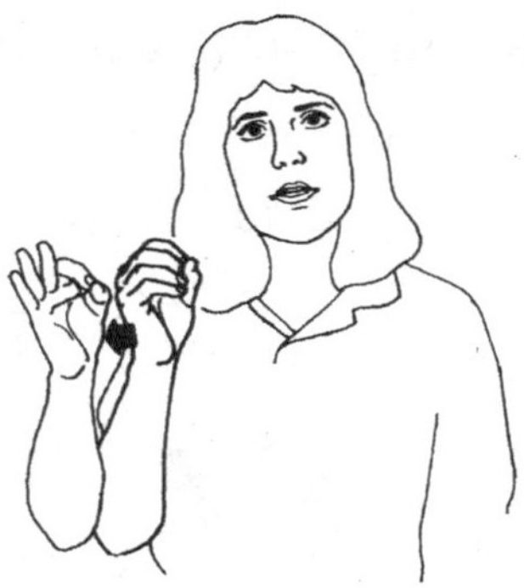

OF

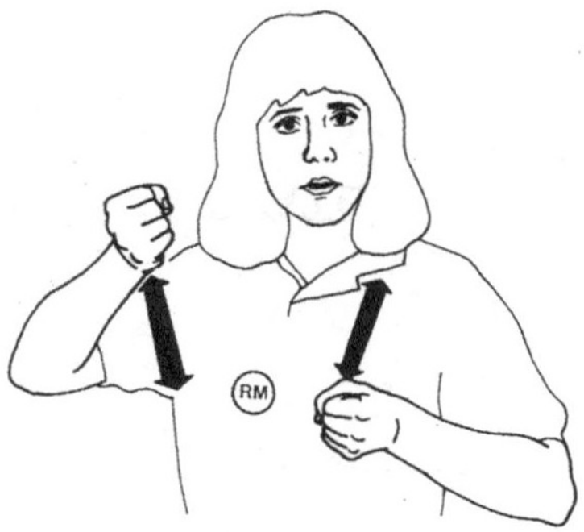

CAR.

Put the girl in front of the car.

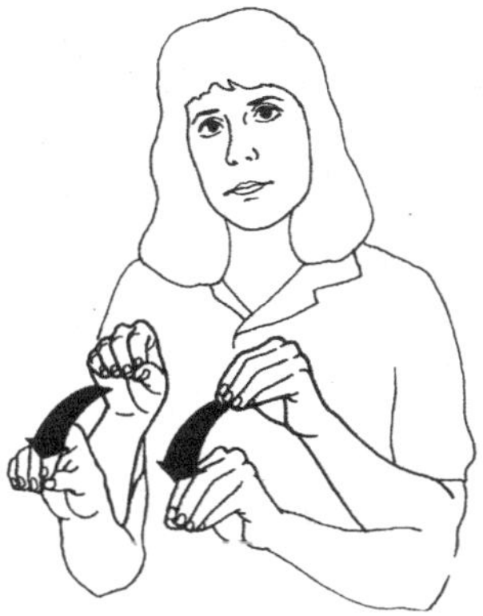

PUT

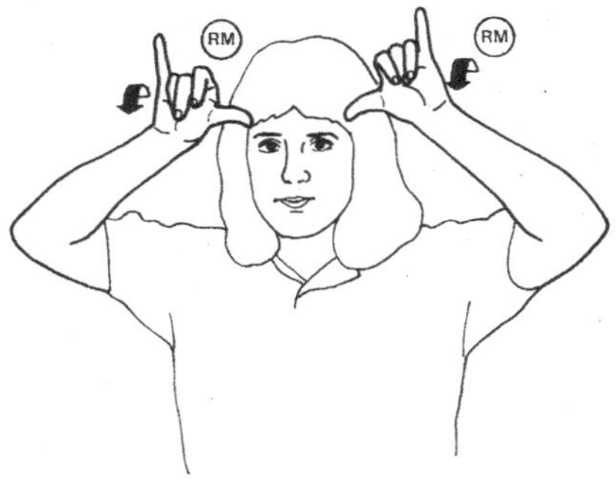

COW

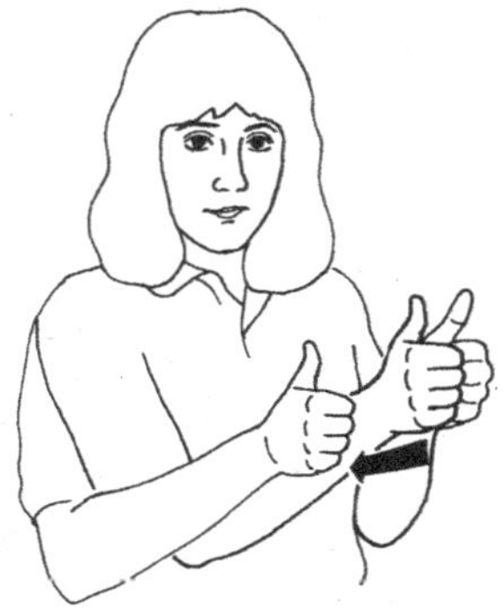

BEHIND

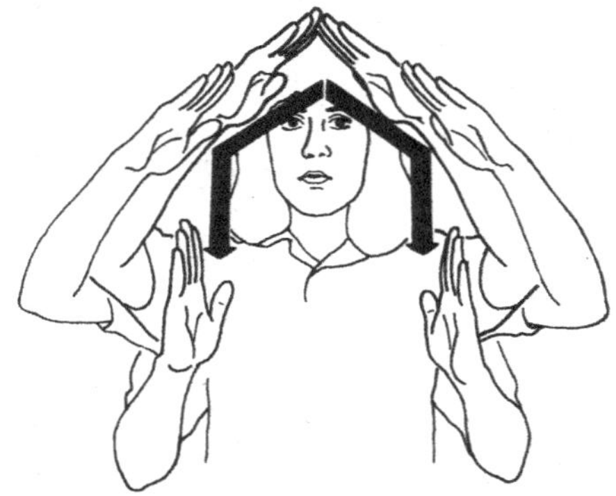

HOUSE.

Put the cow behind the house.

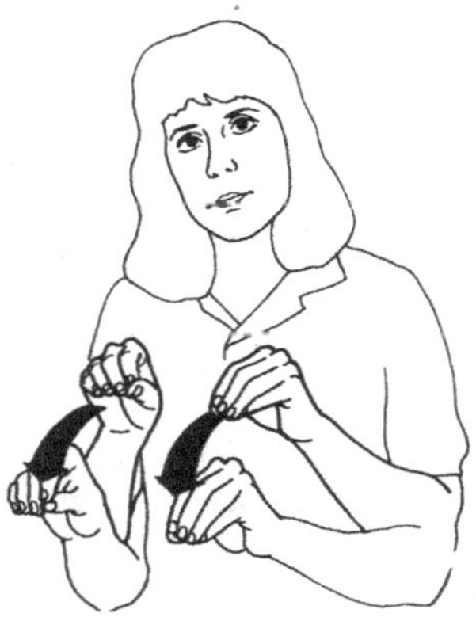

PUT

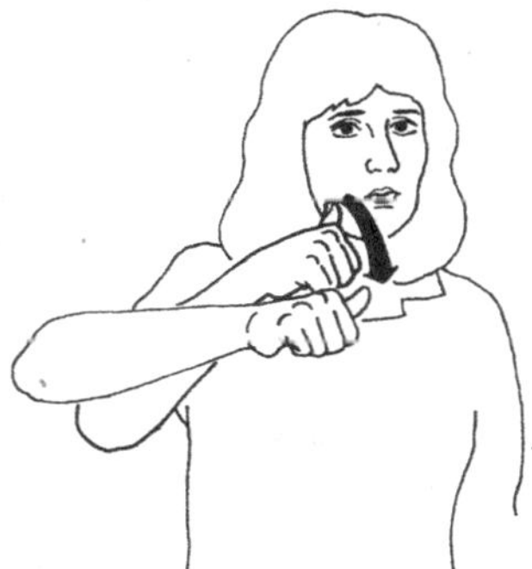

GIRL

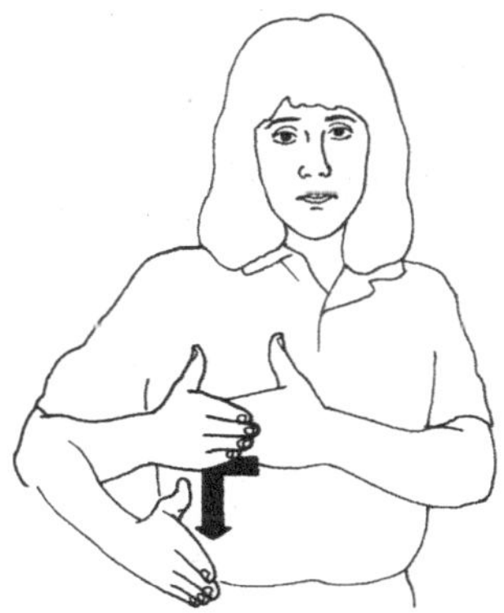

BESIDE

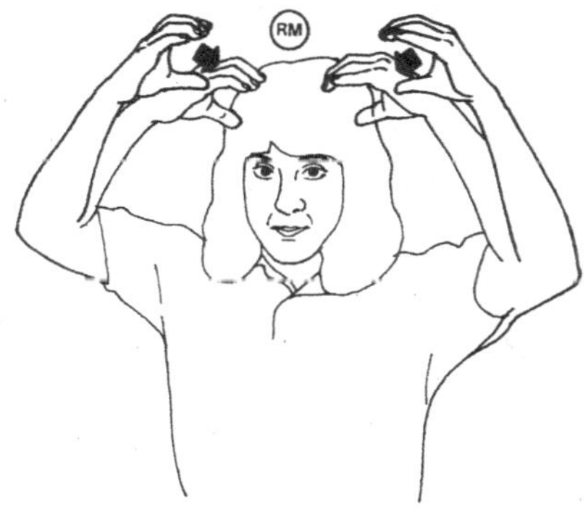

MICKEY-MOUSE.

Put the girl beside Mickey Mouse.

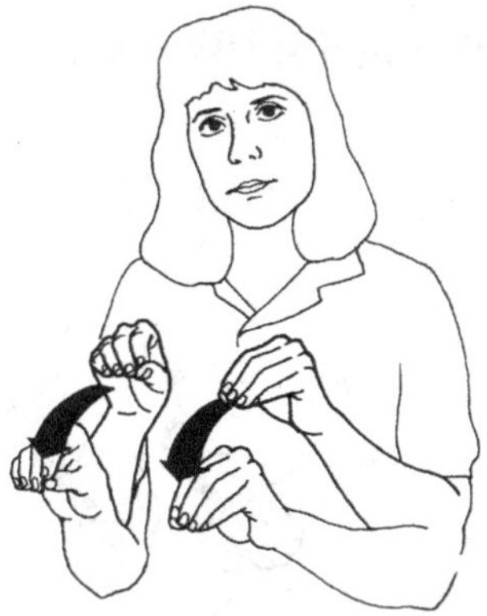

PUT

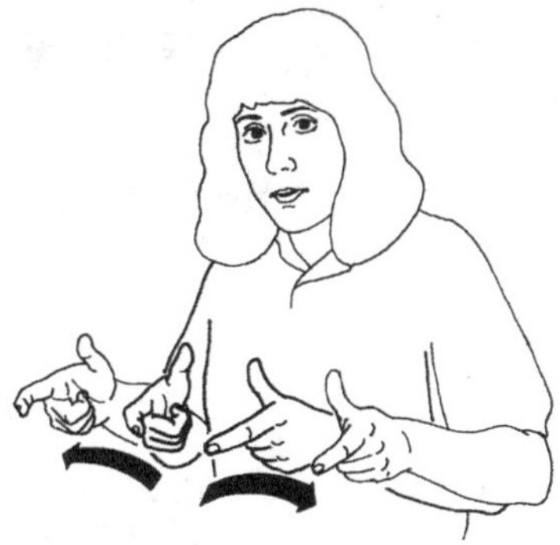

LARGE

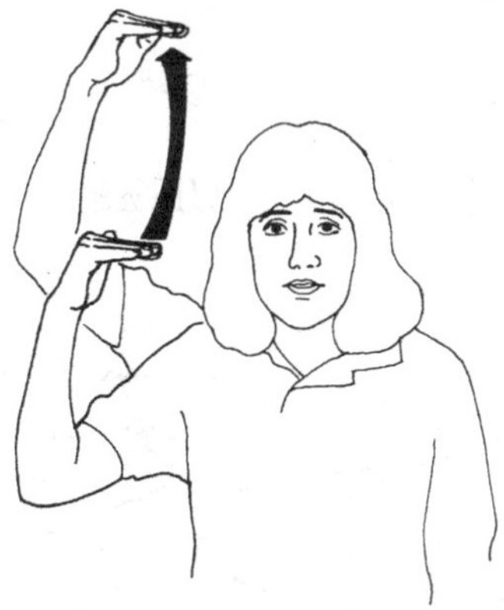

TALL

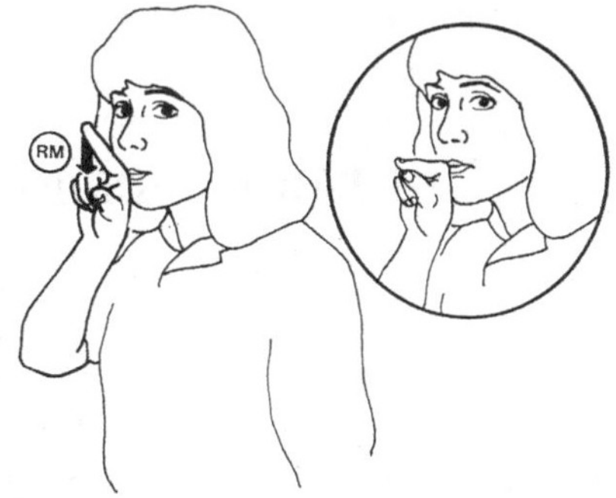

BIRD

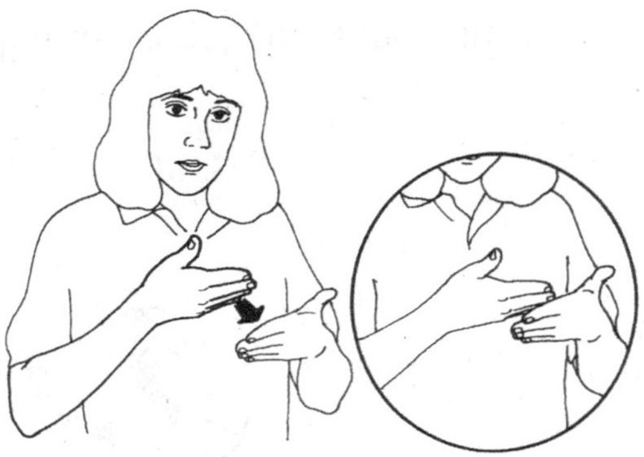

NEAR

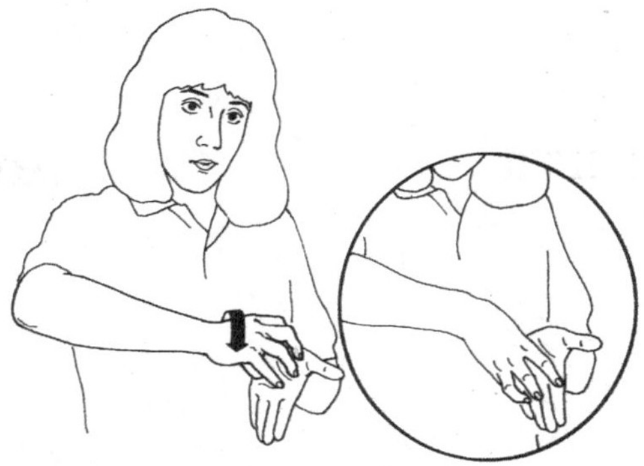

COOKIE

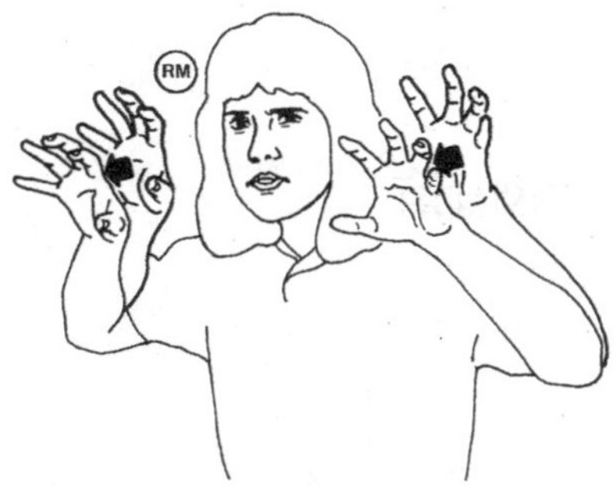

MONSTER.

Put Big Bird near Cookie Monster.

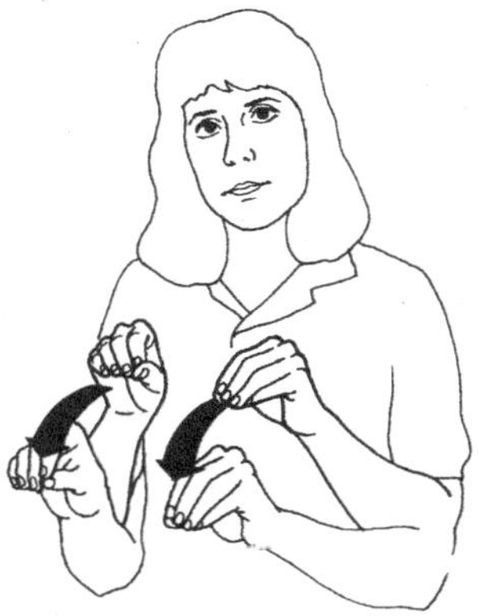

PUT

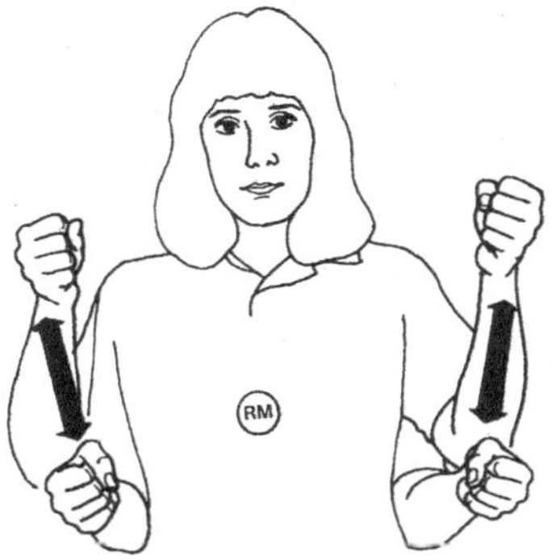

TRUCK

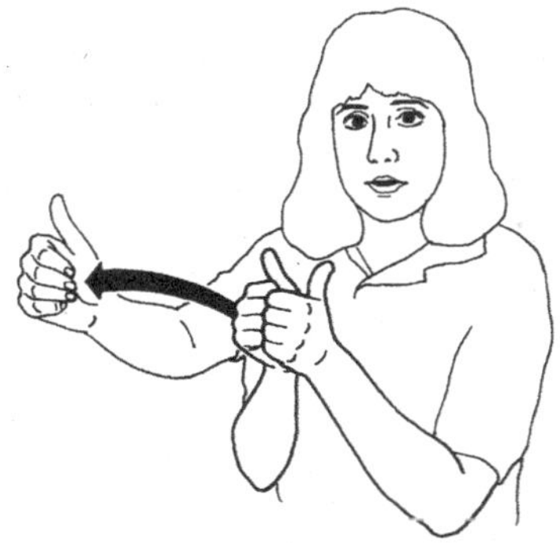

FAR

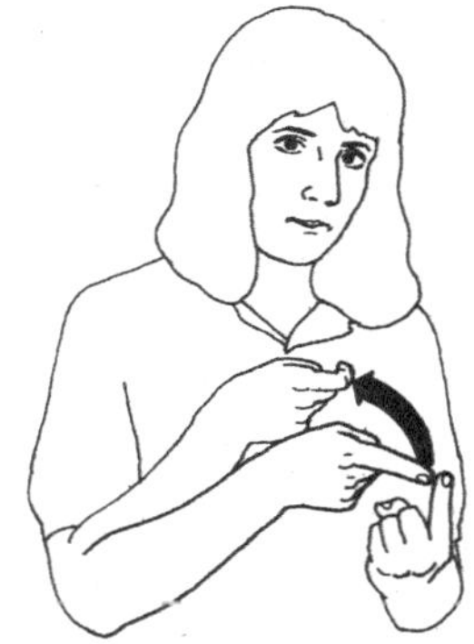

FROM

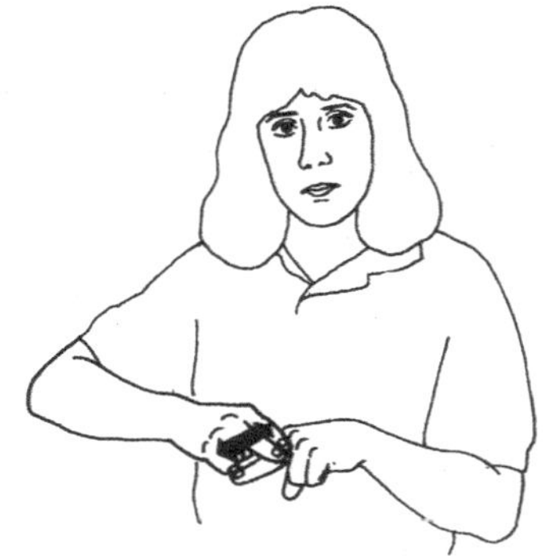

TRAIN.

Put the truck far from the train.

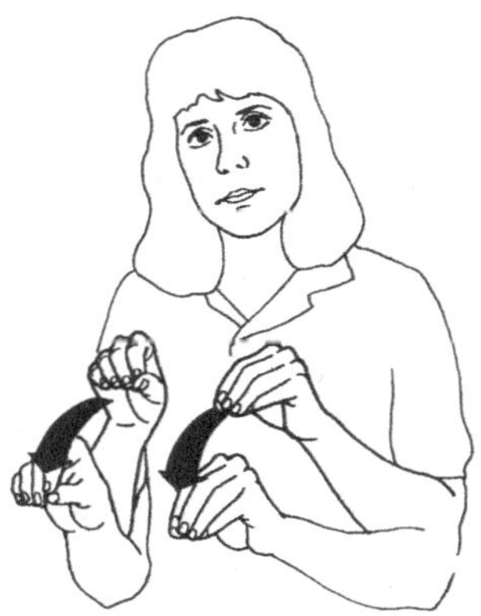

PUT

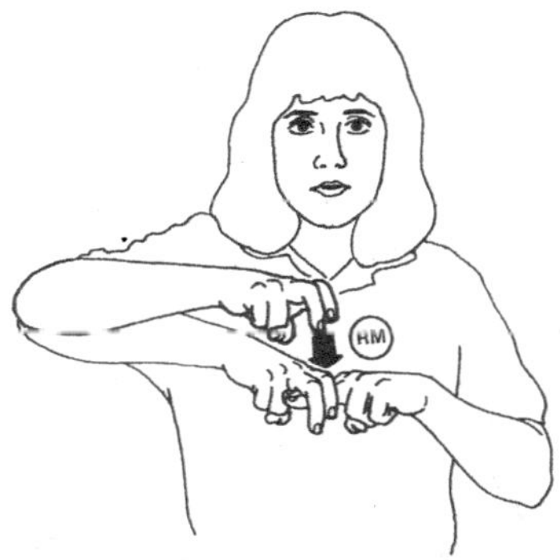

CHAIR

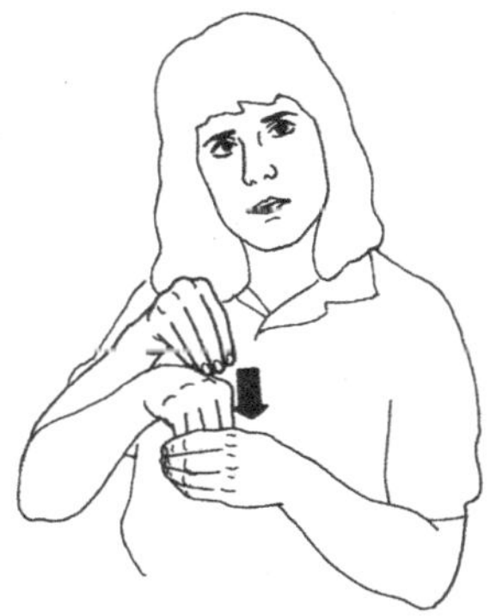

IN

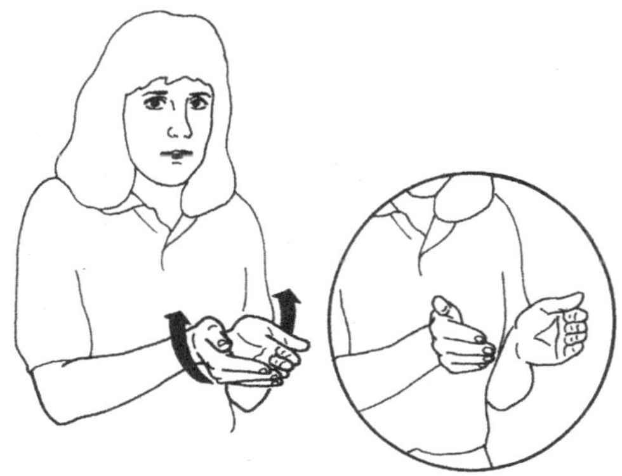

BOWL.

Put the chair in the bowl.

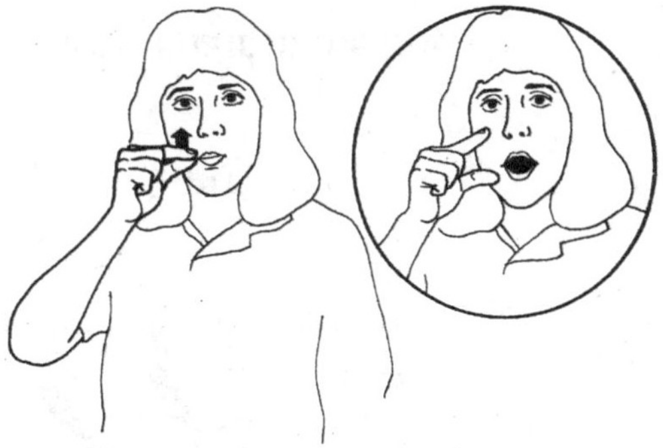

OPEN

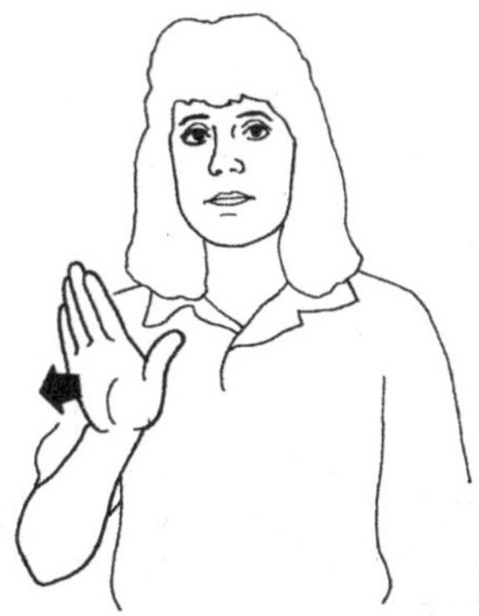

YOUR

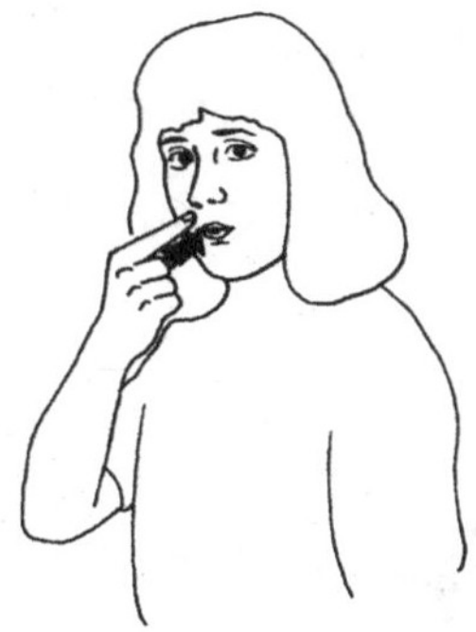

MOUTH.

Open your mouth.

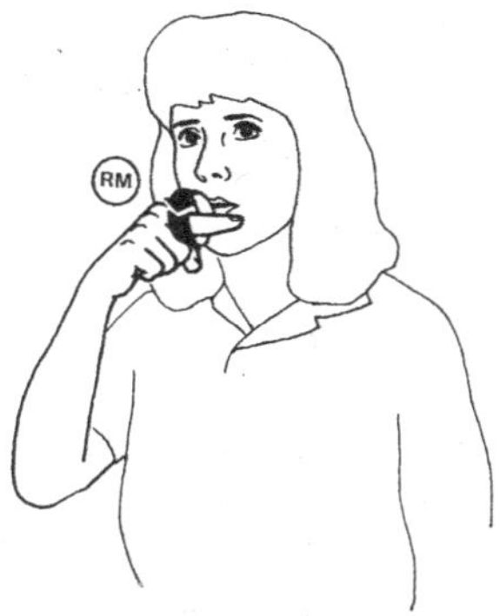

SAY

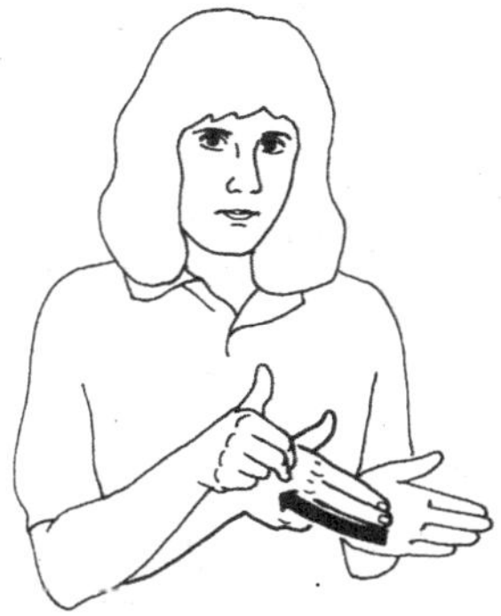

BUTTER

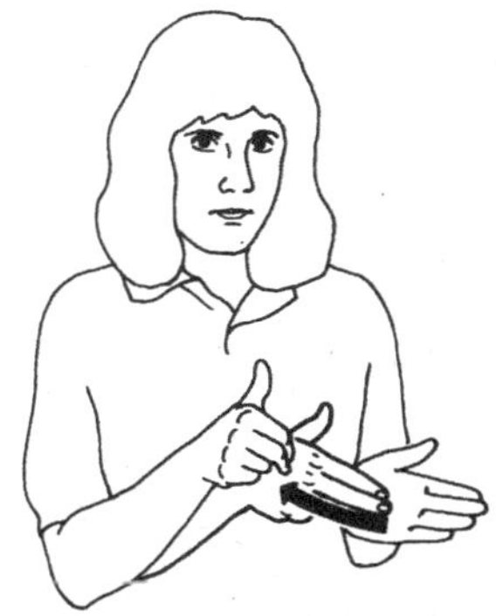

BUTTER

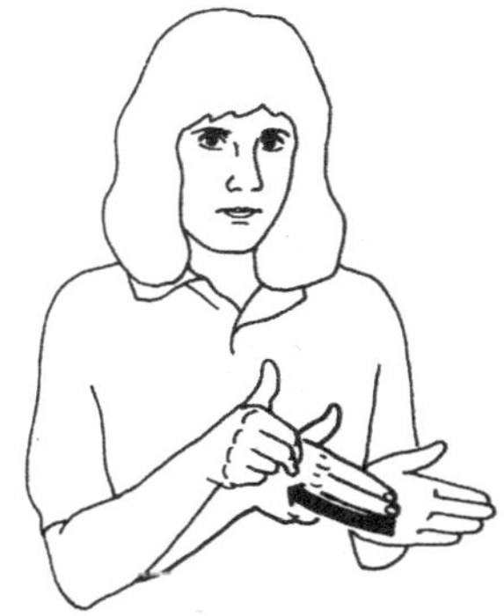

BUTTER

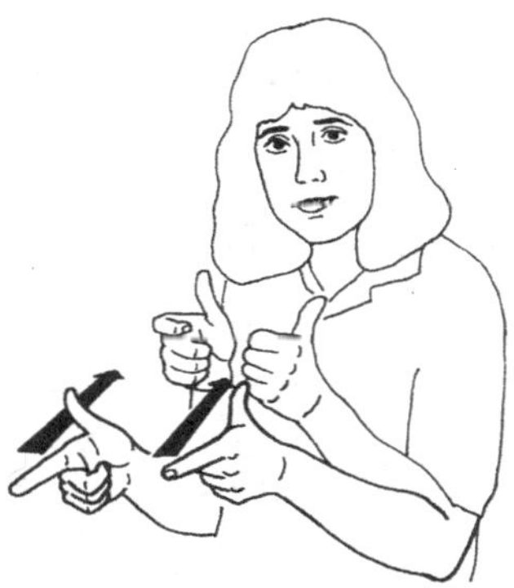

FAST

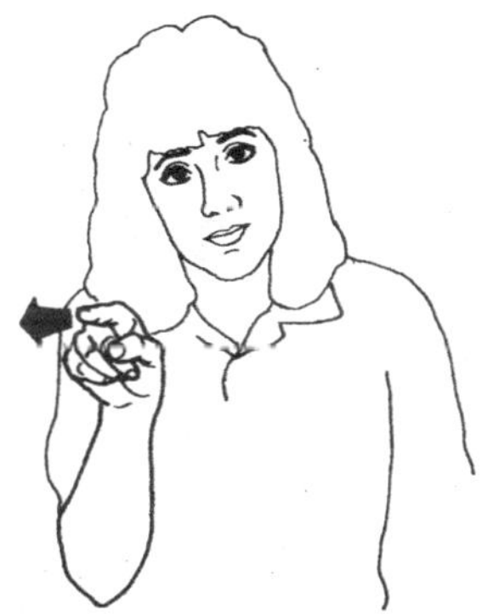

YOU

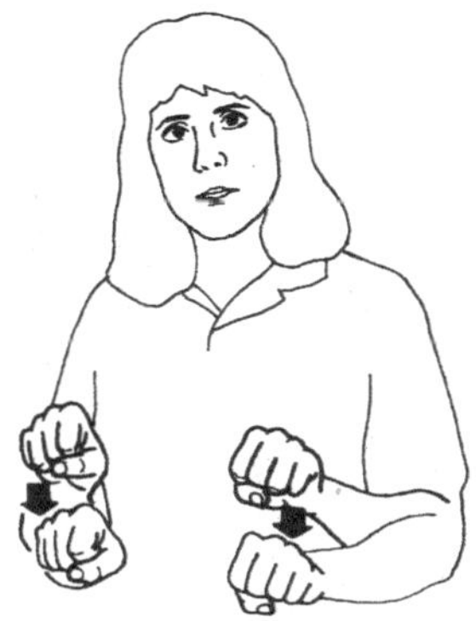

CAN.

Say butter-butter-butter as fast as you can.

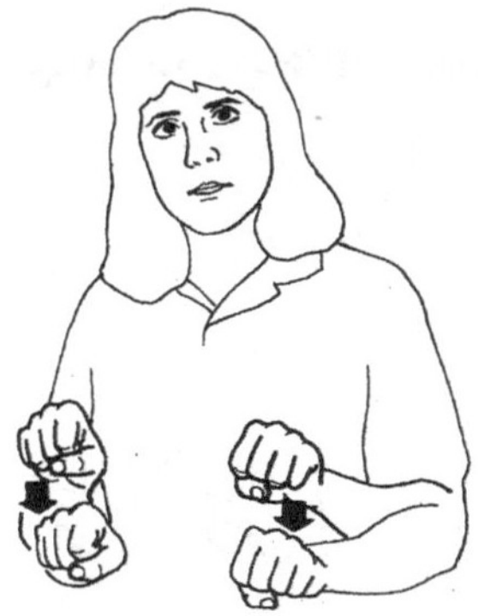

CAN

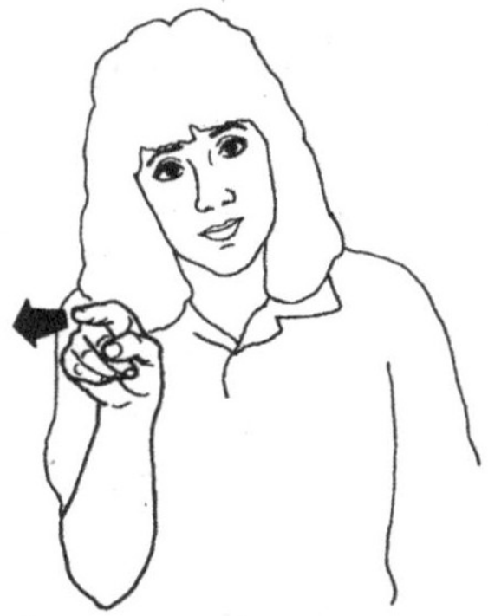

YOU

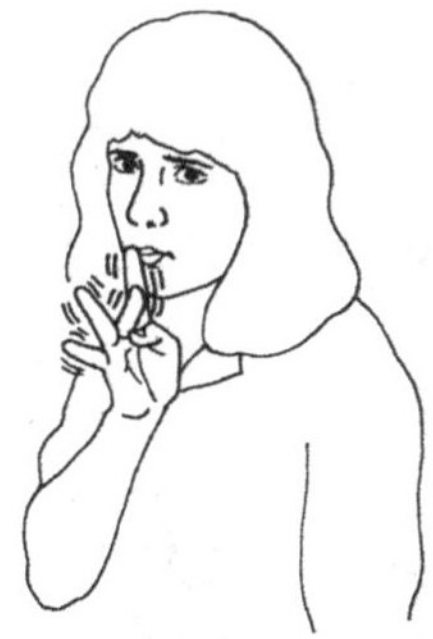

WHISPER?

Can you whisper?

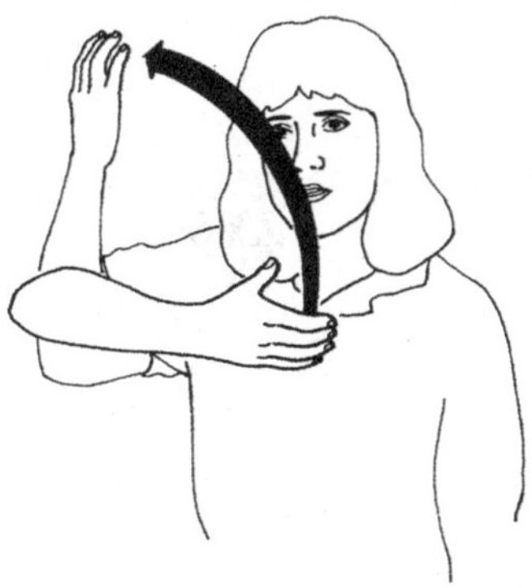

YELL

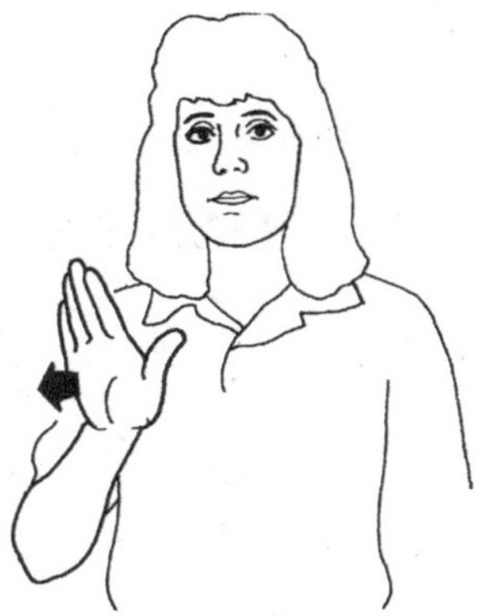

YOUR

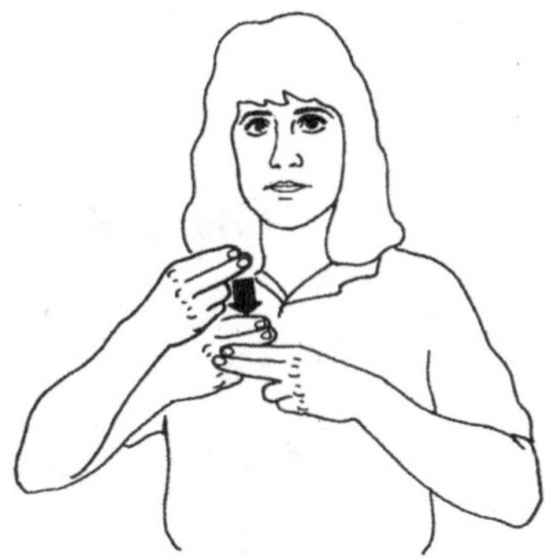

NAME.

Yell your name.

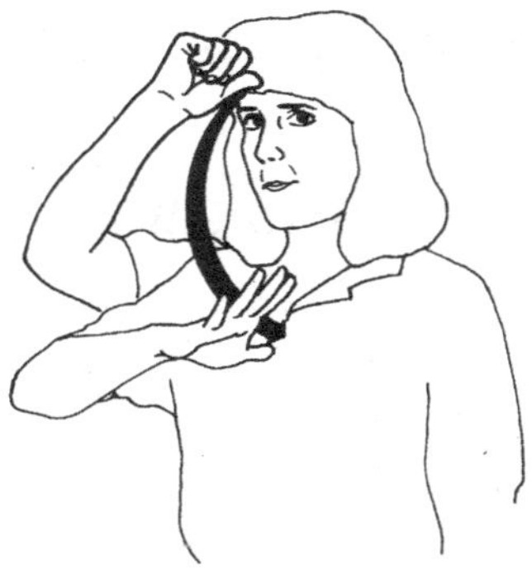

MAN

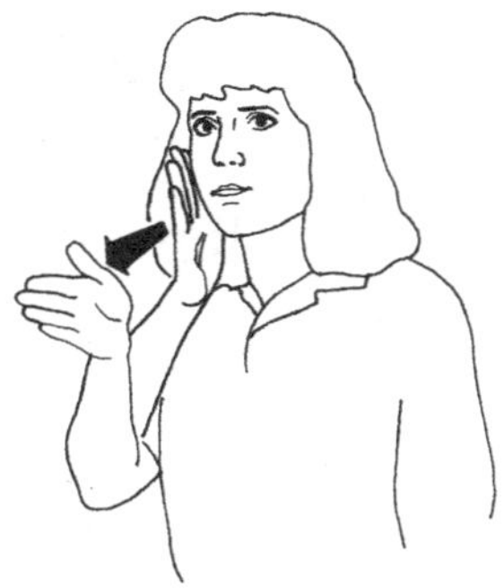

WILL

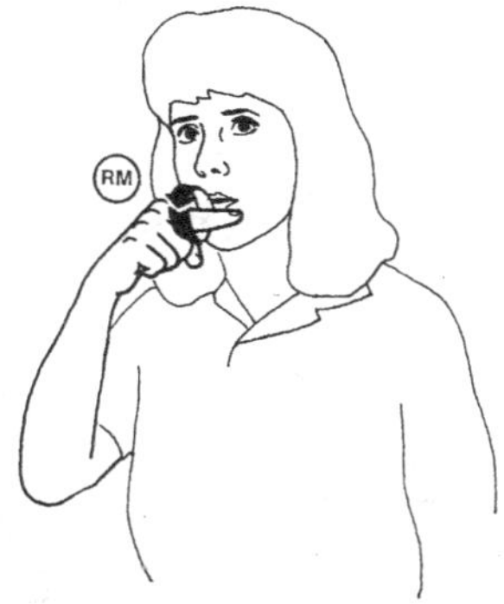

SAY

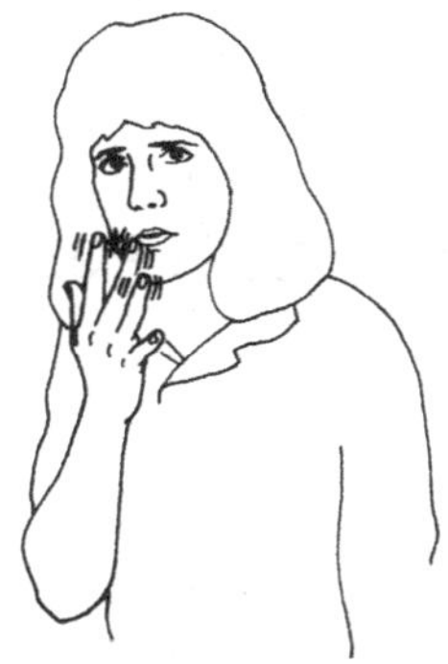

COLOR.

The man will say color.

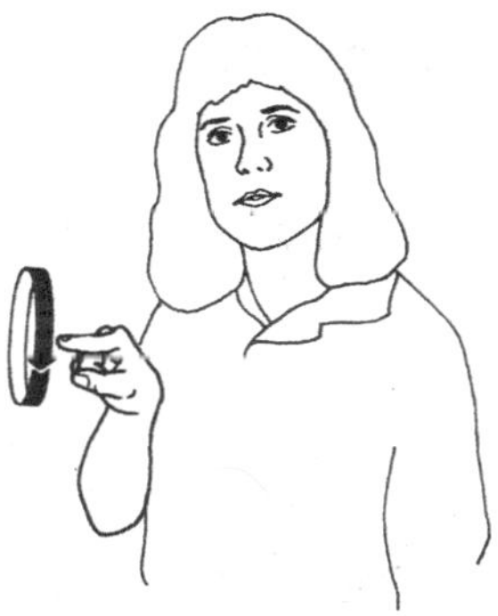

CIRCLE

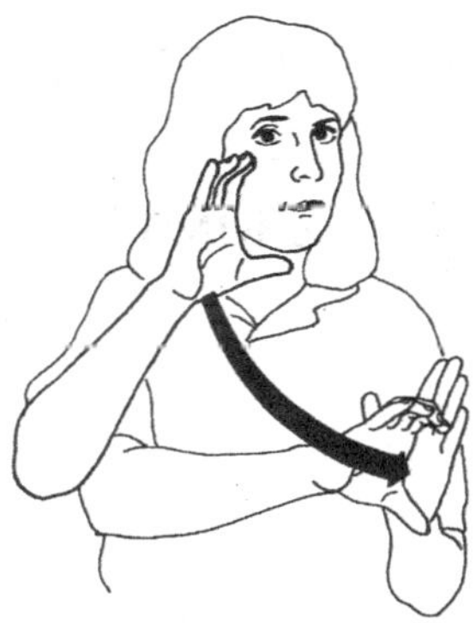

PICTURE

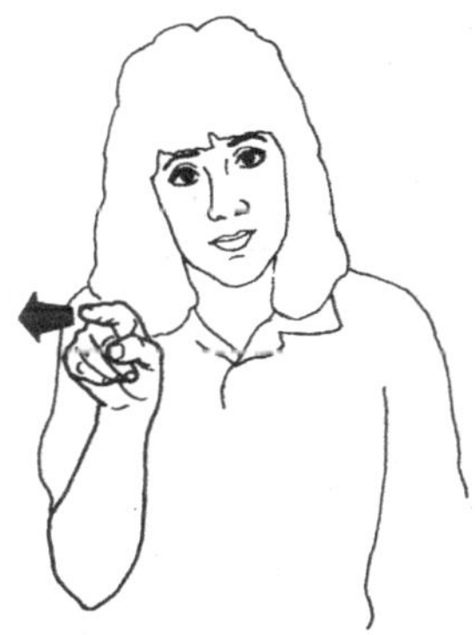

YOU

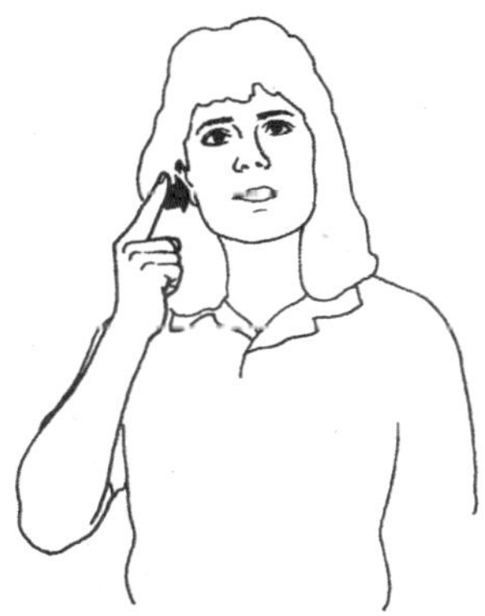

HEAR.

Circle the picture you hear.

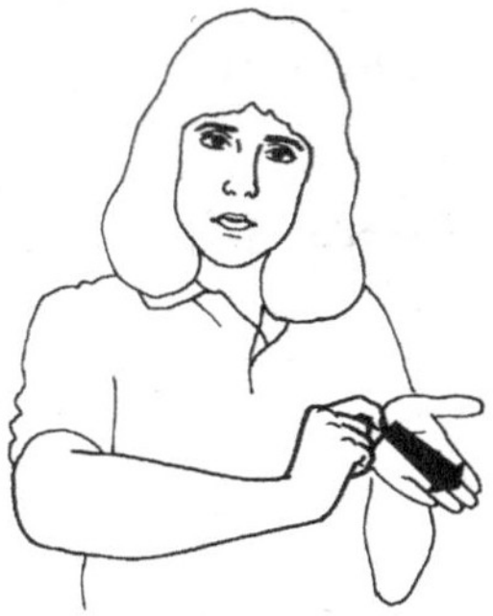

DRAW-LINE

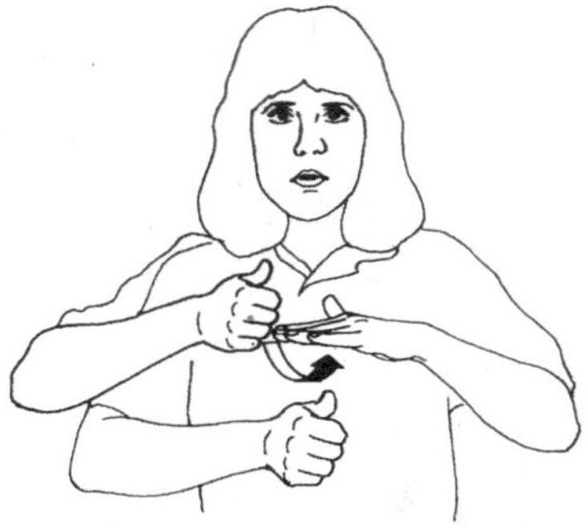

UNDER

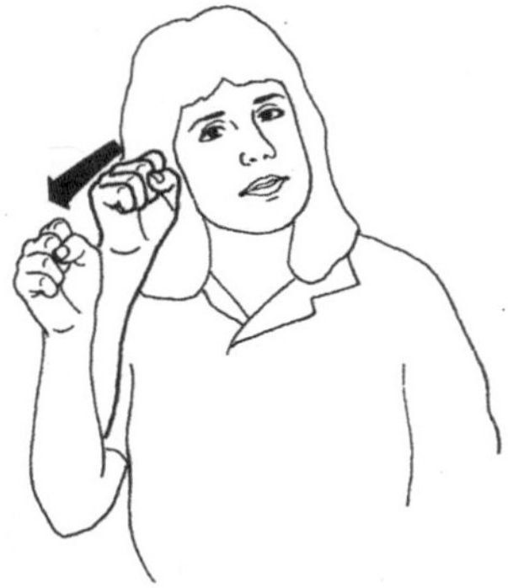

SOUND

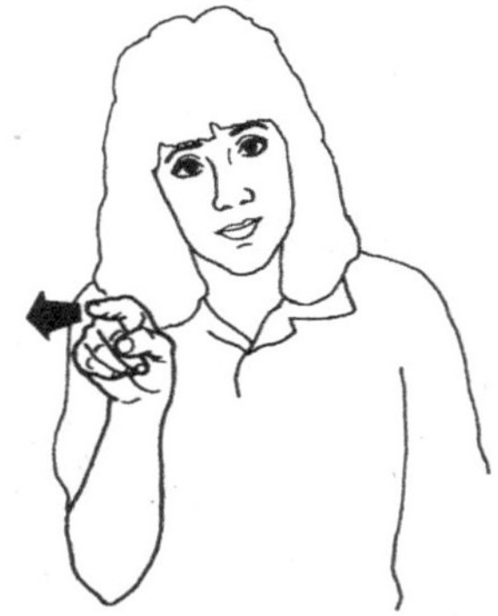

YOU

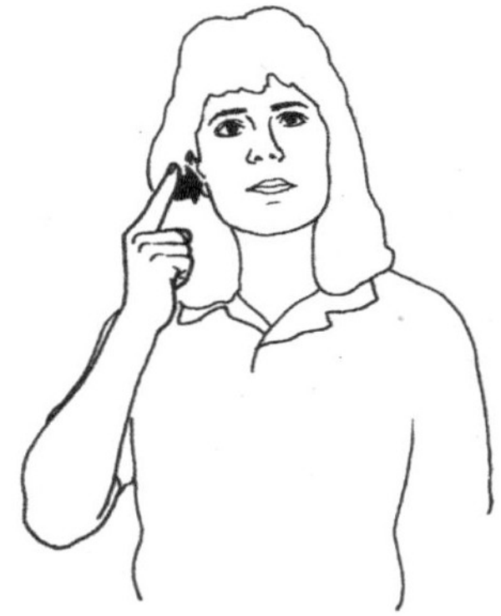

HEAR.

Draw a line under the sound you hear.

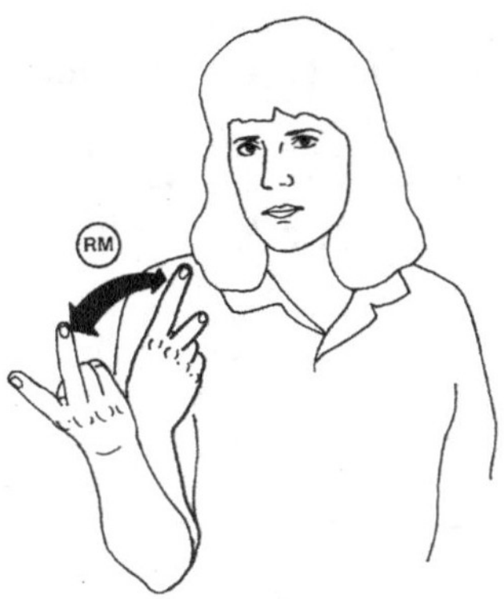

TWO-OF-US

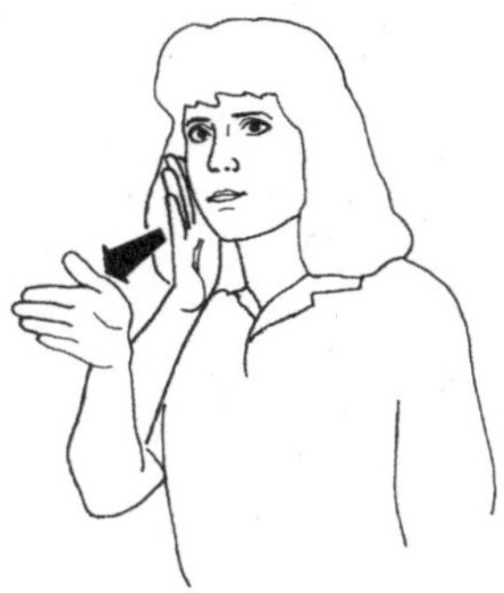

WILL

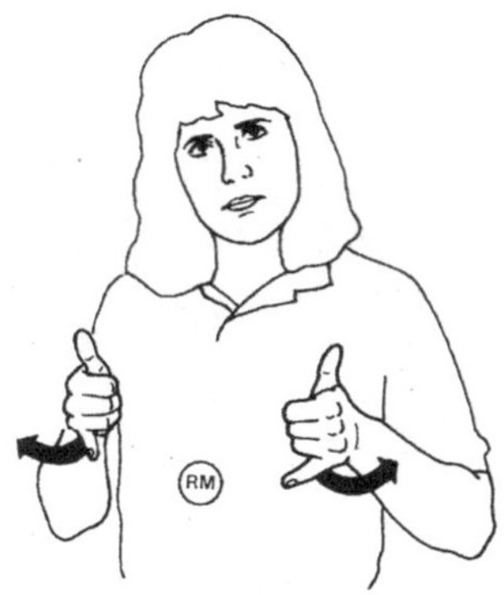

PLAY

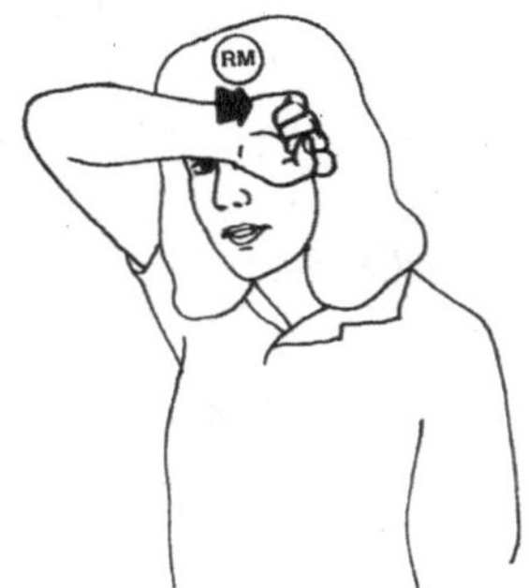

HIDE-SEEK.

Both of us will play hide and seek.

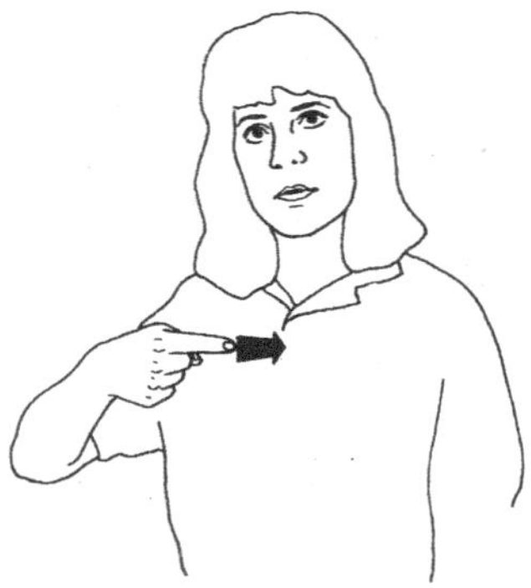

I

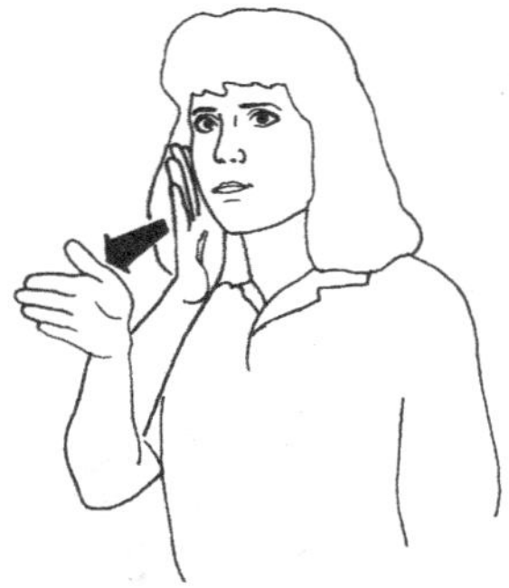

WILL

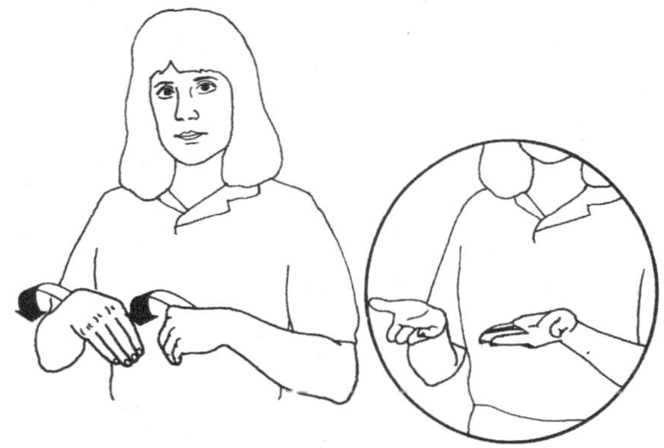

PROVIDE

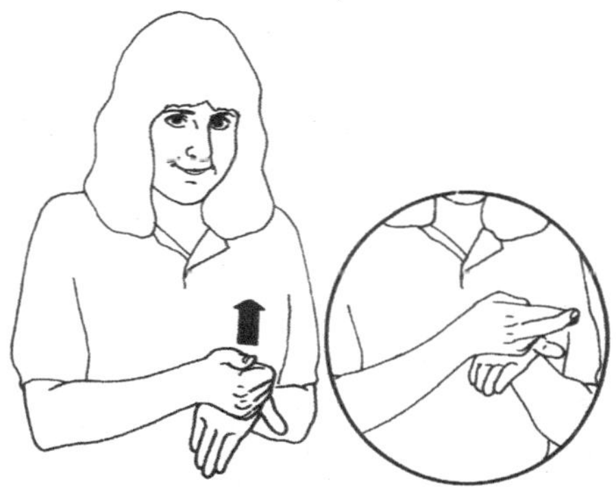

A-R

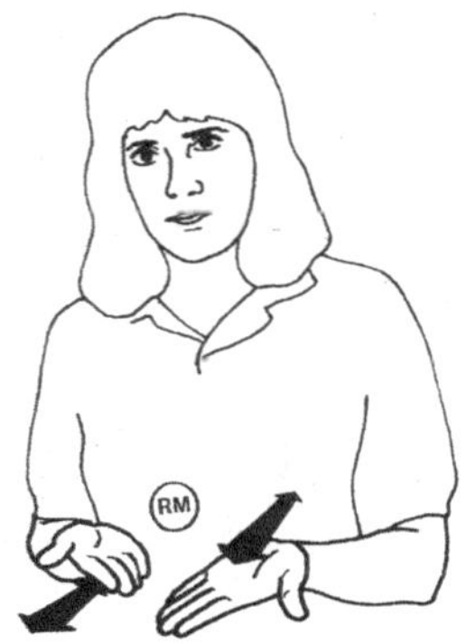

SERVICE.

I will provide aural rehabilitation service.

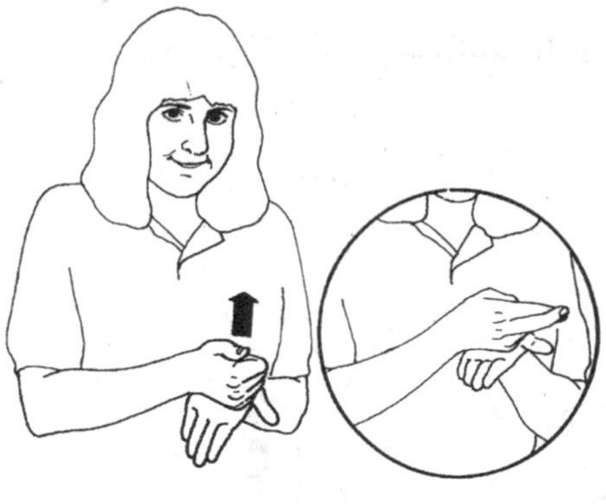

A-R

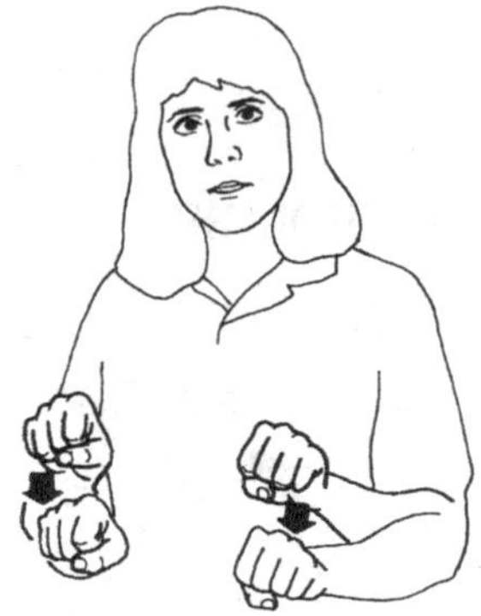

CAN

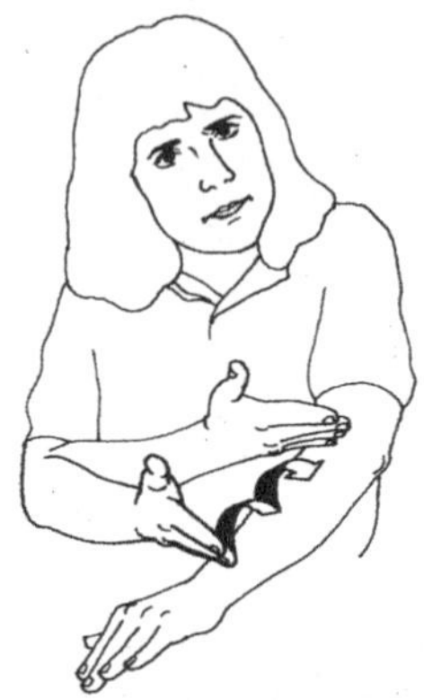

IMPROVE

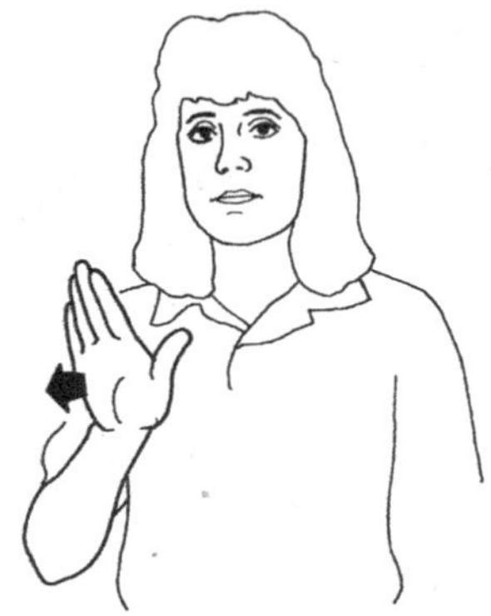

YOUR

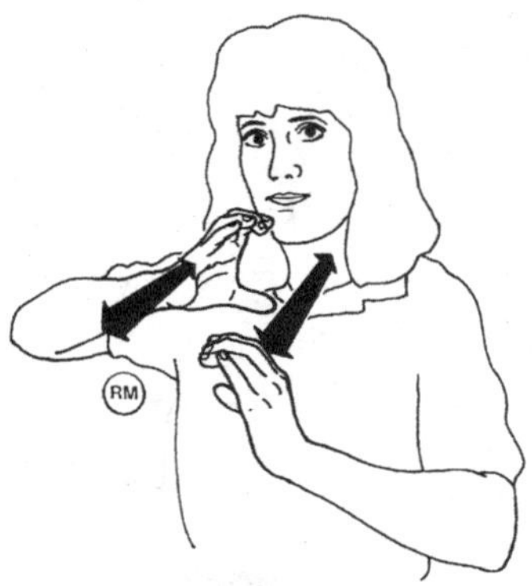

COMMUNICATION

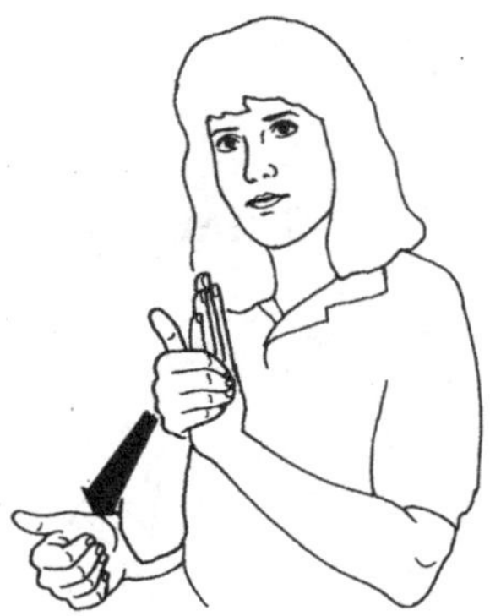

SKILLS

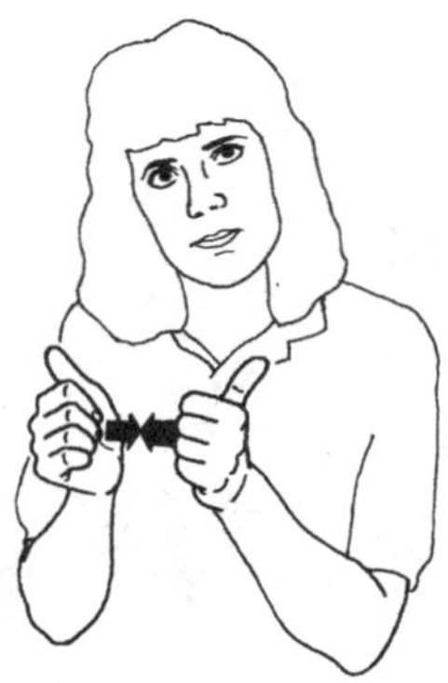

WITH

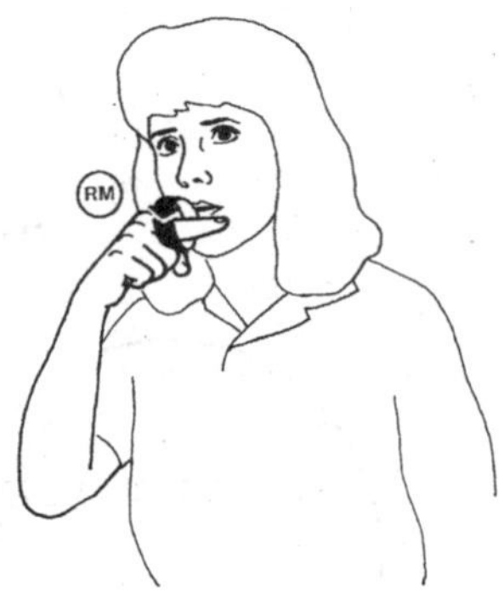

HEARING

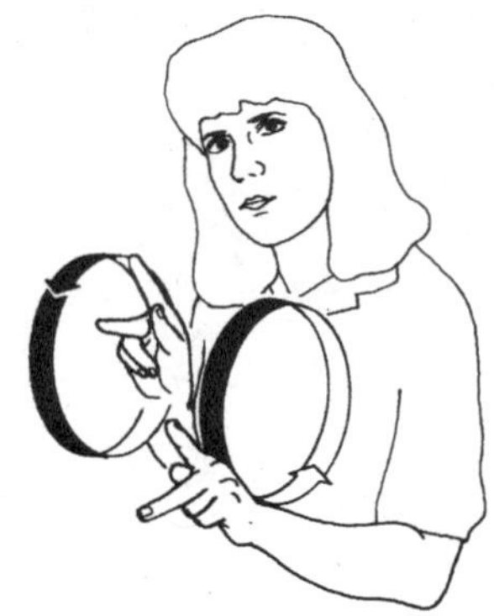

PEOPLE.

Aural rehabilitation can improve your communication skills with hearing people.

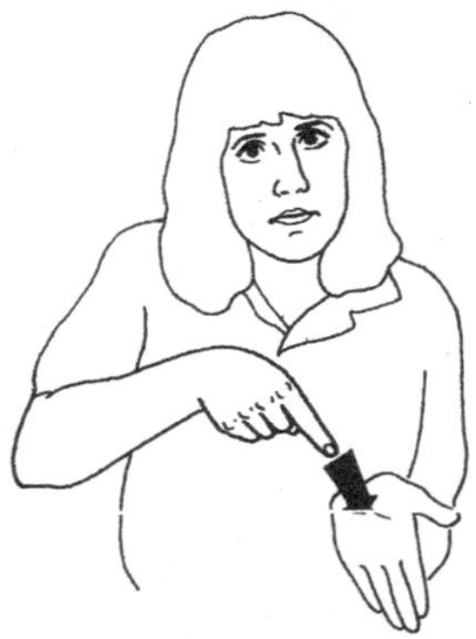

THIS

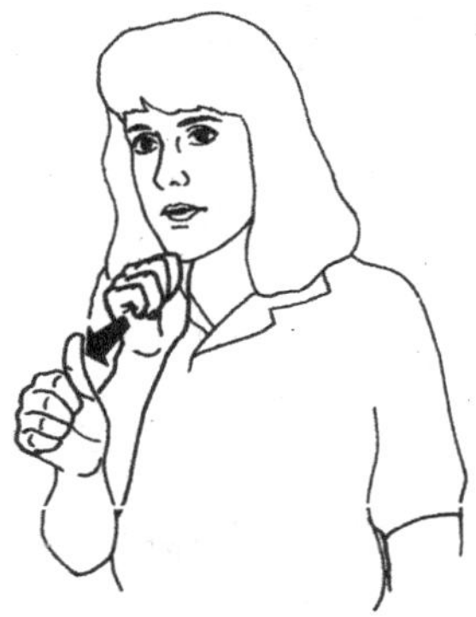

NOT

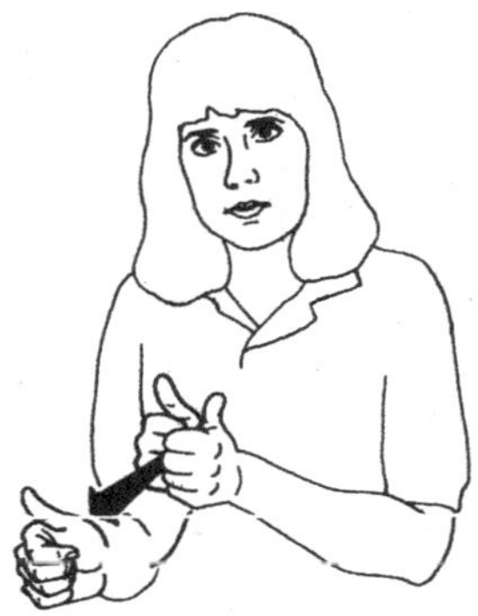

PASS

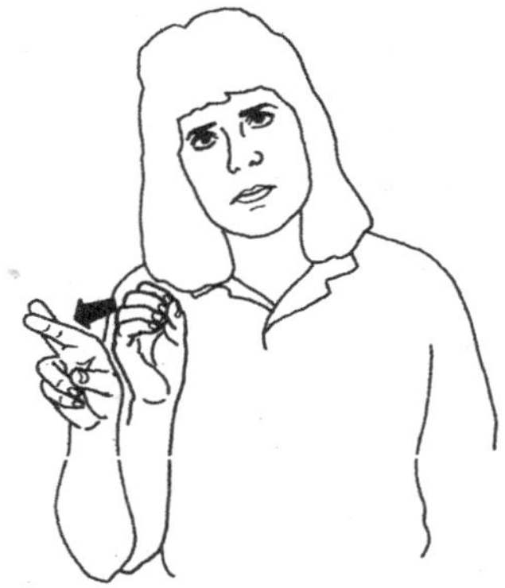

O-R

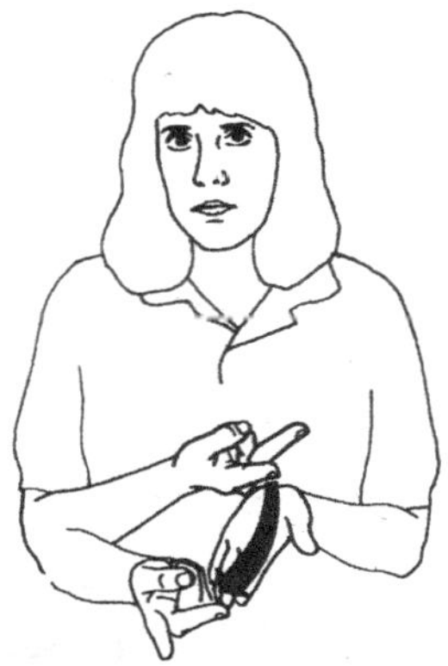

FAIL

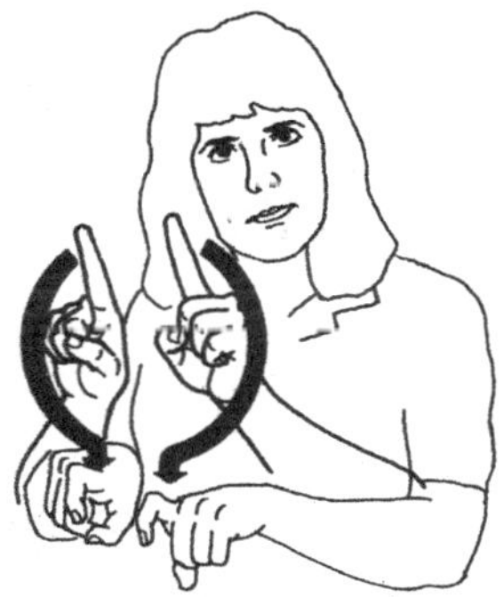

TEST.

This is not a pass or fail test.

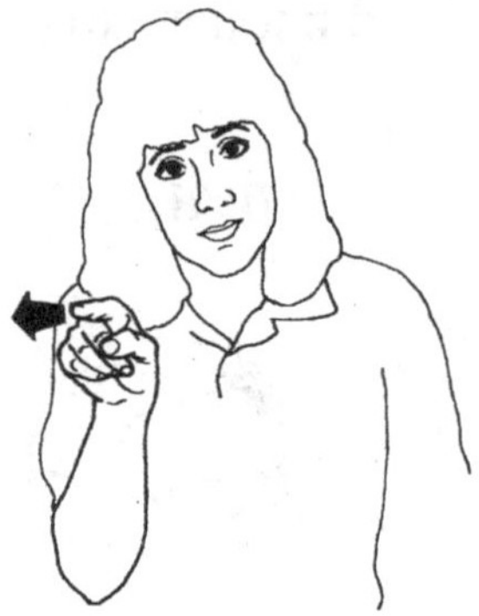

YOU

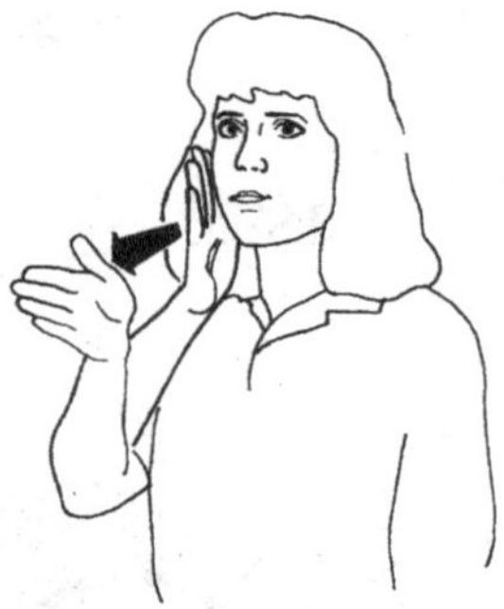

WILL

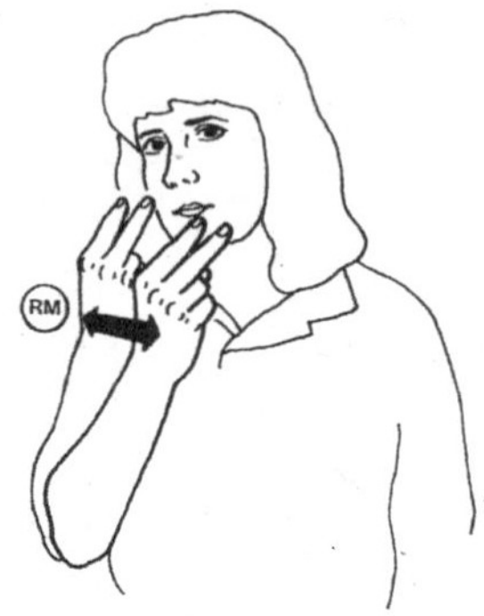

SPEECHREAD

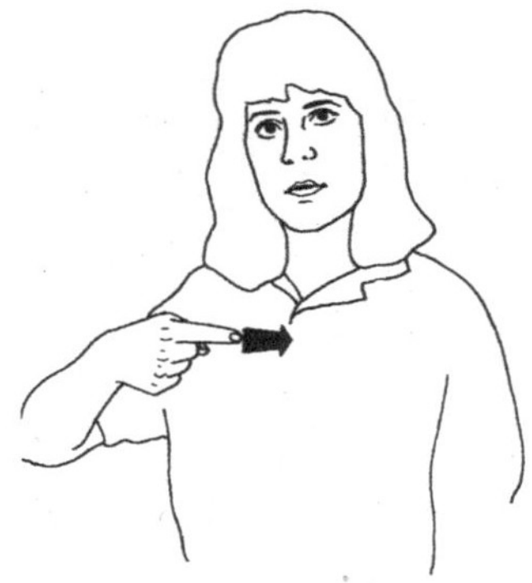

ME

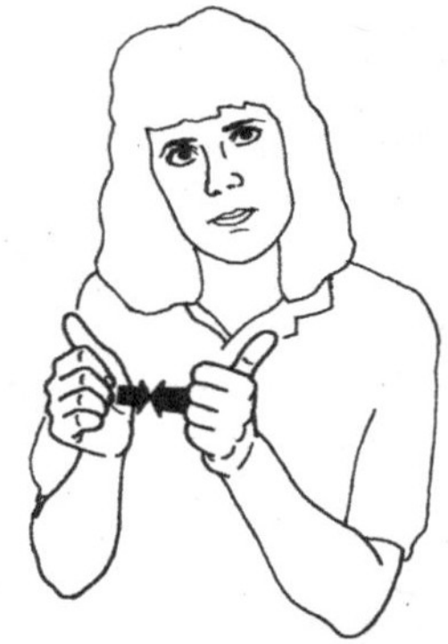

WITH

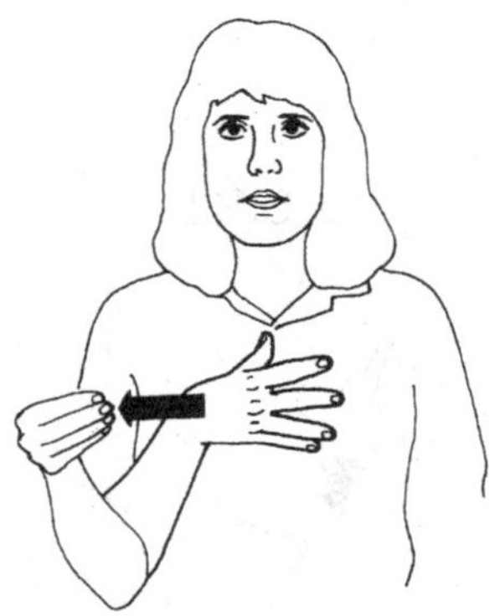

AND

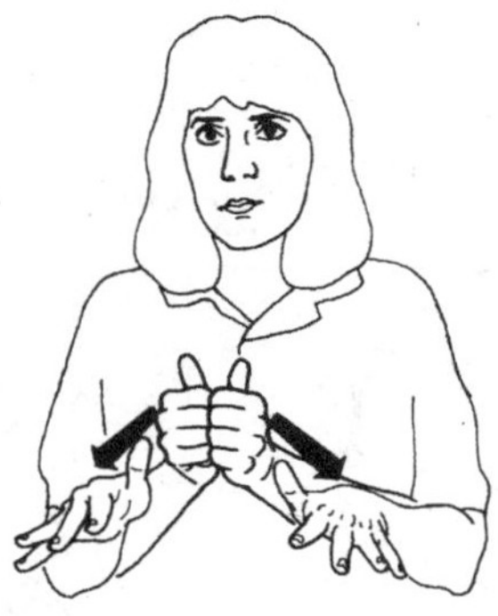

WITHOUT

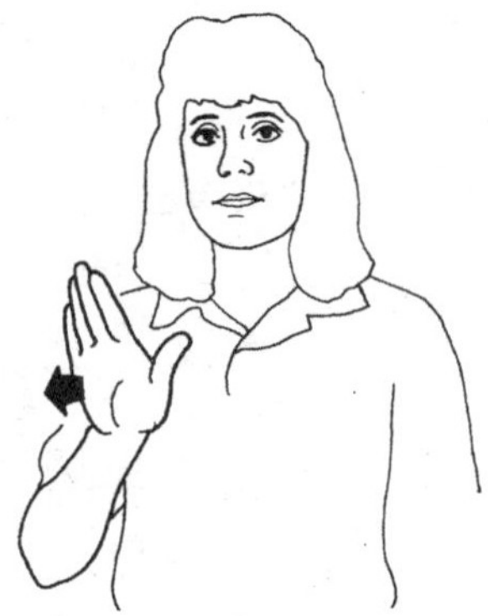

YOUR

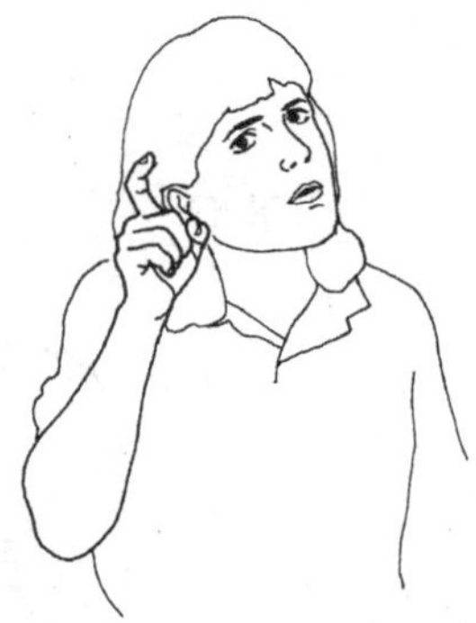

HEARING-AID.

You will speechread me with and without your hearing aid.

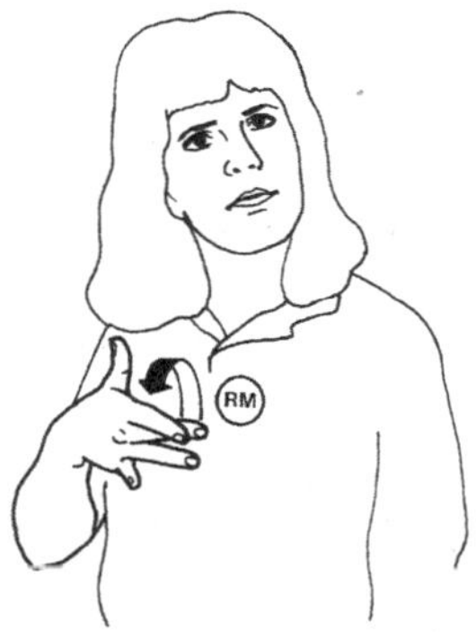

FEEL

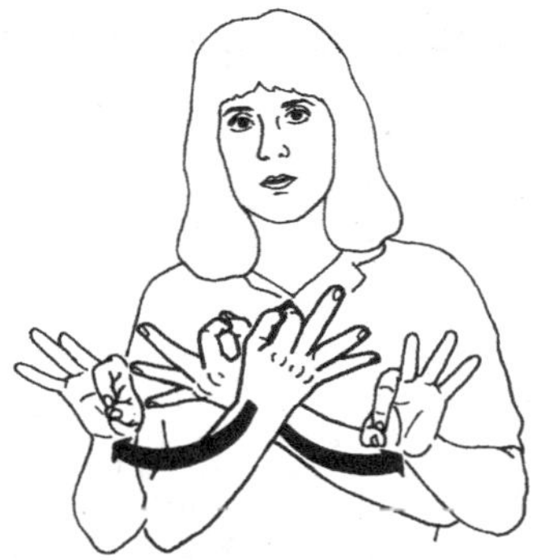

FREE

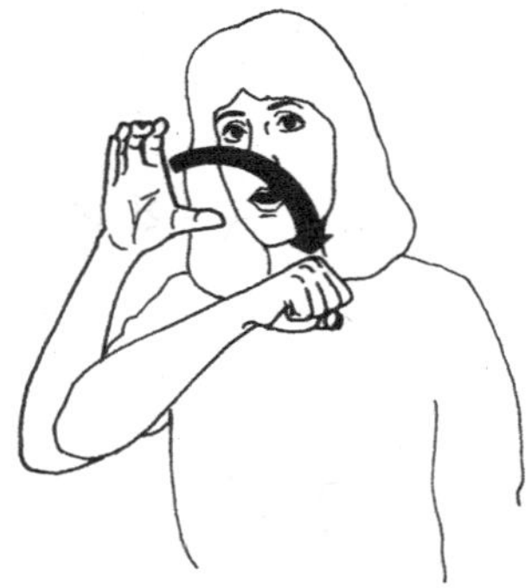

GUESS.

Feel free to guess.

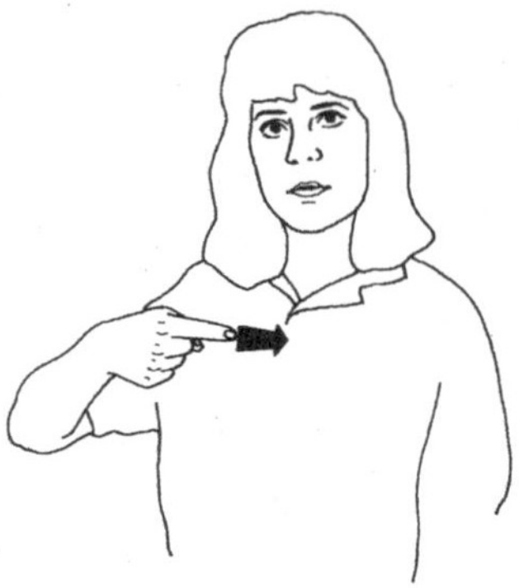

I

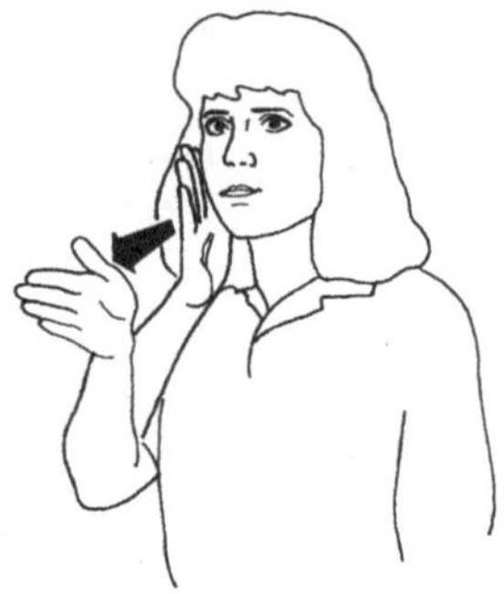

WILL

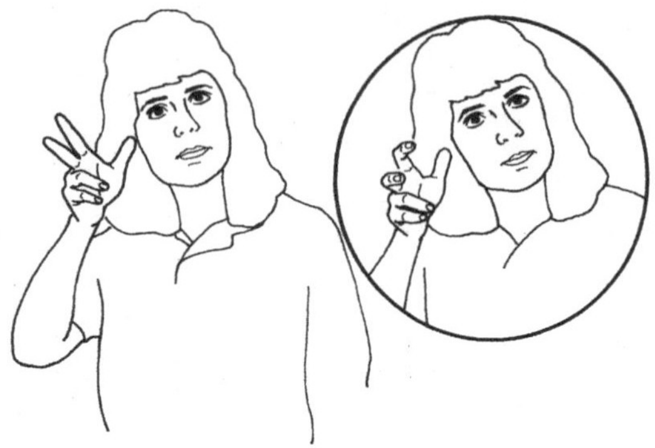

LISTEN

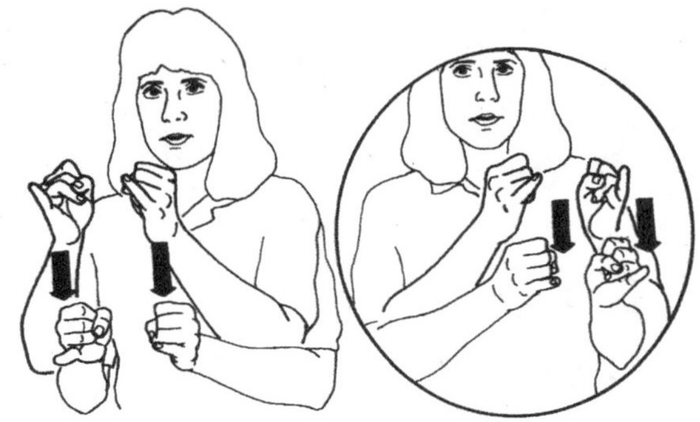

INDIVIDUAL

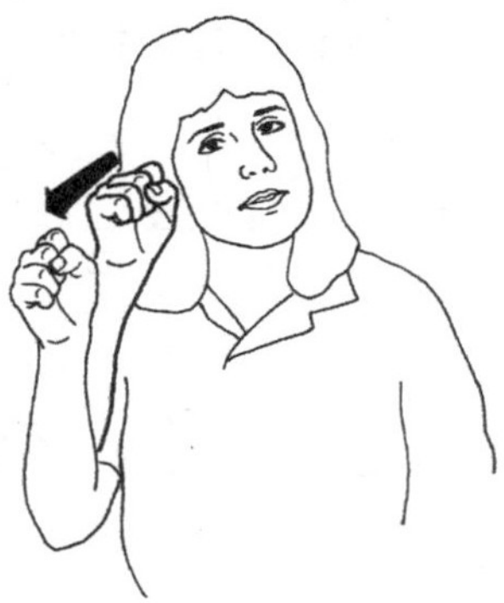

SOUND

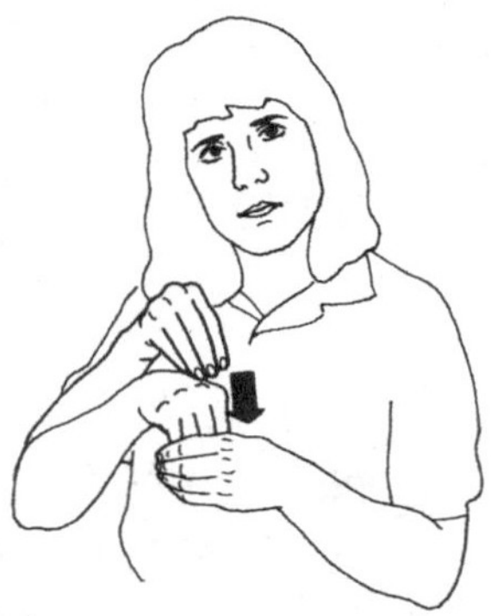

IN

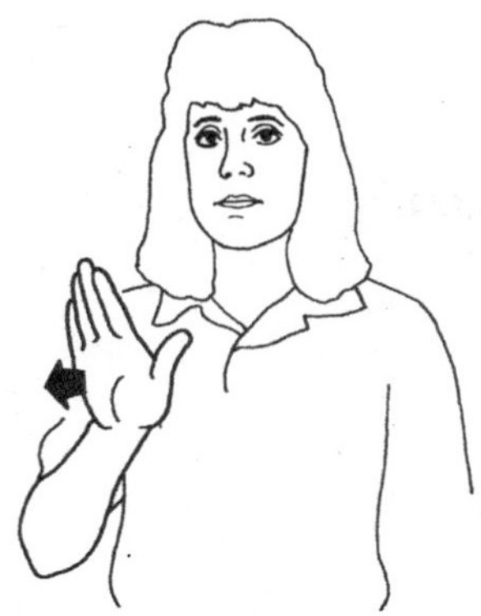

YOUR

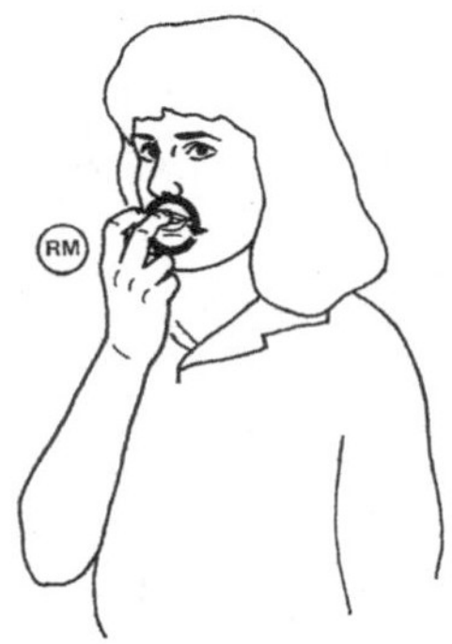

SPEECH.

I will listen to individual sounds in your speech.

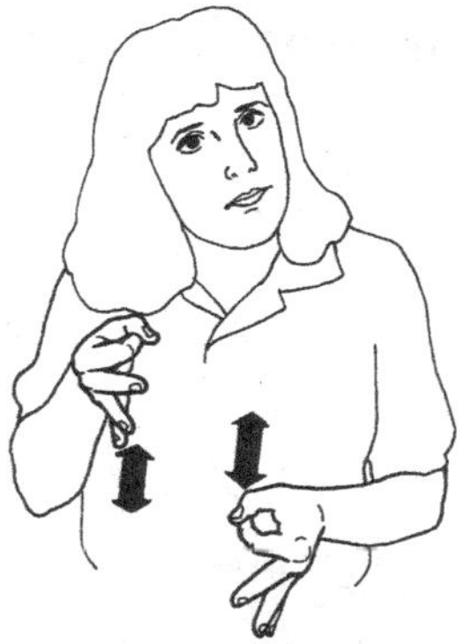

IF

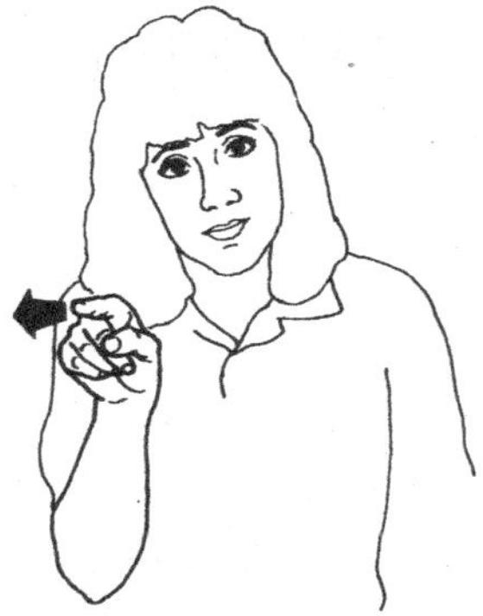

YOU

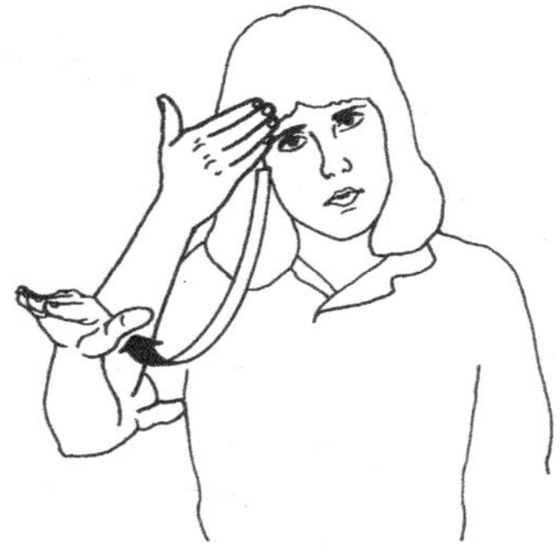

DON'T-KNOW

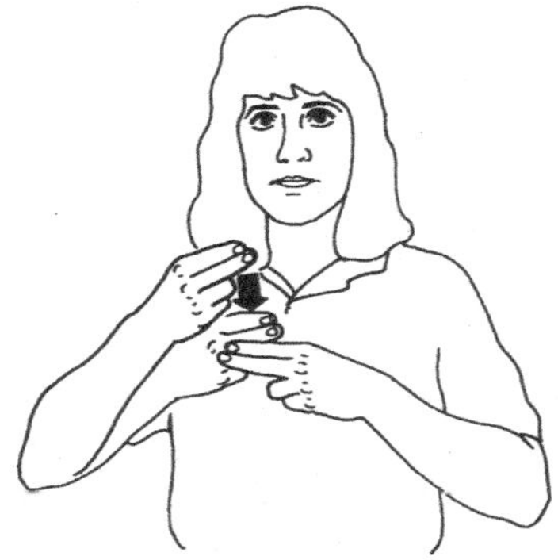

NAME

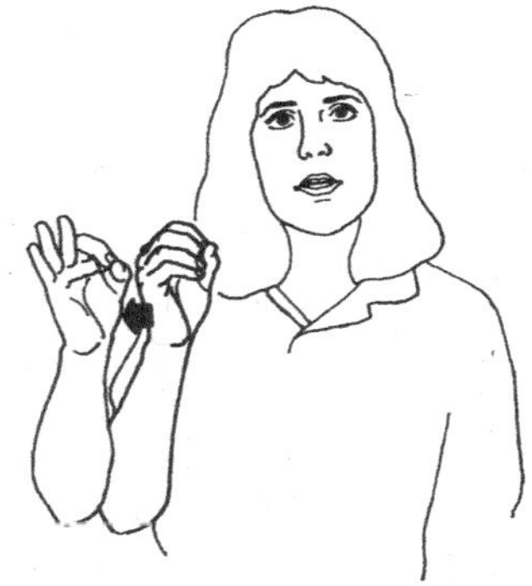

O-F

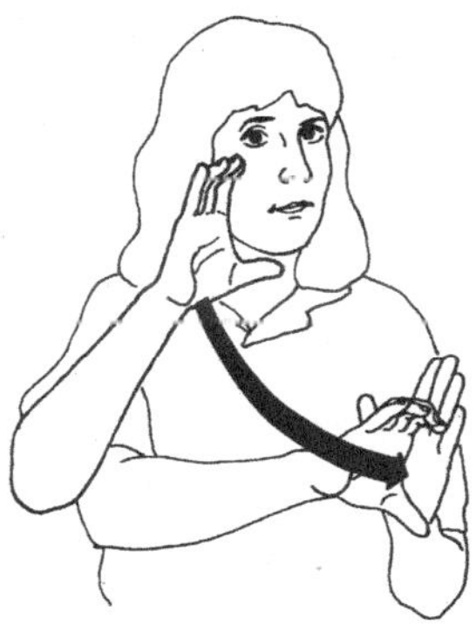

PICTURE

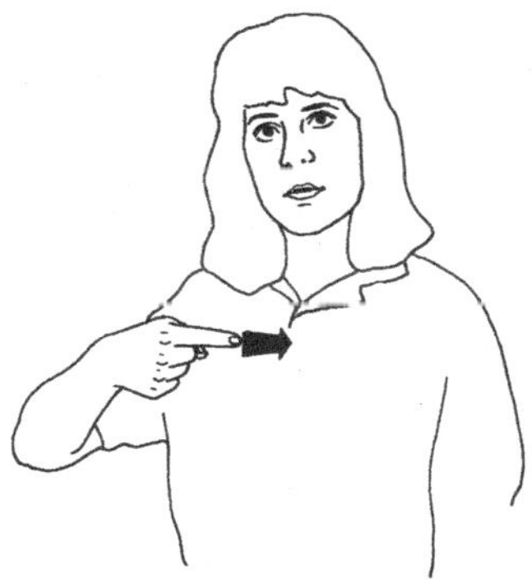

I

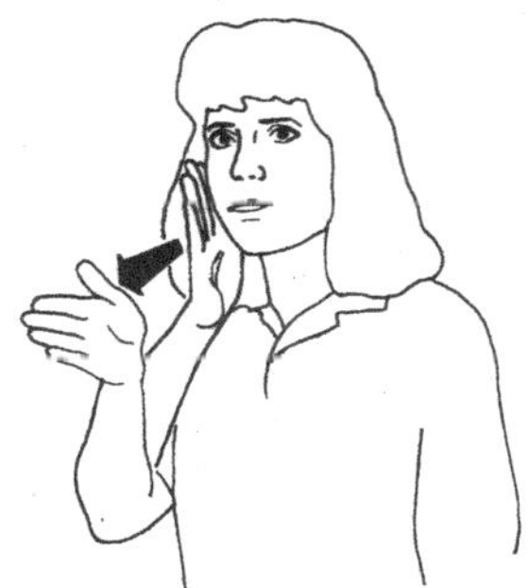

WILL

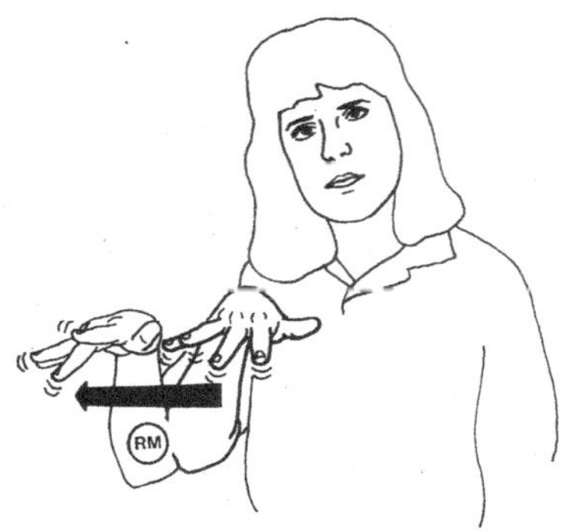

FINGERSPELL

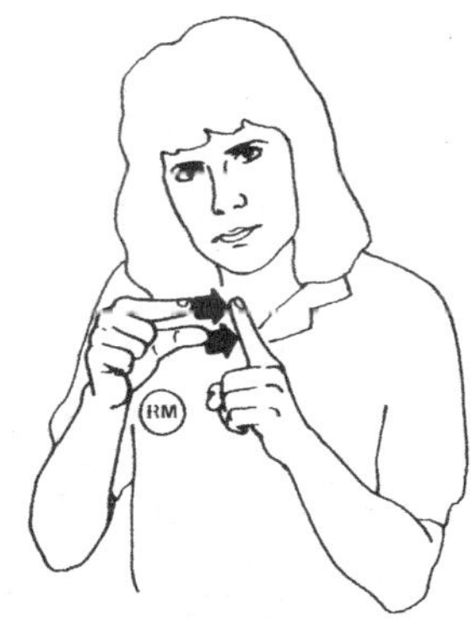

WORD.

If you don't know the name of the picture, I will fingerspell the word.

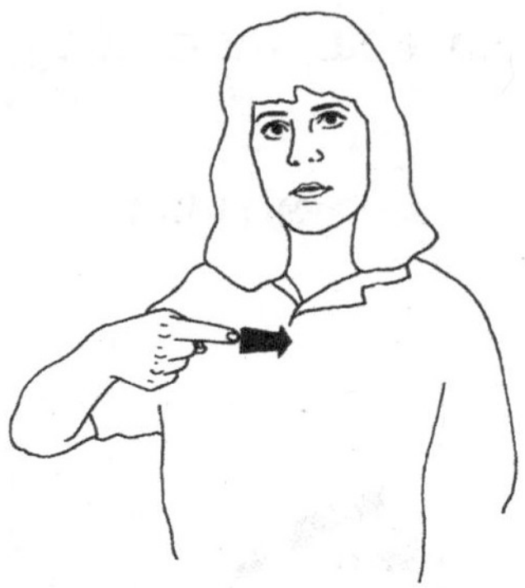

I

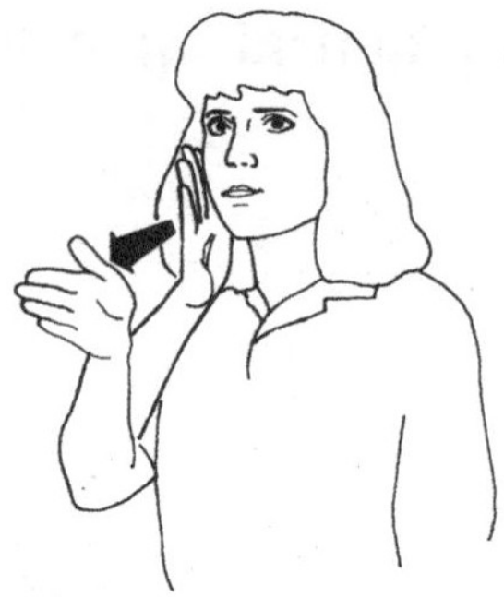

WILL

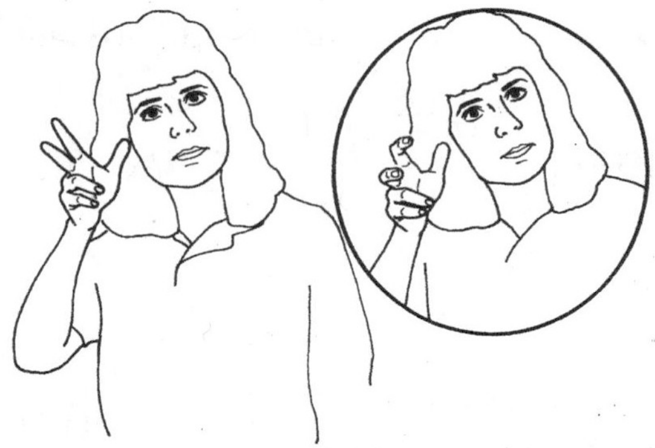

LISTEN

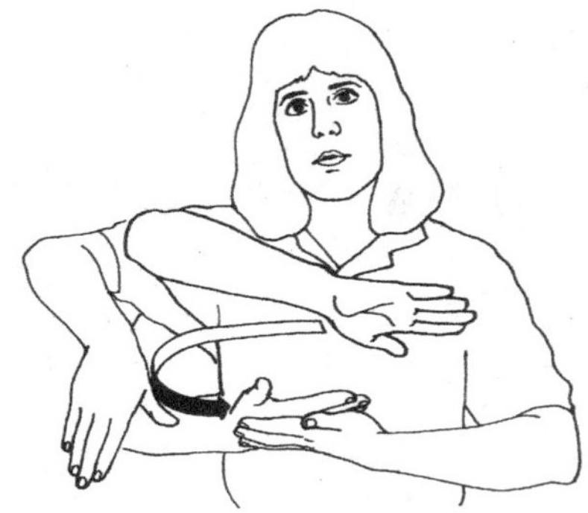

OVERALL

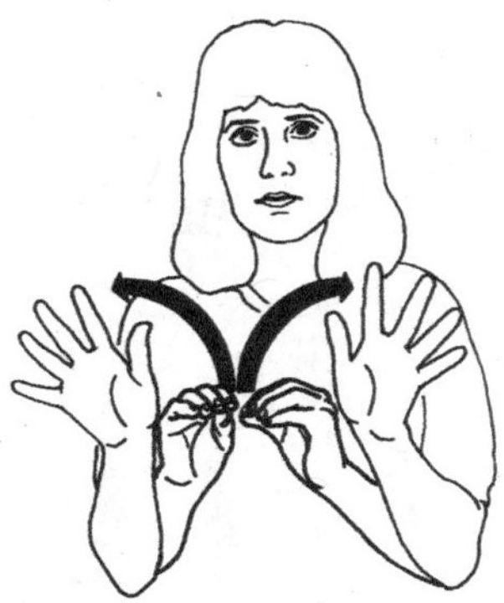

CLARITY

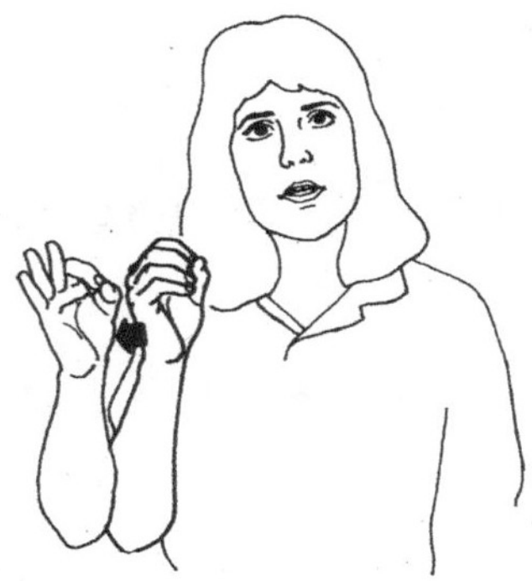

O-F

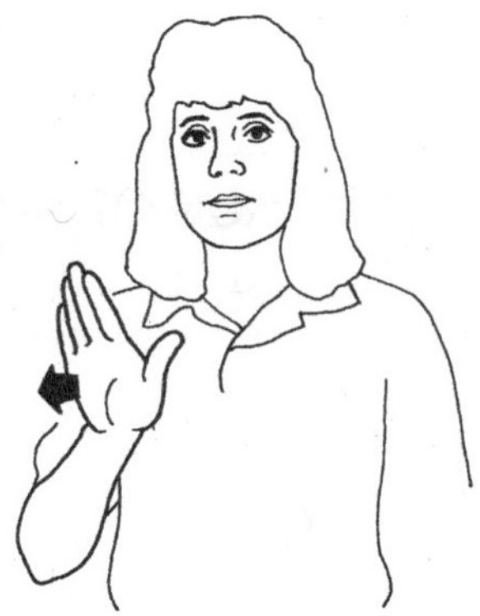

YOUR

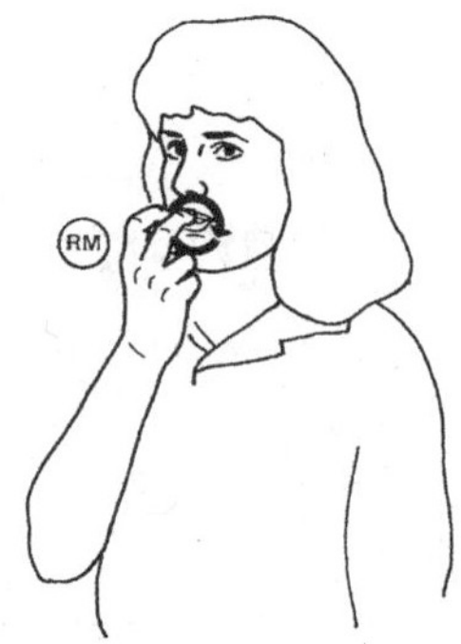

SPEECH.

I will listen to the overall clarity of your speech.

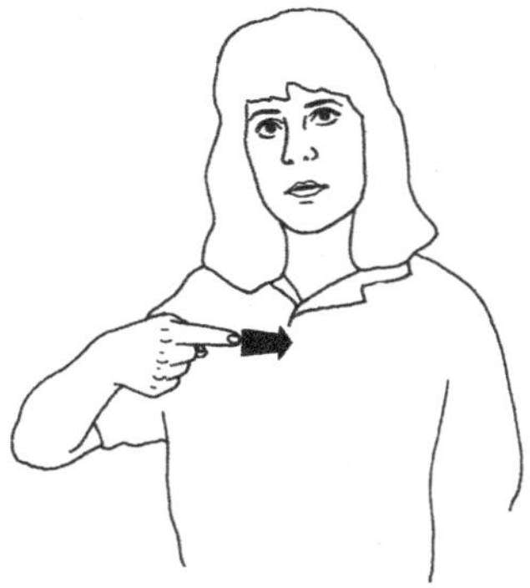

I

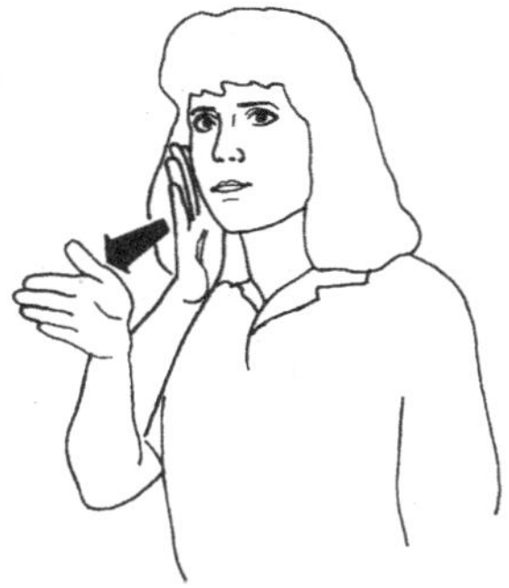

WILL

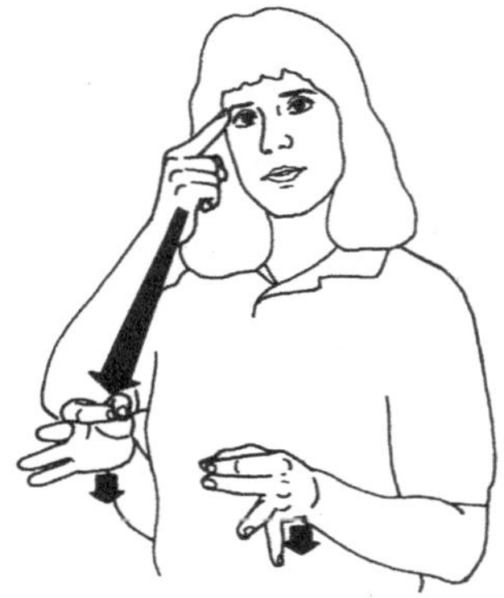

DETERMINE

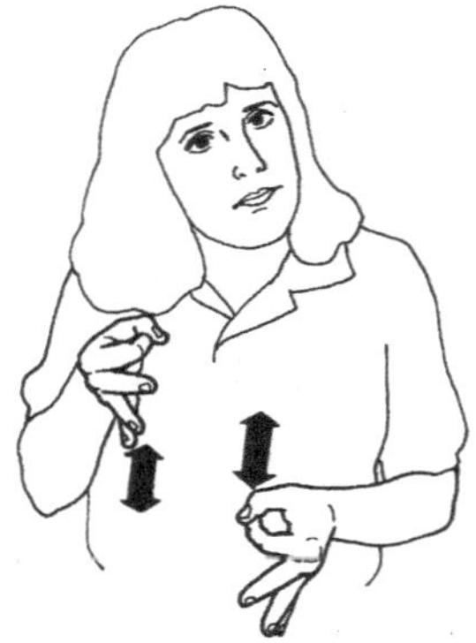

IF

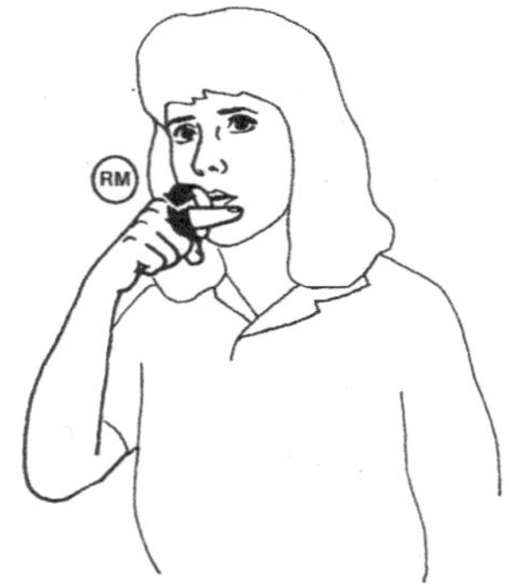

HEARING

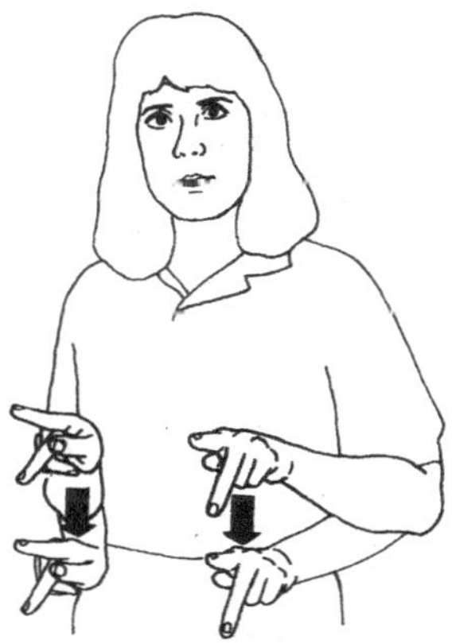

PERSON

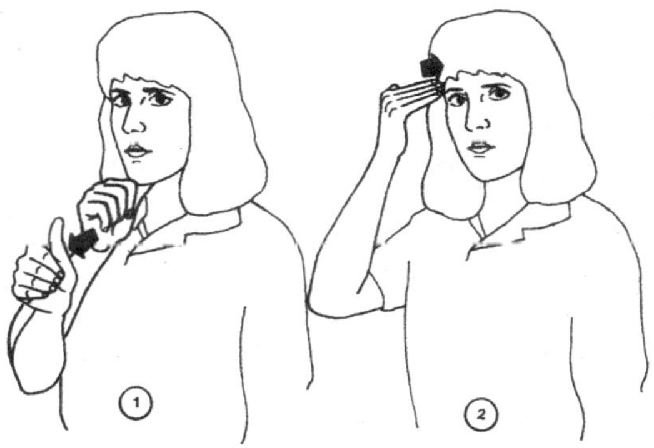

UNFAMILIAR

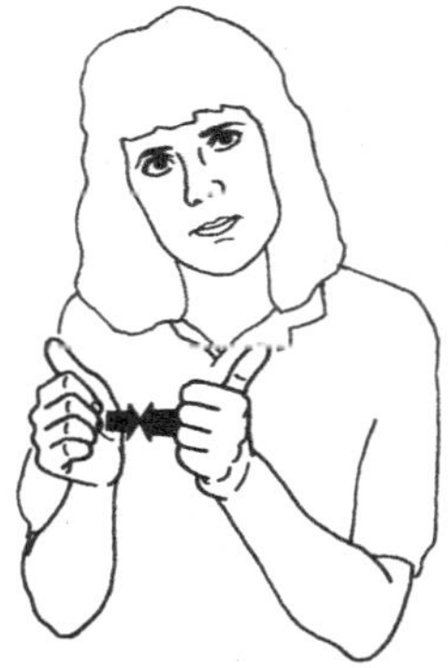

WITH

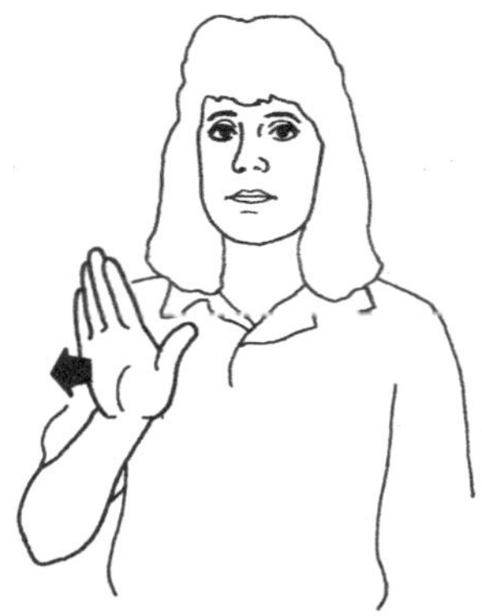

YOUR

I will determine if a hearing person, unfamiliar with your speech, could understand you.

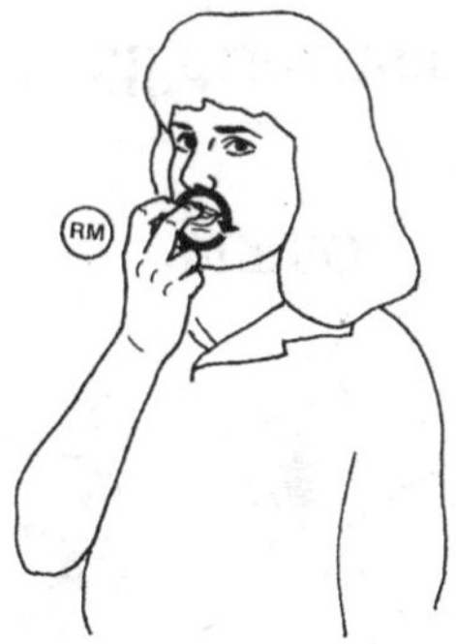

SPEECH

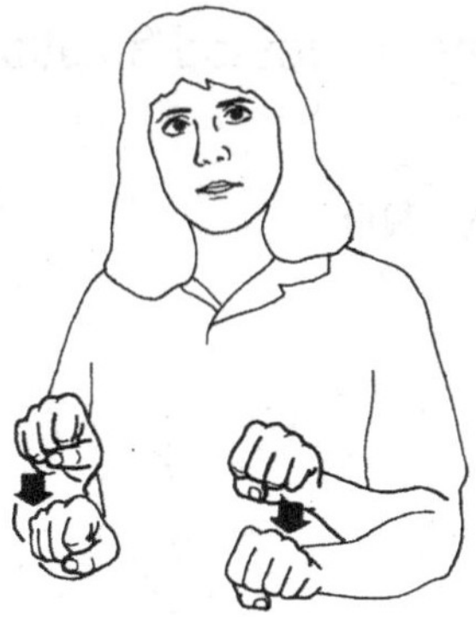

CAN

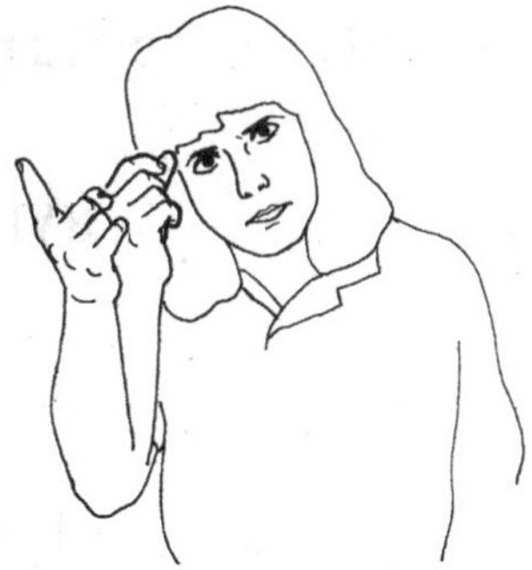

UNDERSTAND

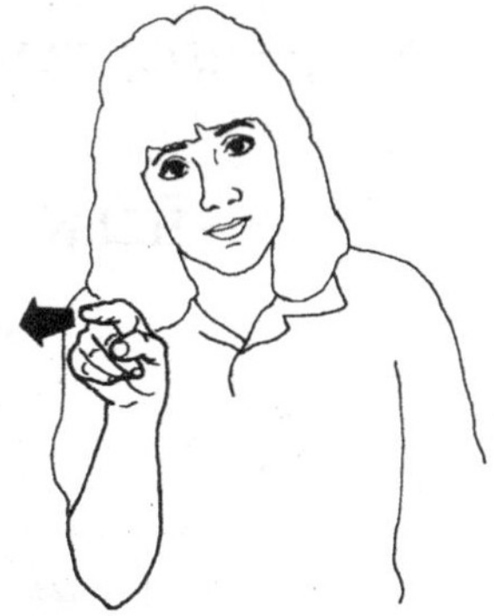

YOU.

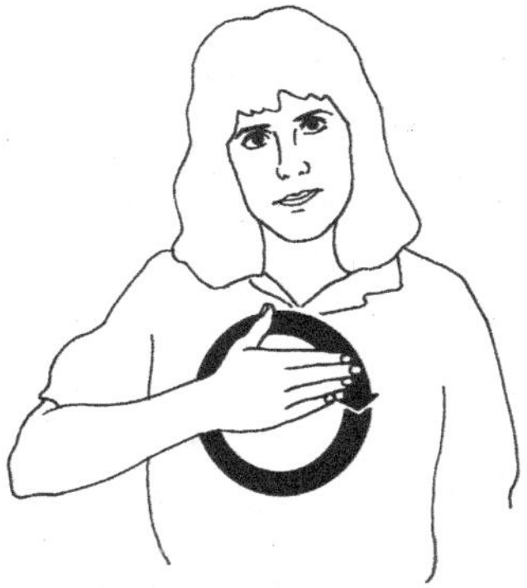

PLEASE

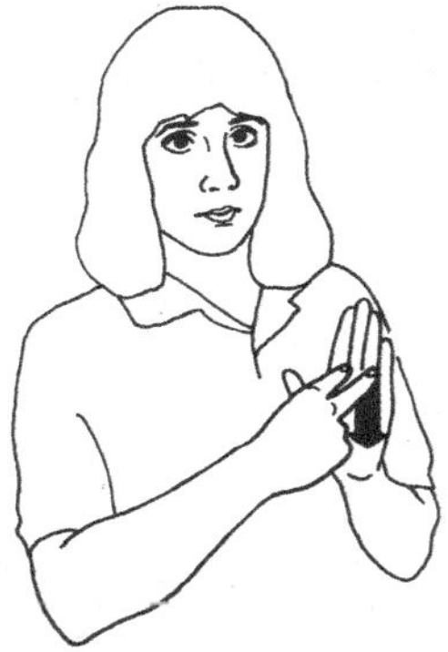

READ

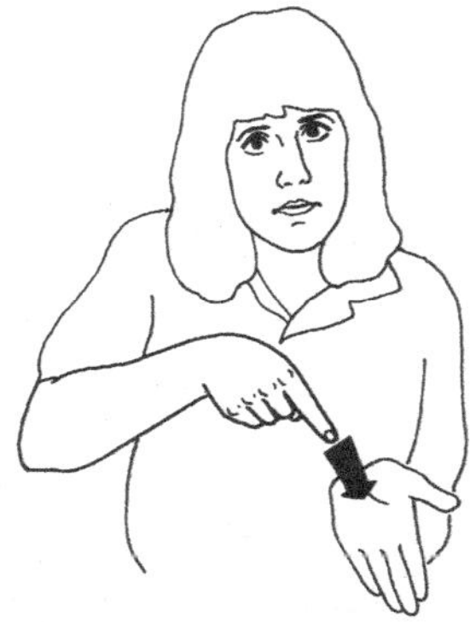

THIS

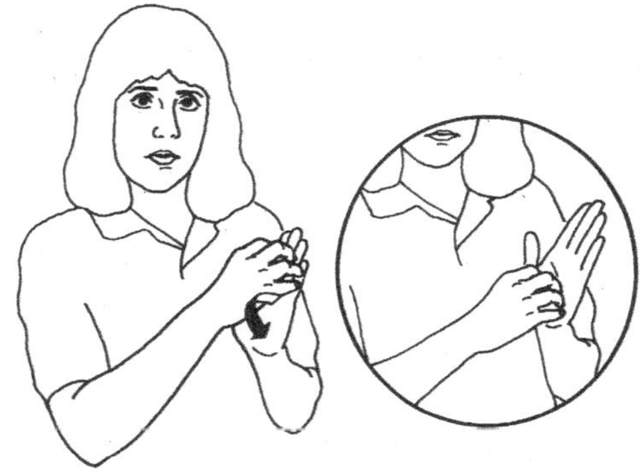

PARAGRAPH

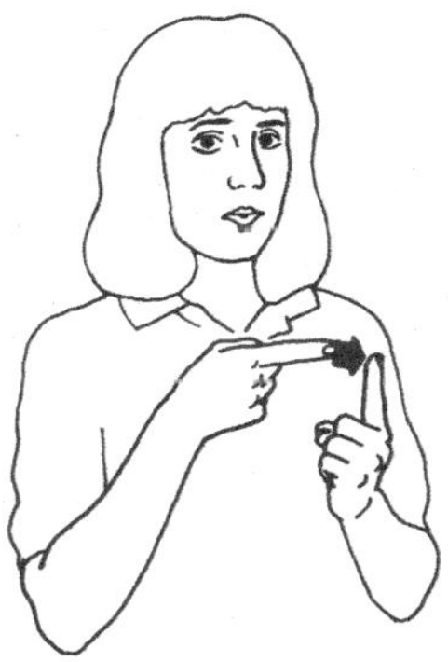

TO

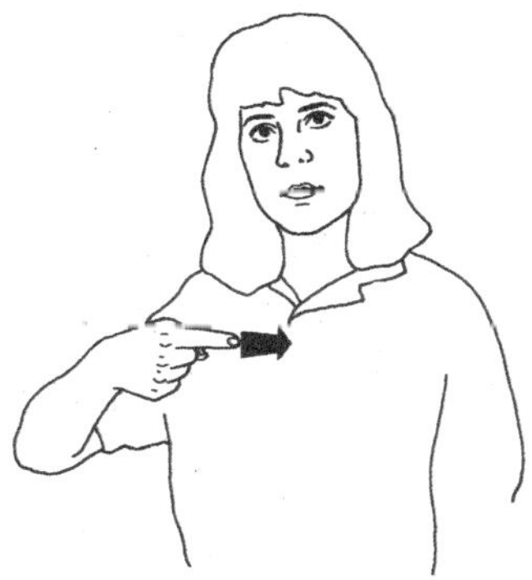

ME.

Please read this paragraph to me.

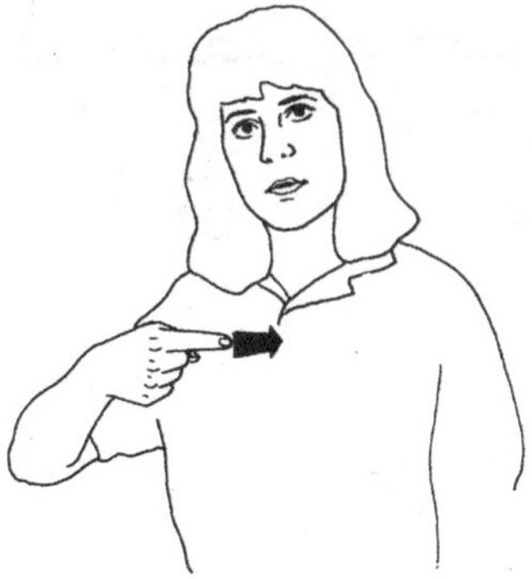

I

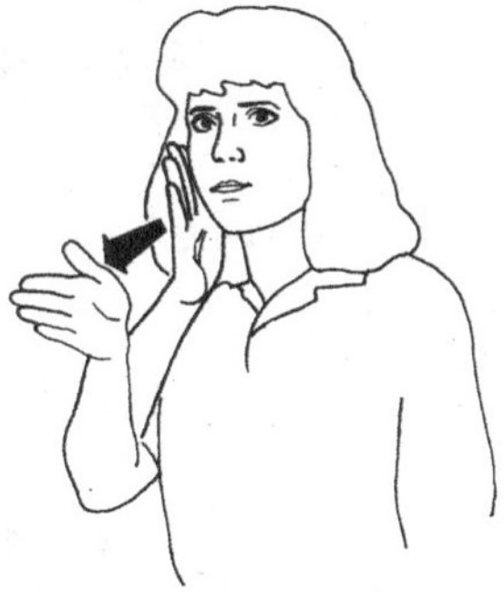

WILL

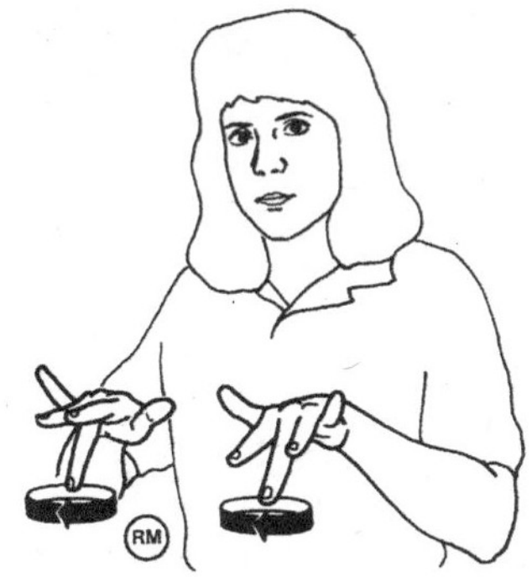

TAPE-RECORD

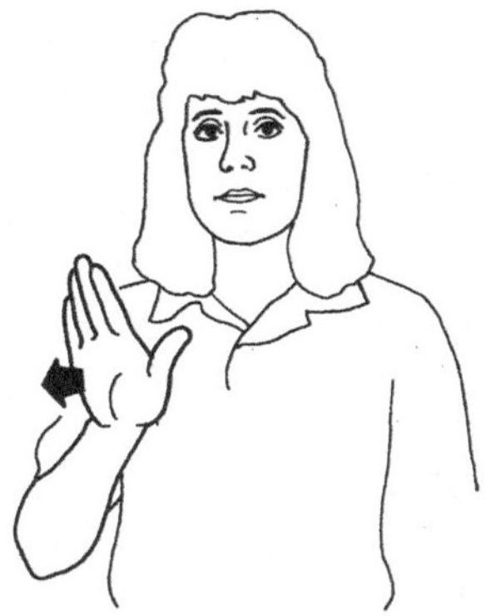

YOUR

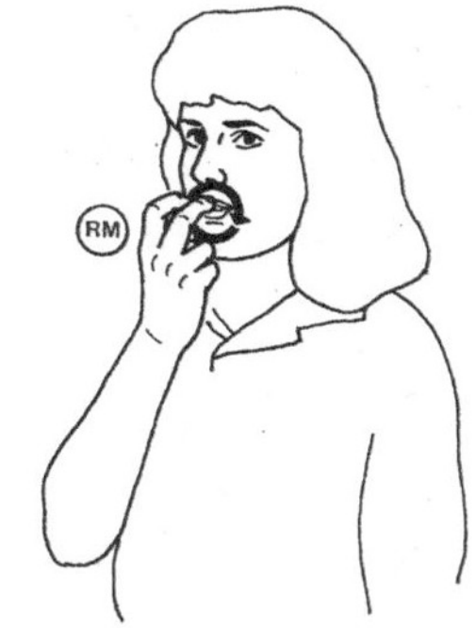

SPEECH

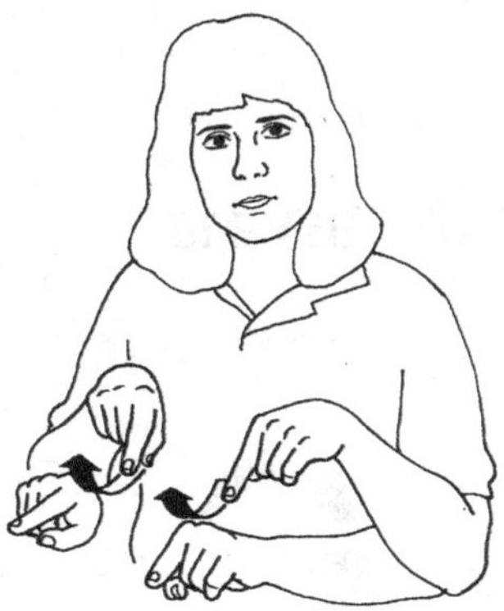

WHILE

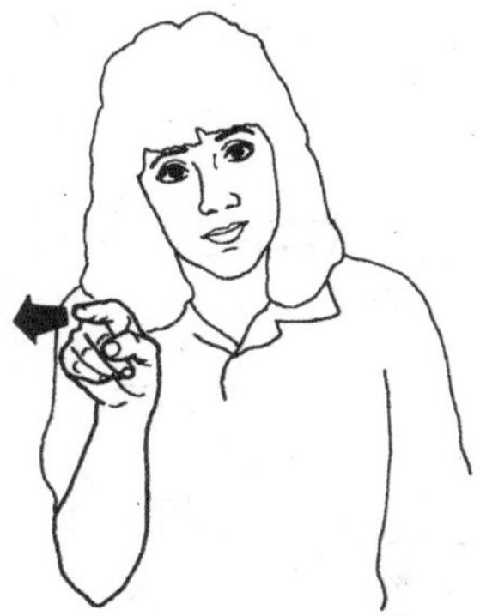

YOU

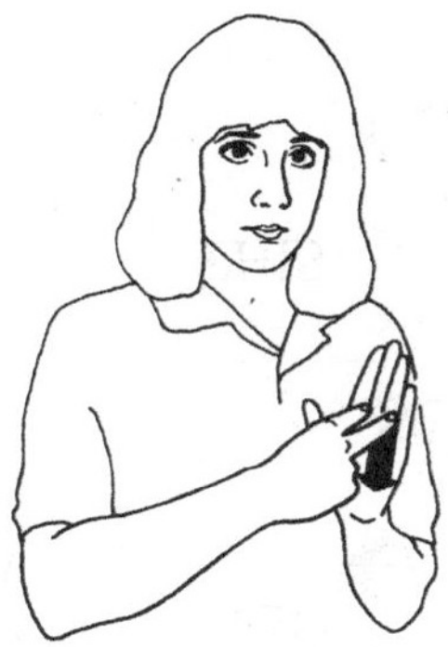

READ.

I will tape record your speech while you read.

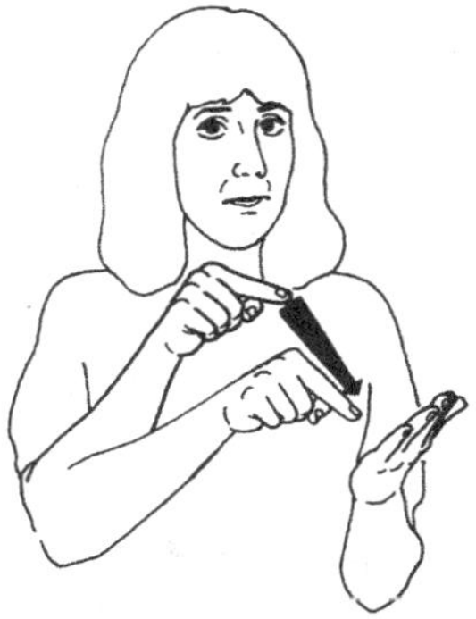

POINT

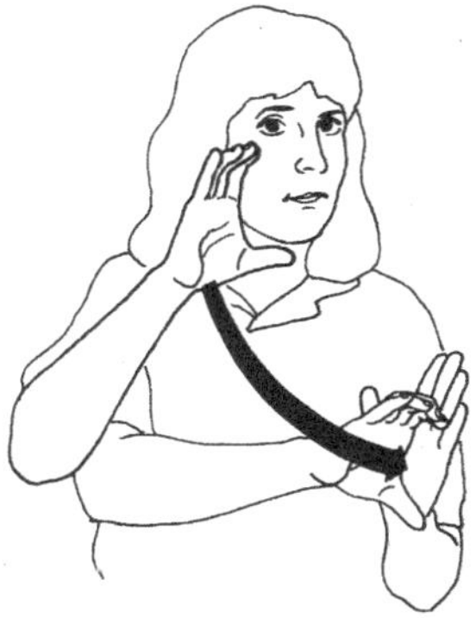

PICTURE

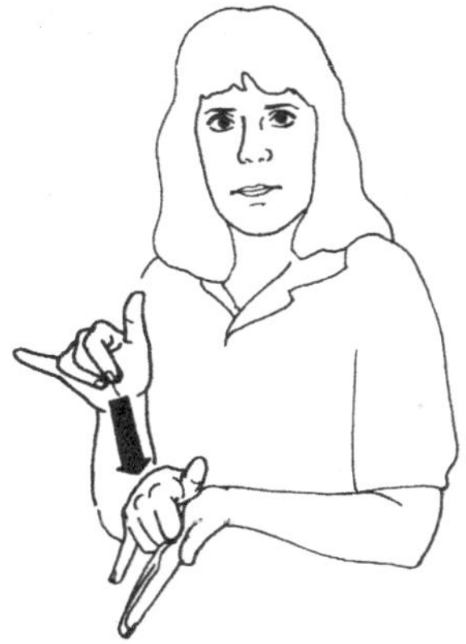

THAT

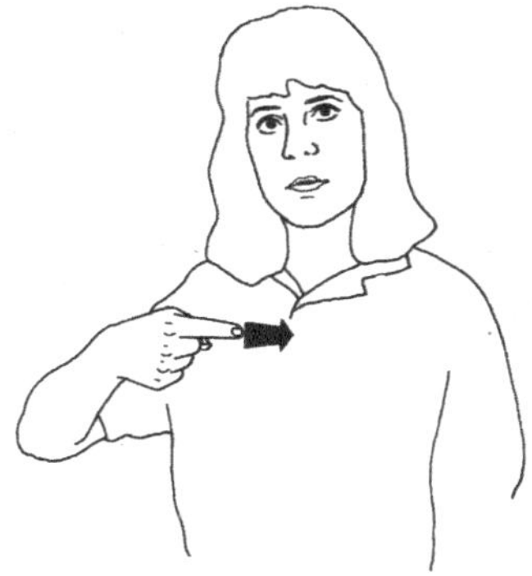

I

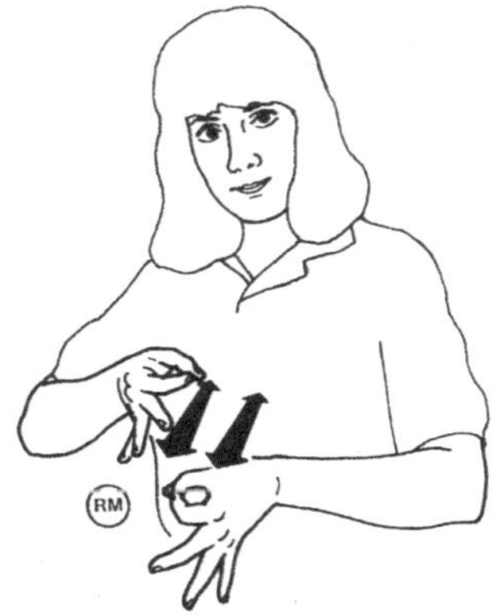

DESCRIBE.

Point to the picture that I describe.

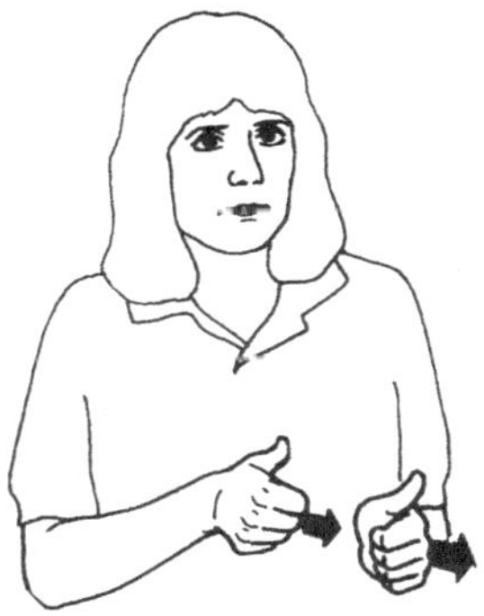

FOLLOW

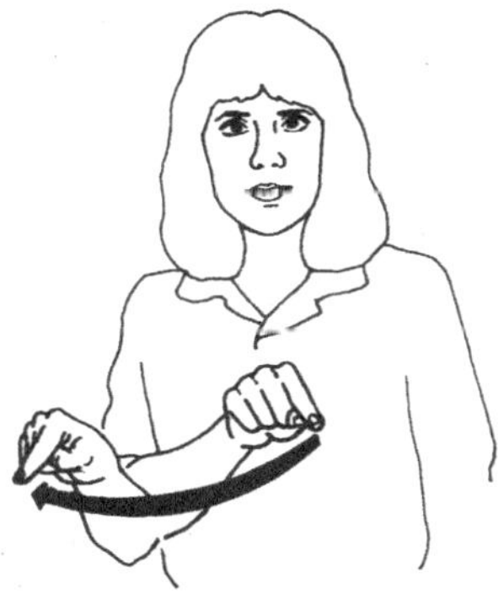

THESE

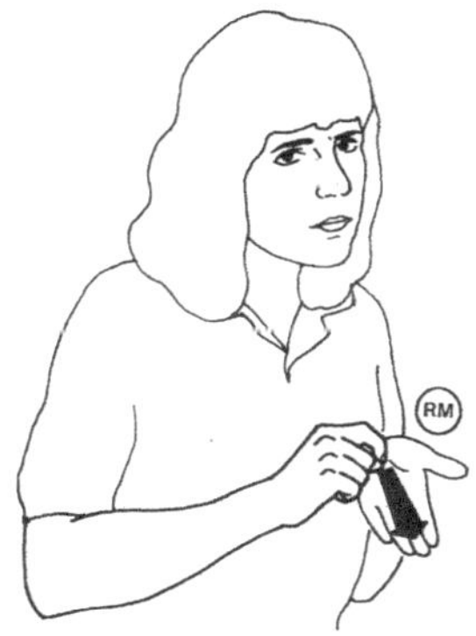

WRITTEN

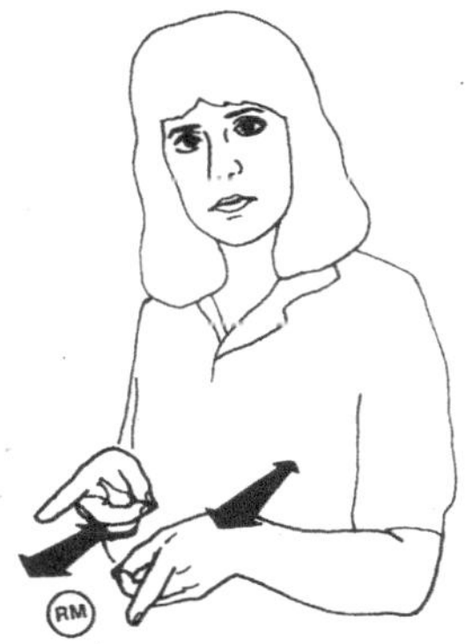

DIRECTION

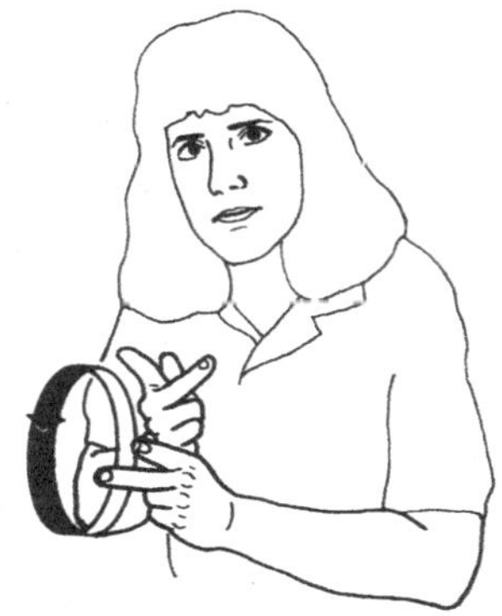

CAREFULLY.

Follow these written directions carefully.

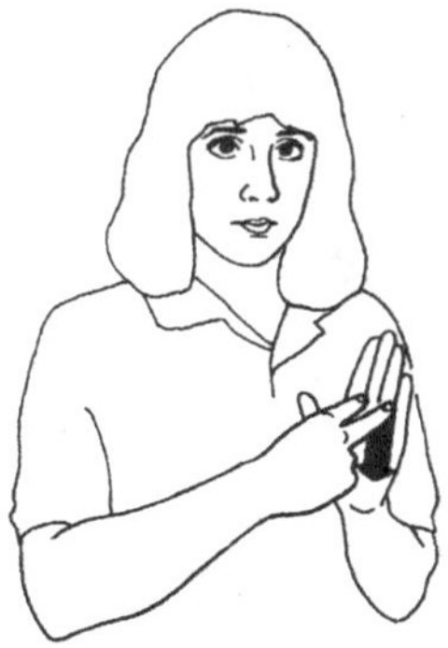

READ

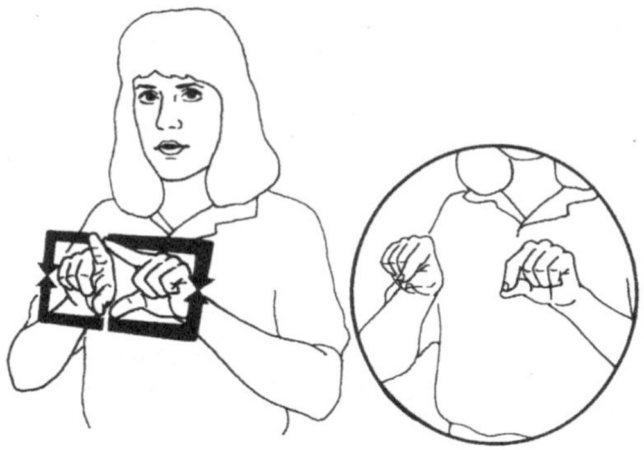

CARD

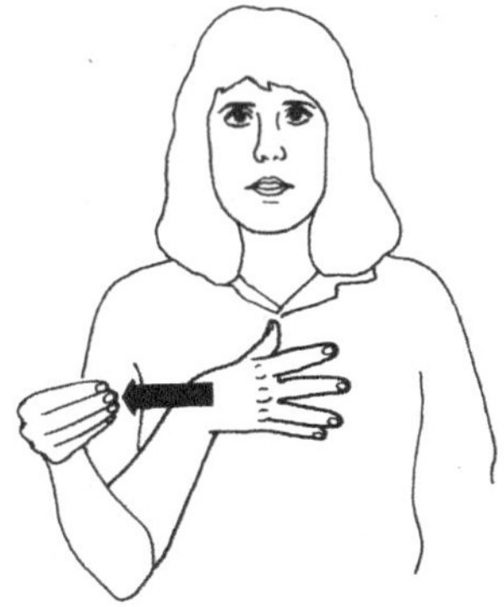

AND

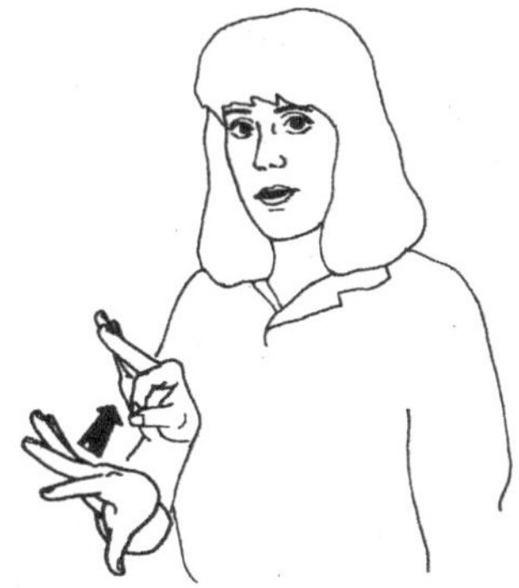

FIND

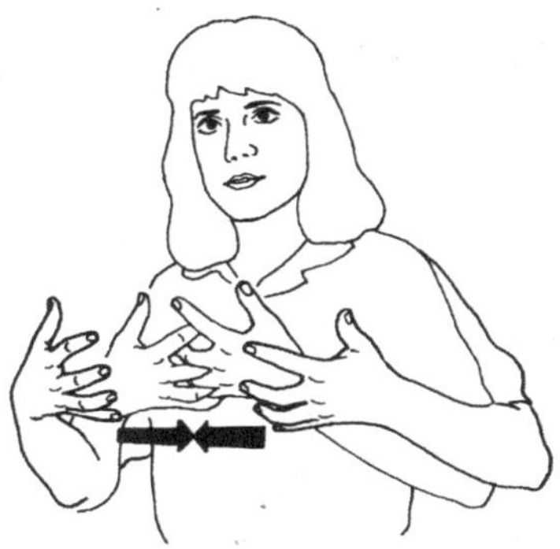

MATCH

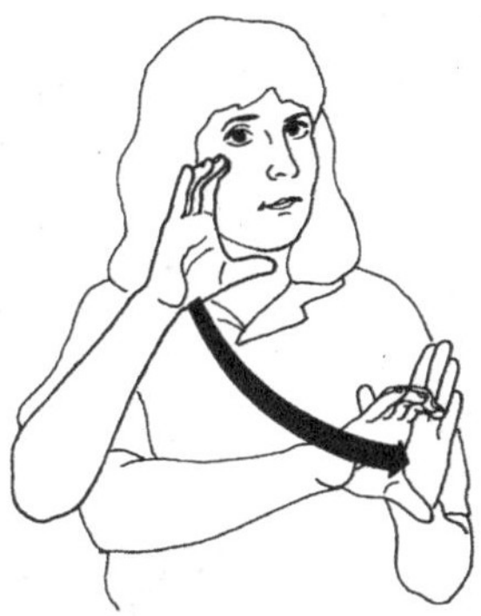

PICTURE.

Read the card and find the matching picture.

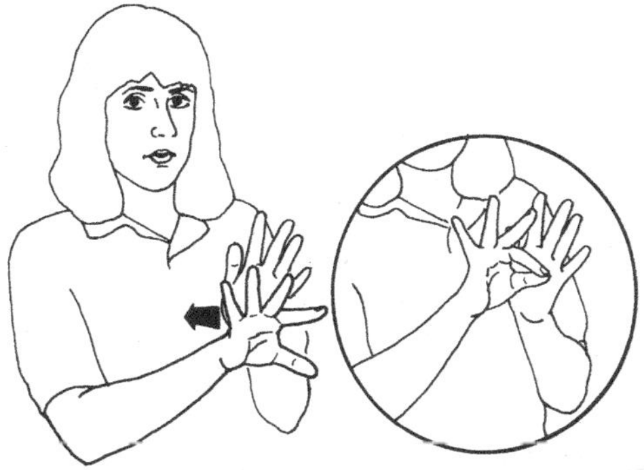

CHOOSE

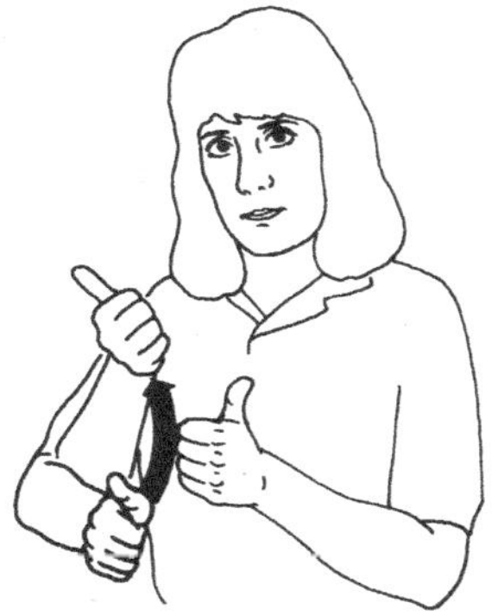

MOST

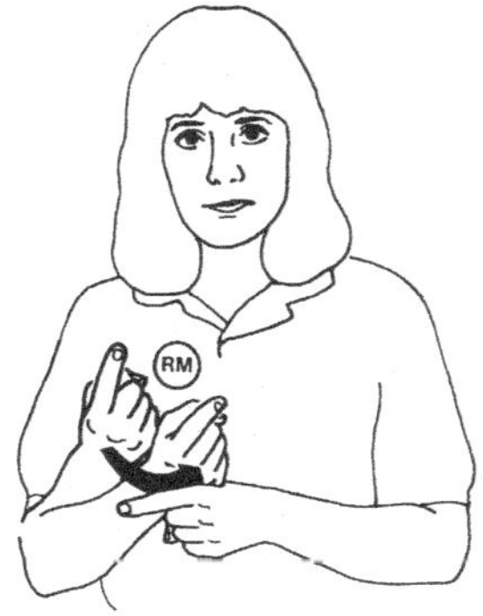

APPROPRIATE

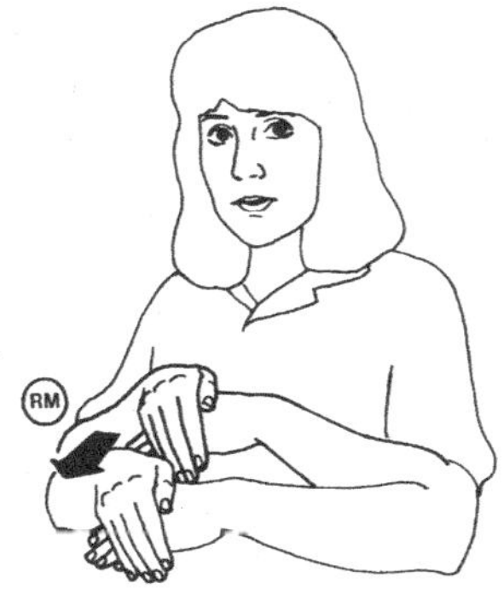

ENGLISH

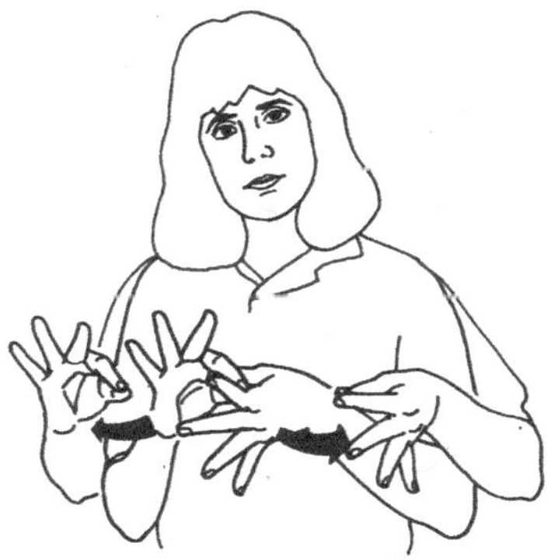

SENTENCE.

Choose the most appropriate English sentence.

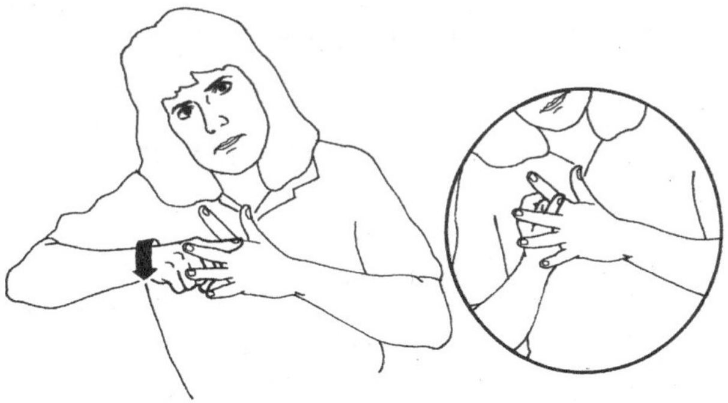

BEGIN

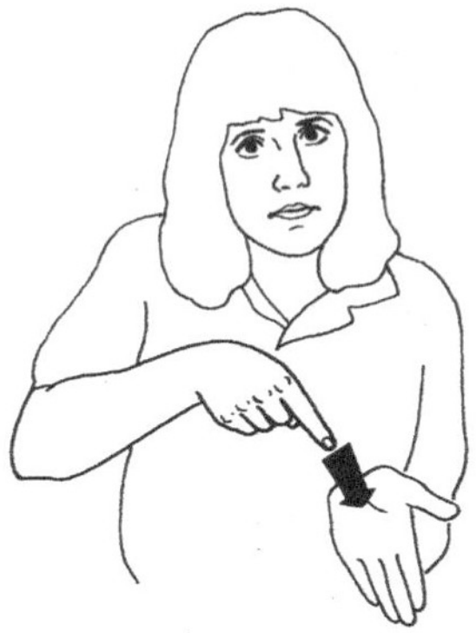

THIS

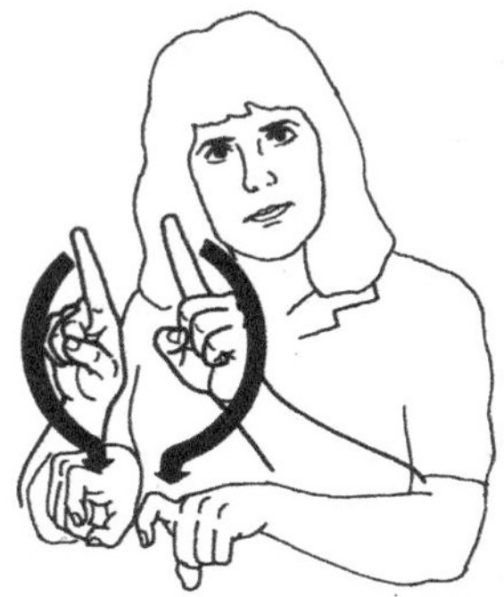

TEST

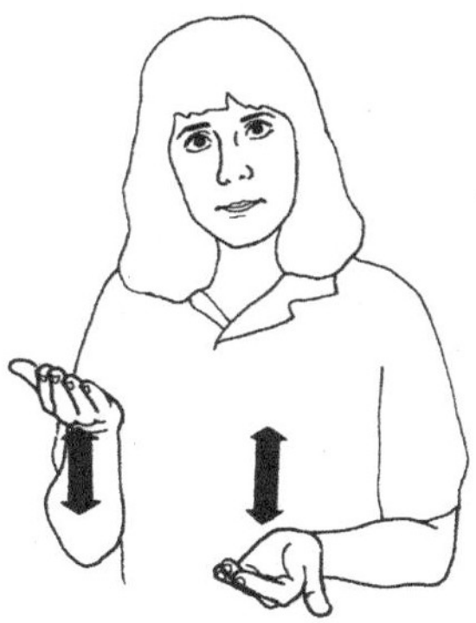

MAYBE

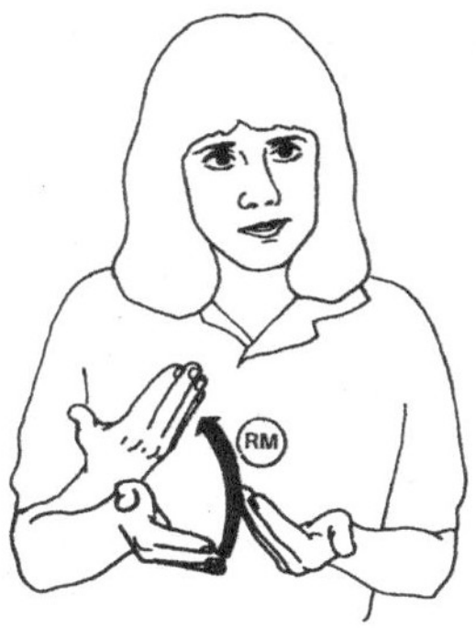

EASY

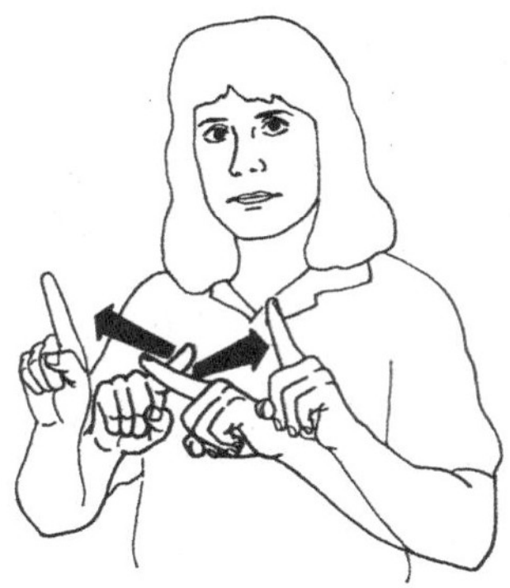

BUT

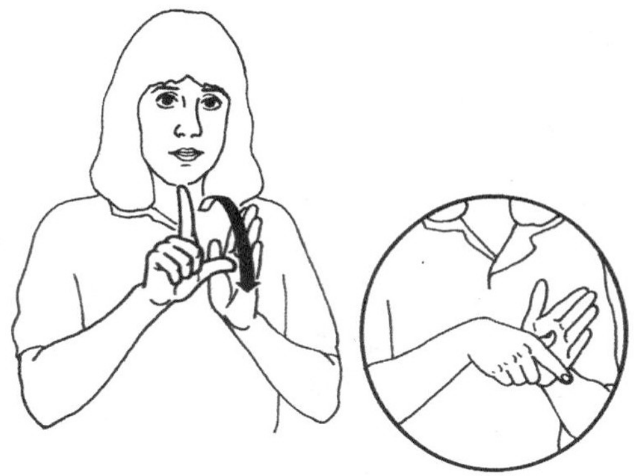

LATER

In the beginning this test might be easy, but later it becomes increasingly complex.

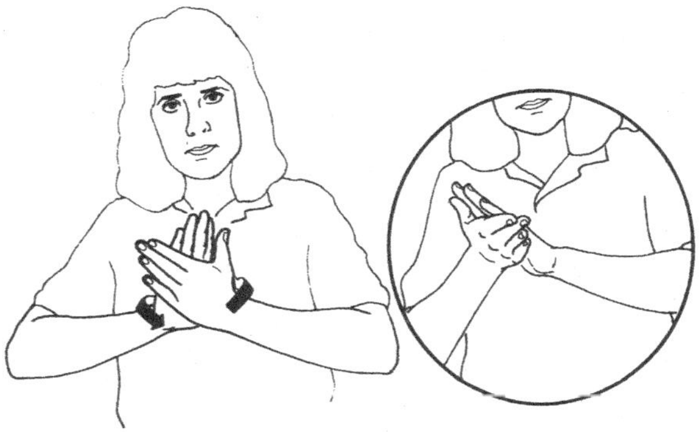

BECOME

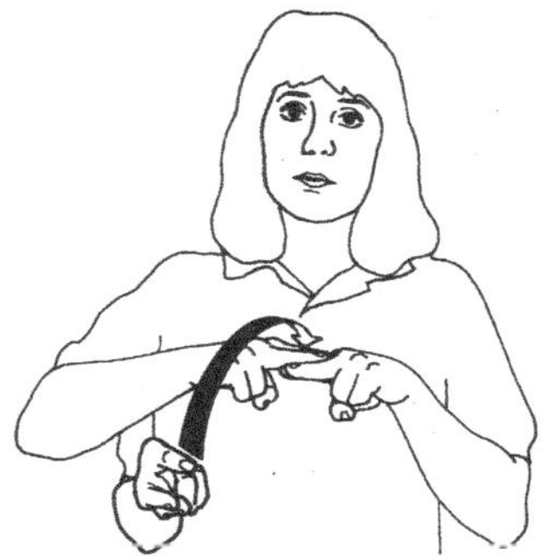

INCREASE

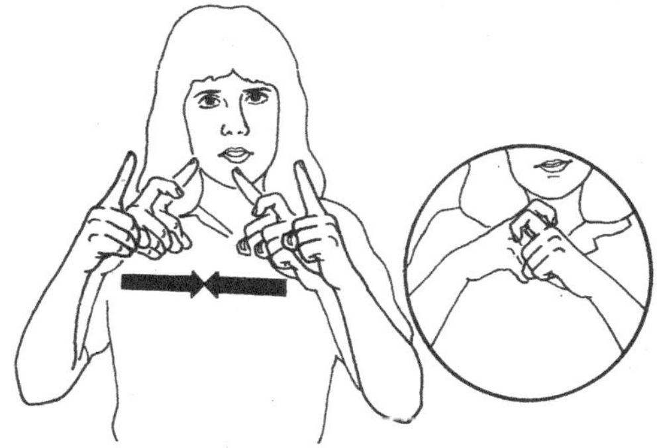

COMPLEX.

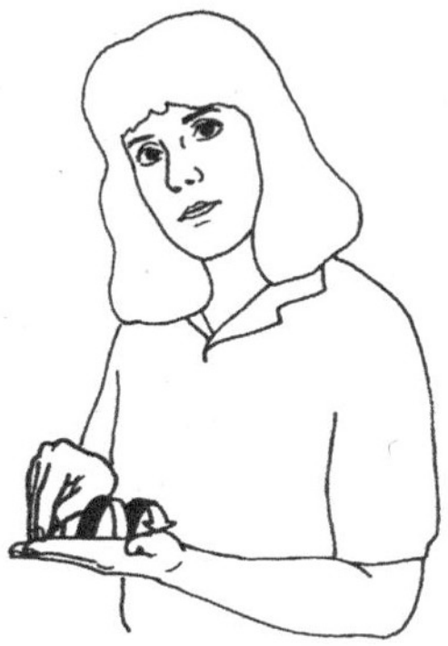

FILL-IN

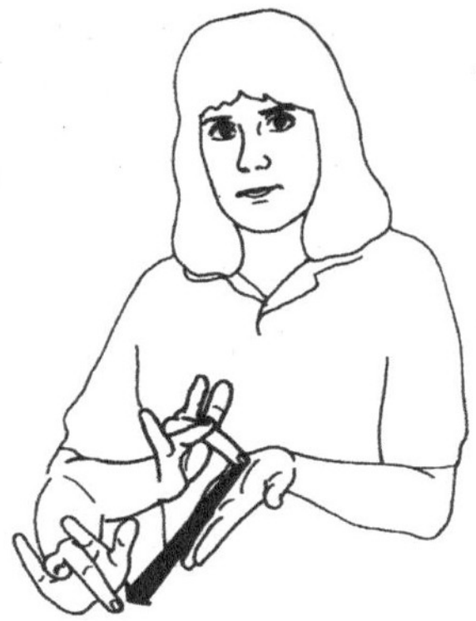

BLANK

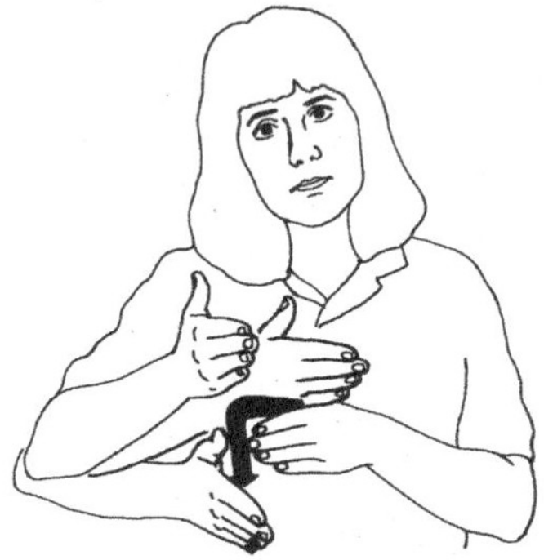

COMPLETE

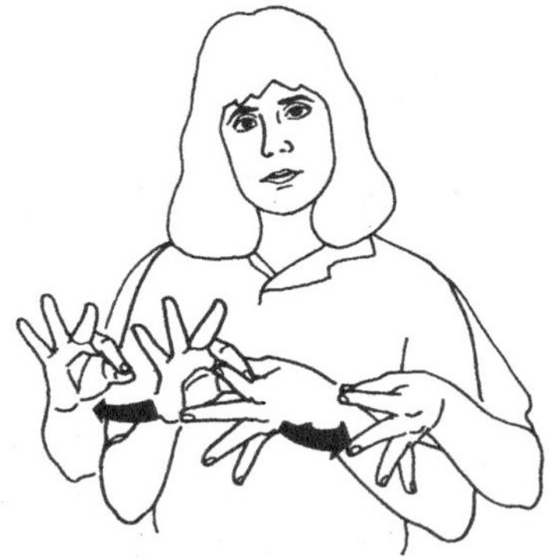

SENTENCE.

Fill in the blank to complete the sentence.

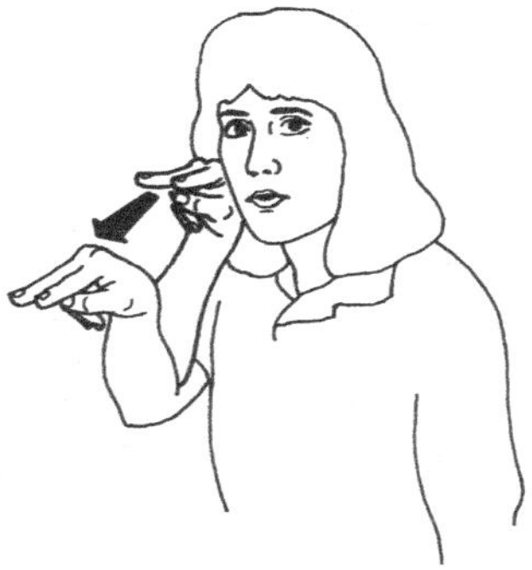

LOOK-AT

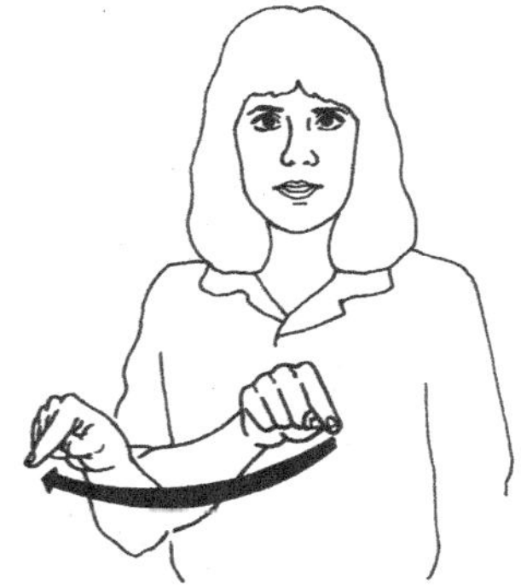

THESE

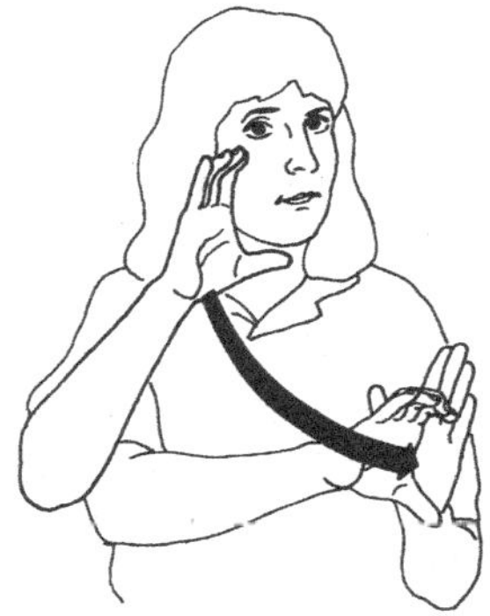

PICTURE

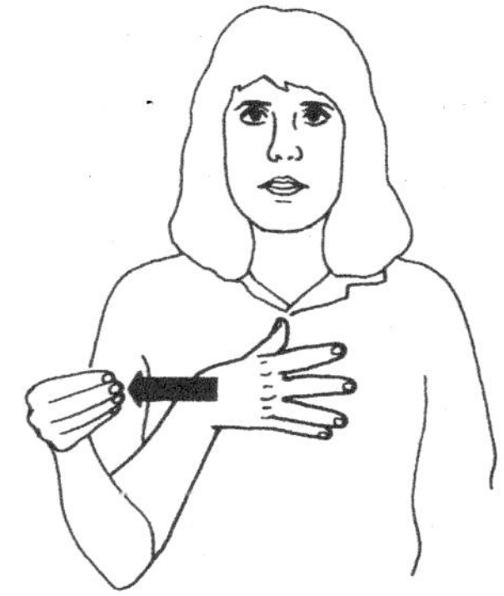

AND

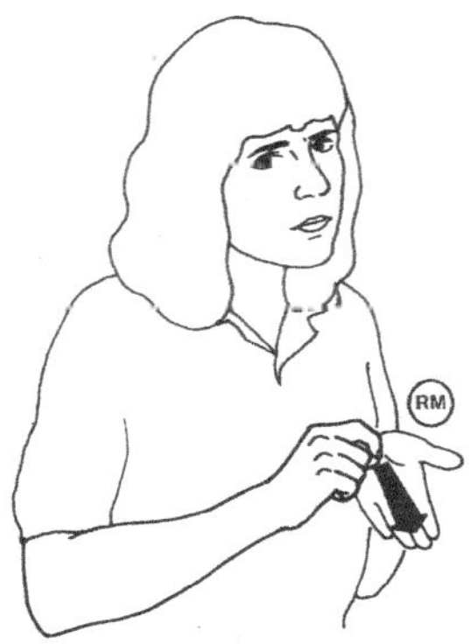

WRITE

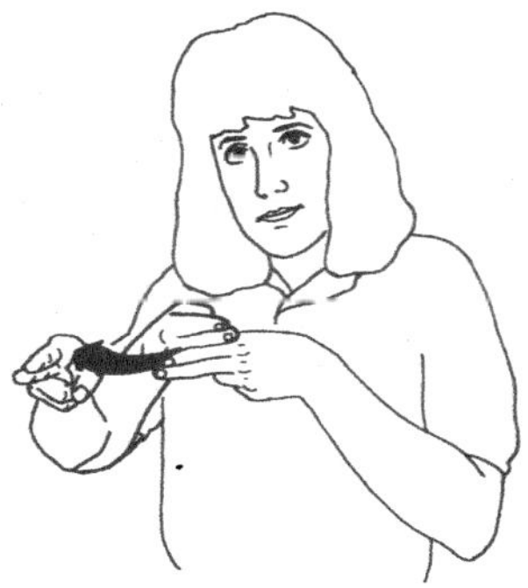

SHORT

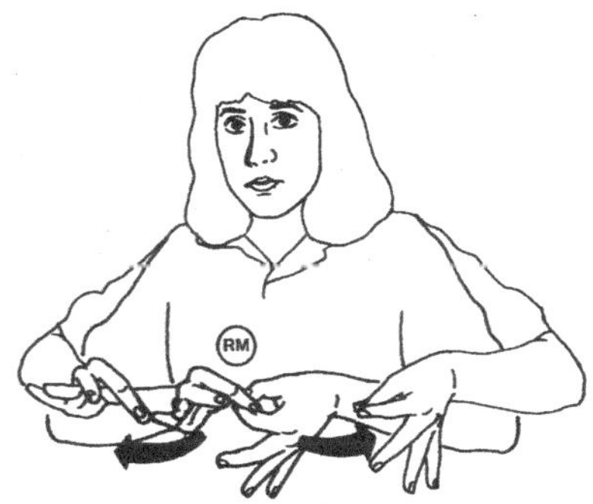

STORY.

Look at these pictures and write a short story.

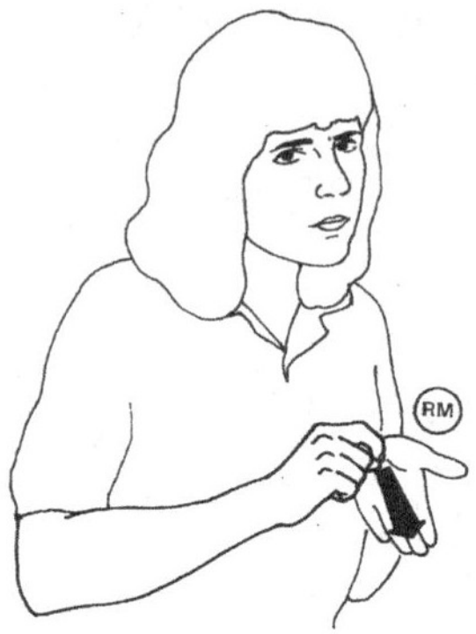

WRITE

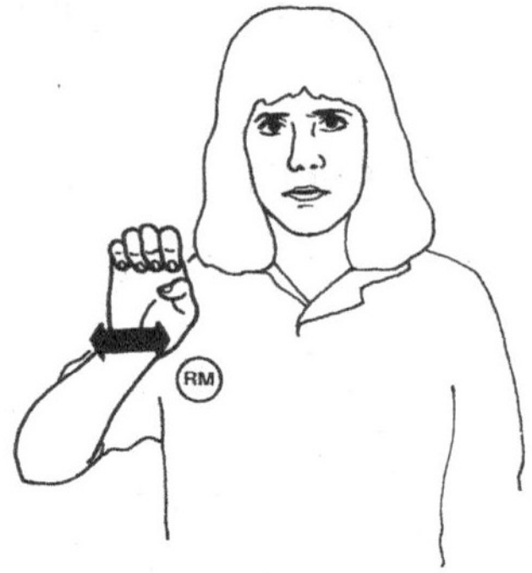

EMERGENCY

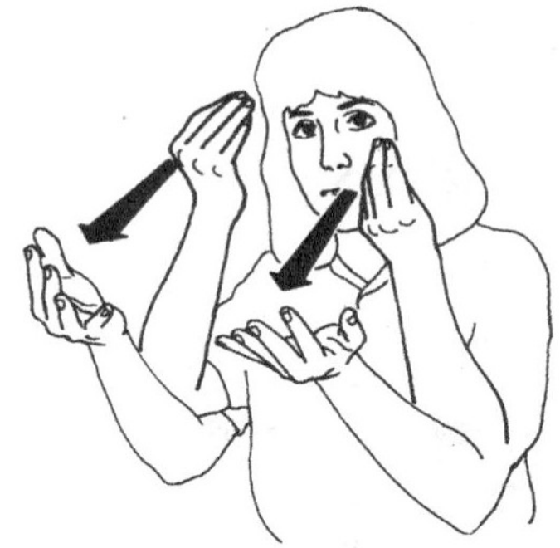

INFORMATION

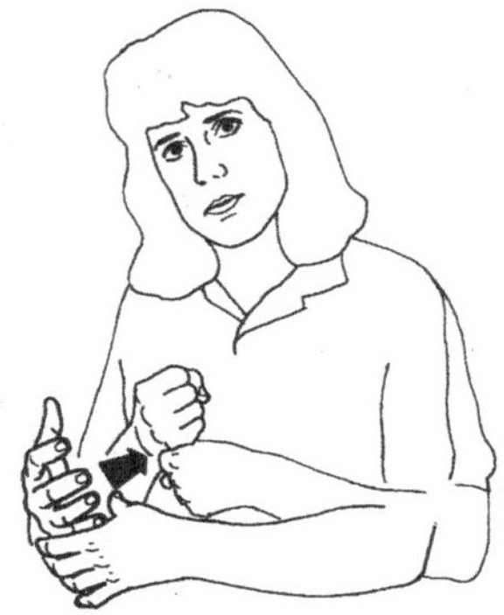

GET

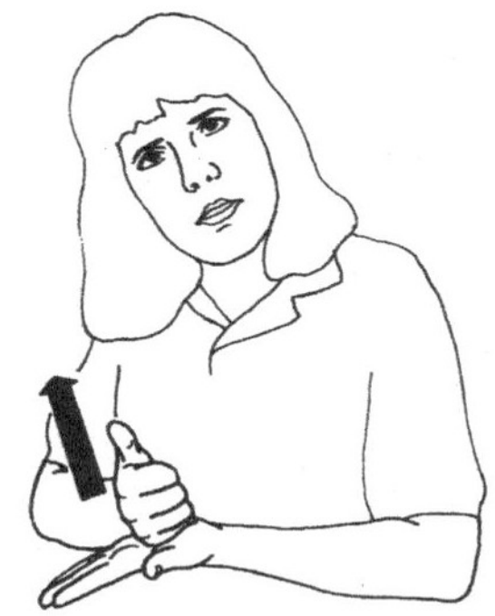

HELP

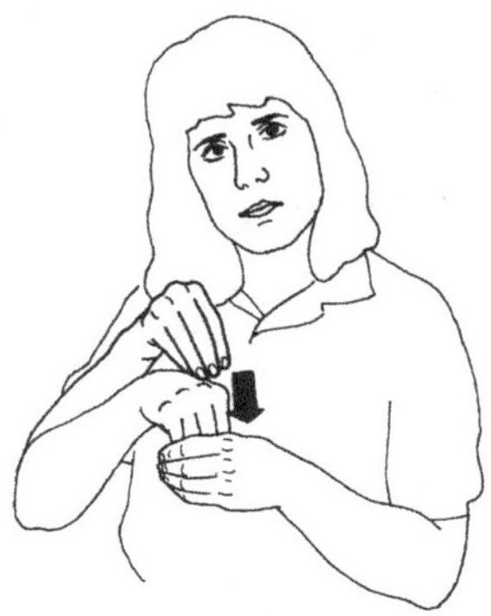

IN

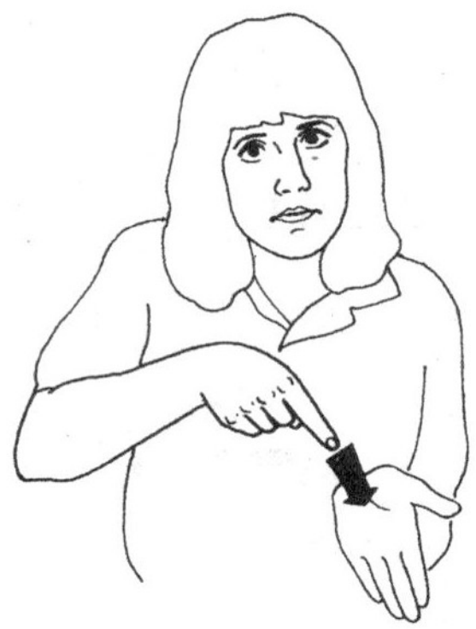

THIS

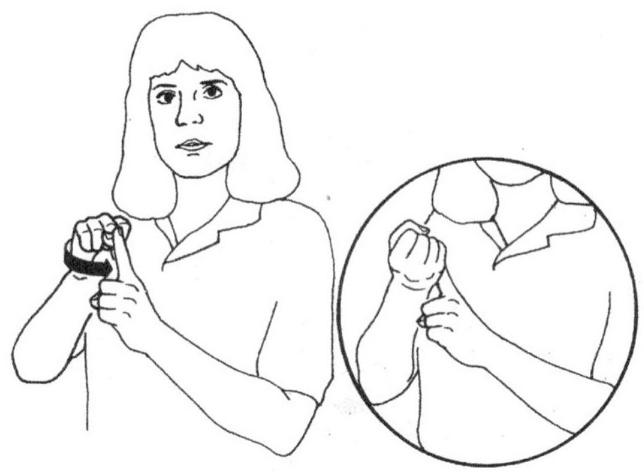

SITUATION.

Write an emergency message to get help in this situation.

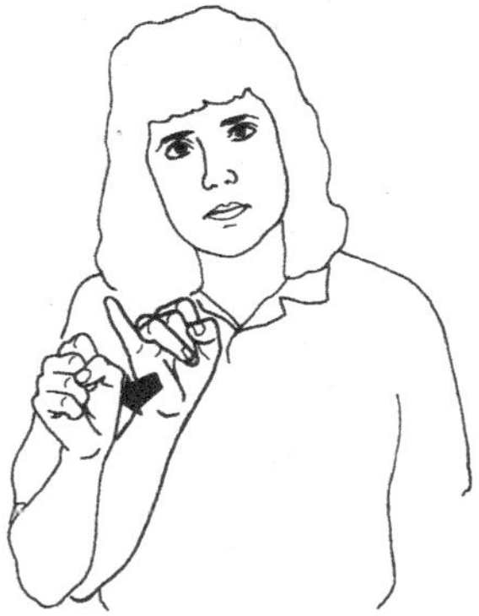

I-S

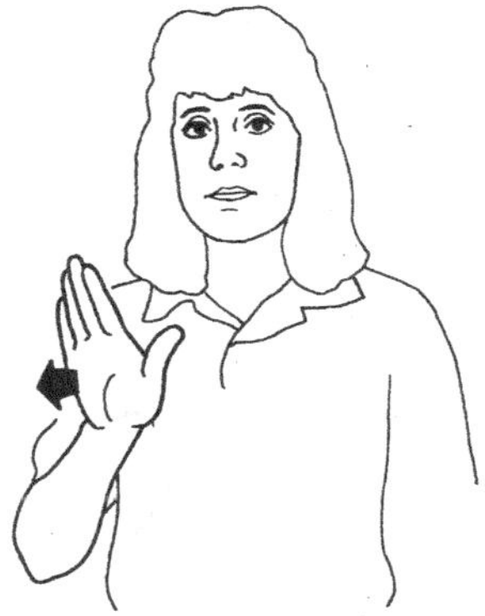

YOUR

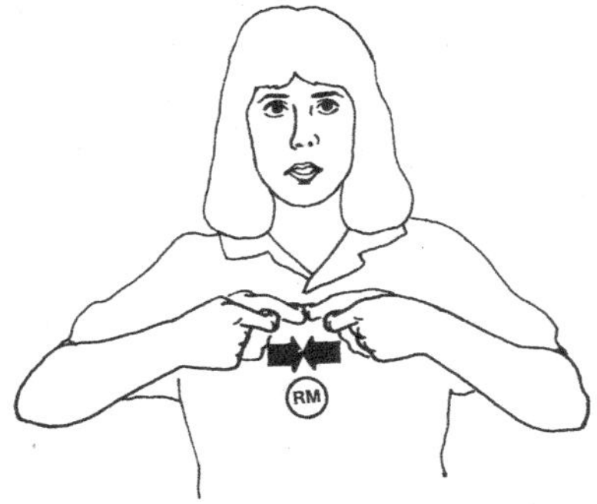

BATTERY

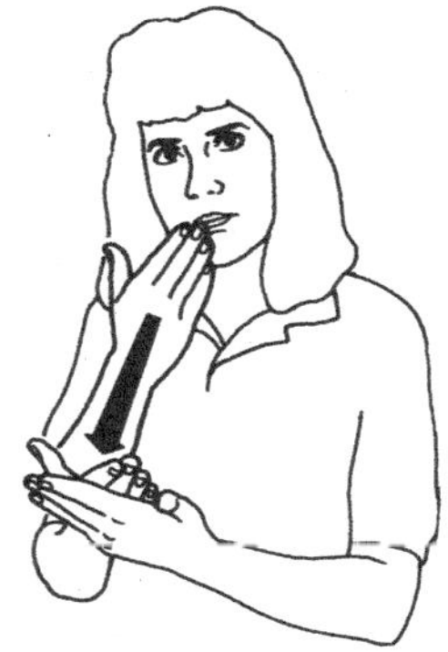

GOOD?

Is your battery good?

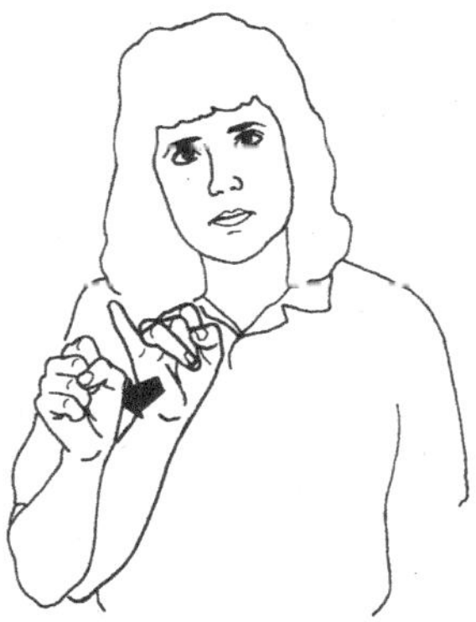

I-S

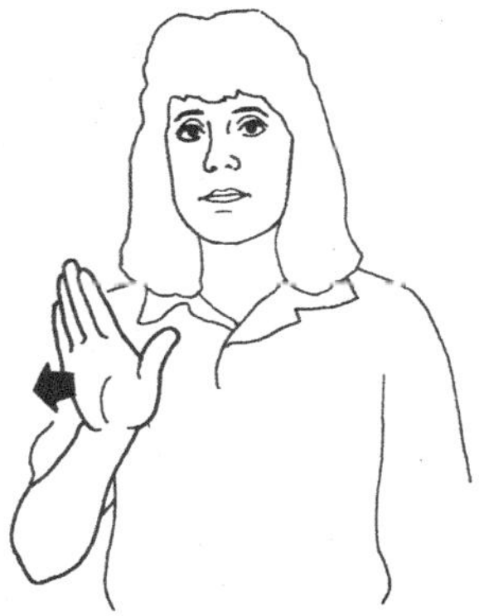

YOUR

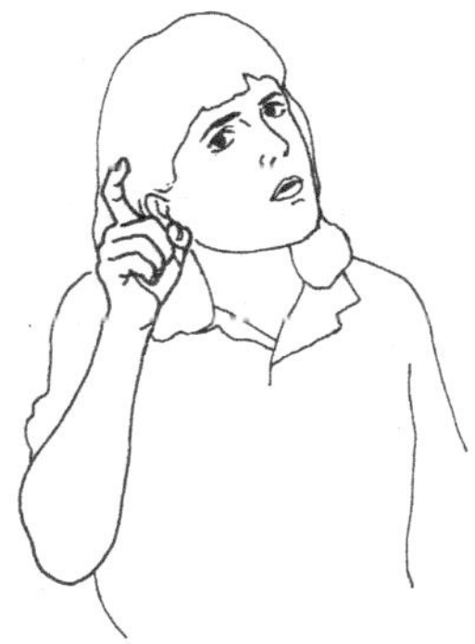

HEARING-AID

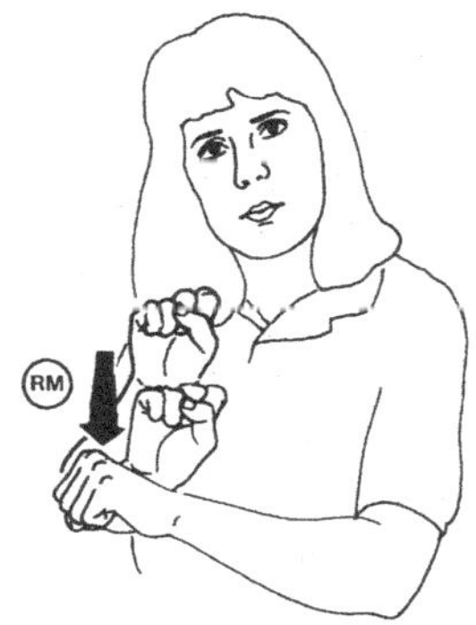

WORK

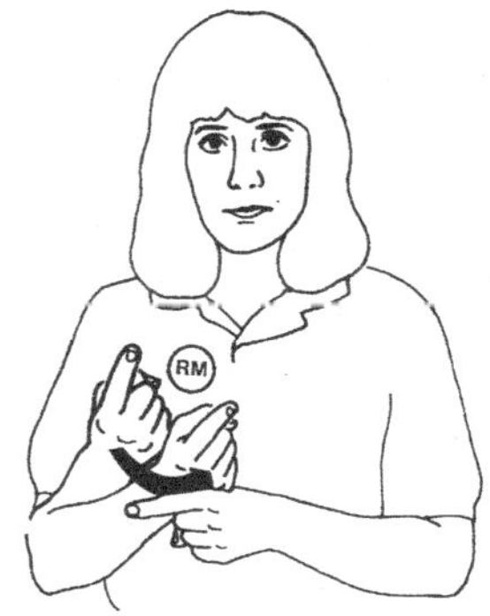

PROPER?

Is your hearing aid working properly?

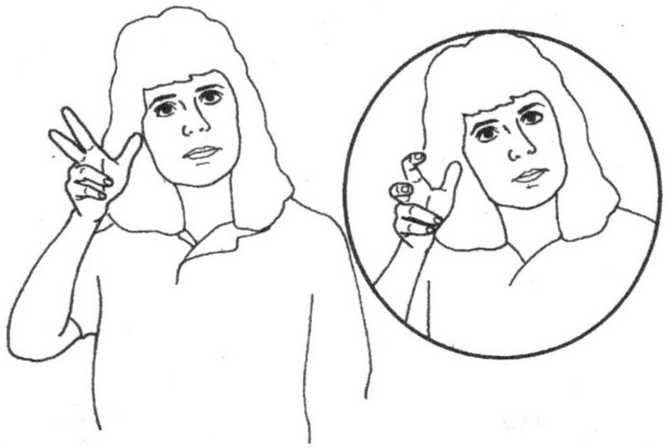

LISTEN

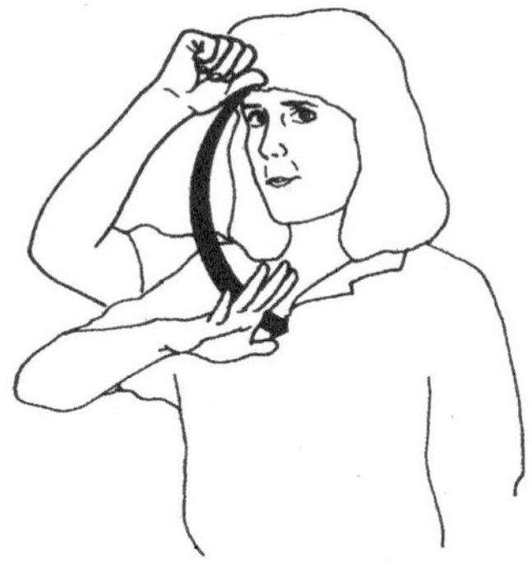

MAN

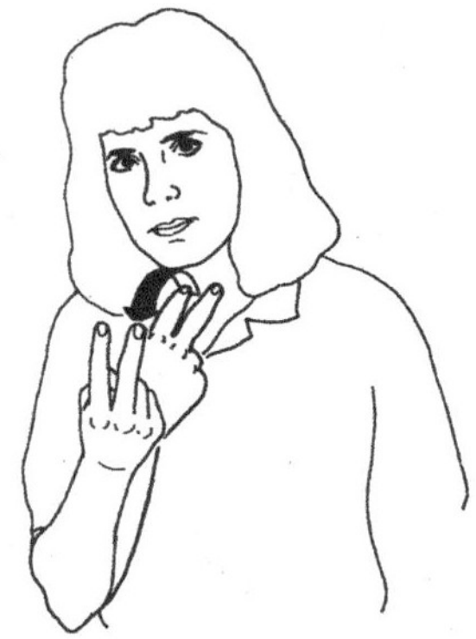

VOICE

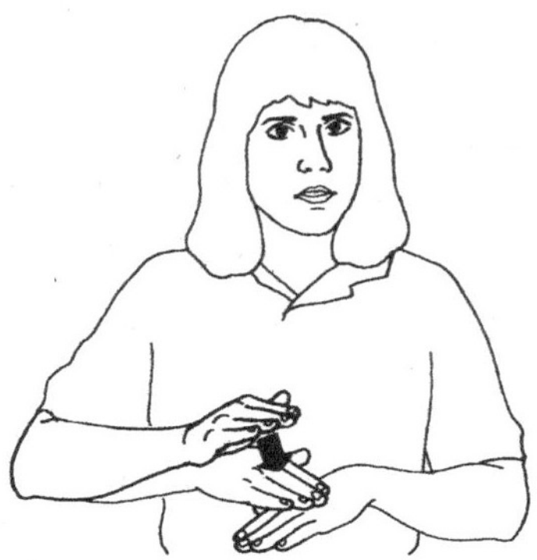

ON

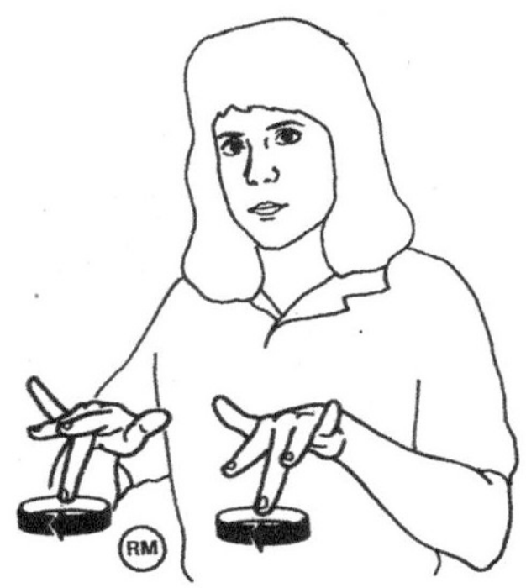

TAPE.

Listen to the man's voice on the tape.

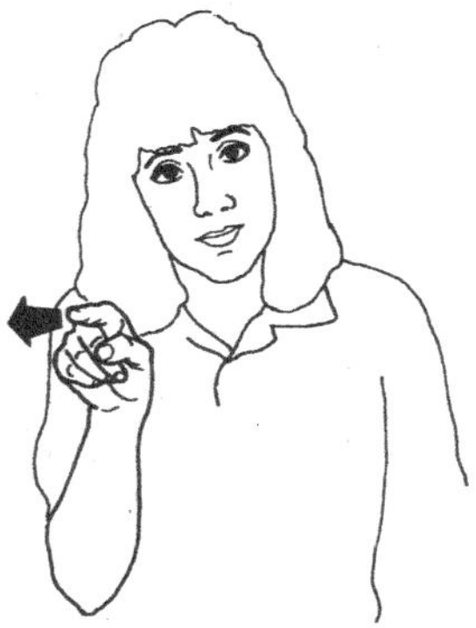

YOU

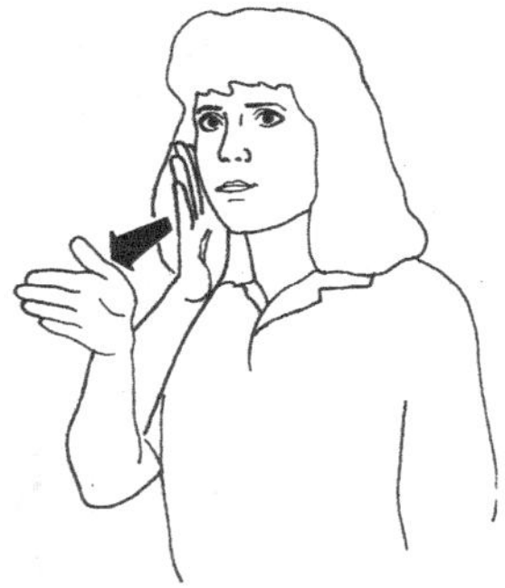

WILL

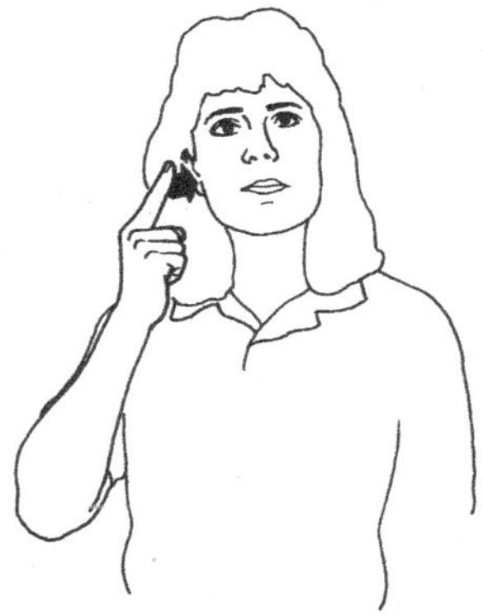

HEAR

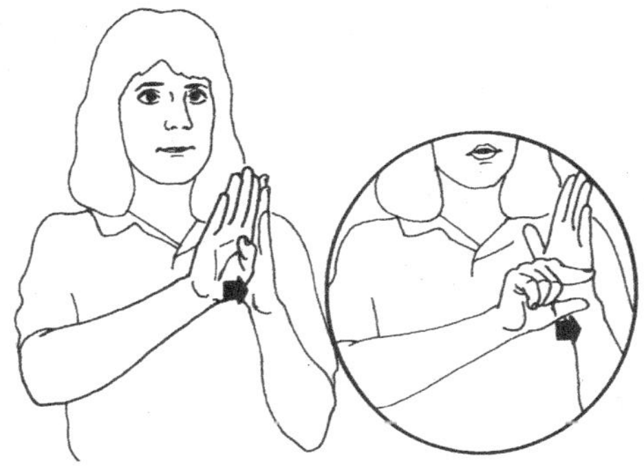

BACKGROUND

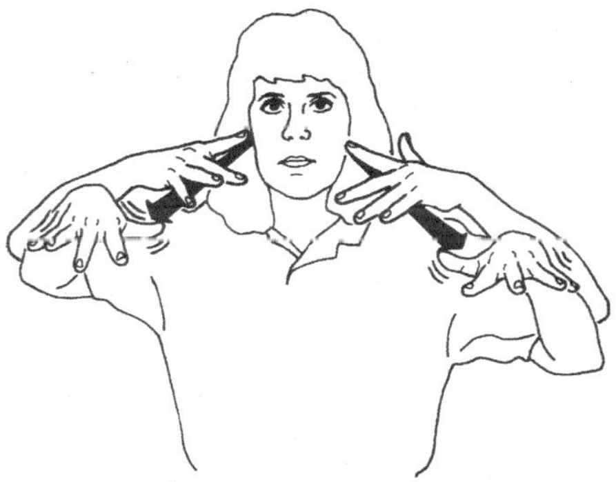

NOISE

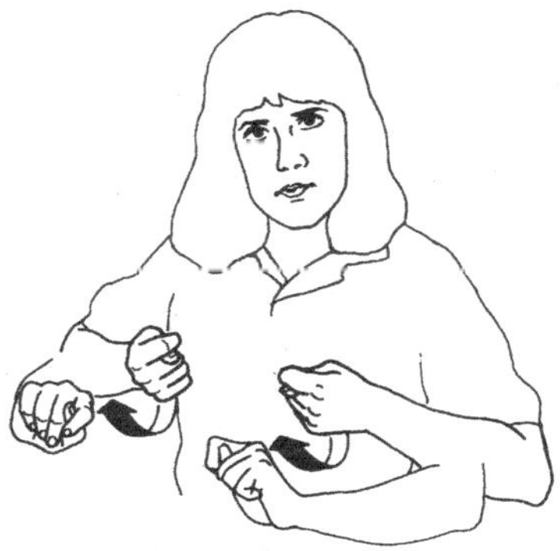

TRY

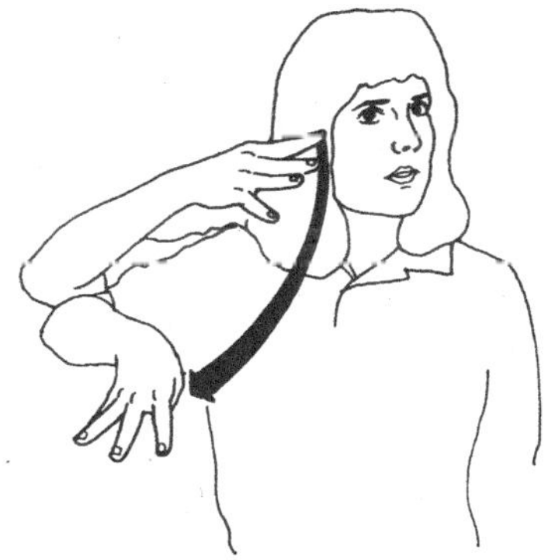

IGNORE.

You will hear background noise; try to ignore it.

Chapter 5

Aural Rehabilitation

Strategies

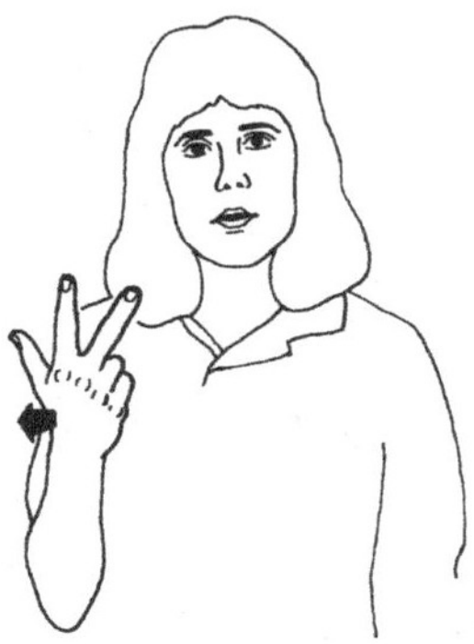

THREE

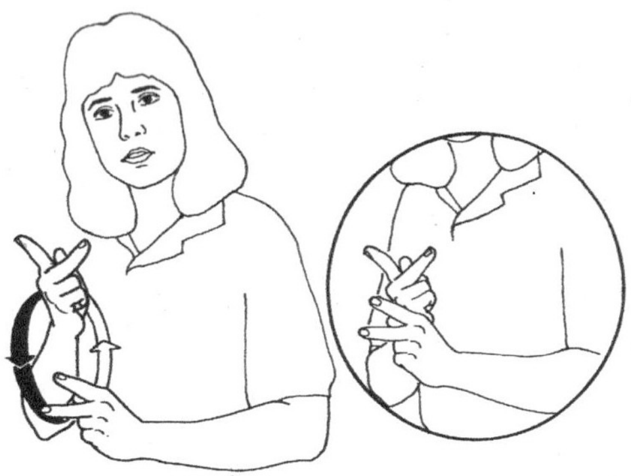

TYPE

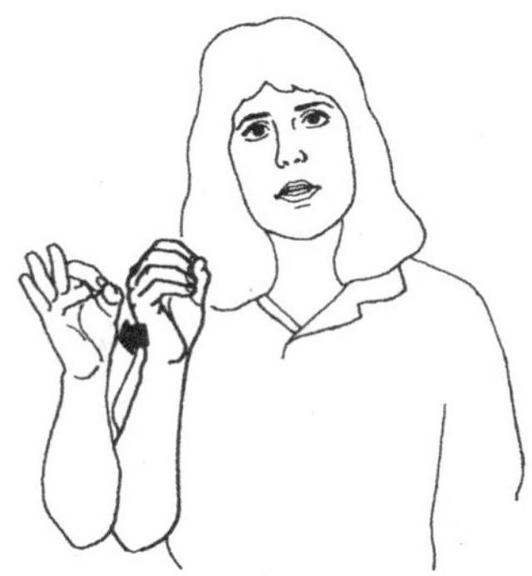

O-F

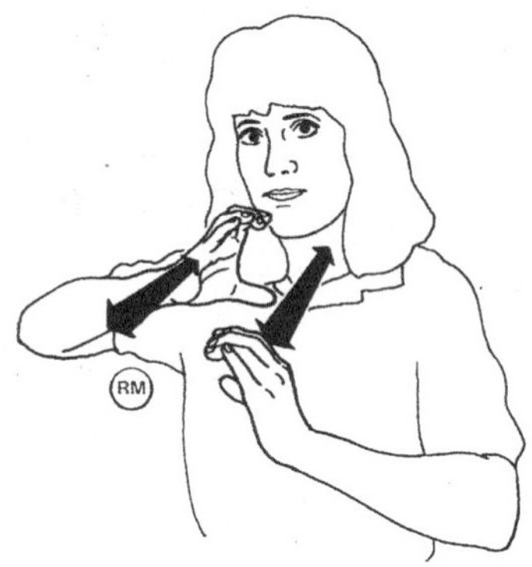

COMMUNICATION

The three types of communication behaviors are passive, assertive, and aggressive.

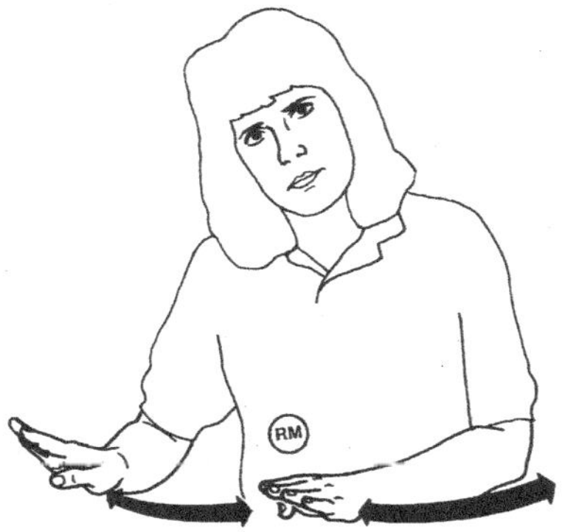

BEHAVIOR

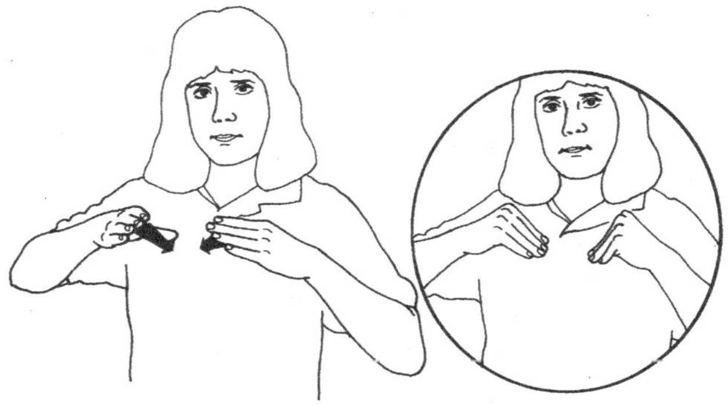

PASSIVE

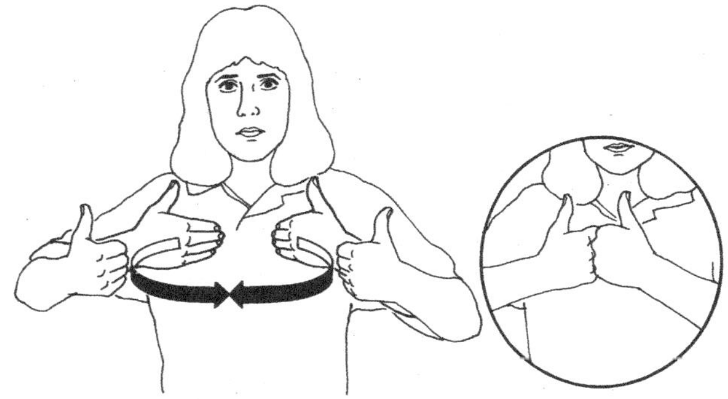

ASSERTIVE

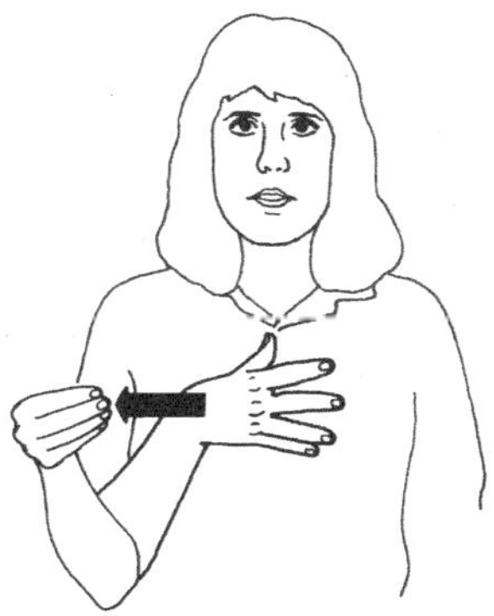

AND

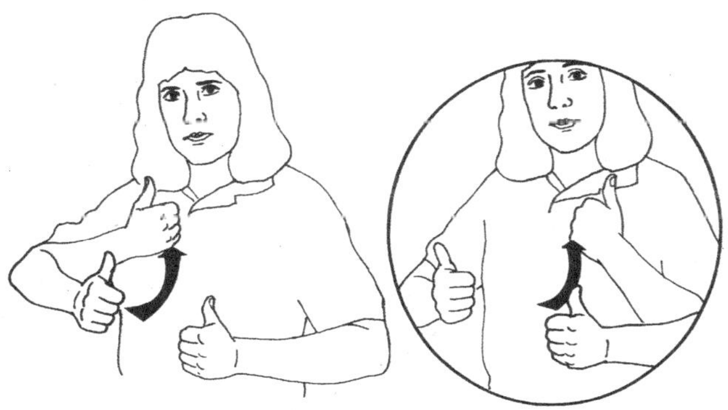

AGGRESSIVE.

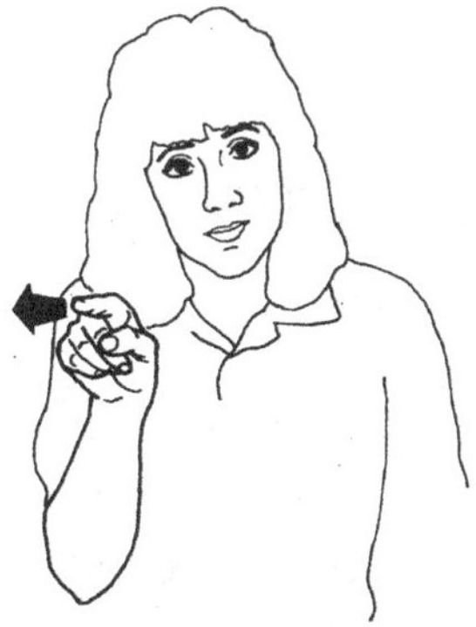

YOU

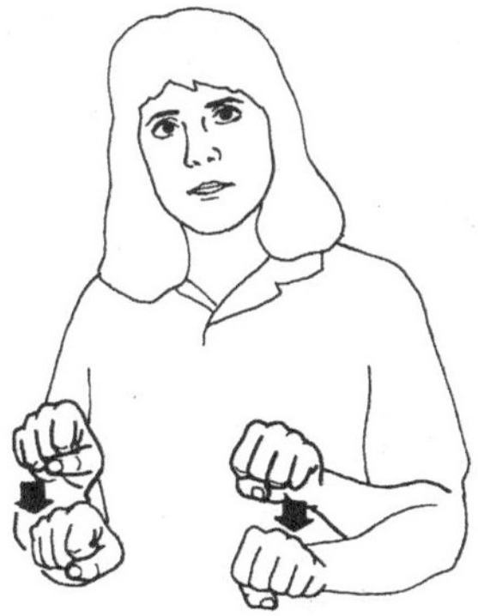

CAN

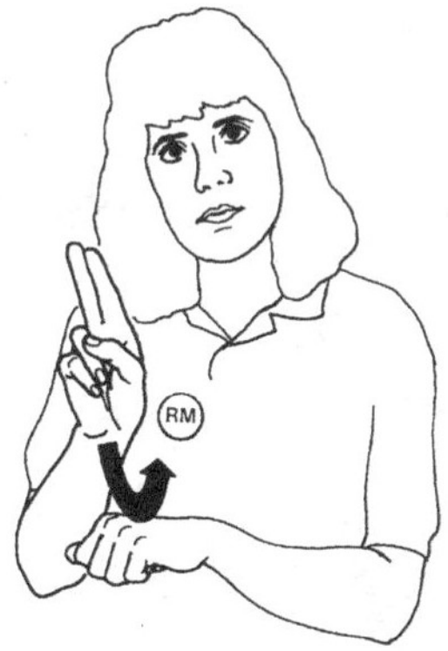

USE

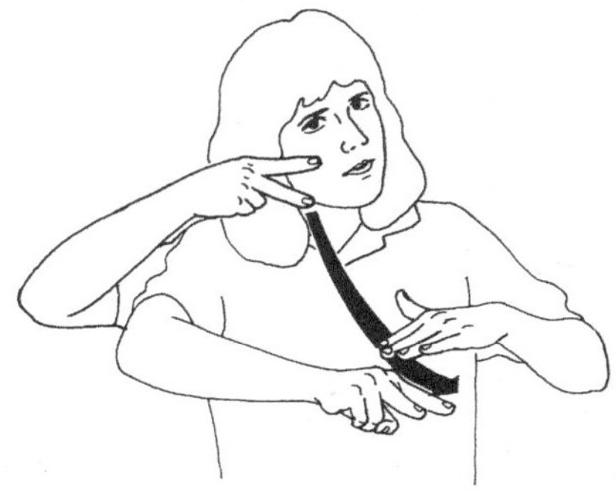

ANTICIPATORY

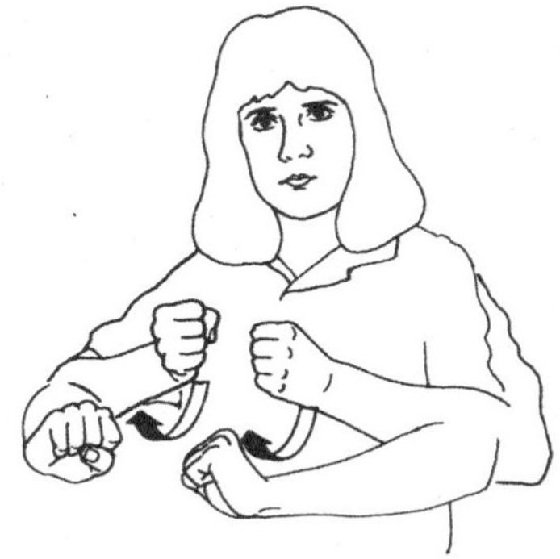

STRATEGIES

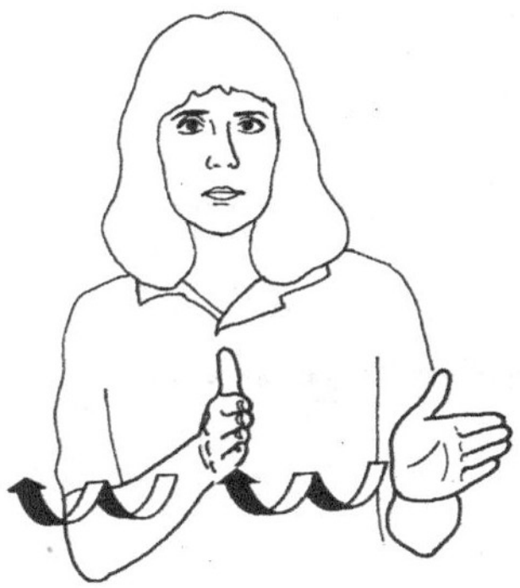

PREPARE

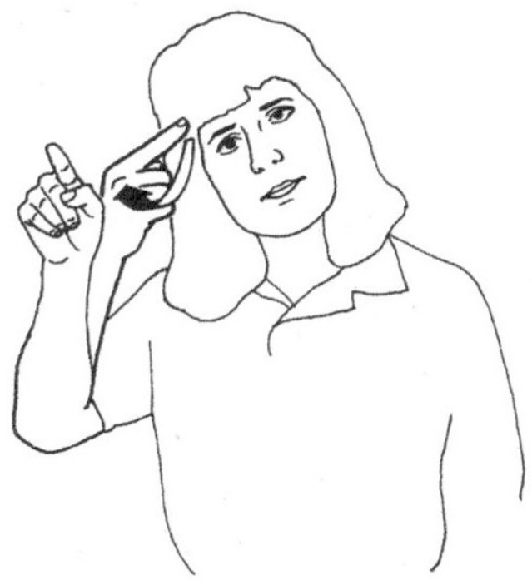

FOR

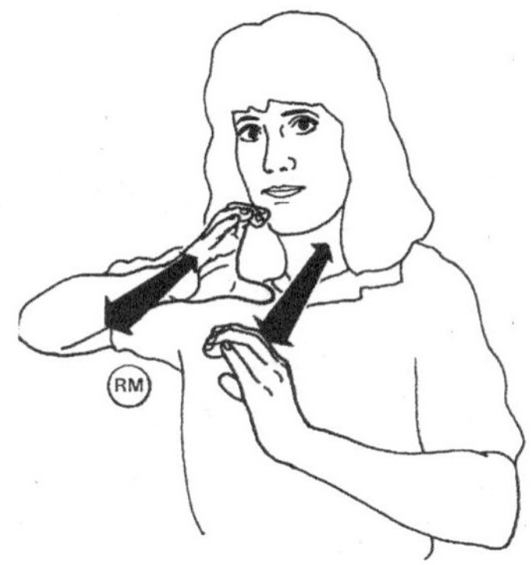

COMMUNICATION

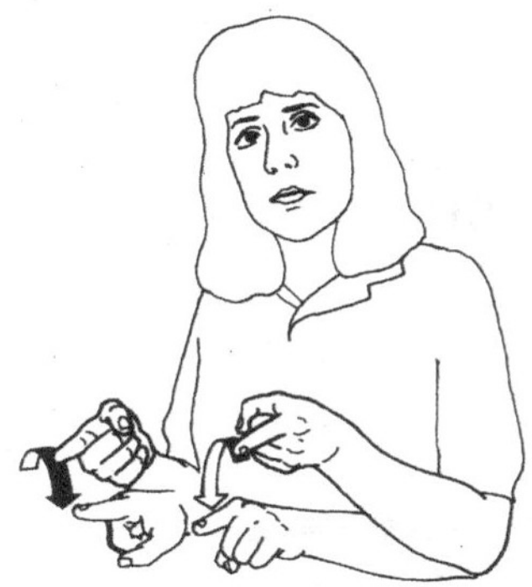

EVENT.

You can use anticipatory strategies to prepare for communication events.

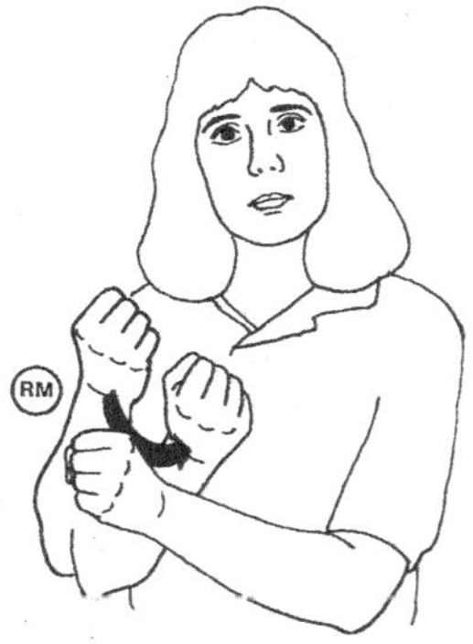

REPAIR

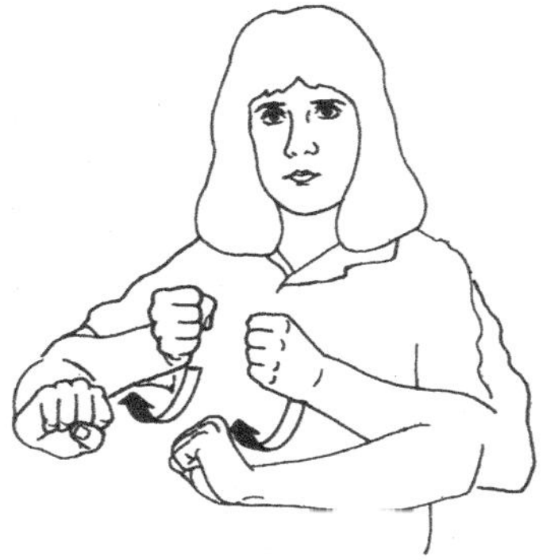

STRATEGIES

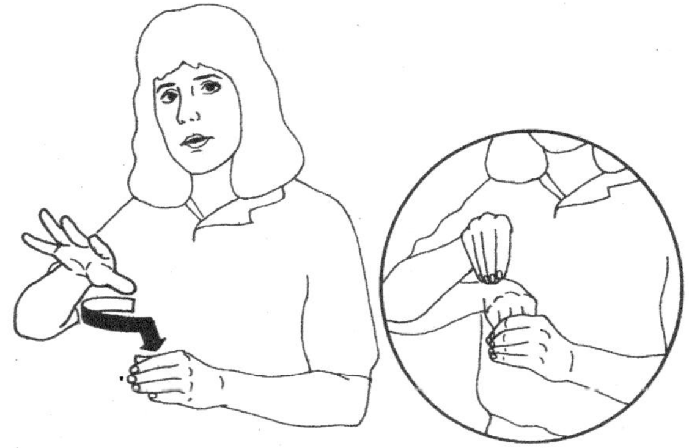

INCLUDE

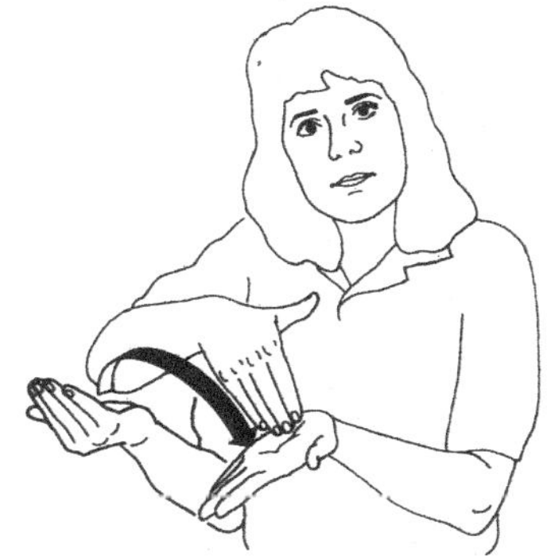

REPEAT

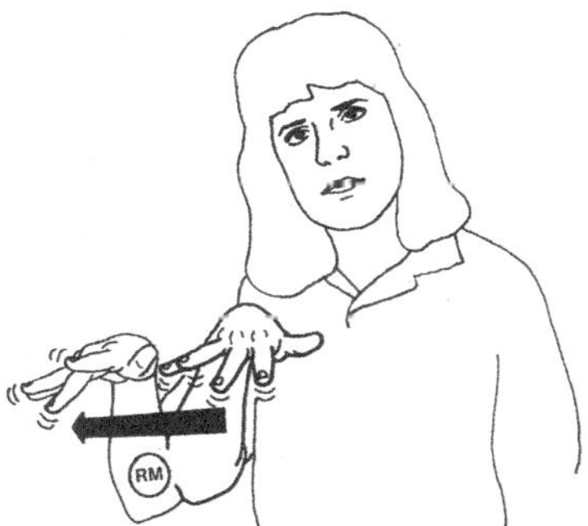

SPELL

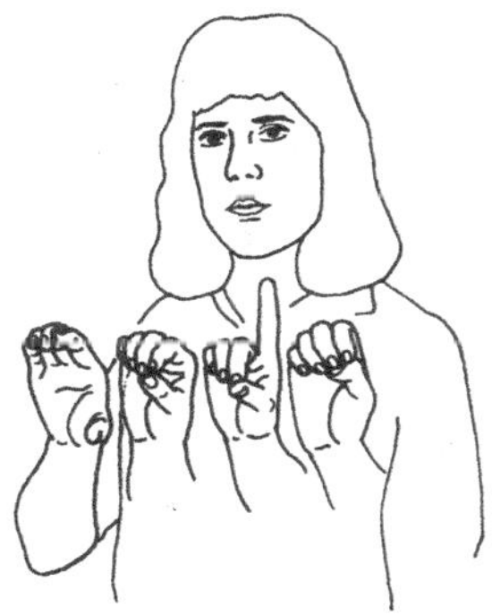

C-O-D-E

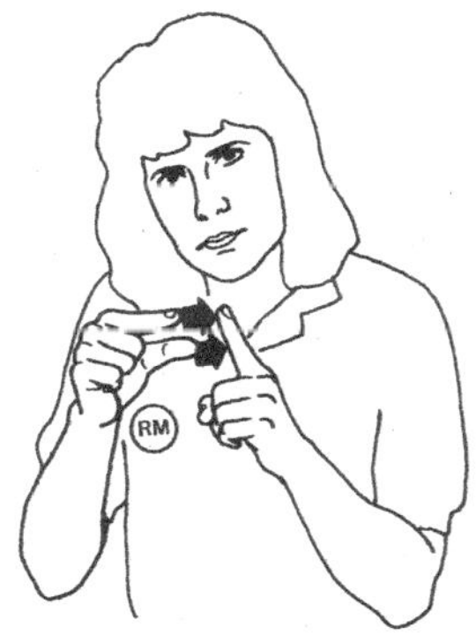

WORD

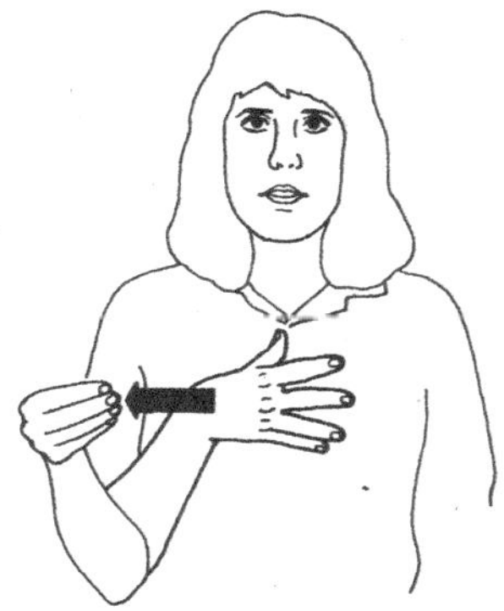

AND

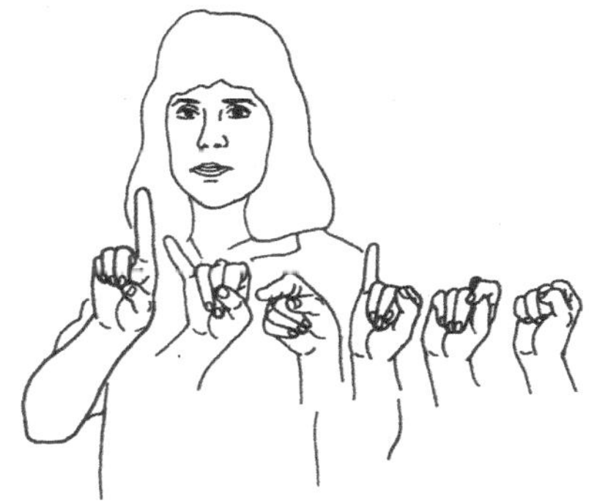

D-I-G-I-T-S.

Repair strategies include repeat, spell, code words, and digits.

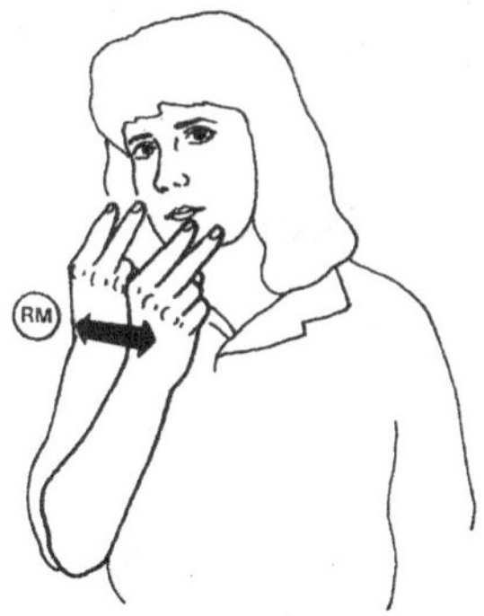

SPEECHREAD

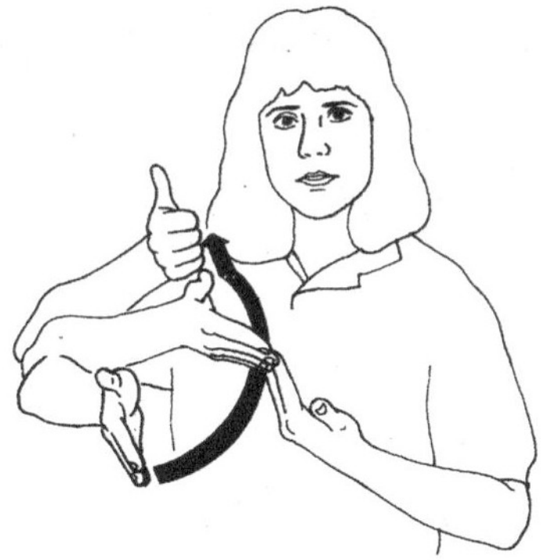

EASIER

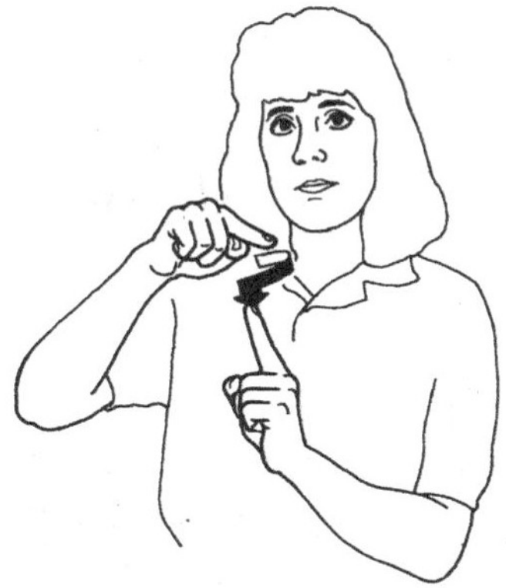

WHEN

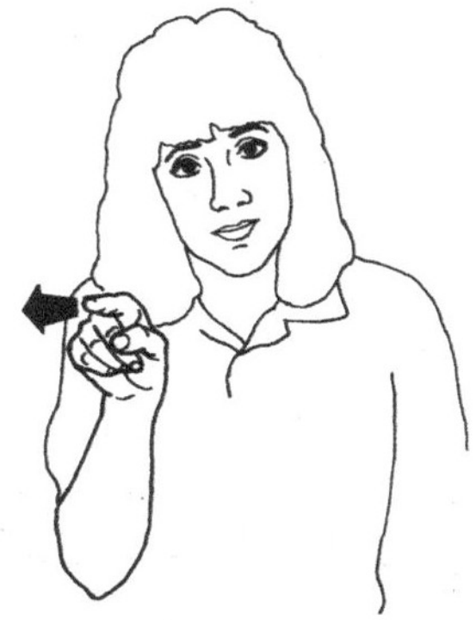

YOU

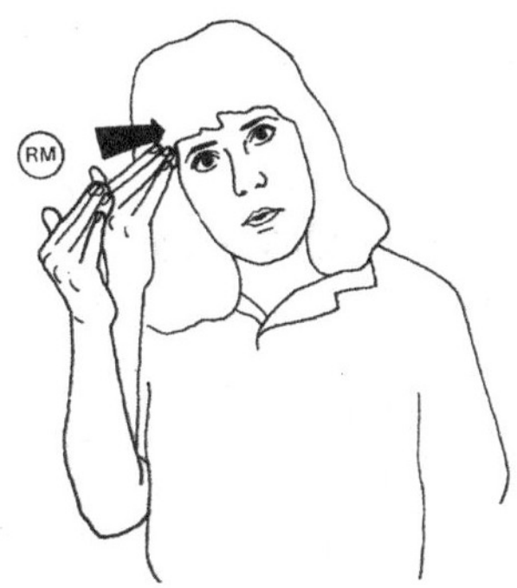

KNOW

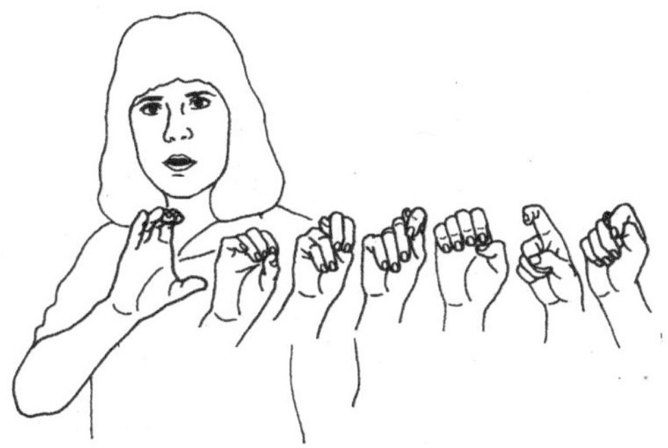

C-O-N-T-E-X-T.

Speechreading is easier when you know the context.

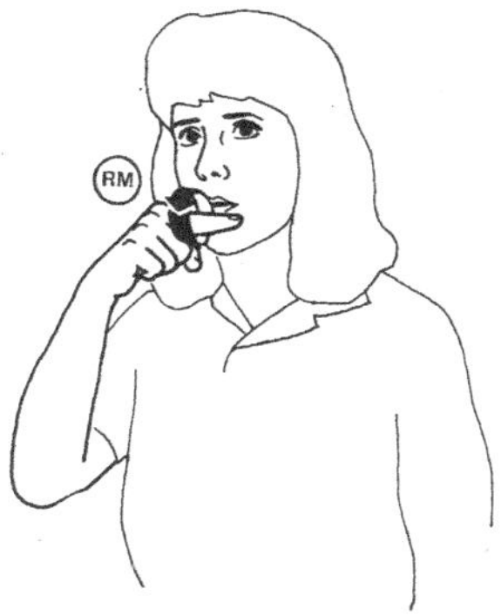

SAY

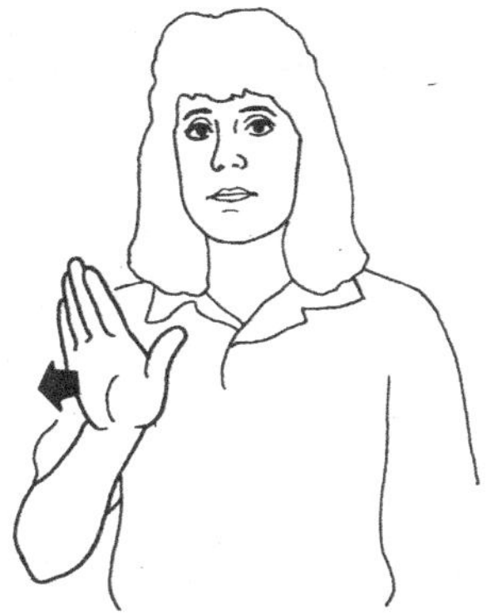

YOUR

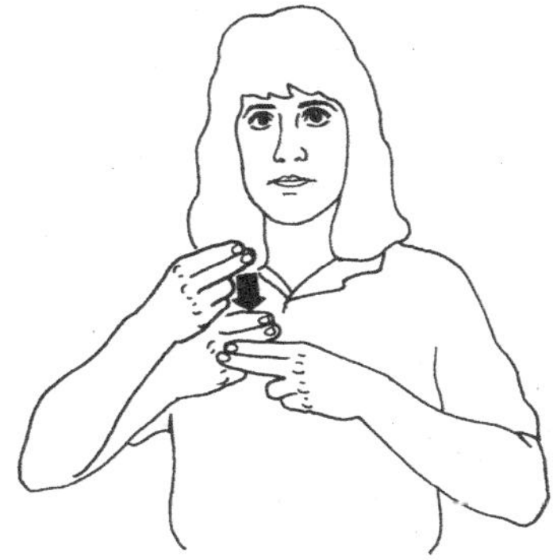

NAME

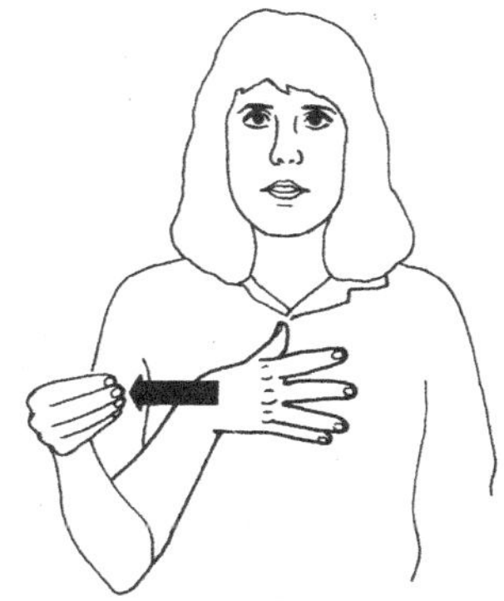

AND

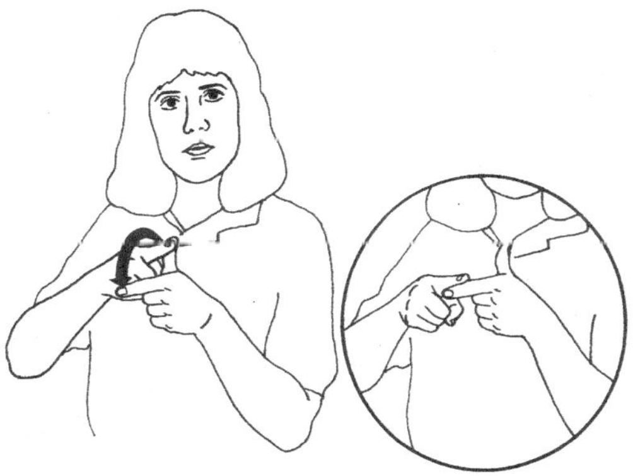

THEN

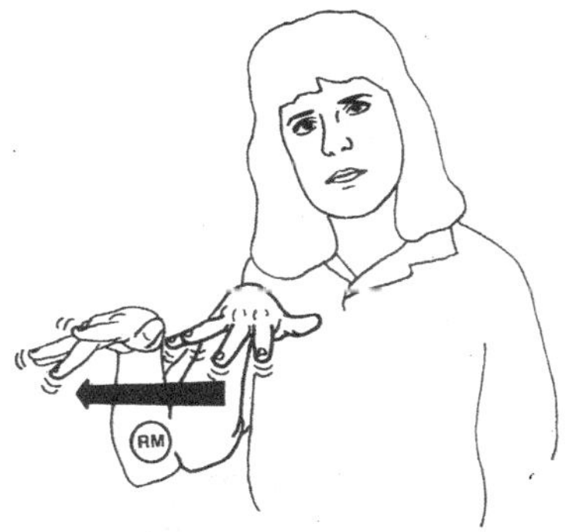

SPELL

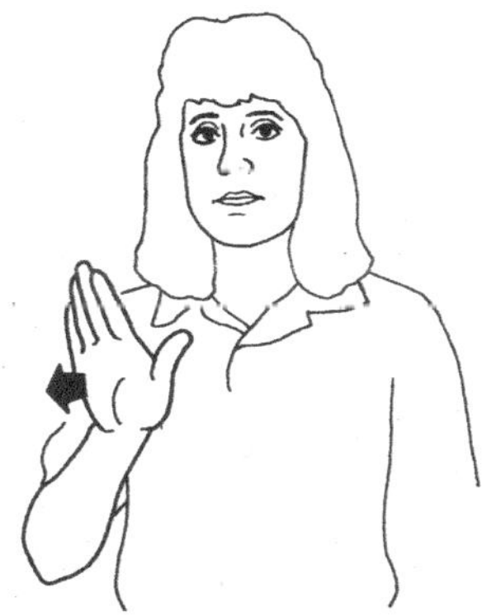

YOUR

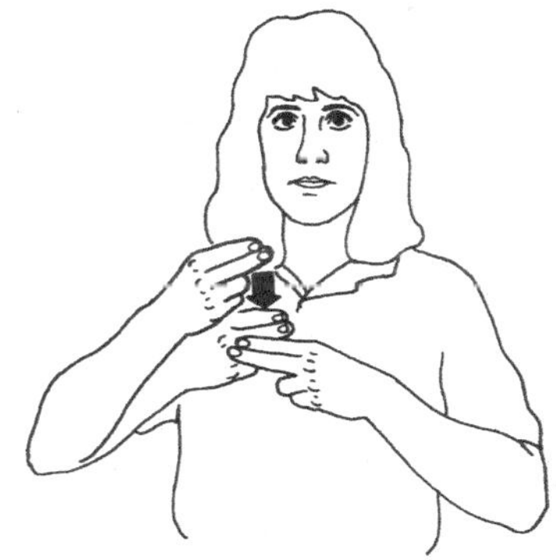

NAME.

Say your name and then spell your name.

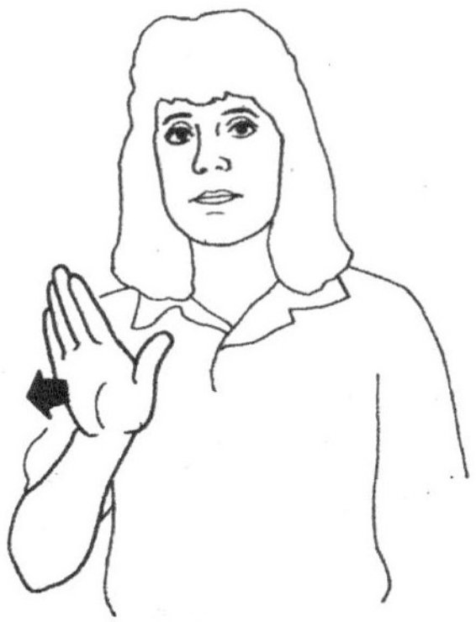

YOUR

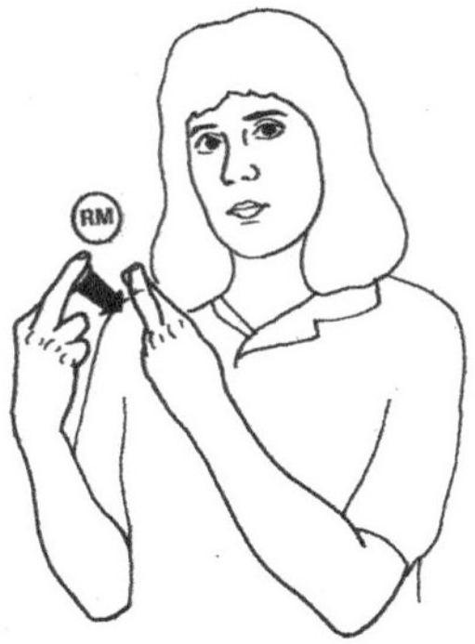

RESPONSIBILITY

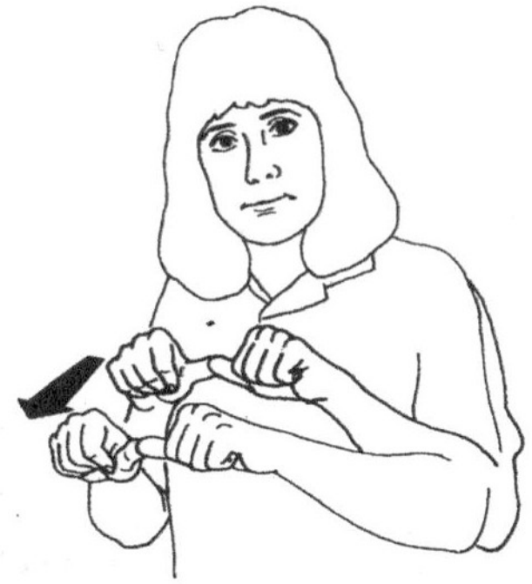

MAINTAIN

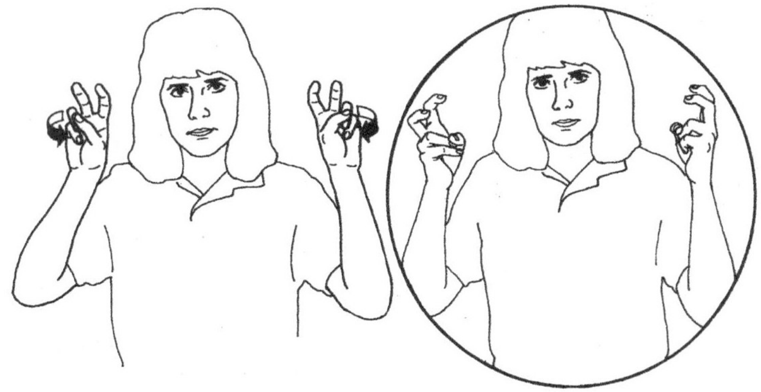

TOPIC

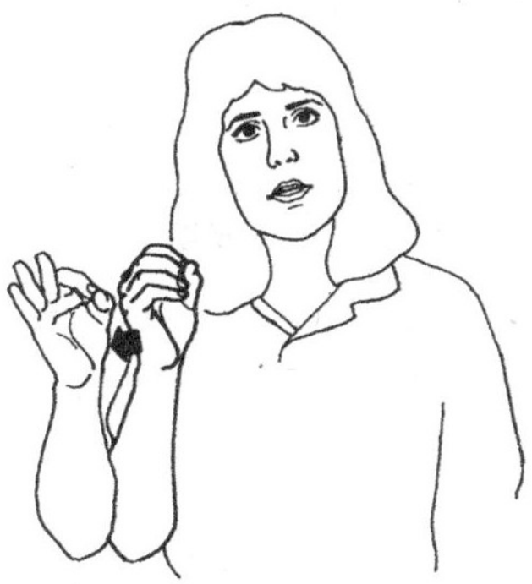

O-F

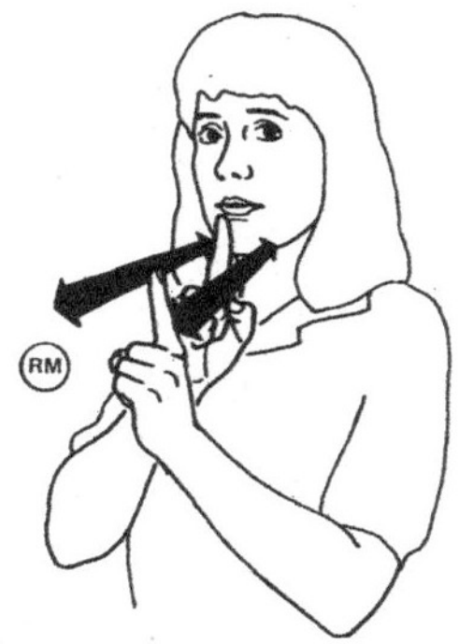

CONVERSATION.

It is your responsibility to maintain the topic of conversation.

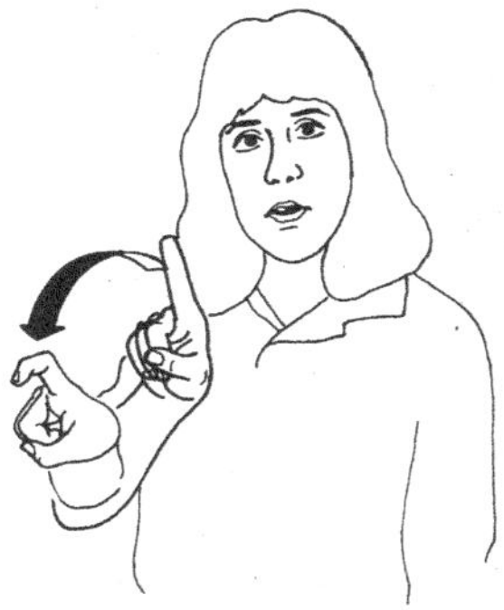

ASK

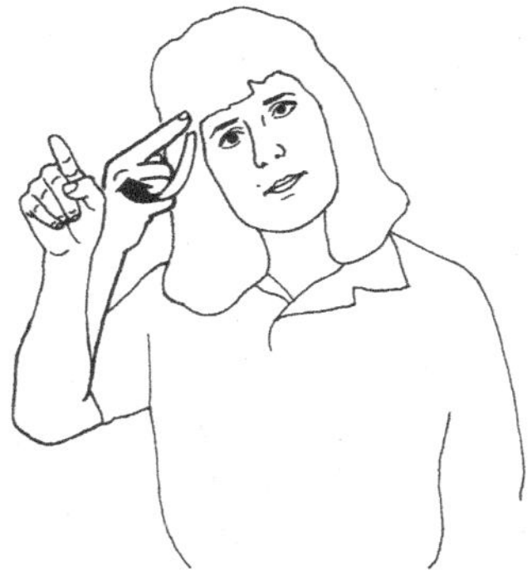

FOR

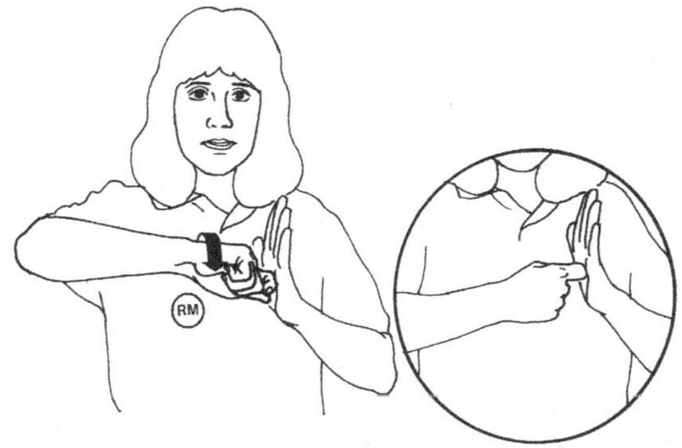

KEY

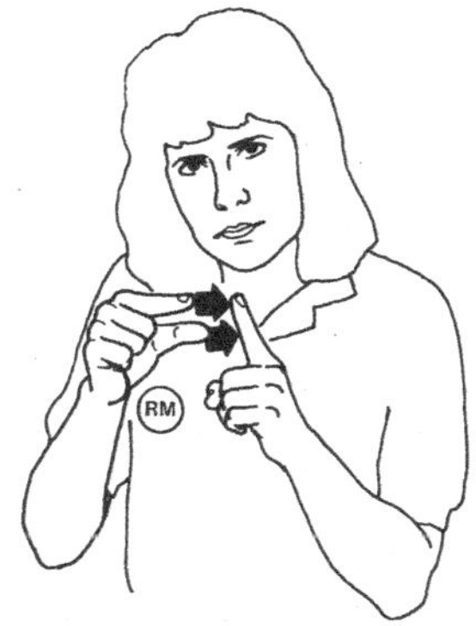

WORD.

Ask for the key word.

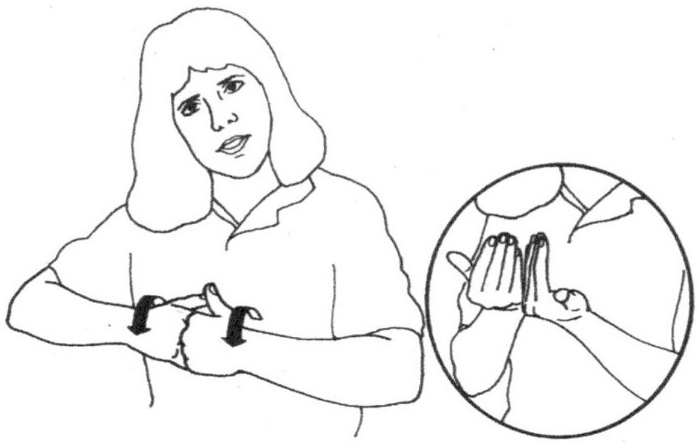

HOW

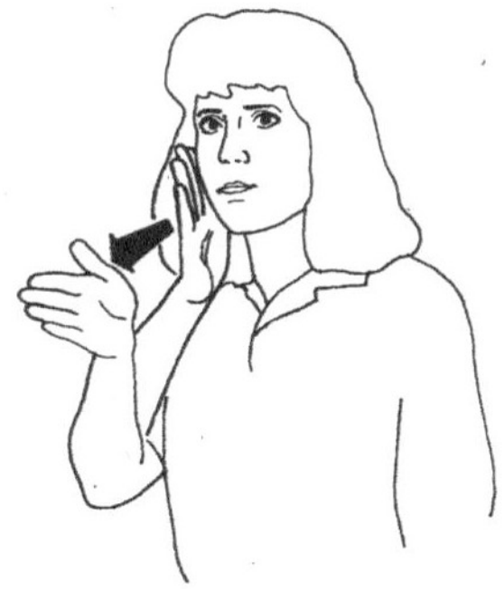

WILL

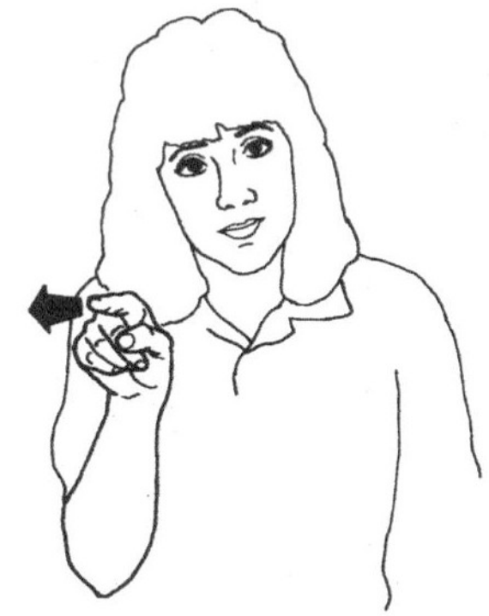

YOU

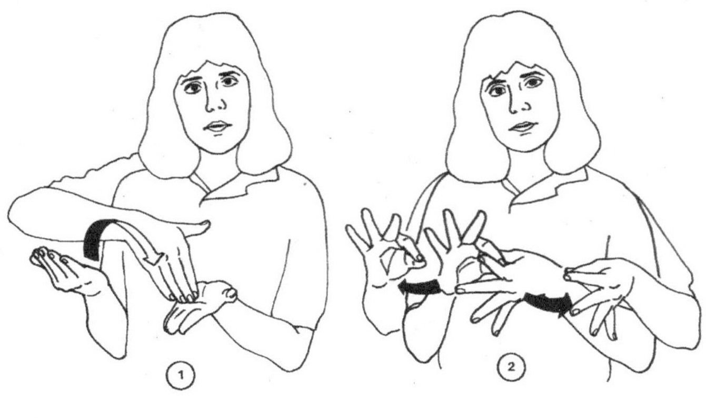

REPHRASE

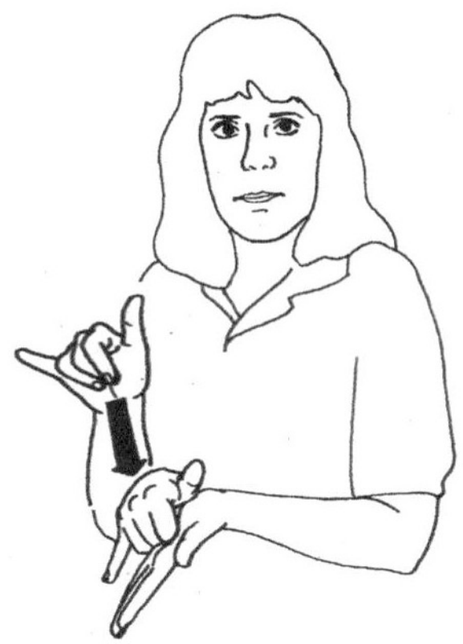

THAT

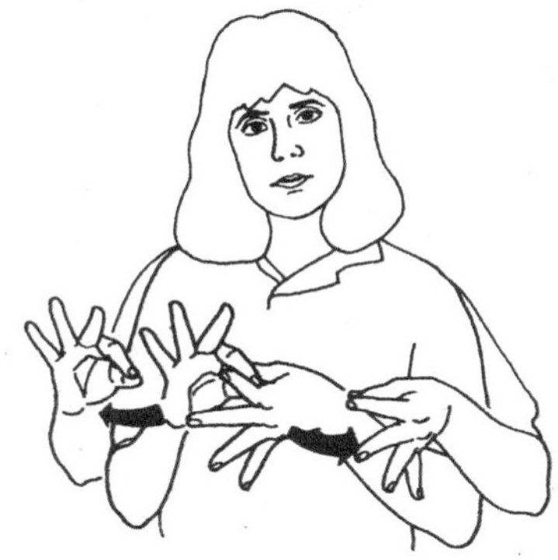

SENTENCE?

How would you rephrase that sentence?

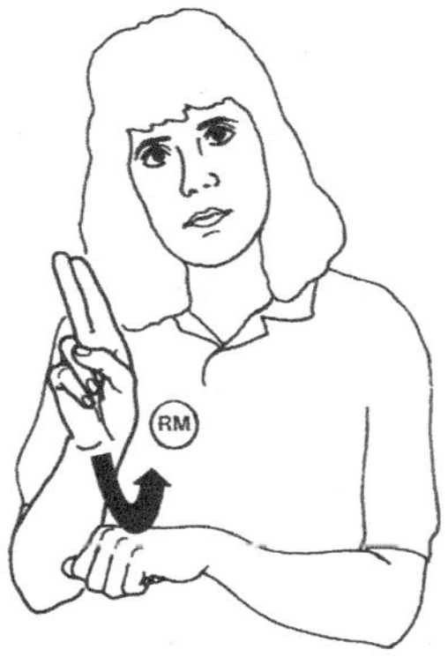

USE

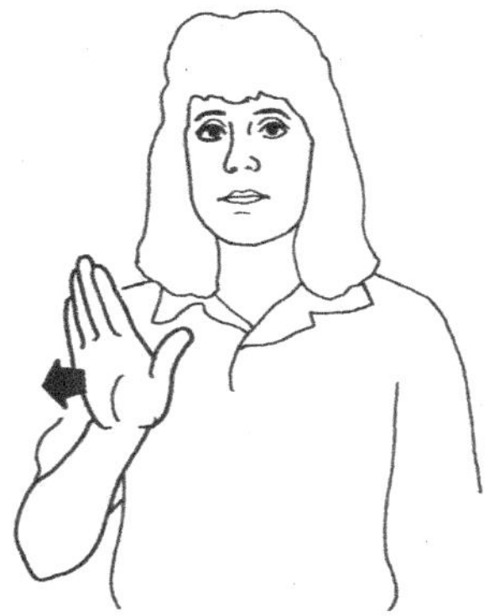

YOUR

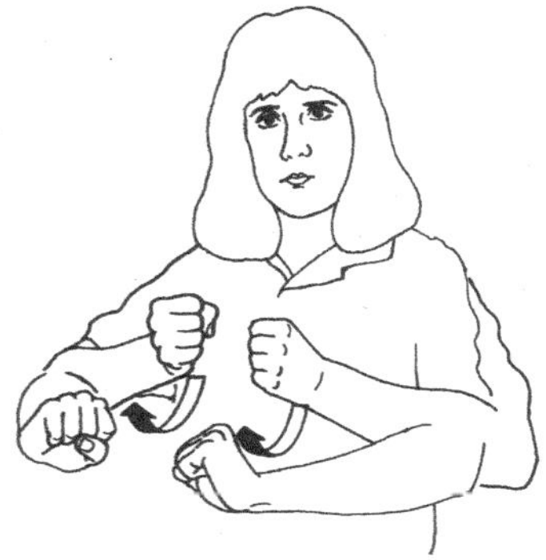

STRATEGIES

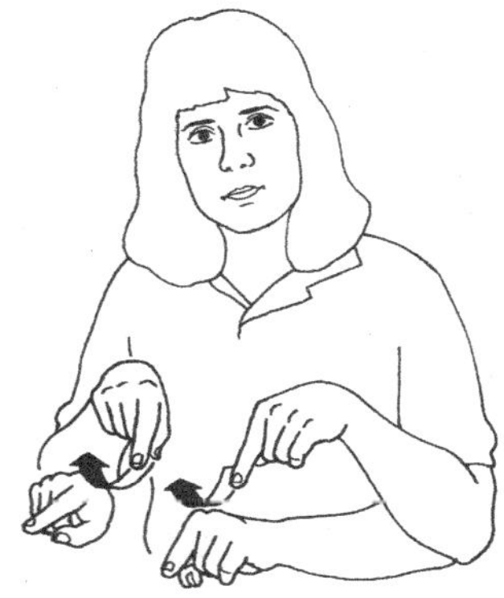

WHILE

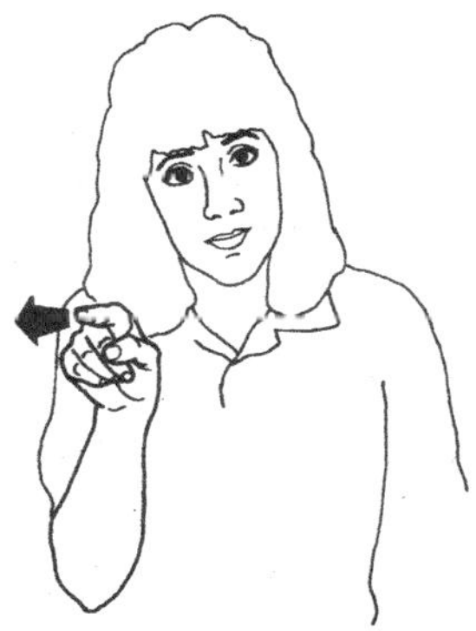

YOU

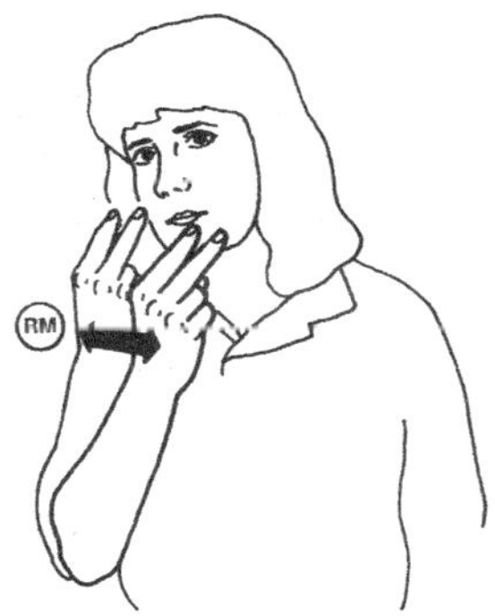

SPEECHREAD.

Use your strategies while you speechread.

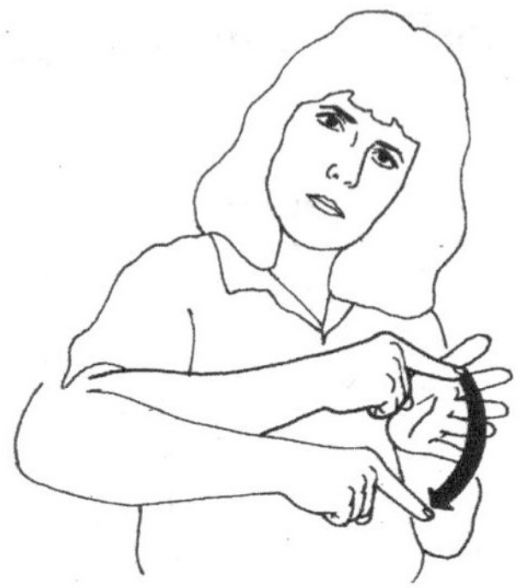

WHAT

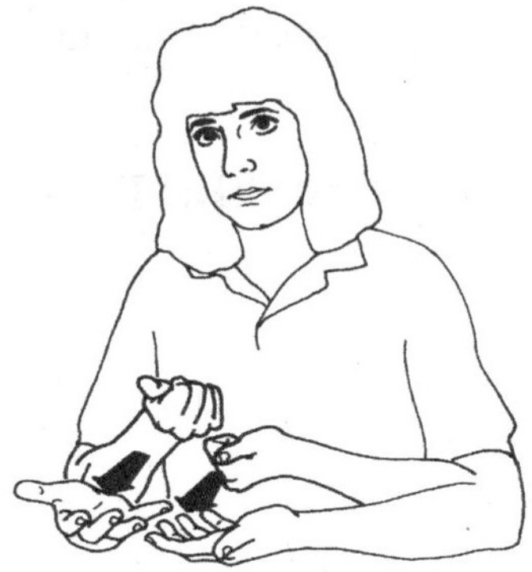

CAUSE

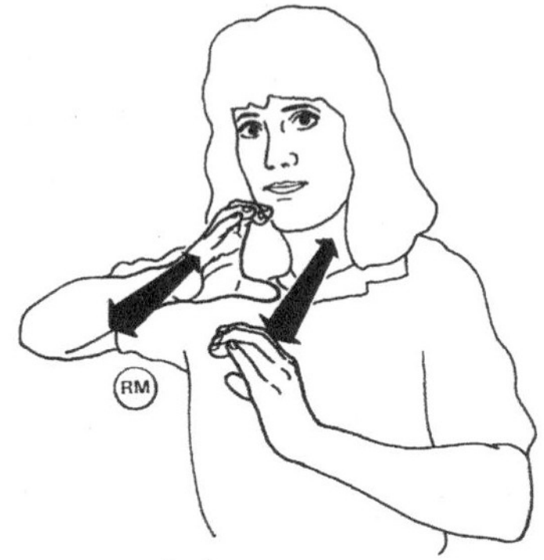

COMMUNICATION

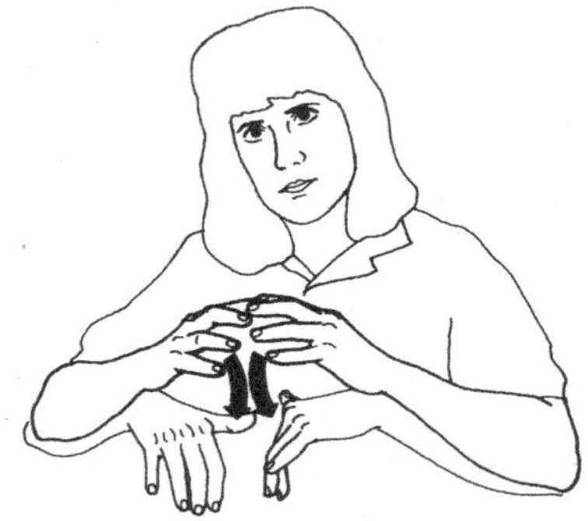

BREAKDOWN?

What caused the communication breakdown?

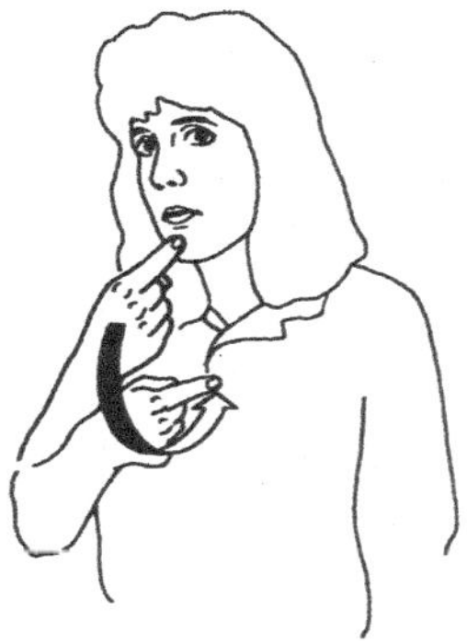

TELL-ME

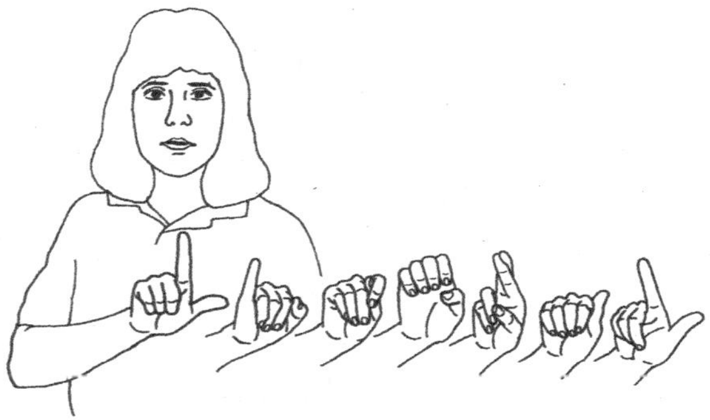

L-I-T-E-R-A-L

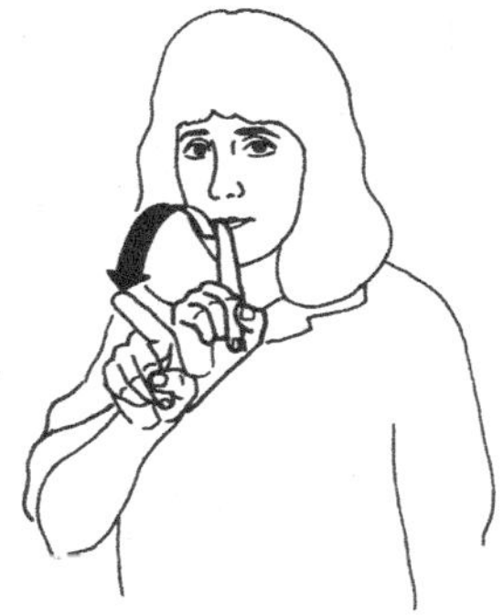

REAL

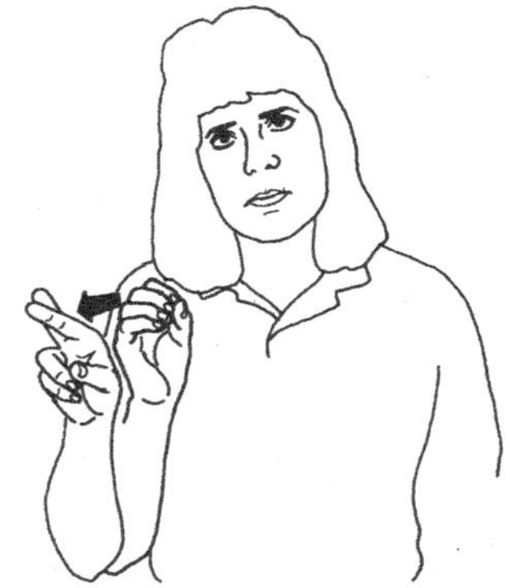

O-R

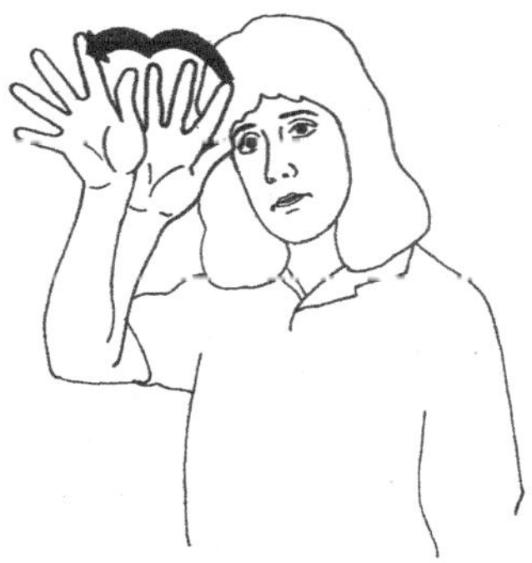

FIGURATIVE

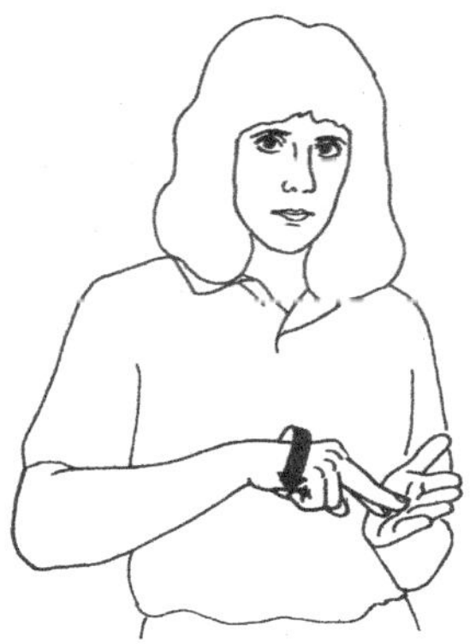

MEANING

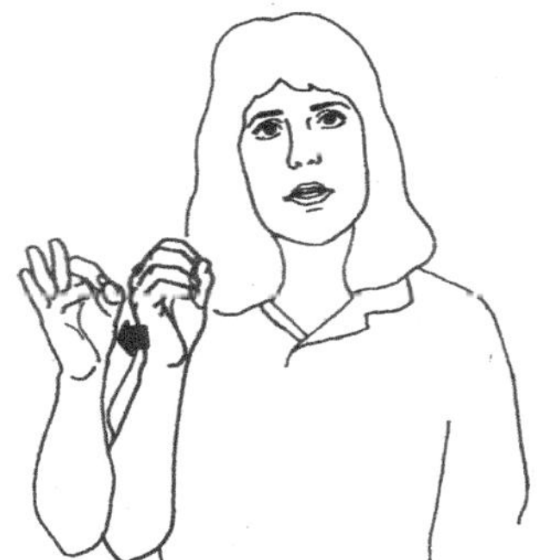

O-F

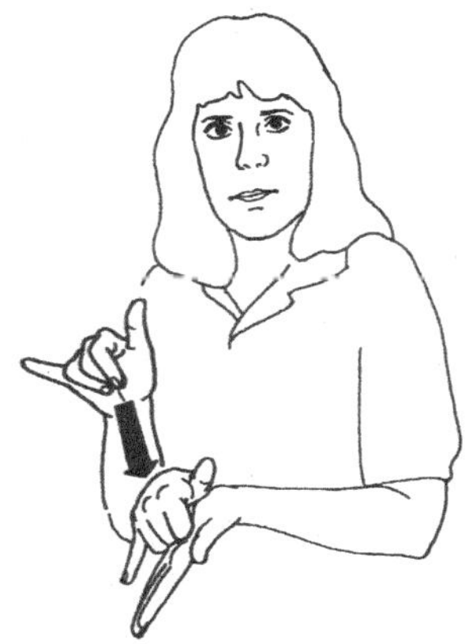

THAT

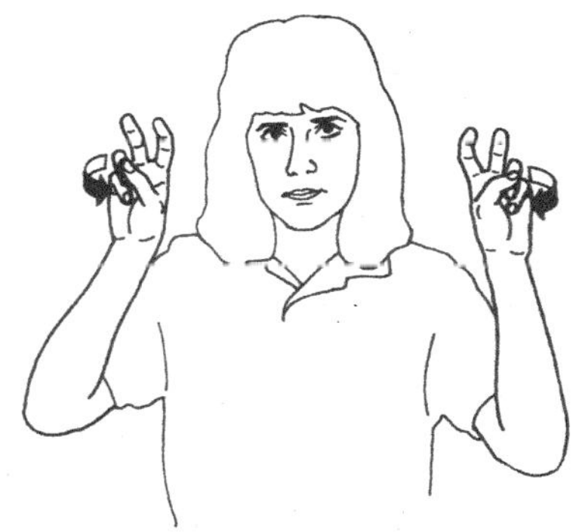

TOPIC.

Tell me the literal or the figurative meaning of that expression.

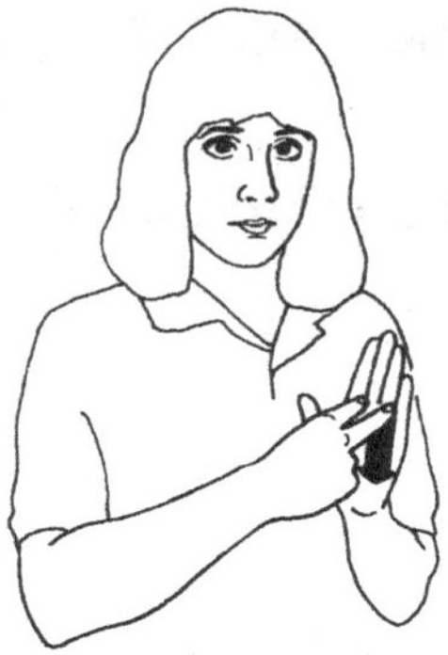

READ

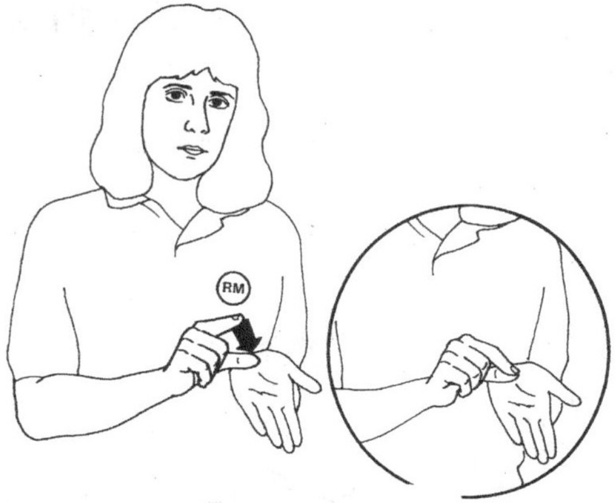

NEWSPAPER

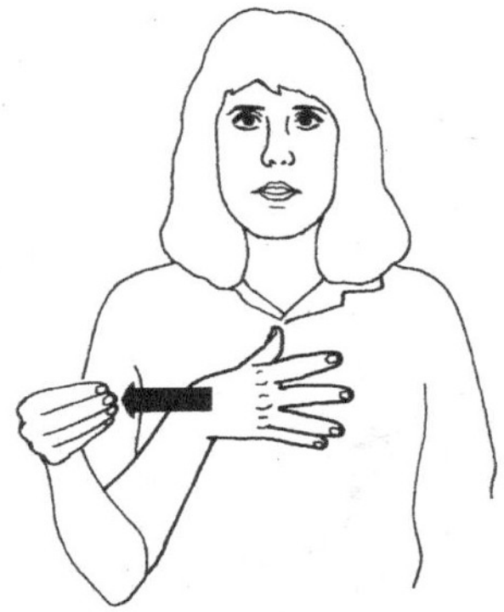

AND

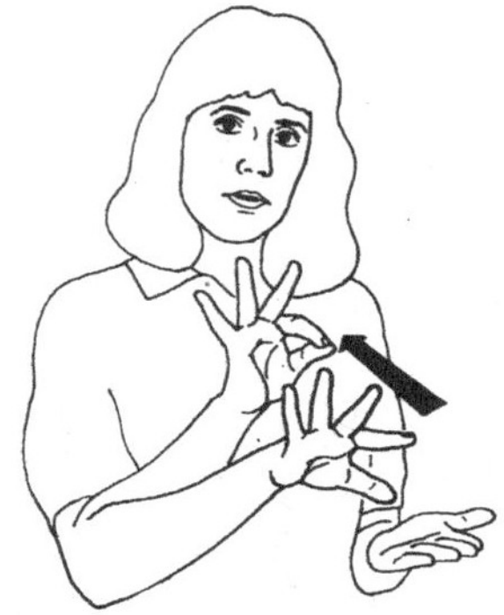

PICK-OUT

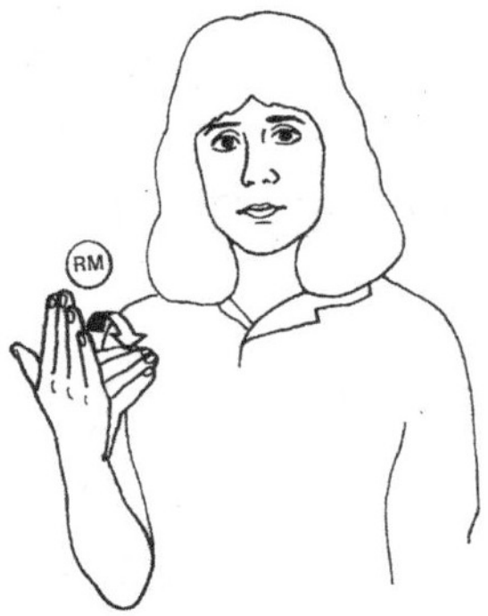

FIFTEEN

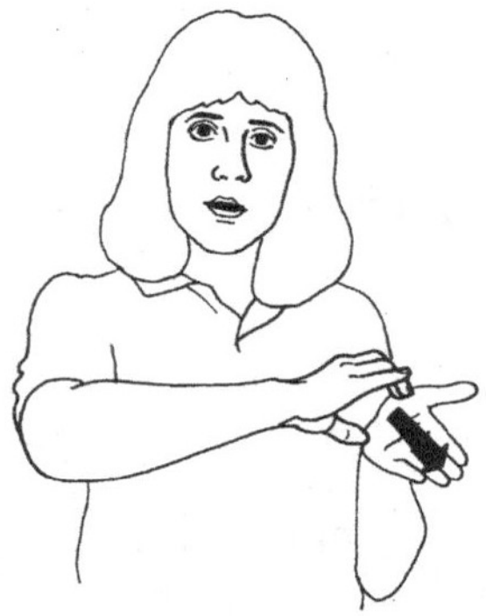

HEADLINES

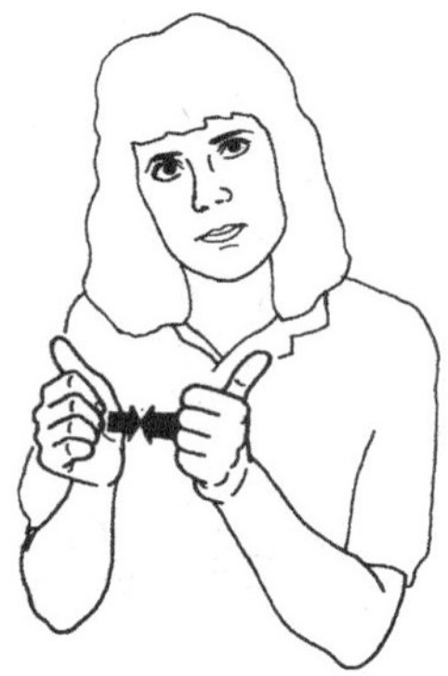

WITH

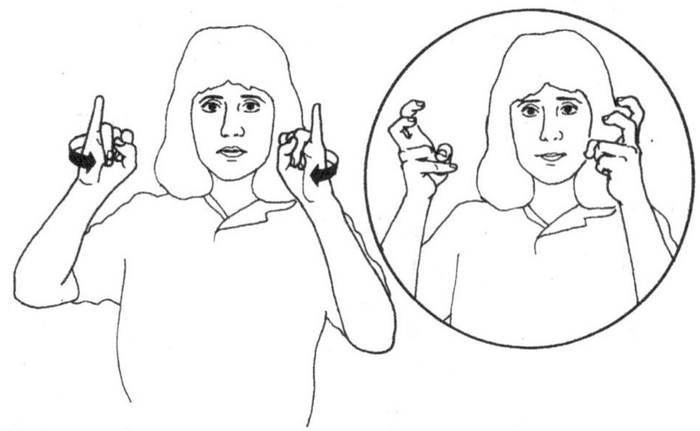

IDIOM.

Read the newspaper and pick out fifteen headlines with idioms.

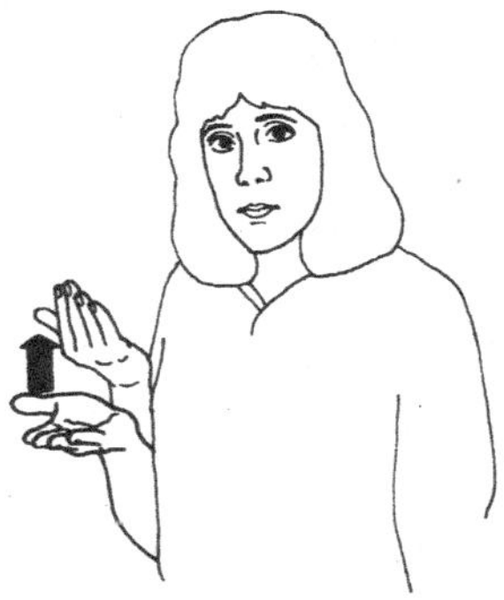

RAISE

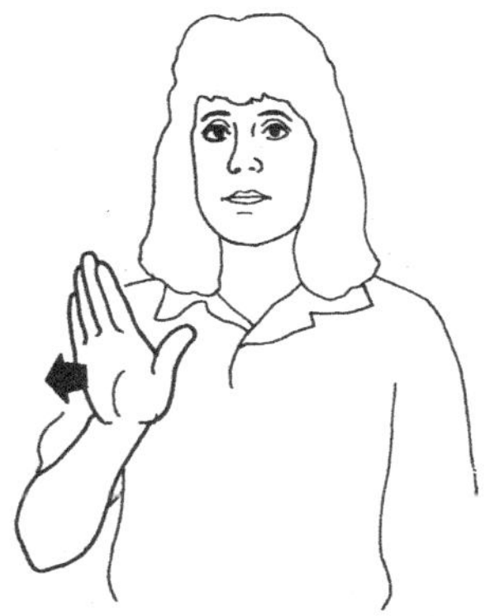

YOUR

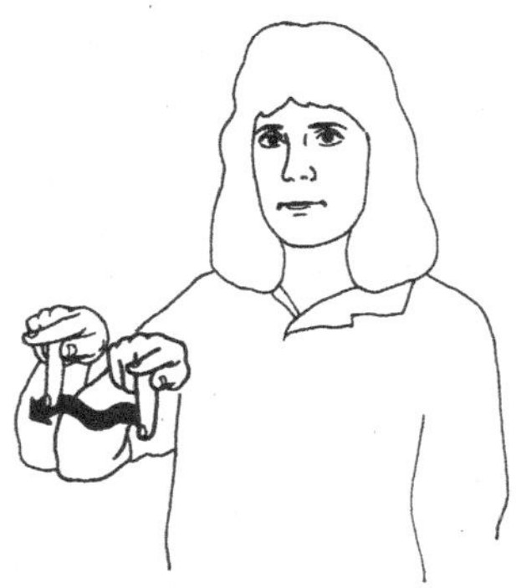

PITCH

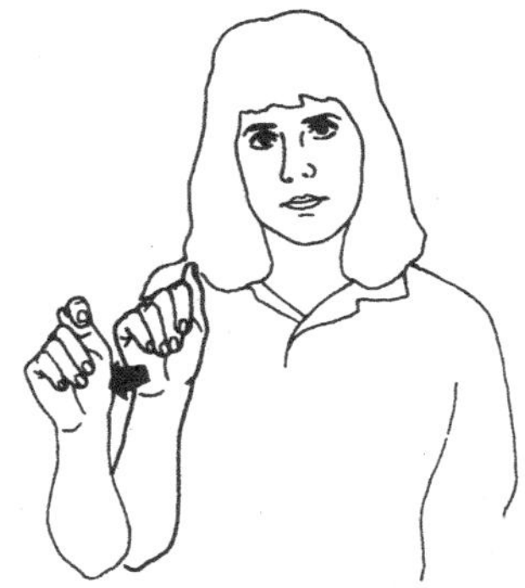

A-T

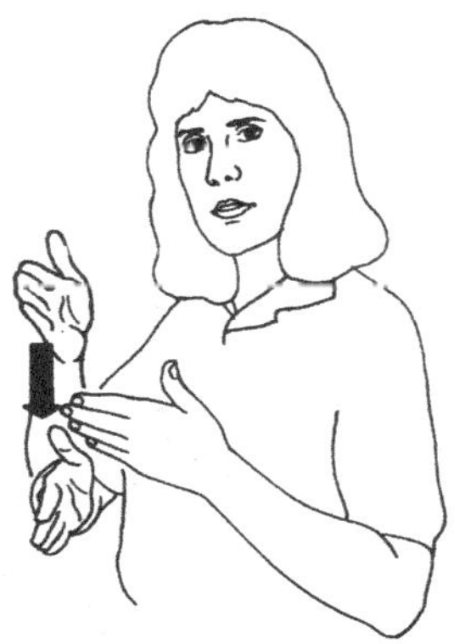

END

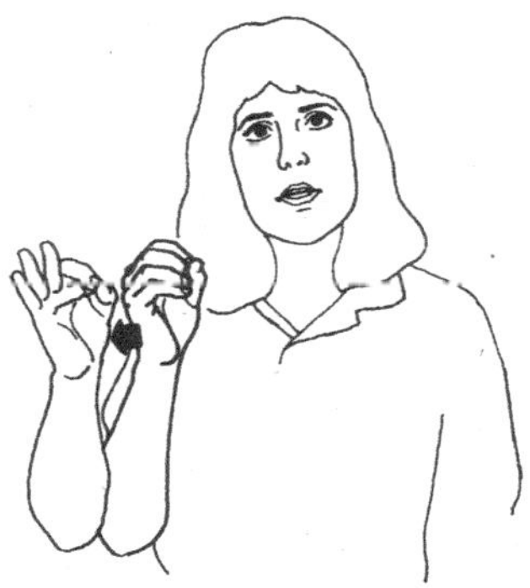

O-F

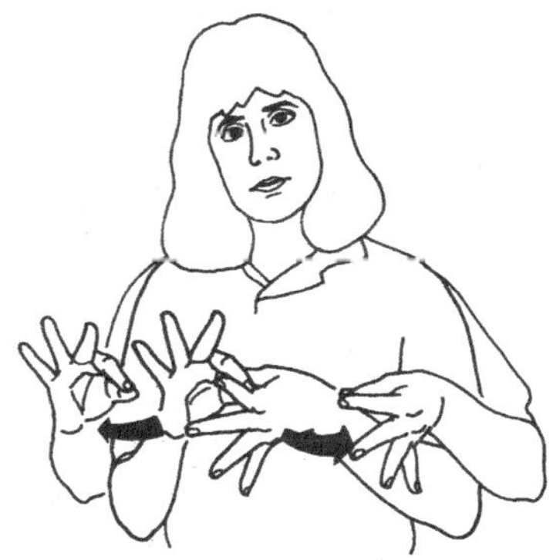

SENTENCE.

Raise your pitch at the end of the sentence.

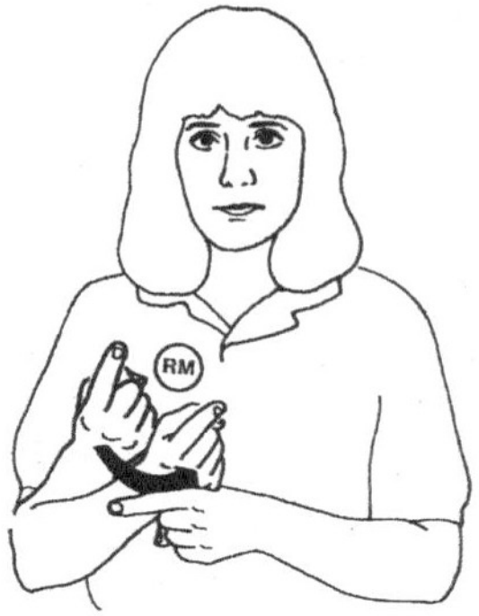

PROPER

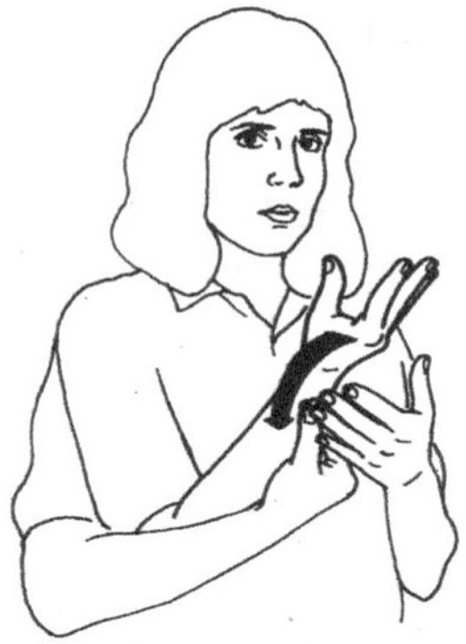

INHALATION

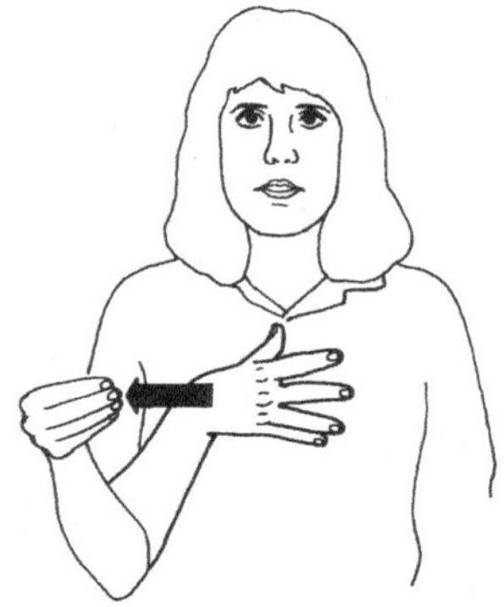

AND

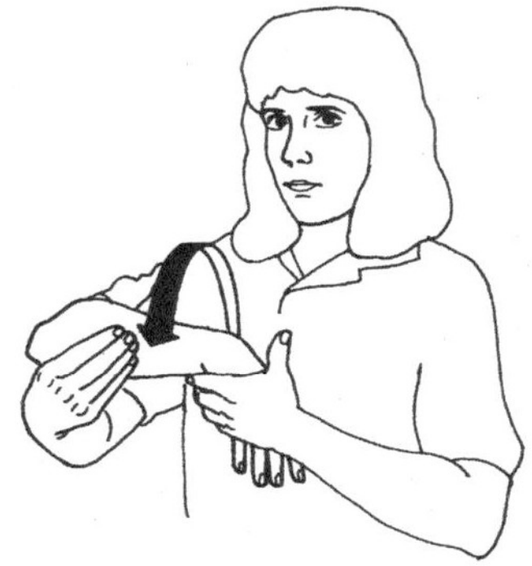

EXHALATION

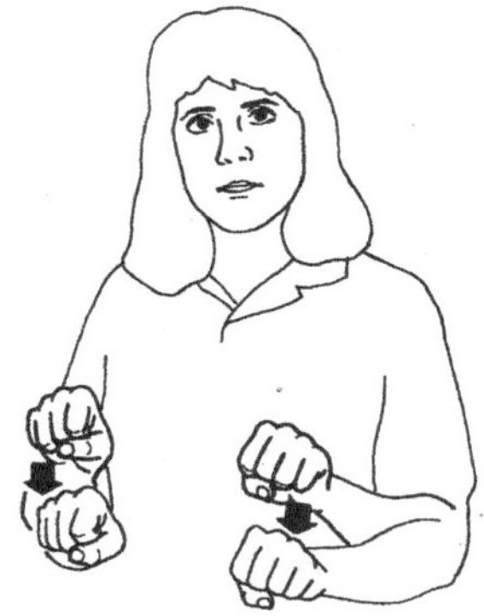

CAN

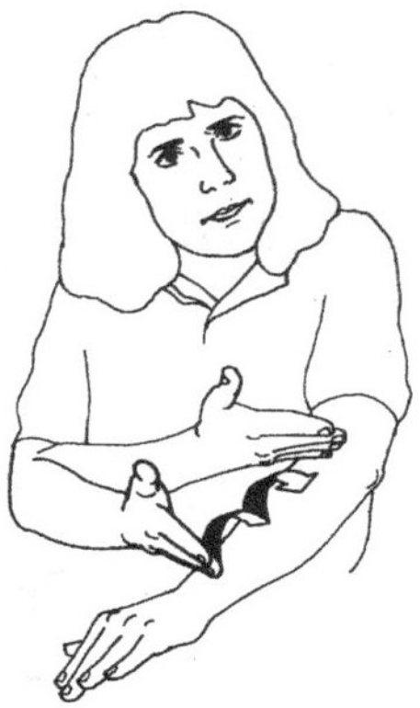

IMPROVE

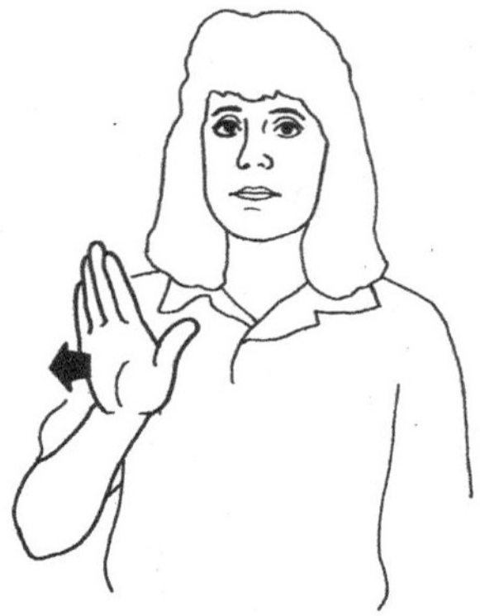

YOUR

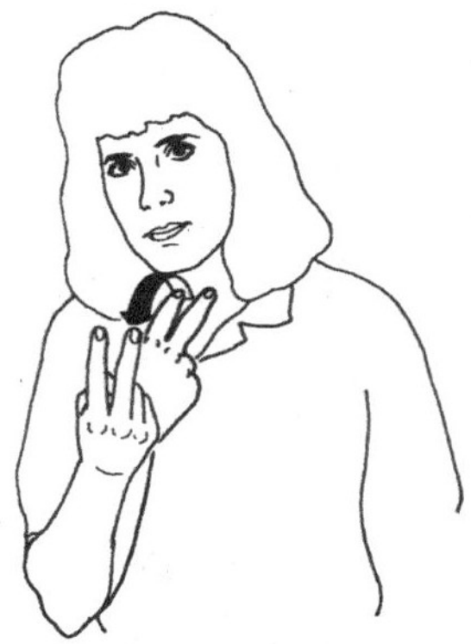

VOICE

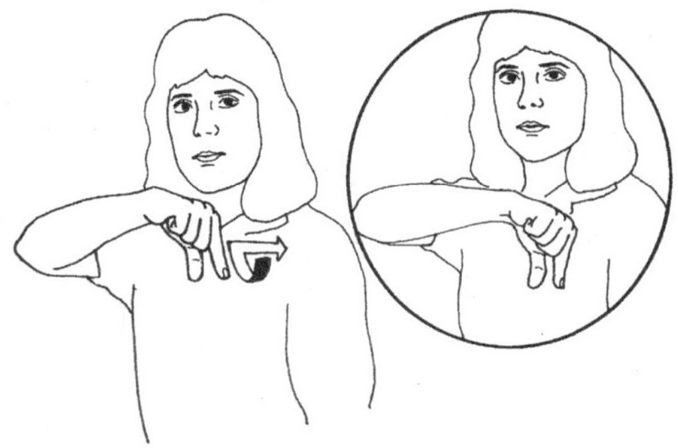

QUALITY.

Proper inhalation and exhalation can improve your voice quality.

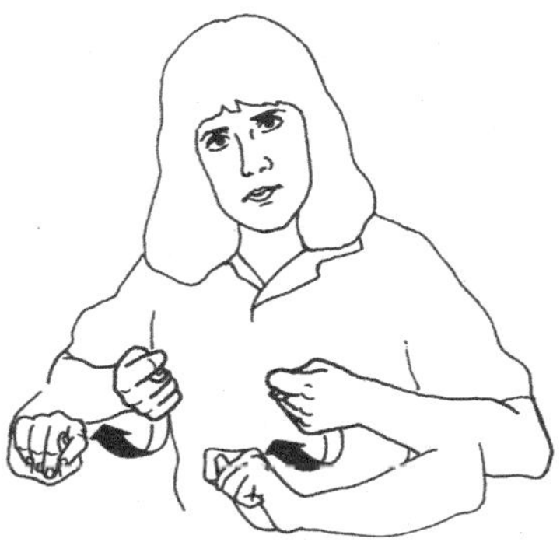

TRY

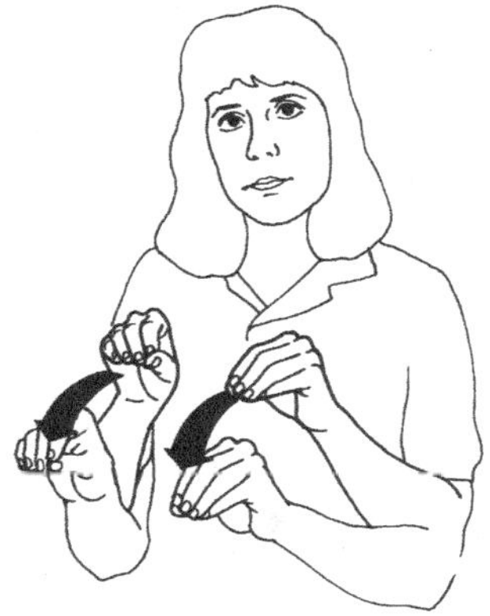

PUT

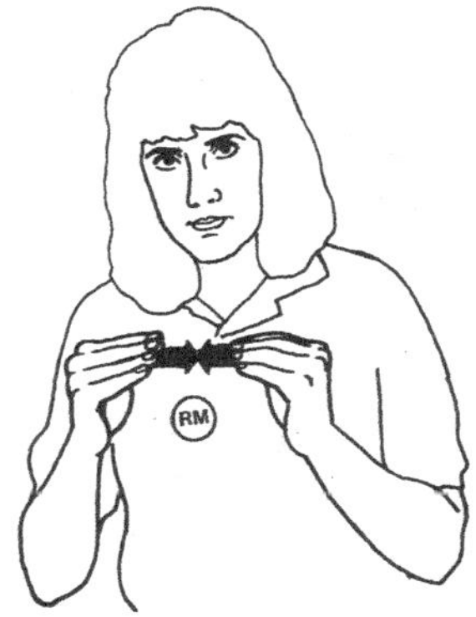

MORE

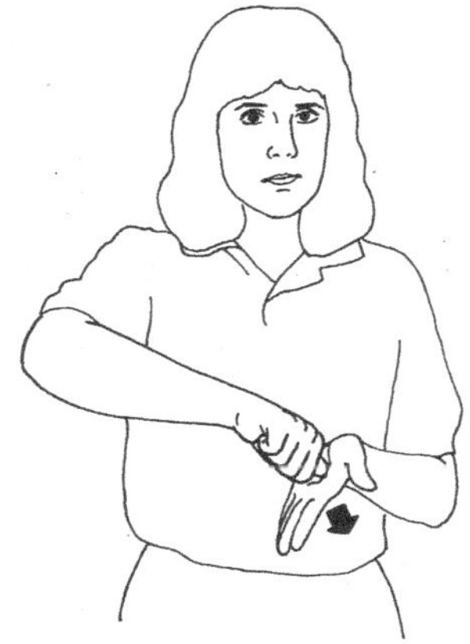

STRESS

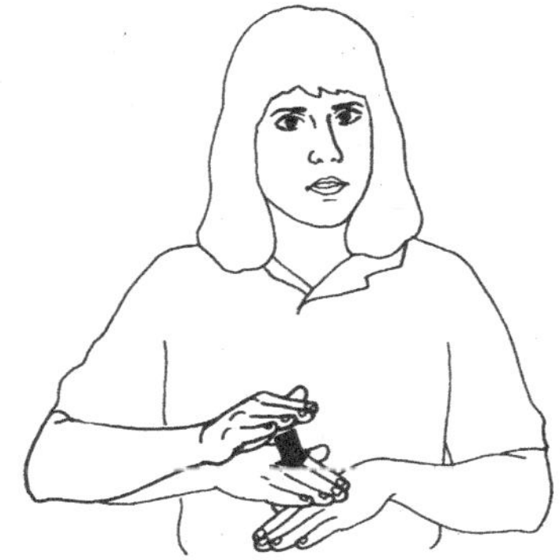

ON

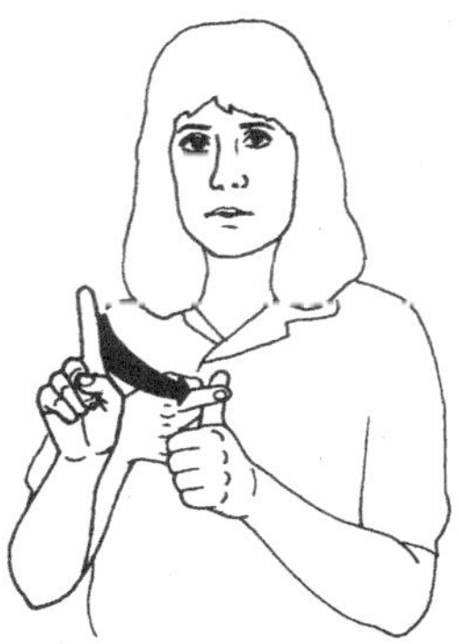

FIRST

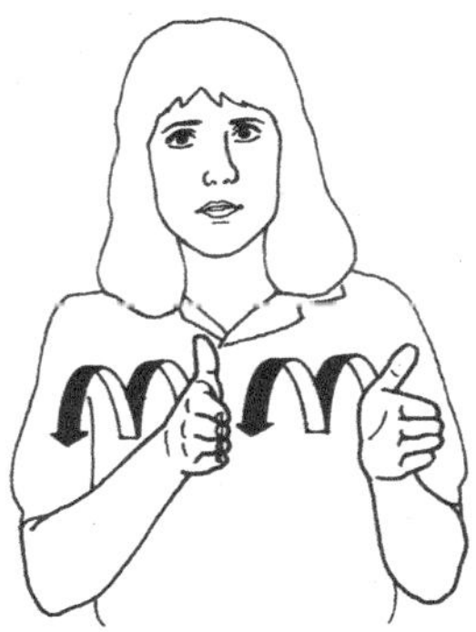

SYLLABLE

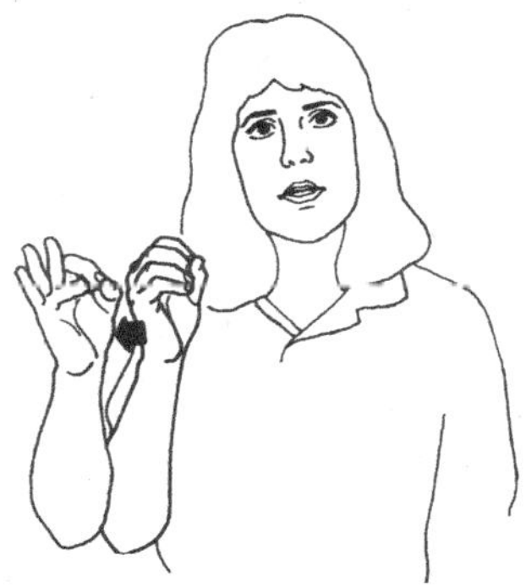

O-F

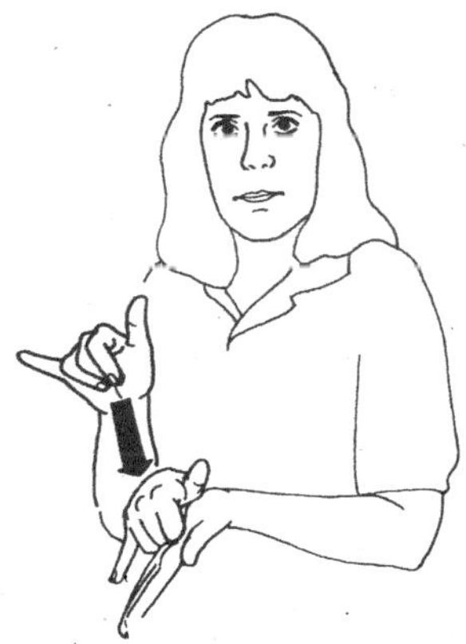

THAT

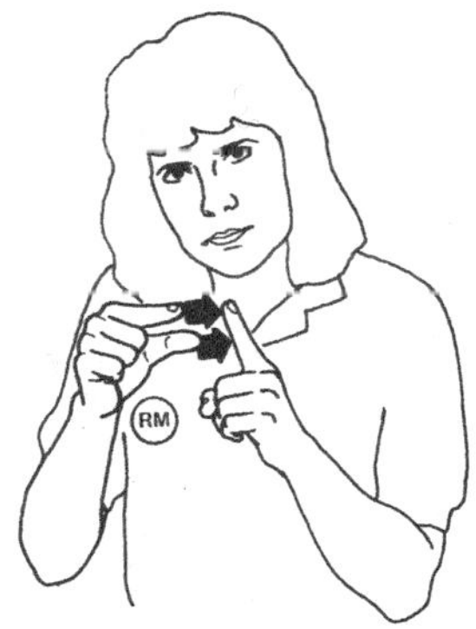

WORD.

Try to put more stress on the first syllable of that word.

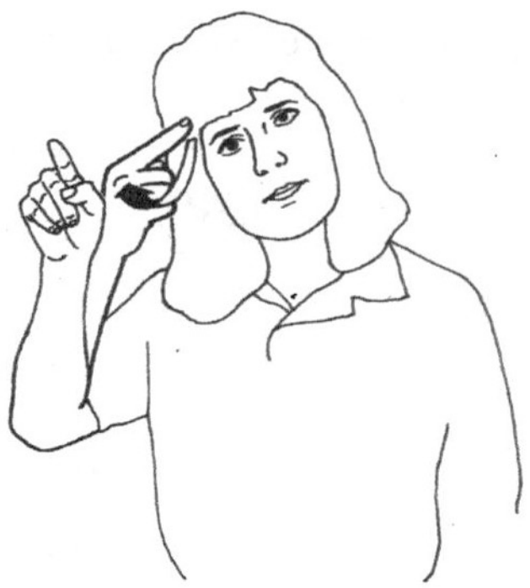

FOR

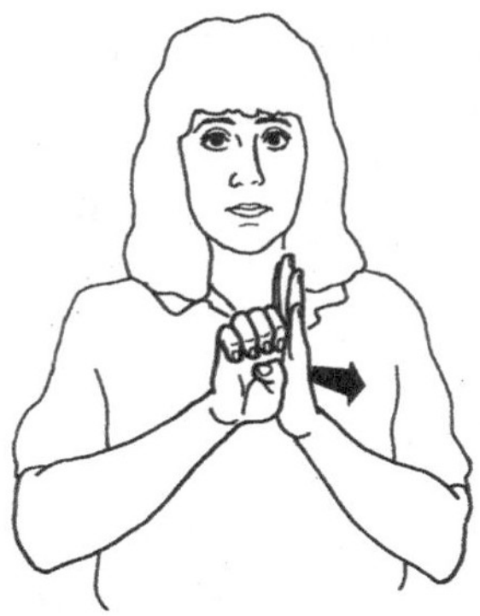

EXAMPLE

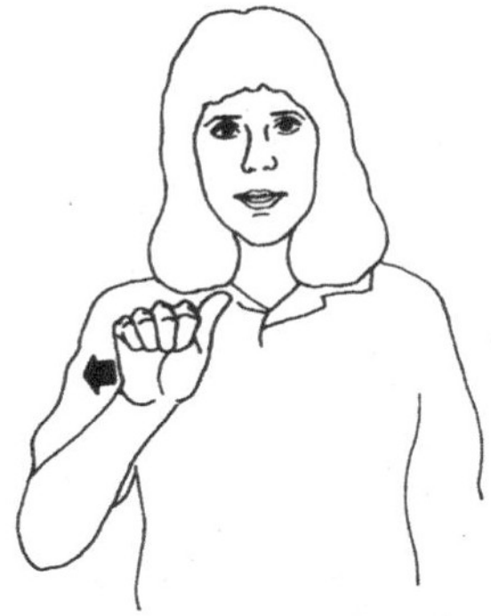

A

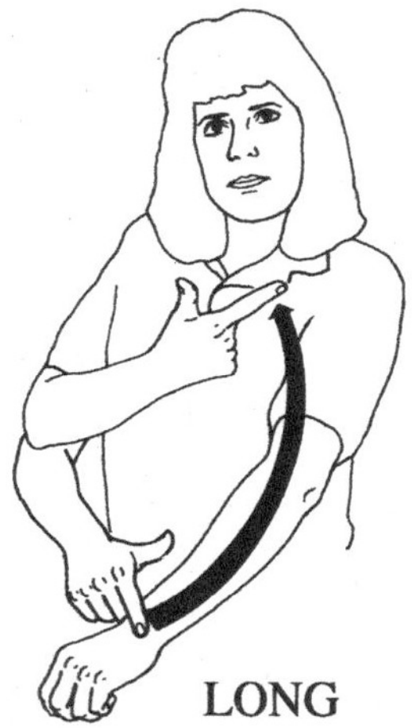

LONG

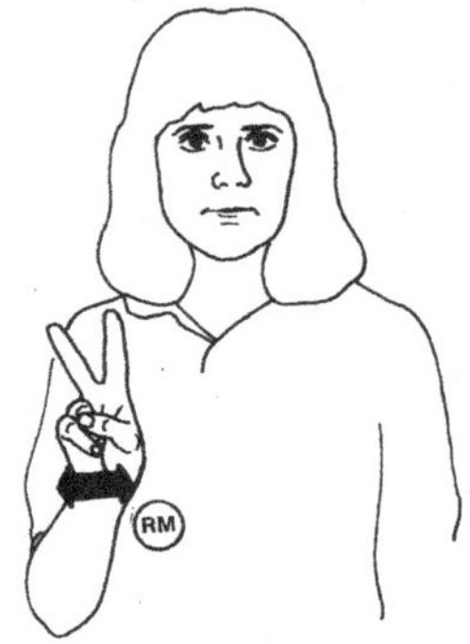

VOWEL.

For example *A* is a long vowel.

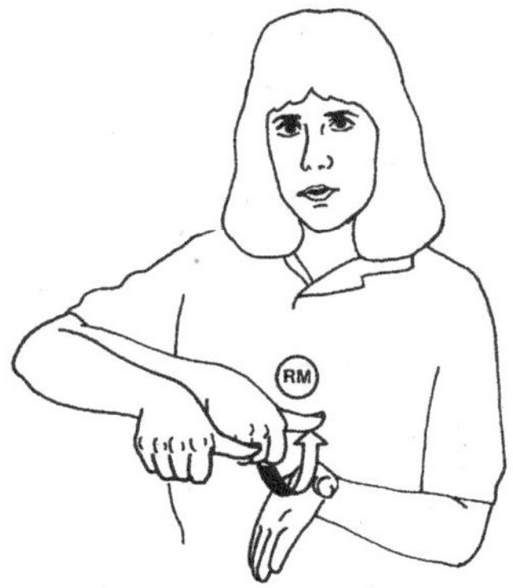

LOOK-UP

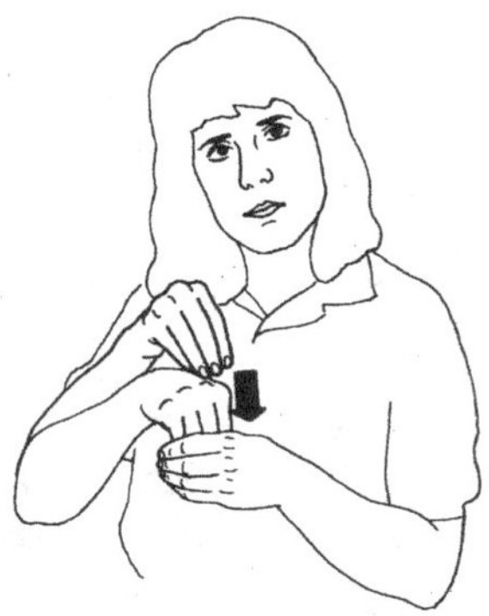

IN

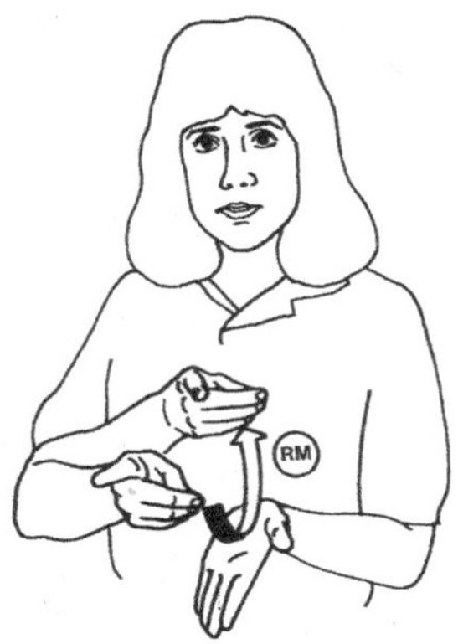

DICTIONARY.

Look it up in the dictionary.

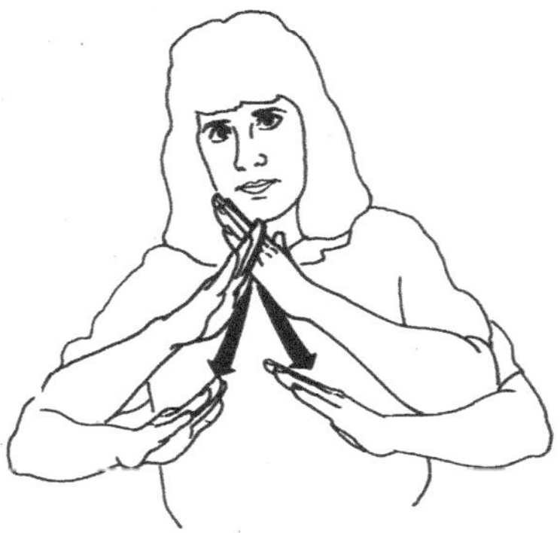

SILENT

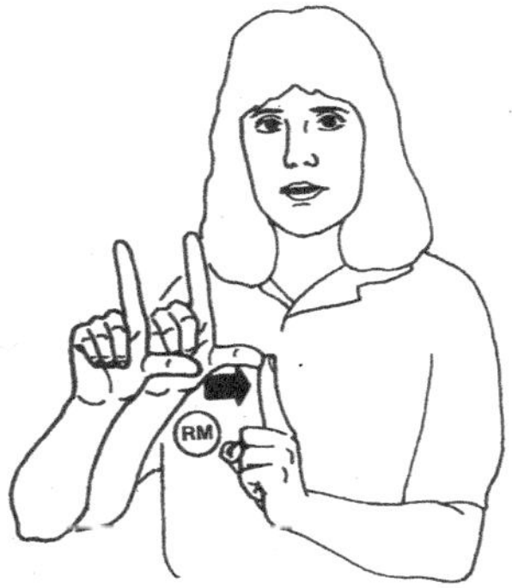

LETTER

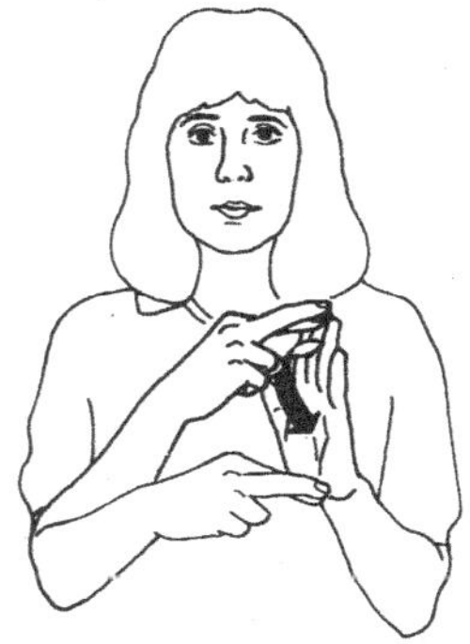

RULE

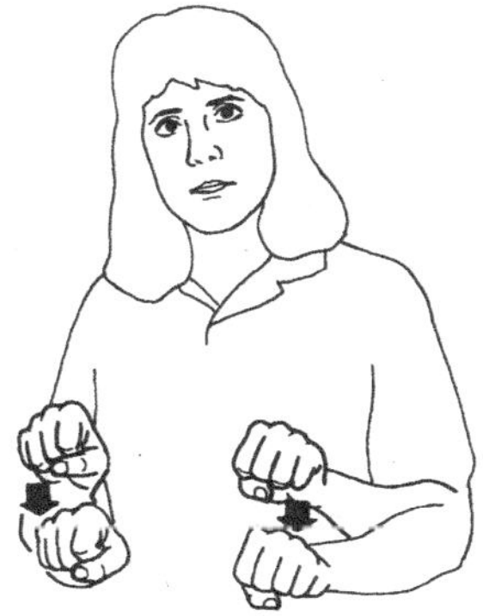

CAN

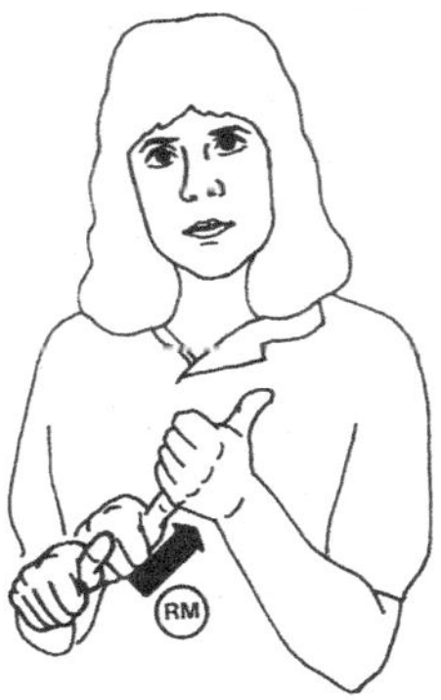

ASSIST

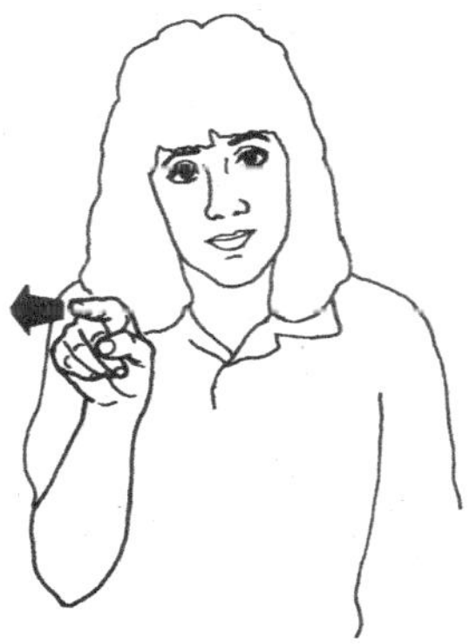

YOU

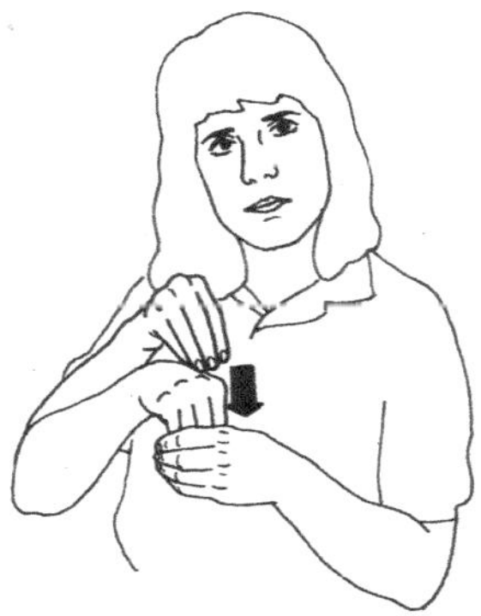

IN

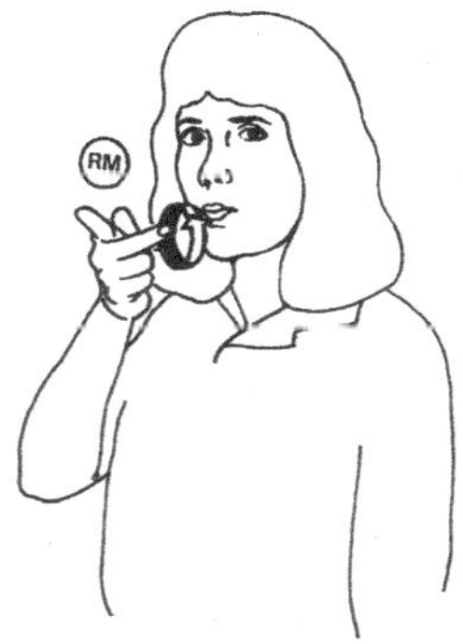

PRONOUNCE

Silent letter rules can assist you in pronouncing multisyllabic words.

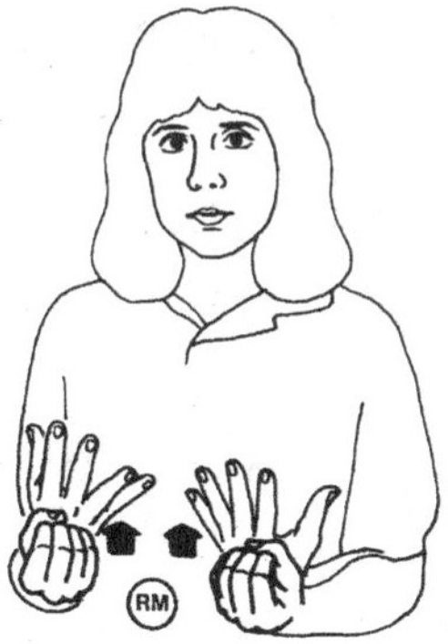

MANY

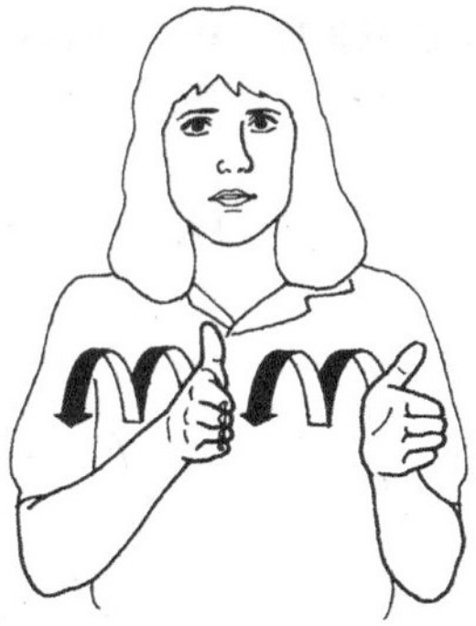

SYLLABLE

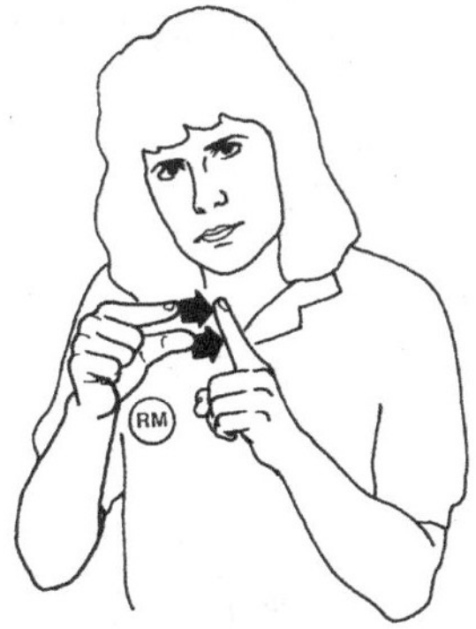

WORD.

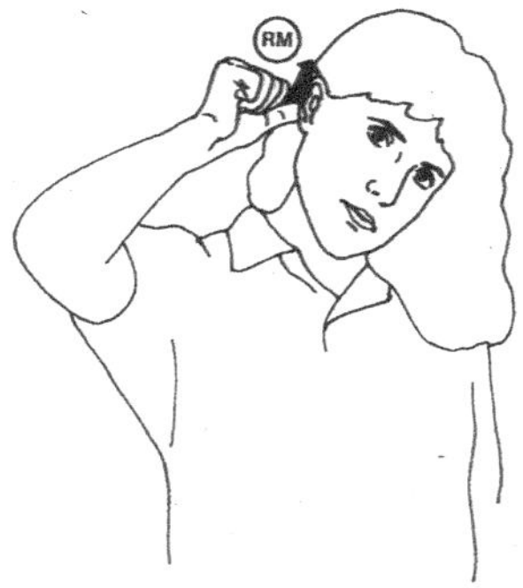

ADJUST-VOLUME

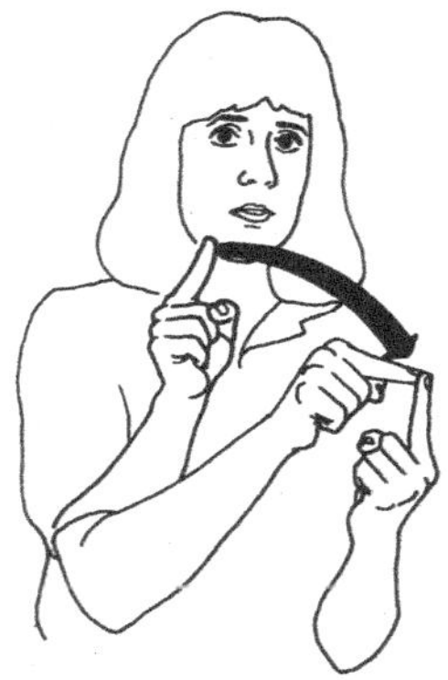

UNTIL

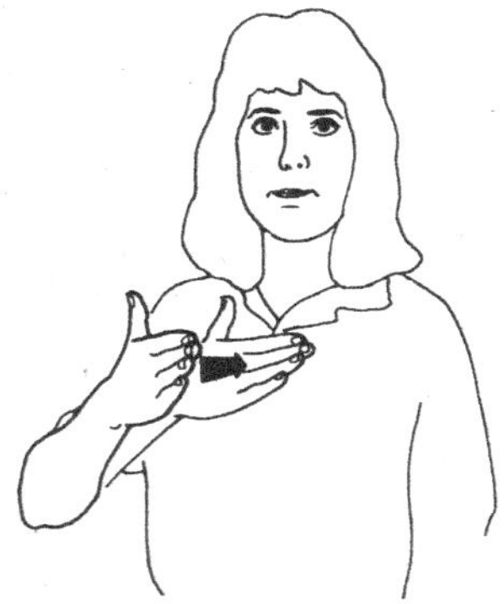

MY

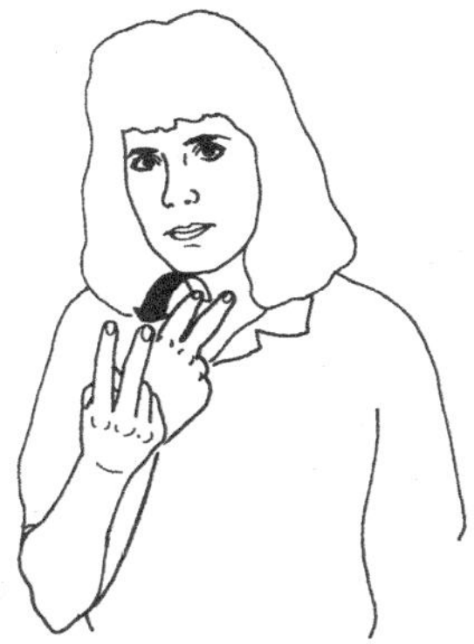

VOICE

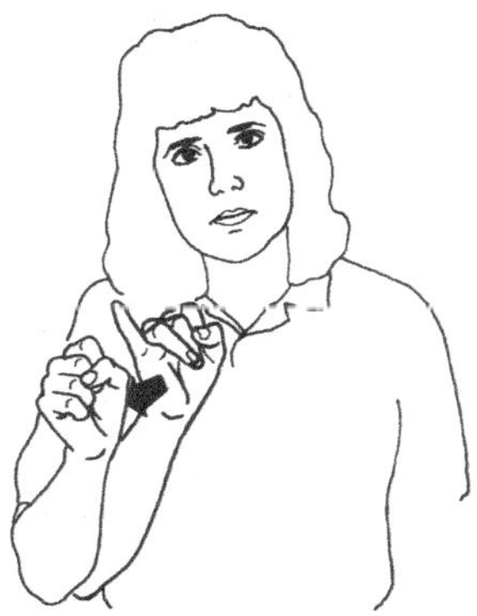

I-S

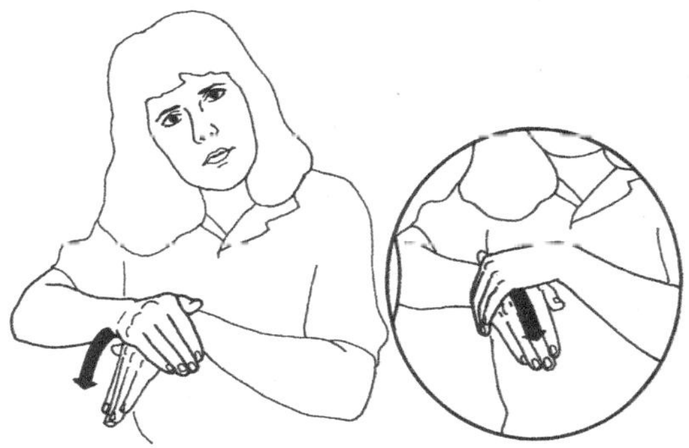

COMFORTABLE.

Adjust the volume until my voice is comfortable.

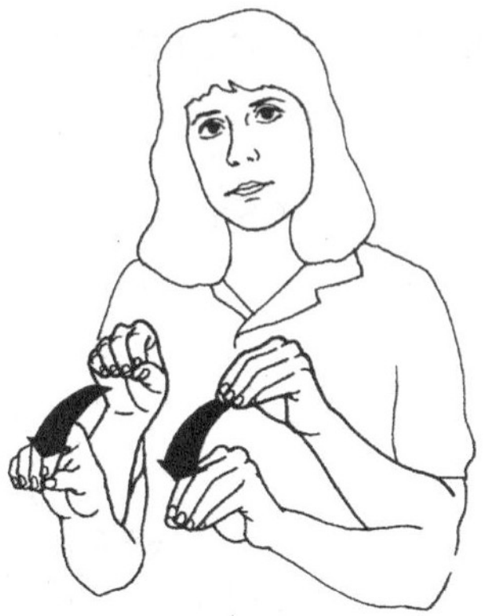

PUT

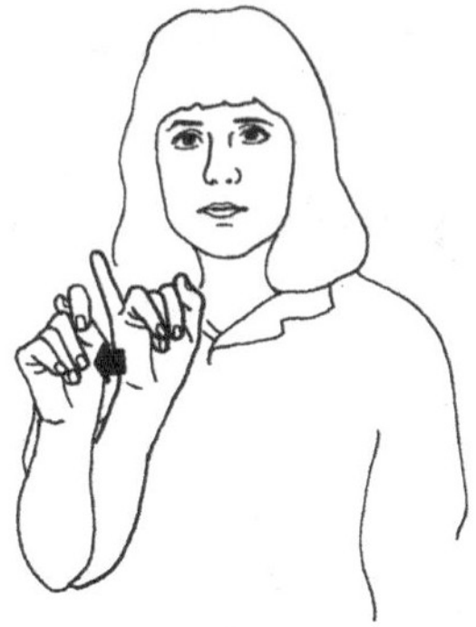

I-T

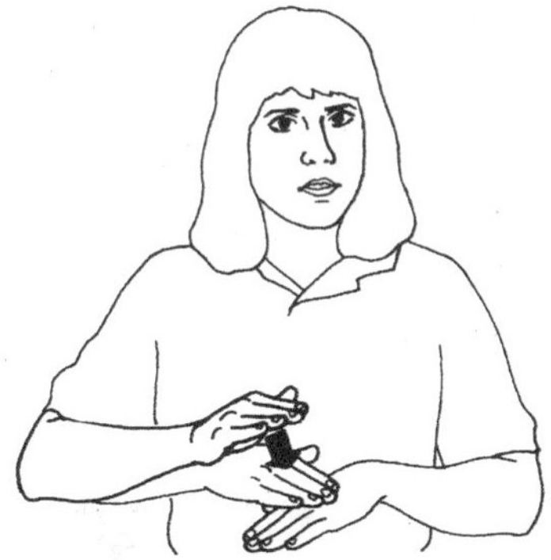

ON

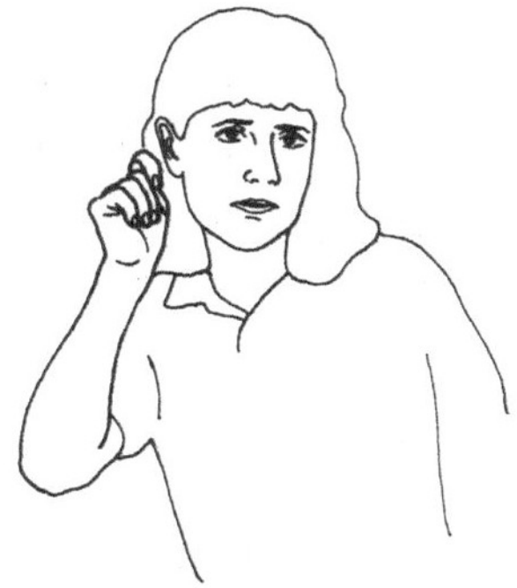

T

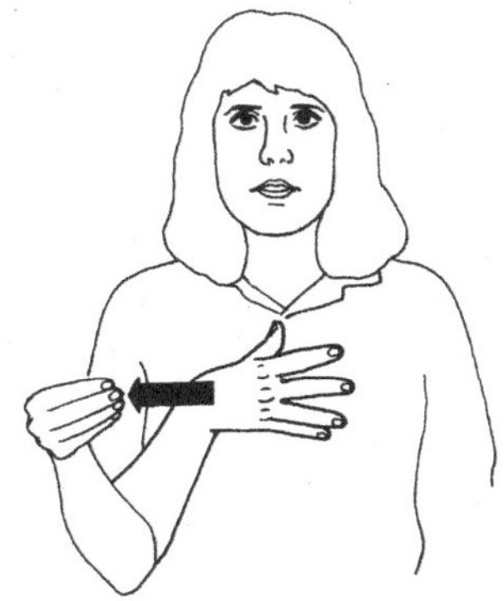

AND

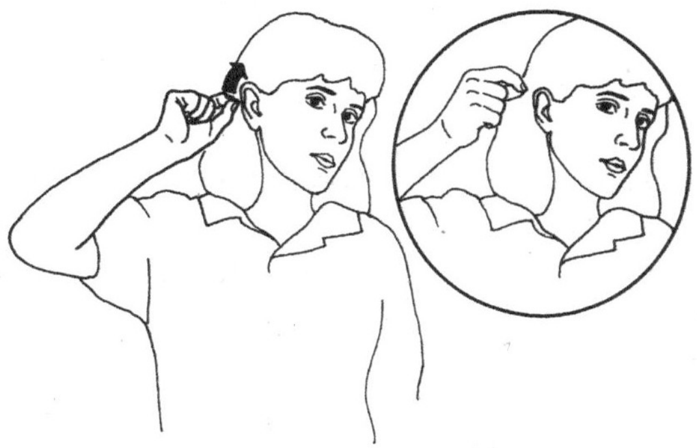

TURN-VOLUME

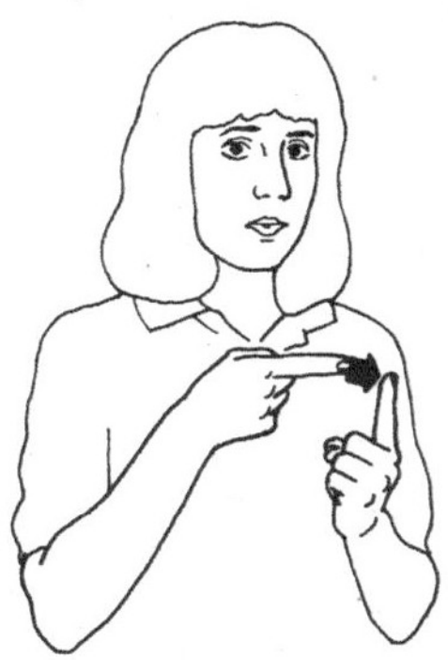

TO

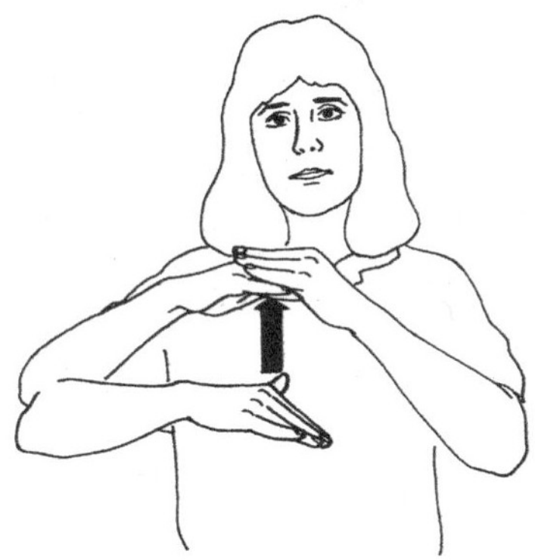

MAXIMUM.

Put it on *T* and turn the volume to its maximum.

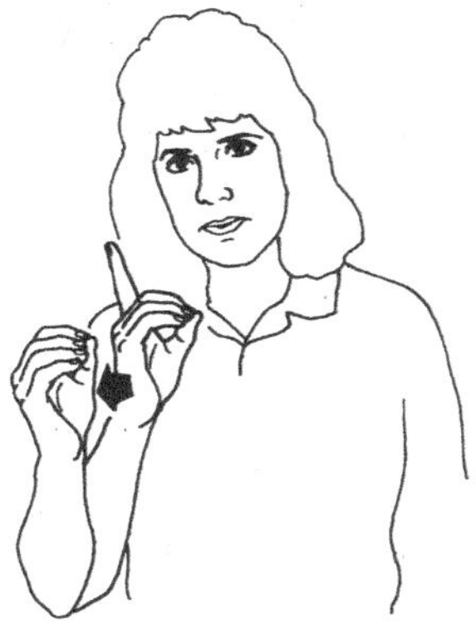

D-O

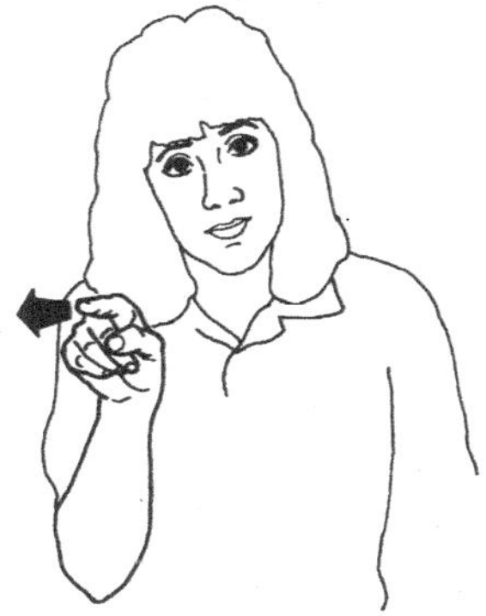

YOU

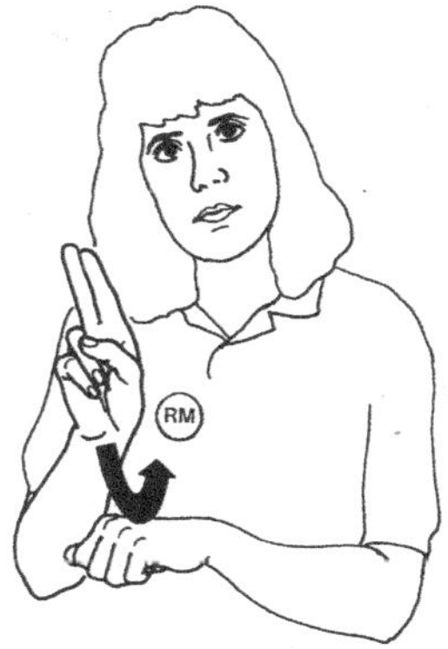

USE

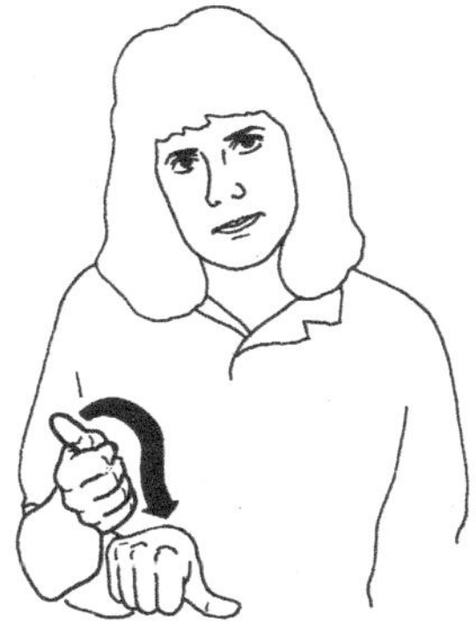

ANY

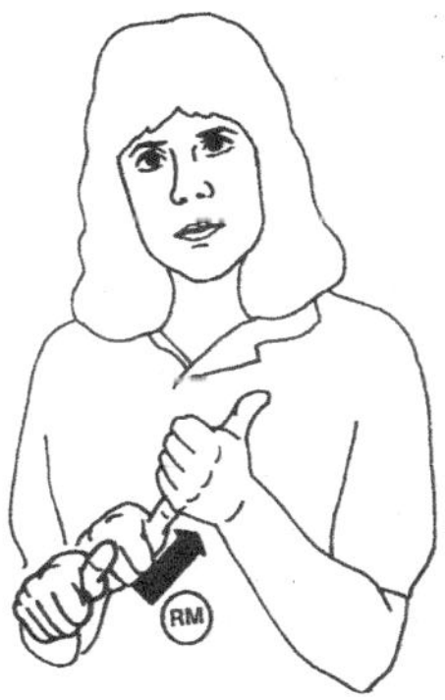

ASSIST

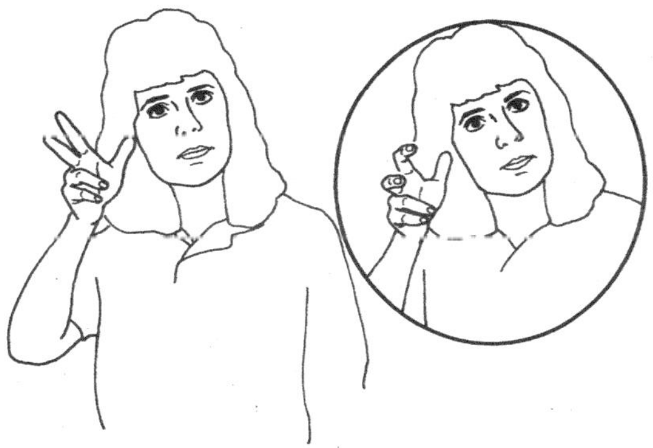

LISTEN

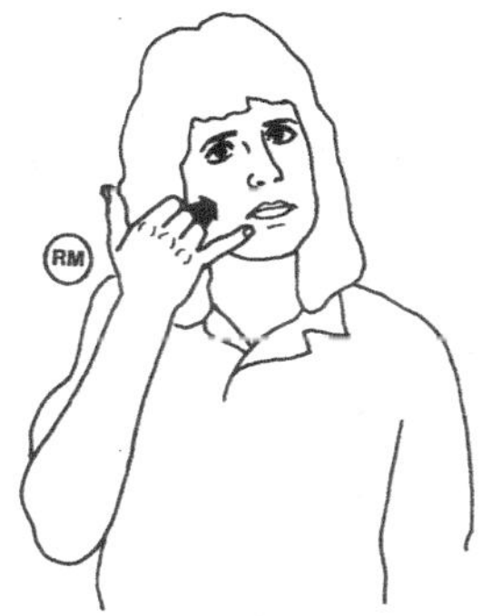

TELEPHONE

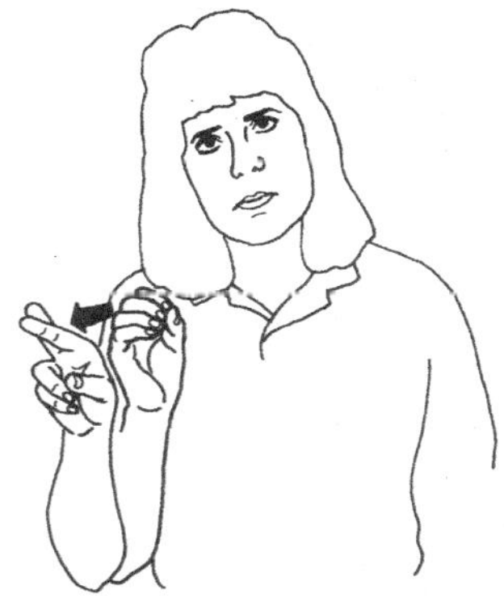

O-R

Do you use any assistive listening, telephone, or alerting devices?

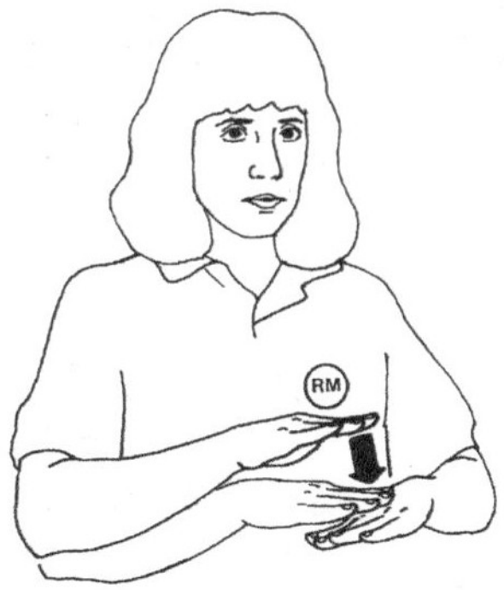

ALERT

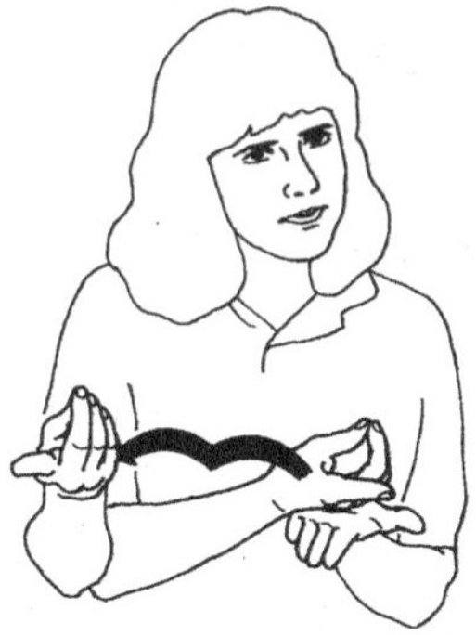

DEVICES?

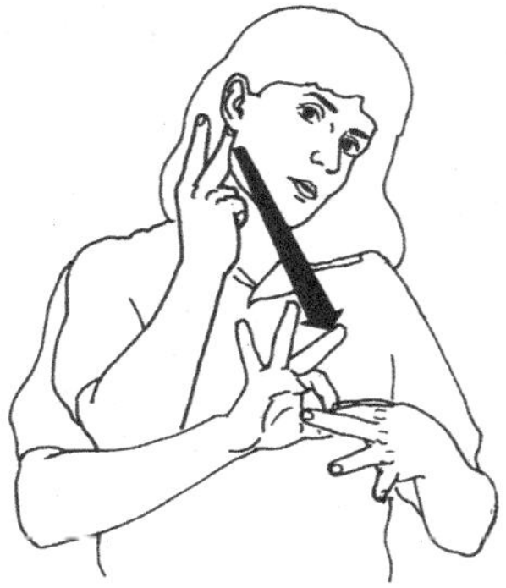

DIRECT-AUDIO-INPUT

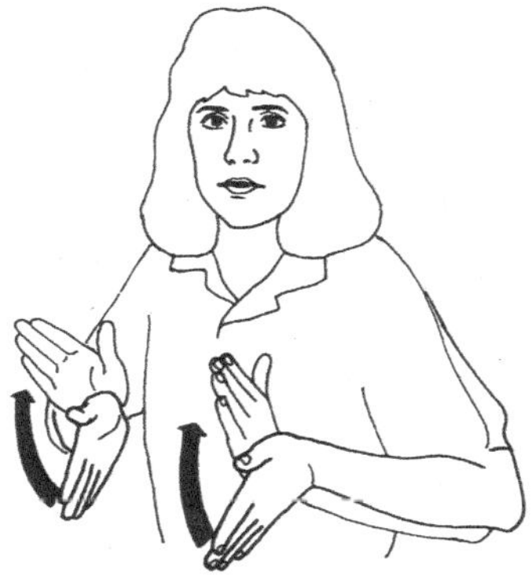

ALLOW

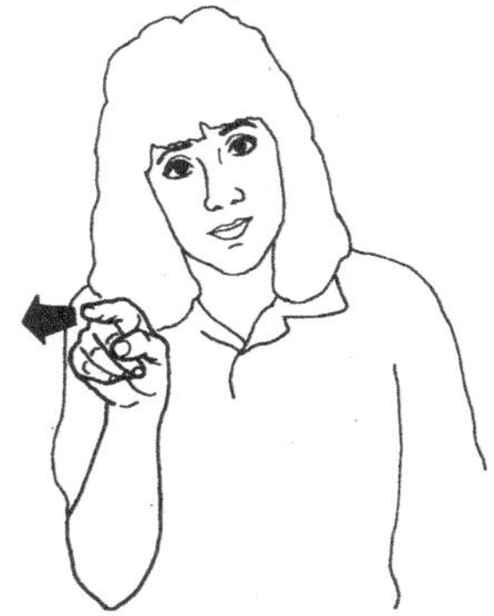

YOU

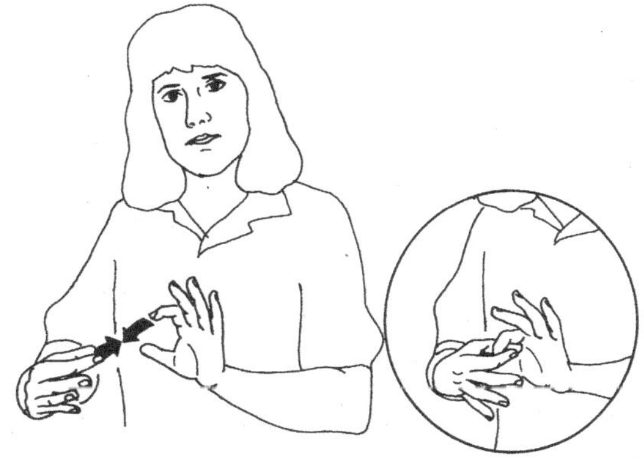

CONNECT

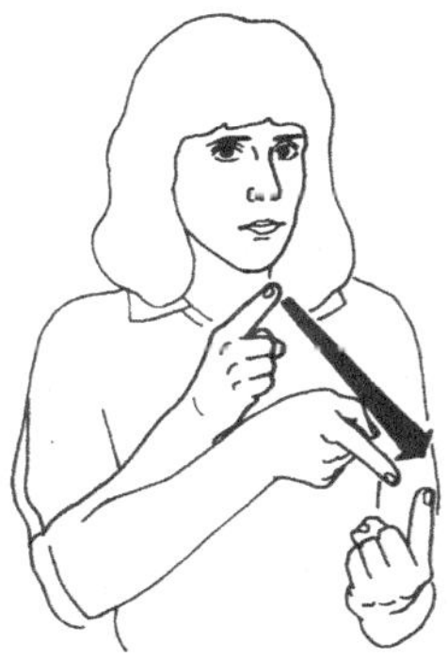

DIRECT-TO

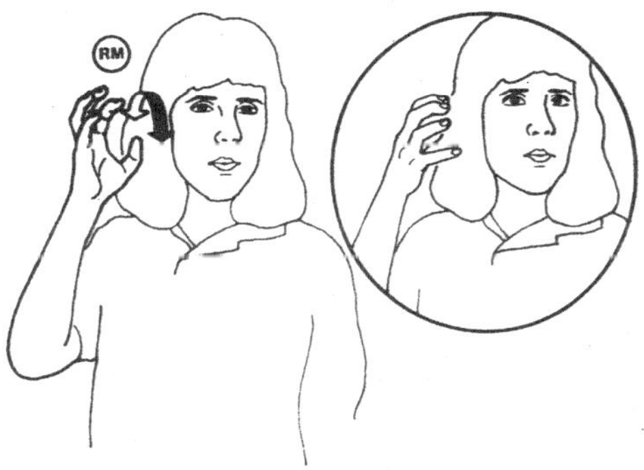

RADIO.

Direct audio input allows you to connect directly to the radio.

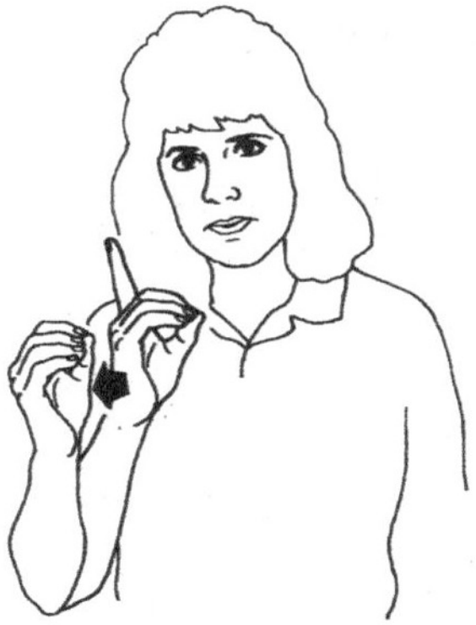

D-O

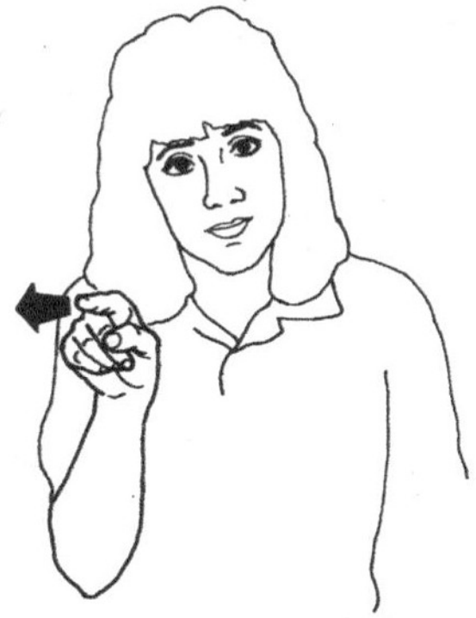

YOU

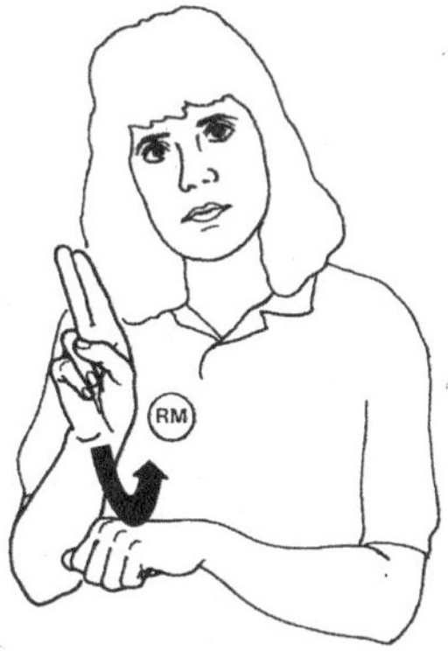

USE

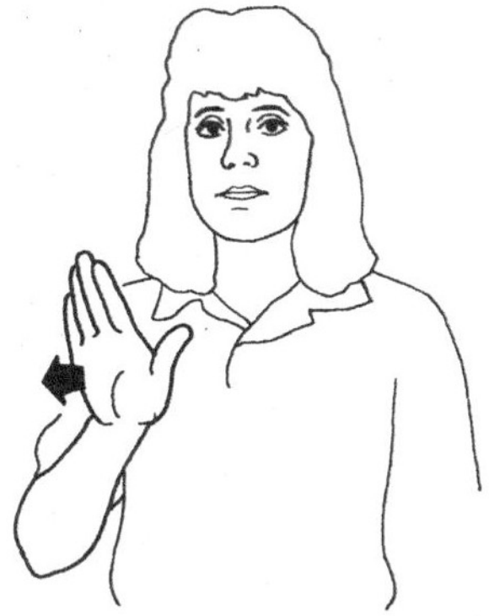

YOUR

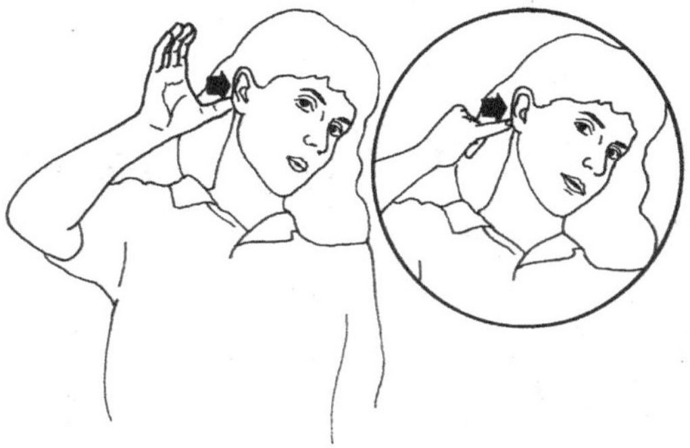

COCHLEAR-IMPLANT

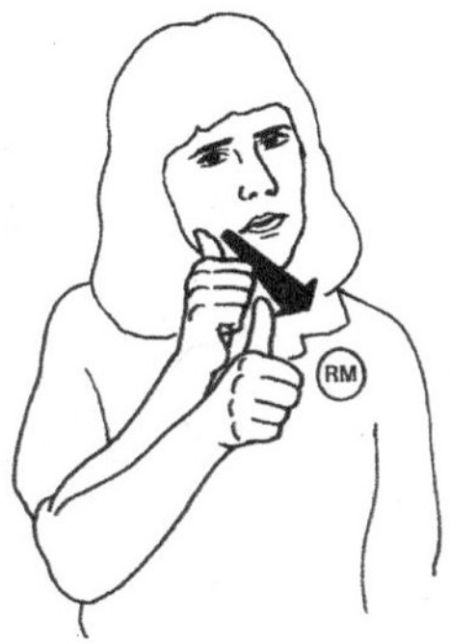

EVERYDAY?

Do you use your cochlear implant every day?

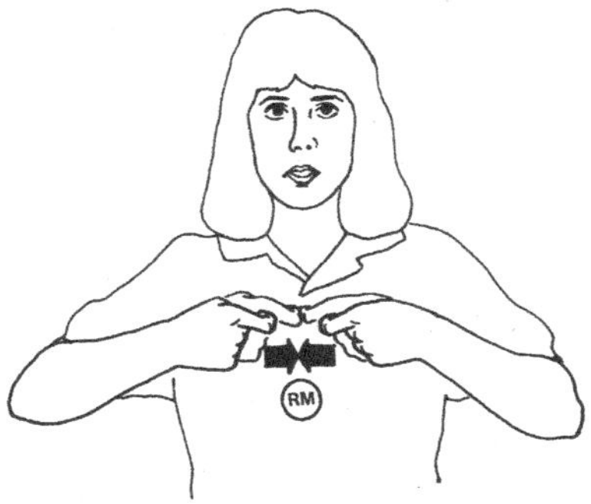

BATTERY

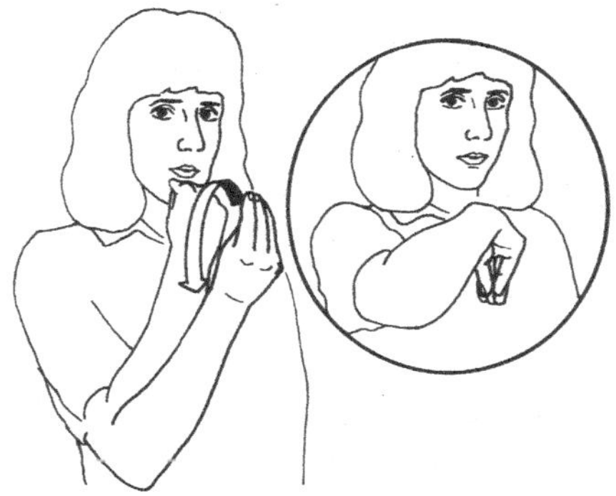

INGESTION

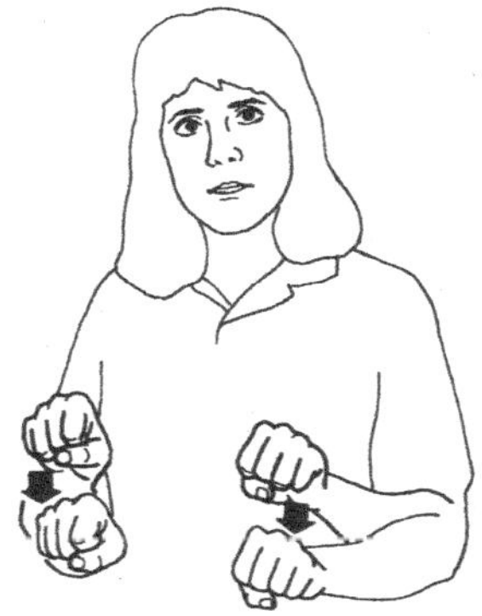

CAN

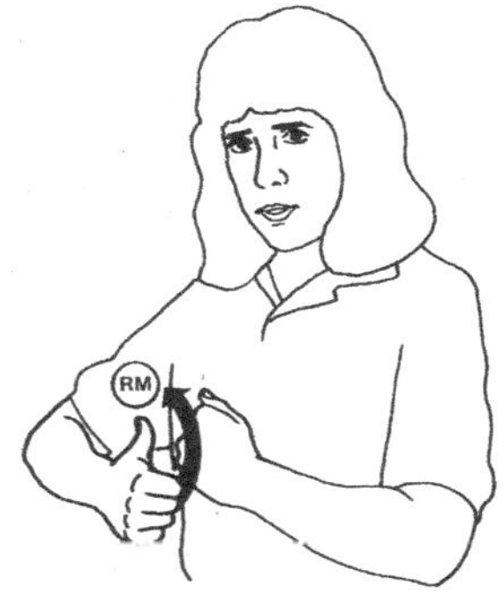

DANGEROUS.

Battery ingestion can be dangerous.

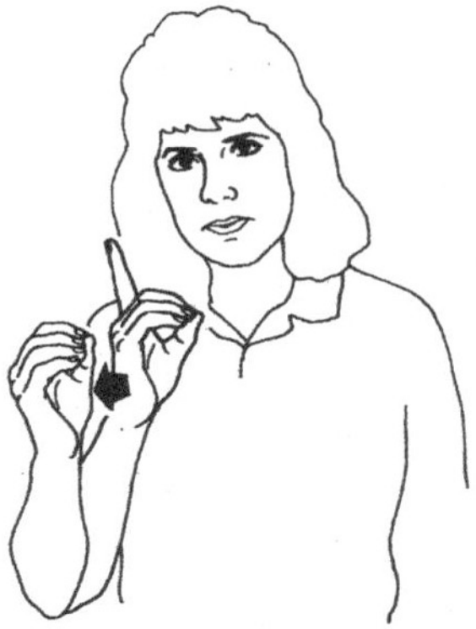

D-O

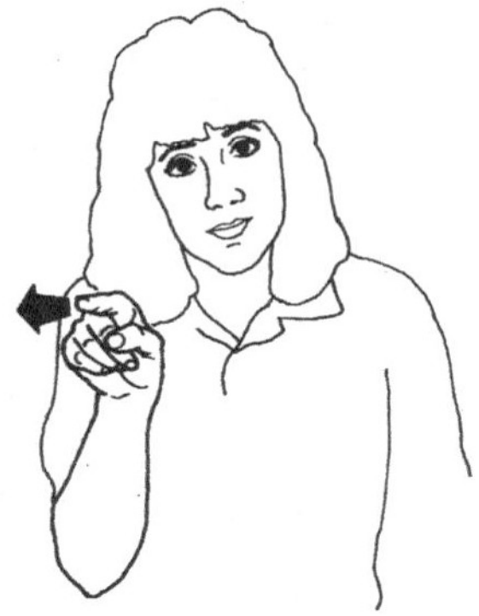

YOU

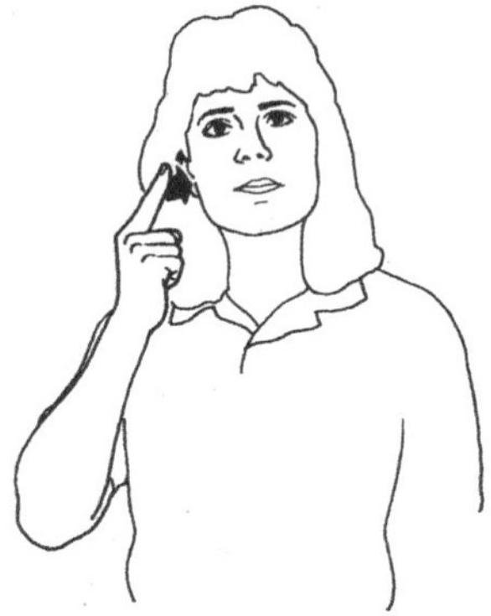

HEAR

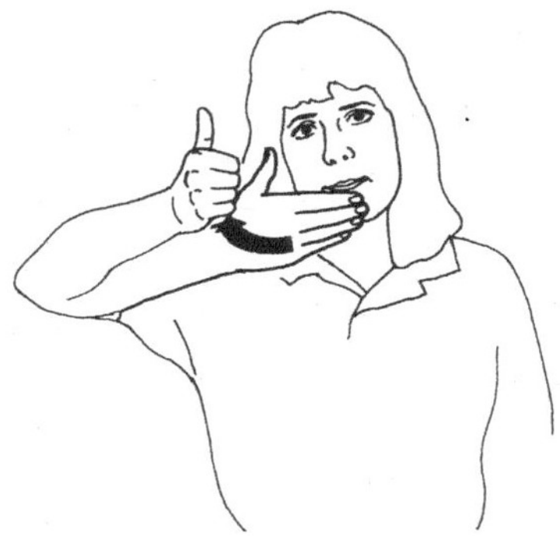

BETTER

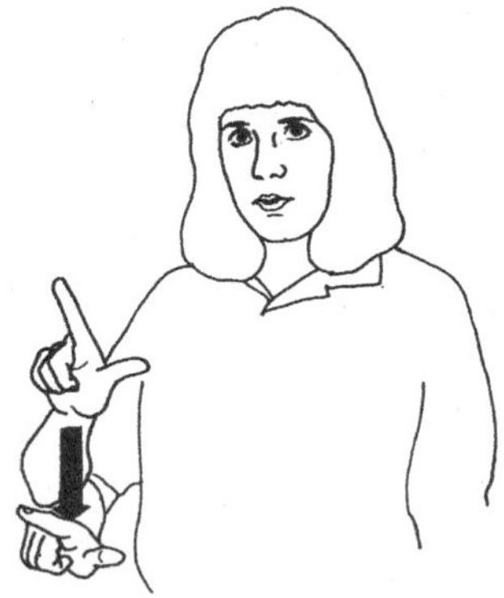

LOW

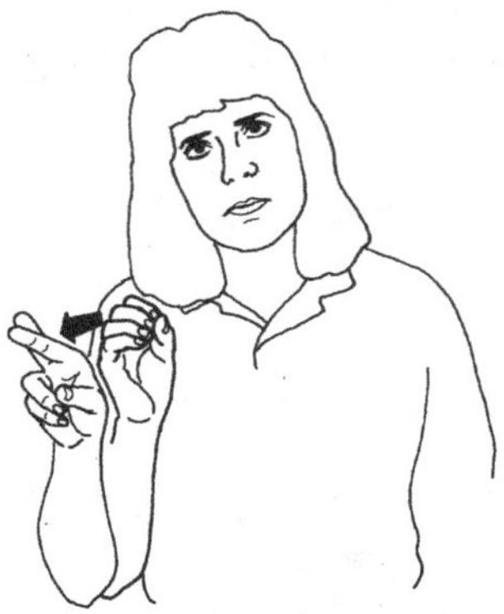

O-R

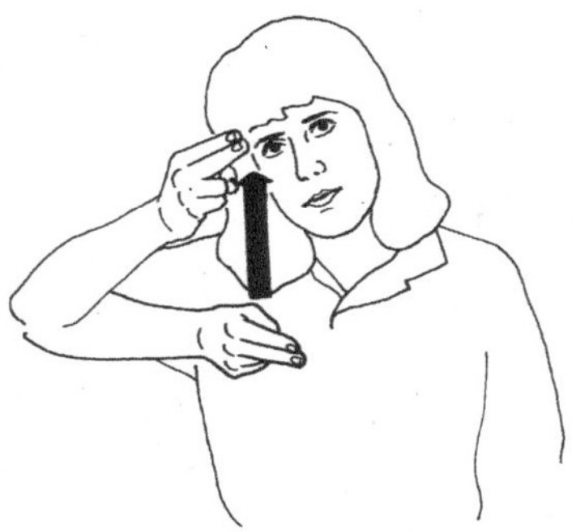

HIGH

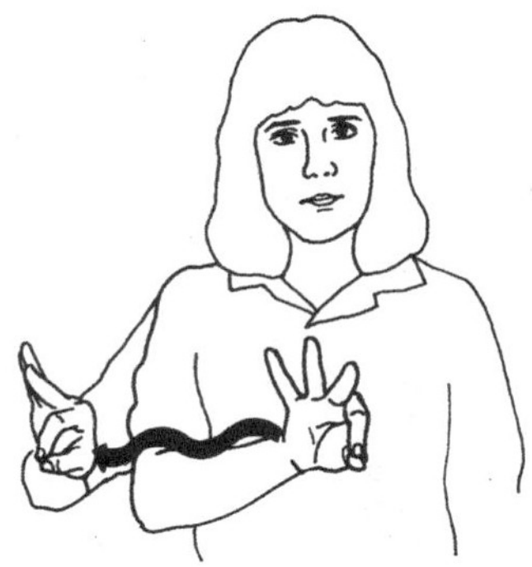

FREQUENCY?

Do you hear better in the low or high frequencies?

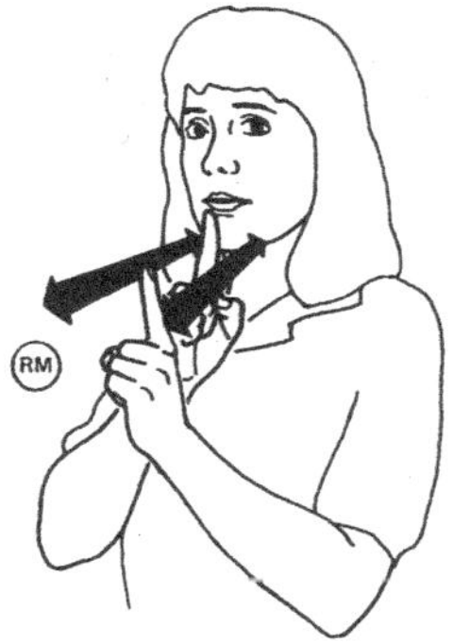

CONVERSATION

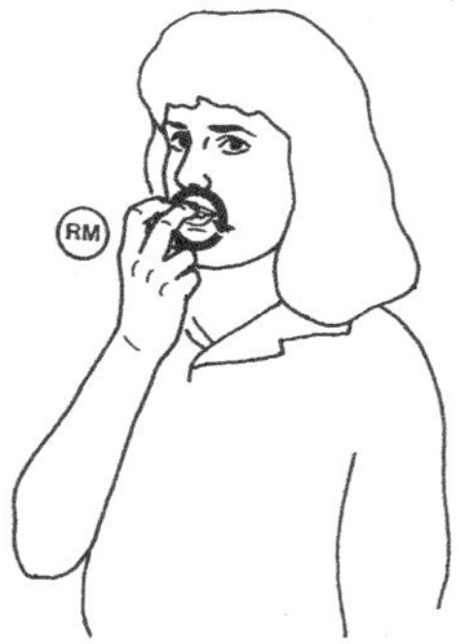

SPEECH

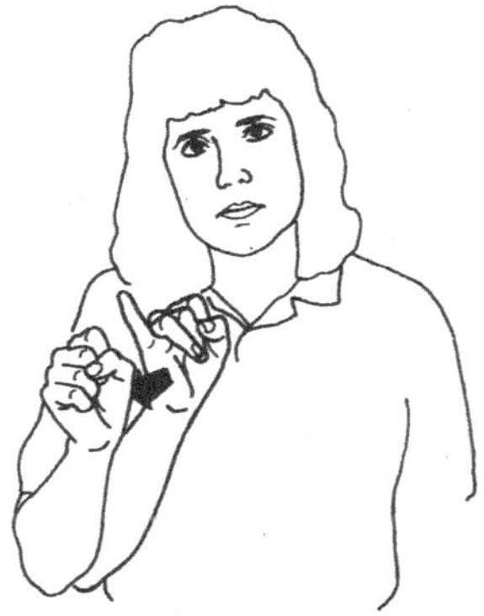

I-S

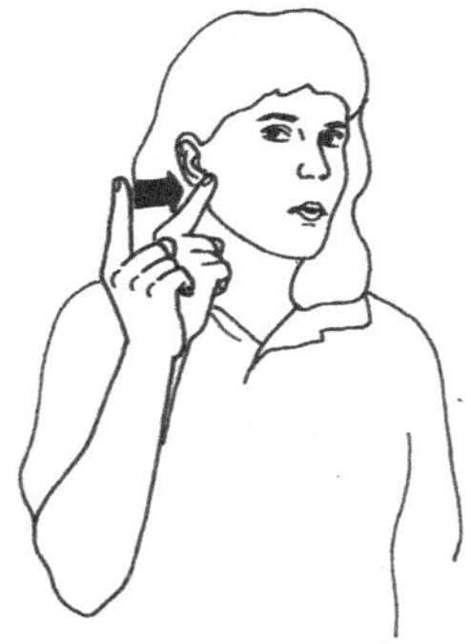

HEARD

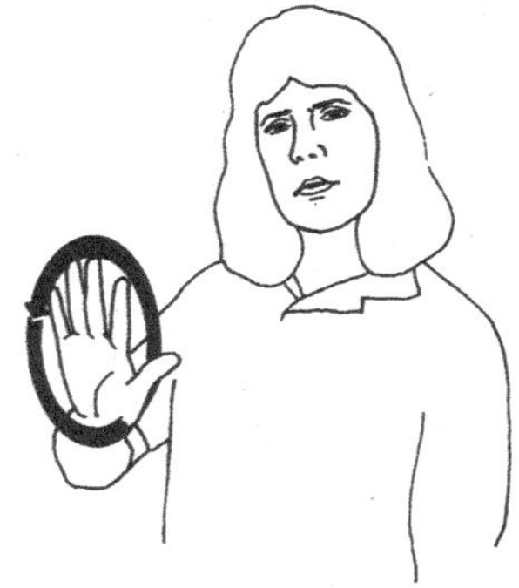

APPROXIMATELY

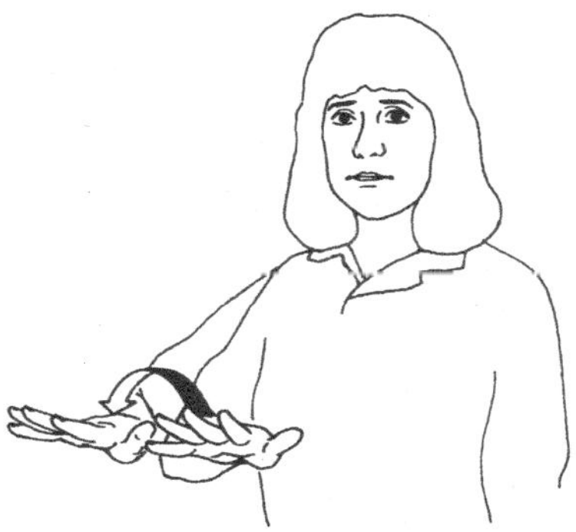

55

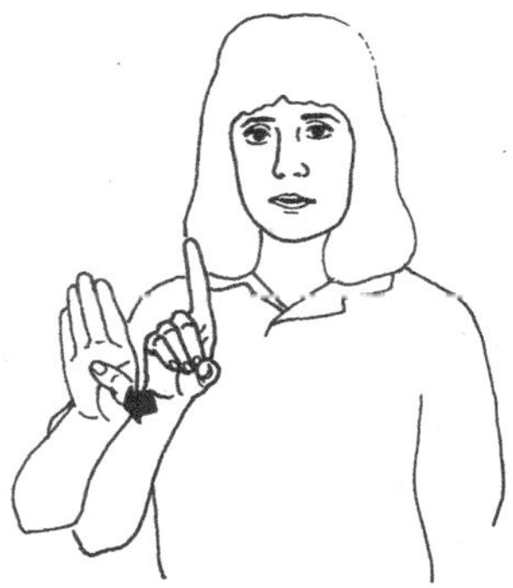

D-B.

Conversational speech is heard at approximately 55 dB.

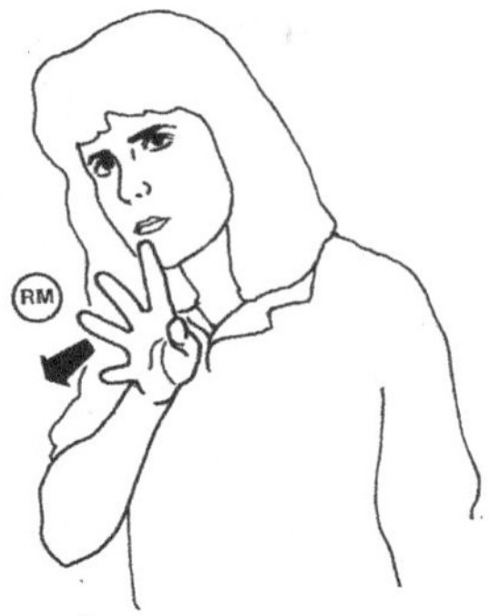

SPEAK

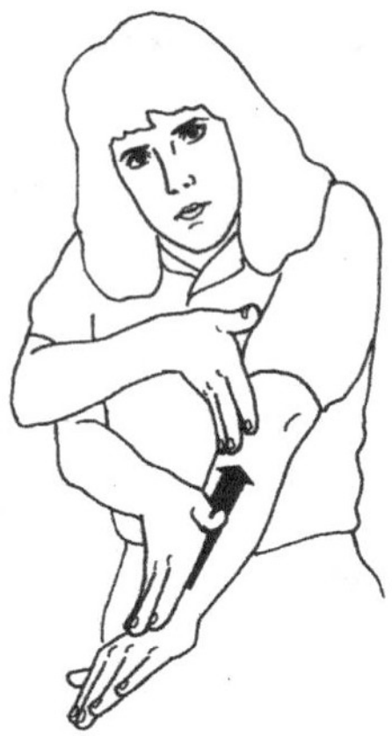

SLOW

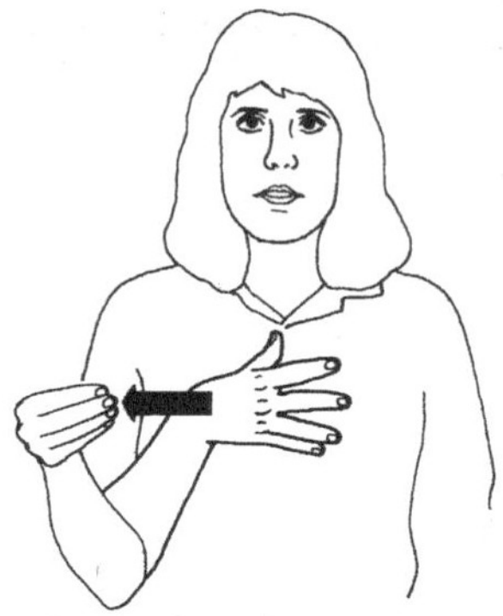

AND

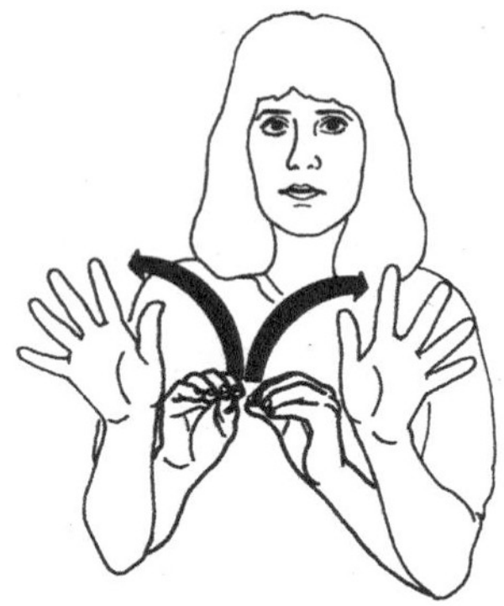

CLEAR.

Speak slowly and clearly.

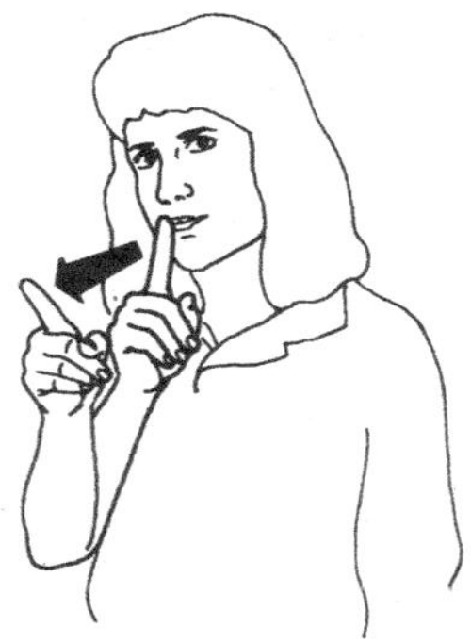

IS

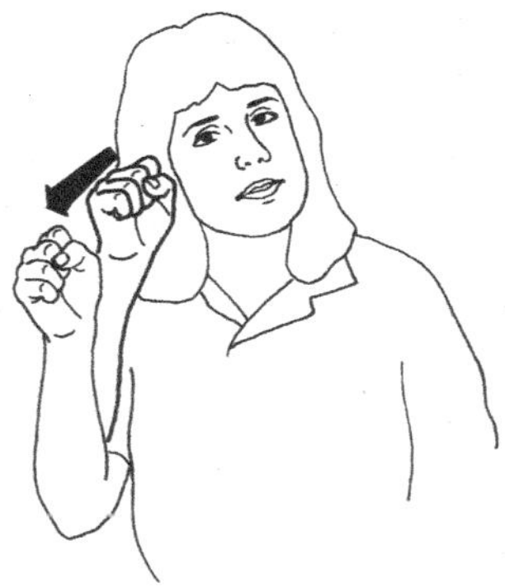

SOUND

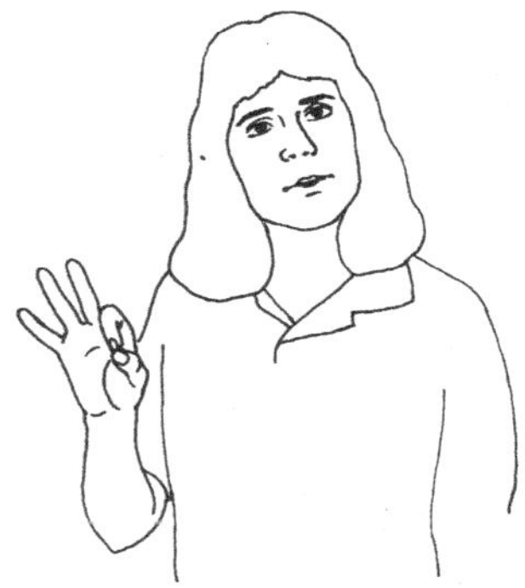

F

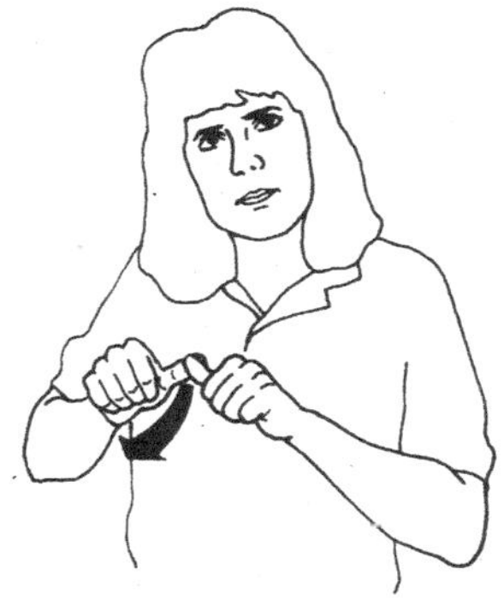

CONTINUE

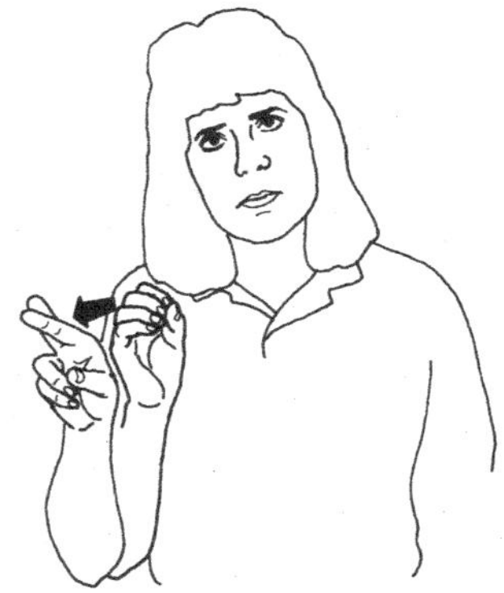

O-R

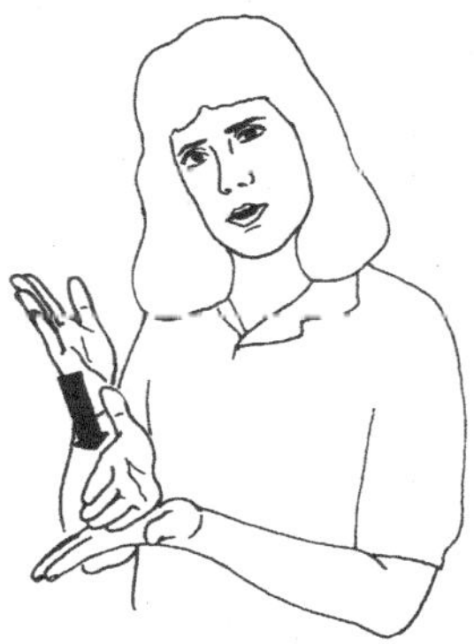

STOP

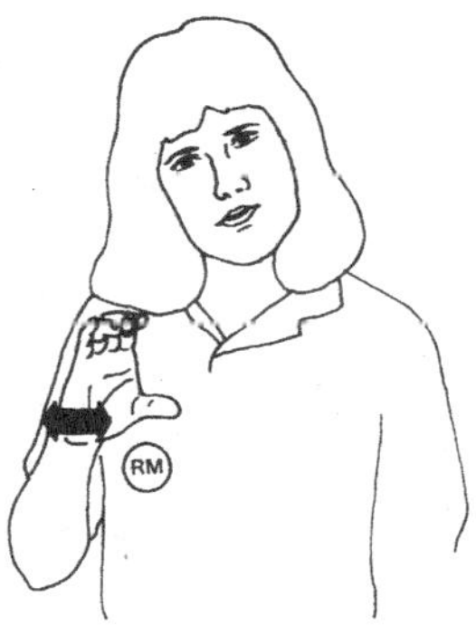

CONSONANT?

Is the sound *F* a continuant or stop consonant?

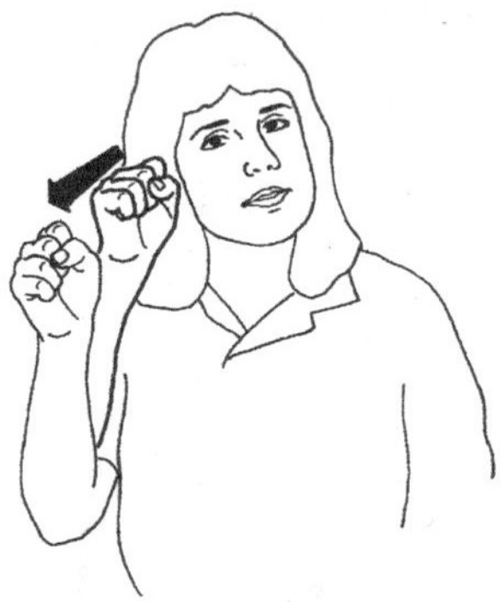

SOUND

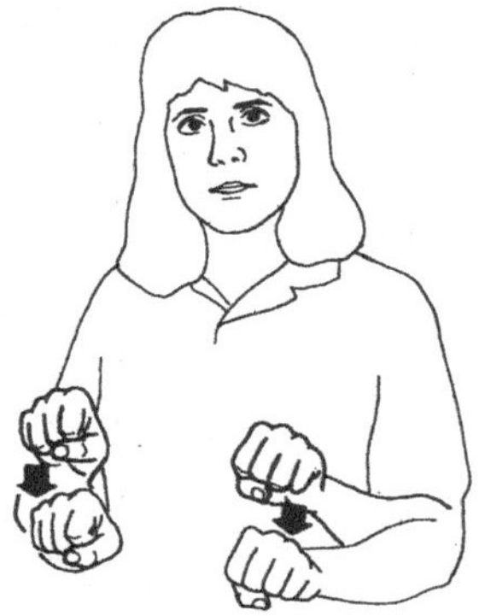

CAN

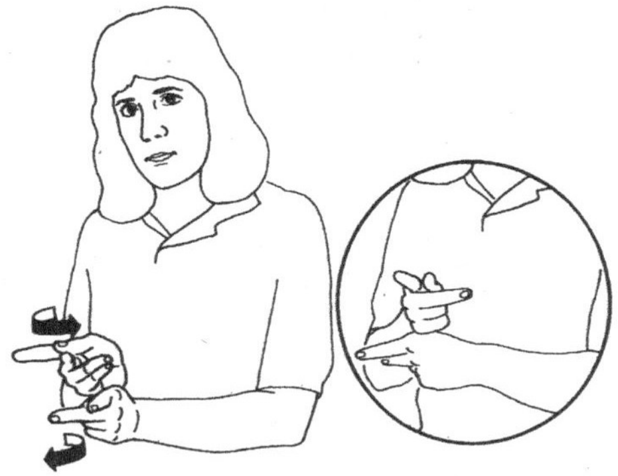

PRODUCE

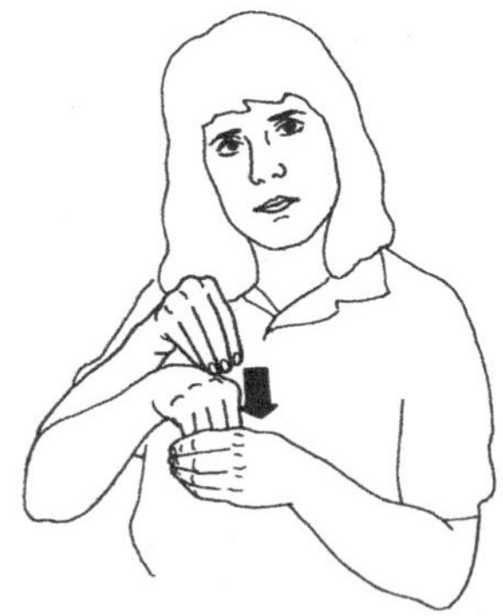

IN

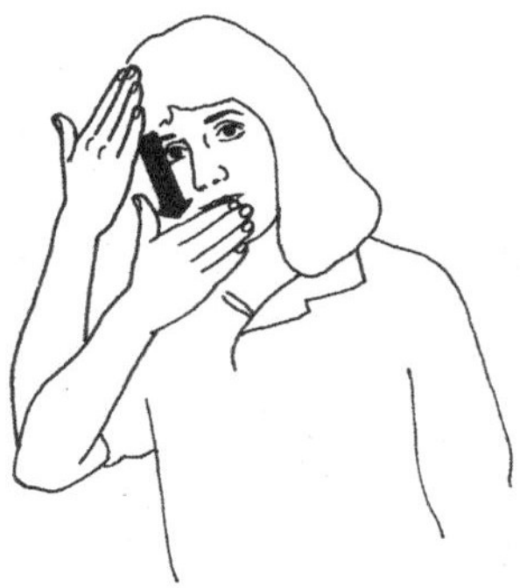

FRONT

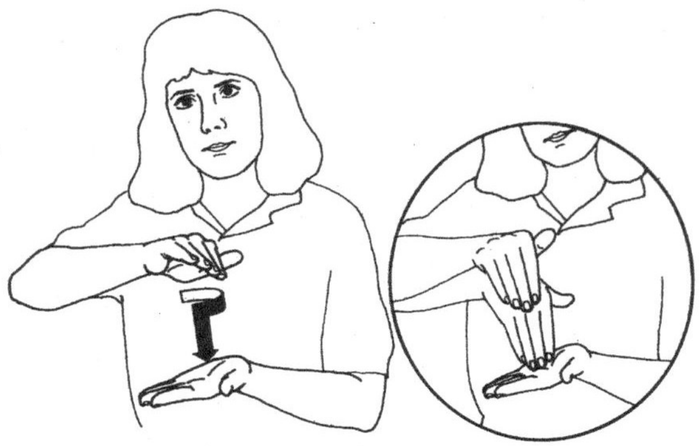

MIDDLE

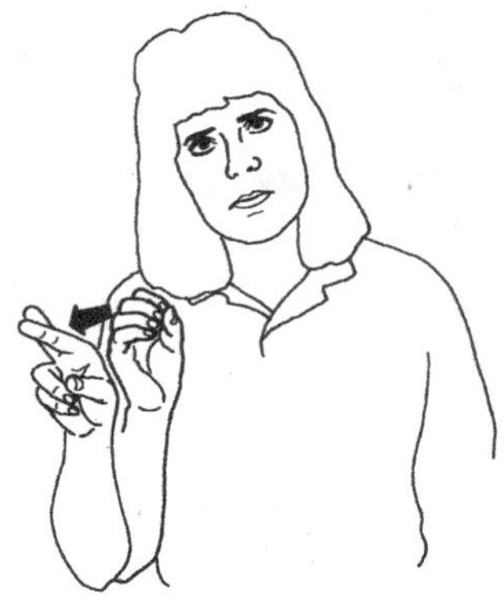

O-R

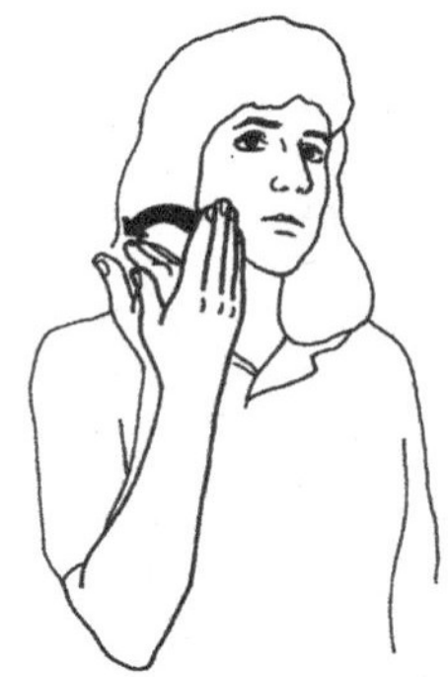

BACK

Sounds can be produced in the front, middle, or back of the mouth.

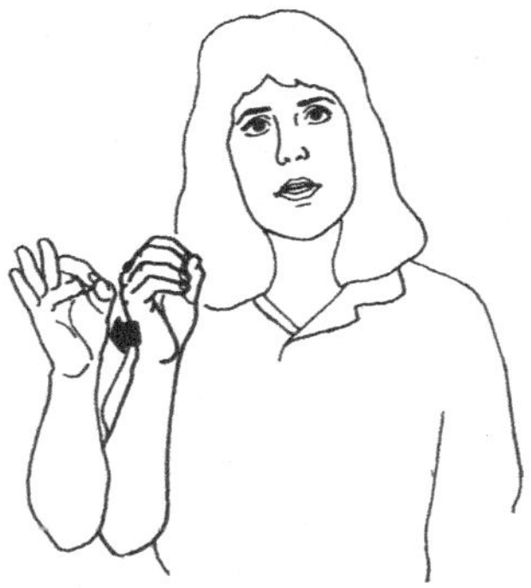

O-F

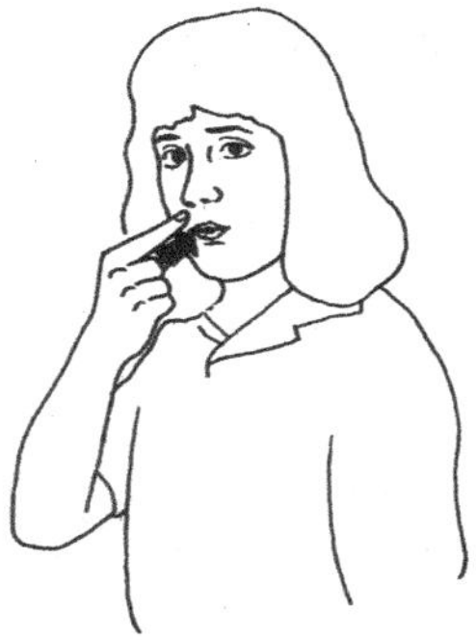

MOUTH.

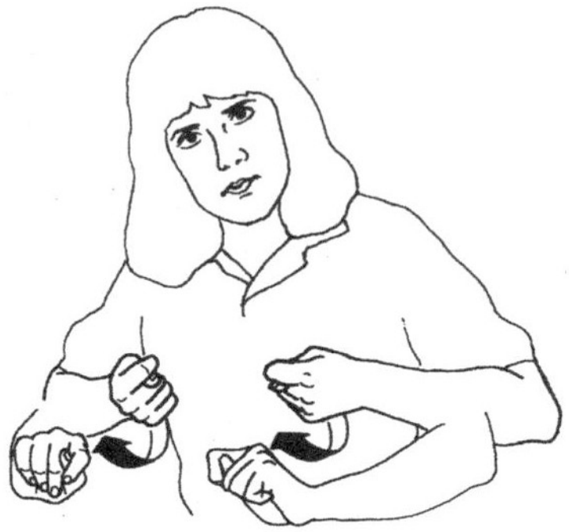

TRY

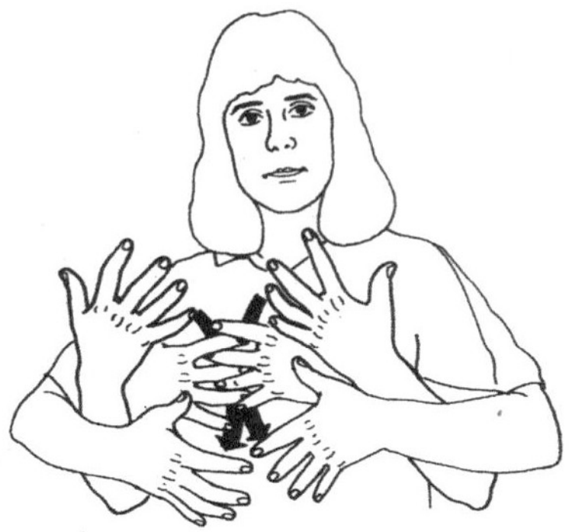

BLEND

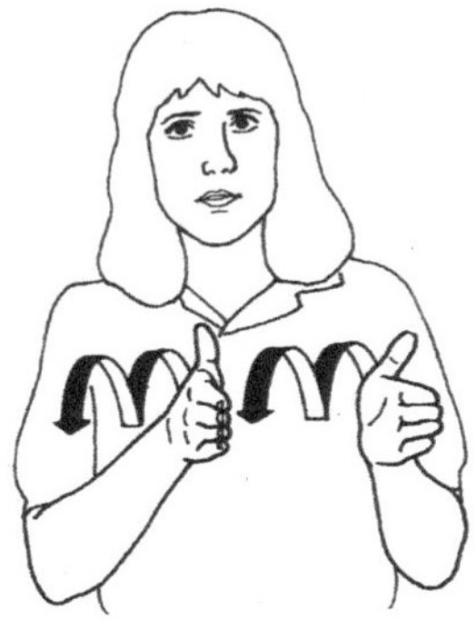

SYLLABLE

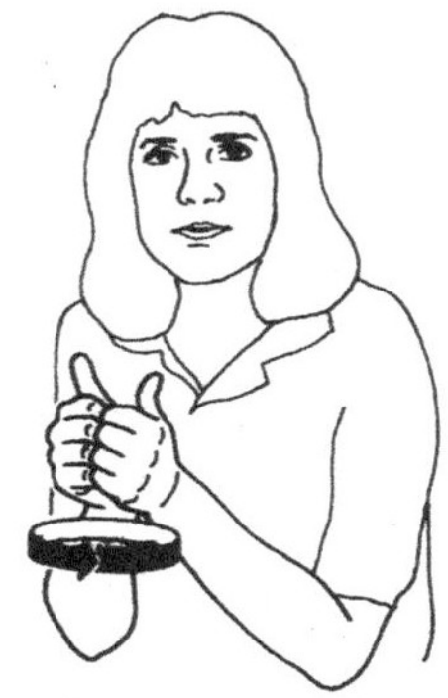

TOGETHER

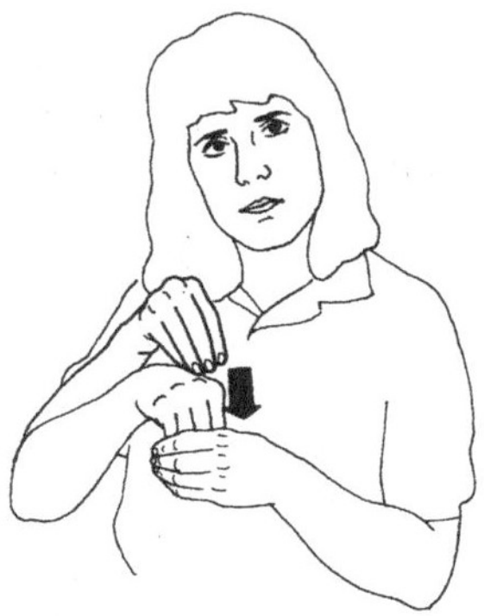

IN

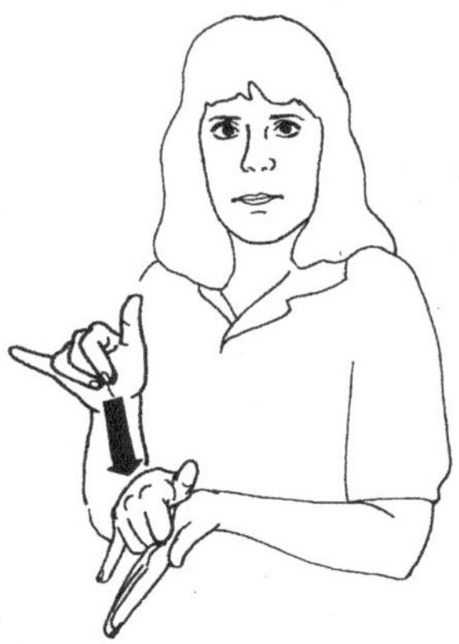

THAT

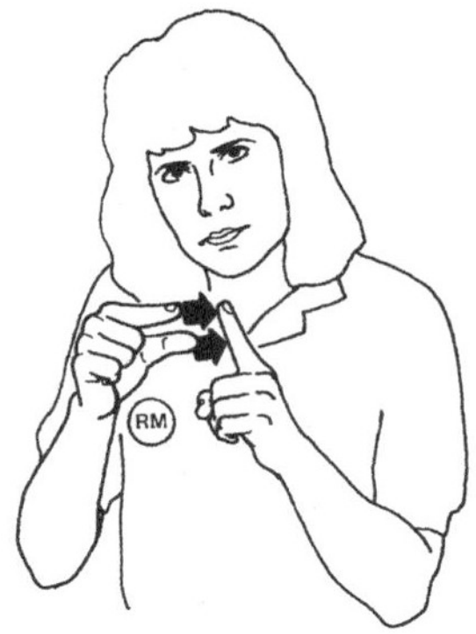

WORD.

Try to blend the syllables together in that word.

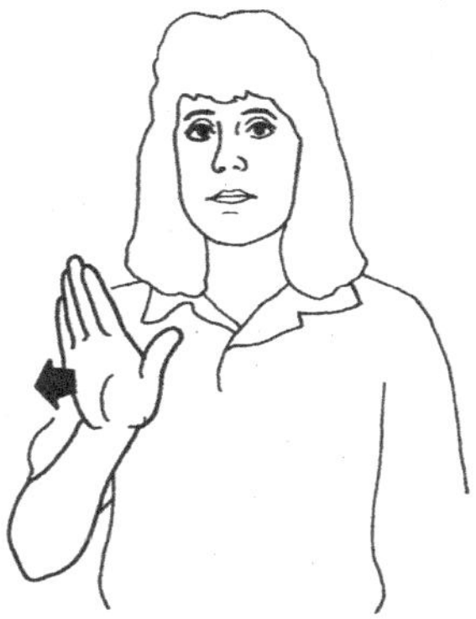

YOUR

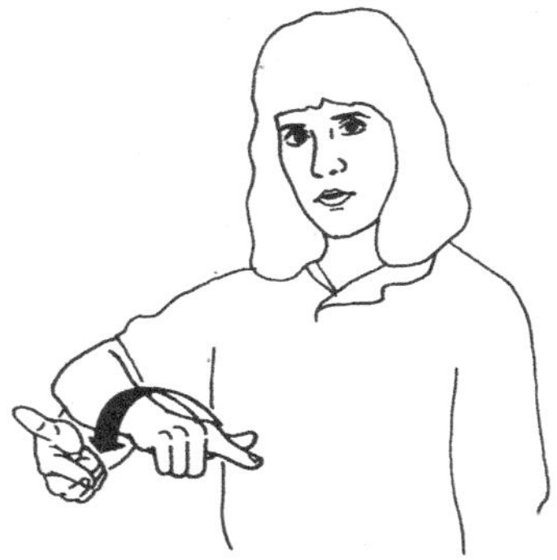

TURN

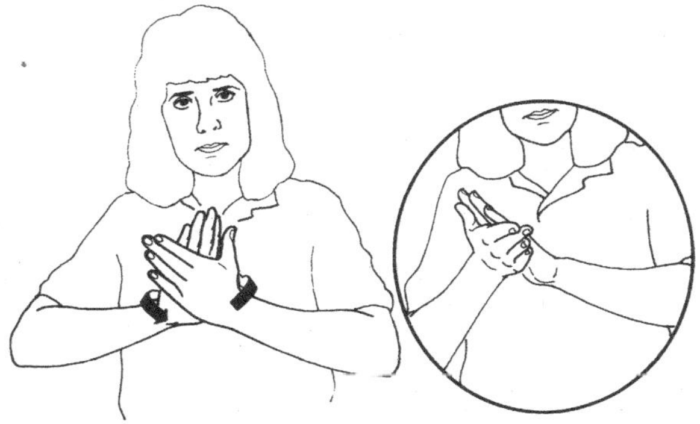

BECOME

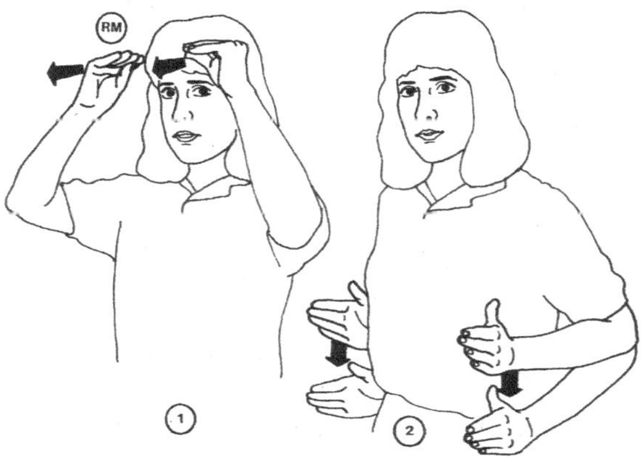

TEACHER.

It's your turn to become the teacher.

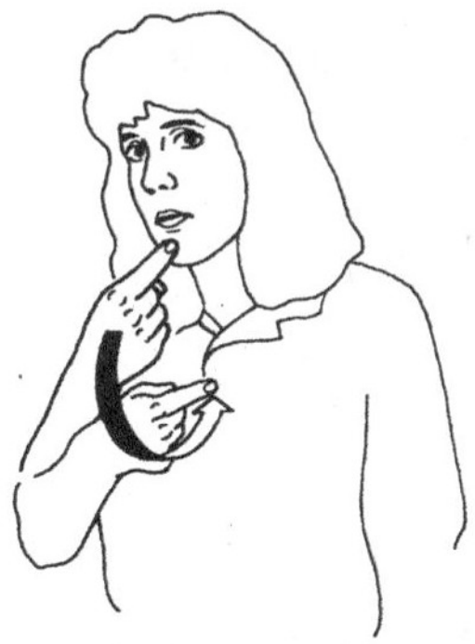

TELL-ME

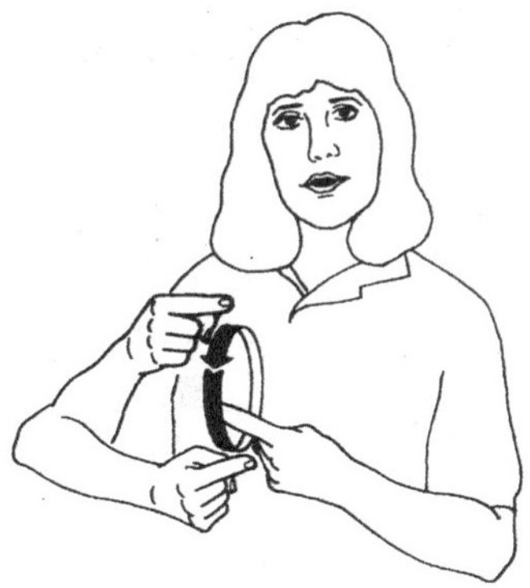

ABOUT

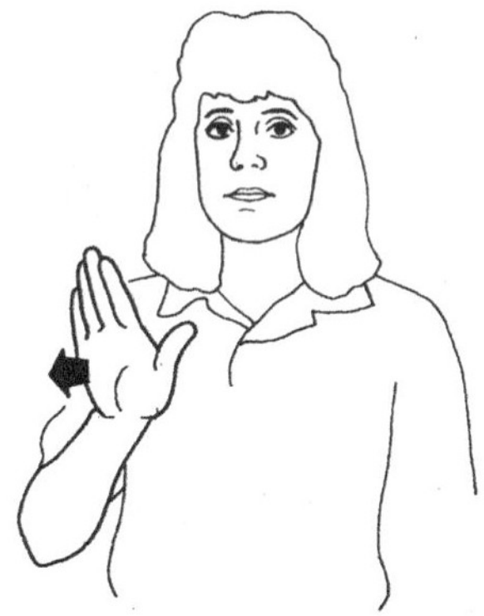

YOUR

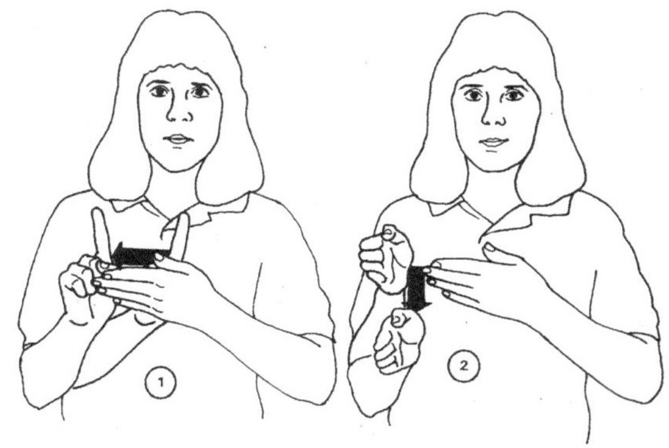

WEEKEND.

Tell me about your weekend.

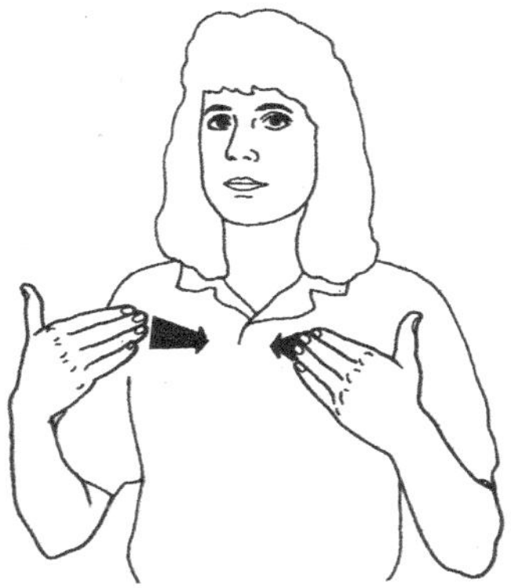

HAVE

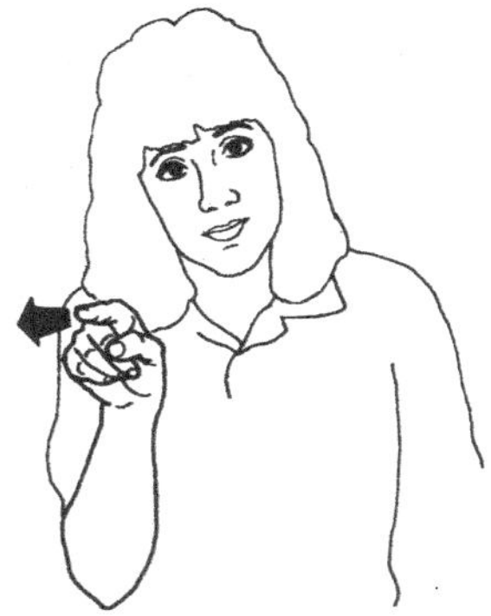

YOU

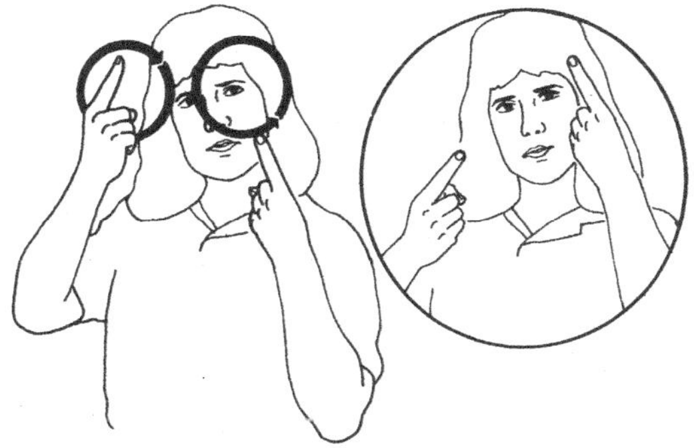

CONSIDER

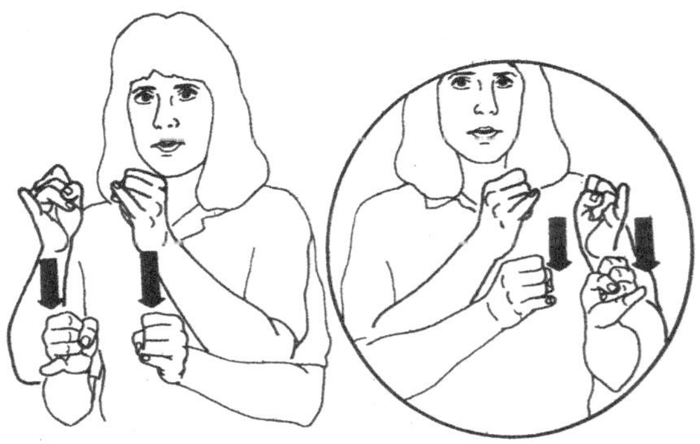

INDIVIDUAL

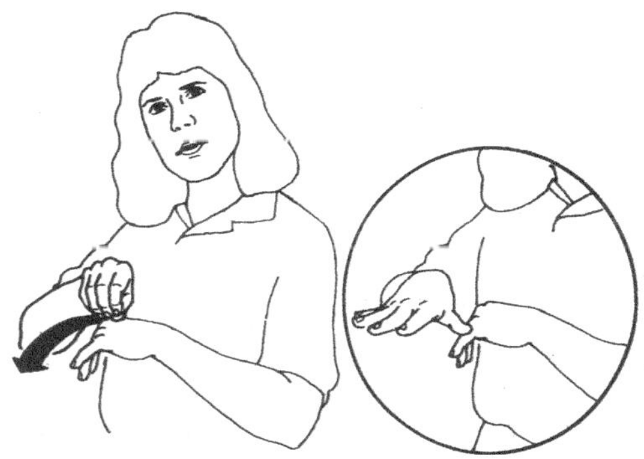

COUNSELING?

Have you considered individual counseling?

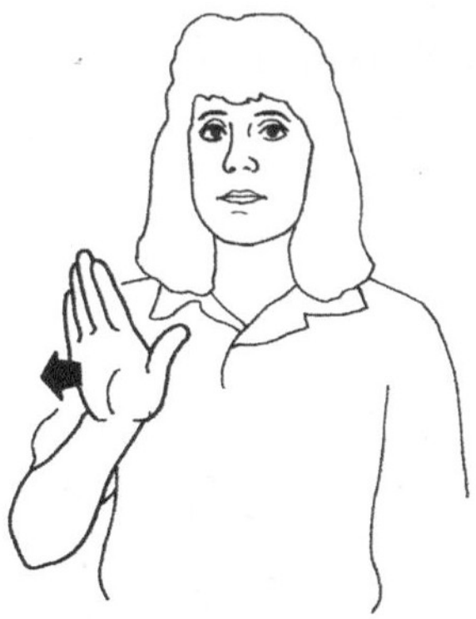

YOUR

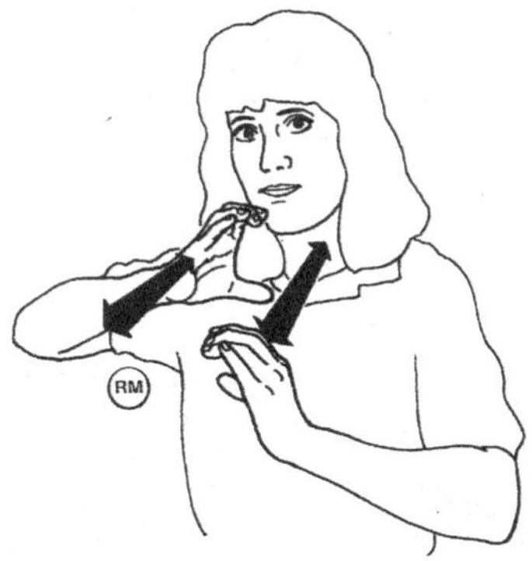

COMMUNICATION

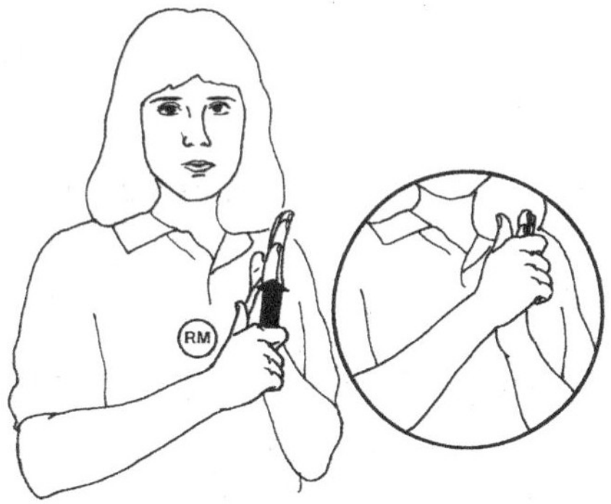

JOURNAL

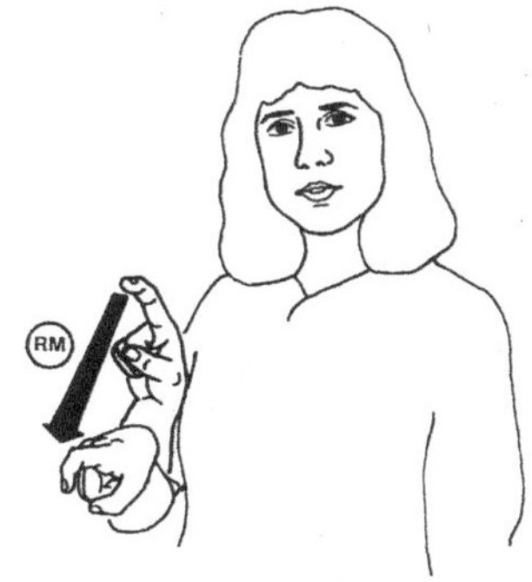

SHOULD

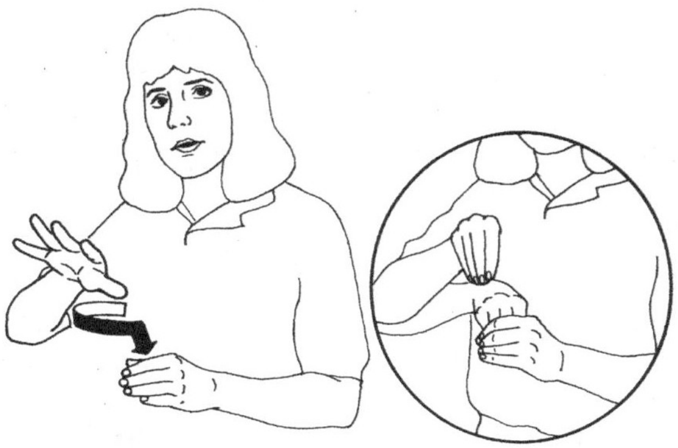

INCLUDE

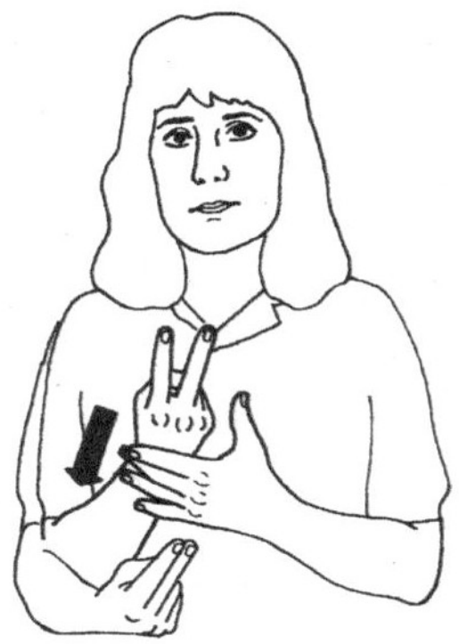

BOTH

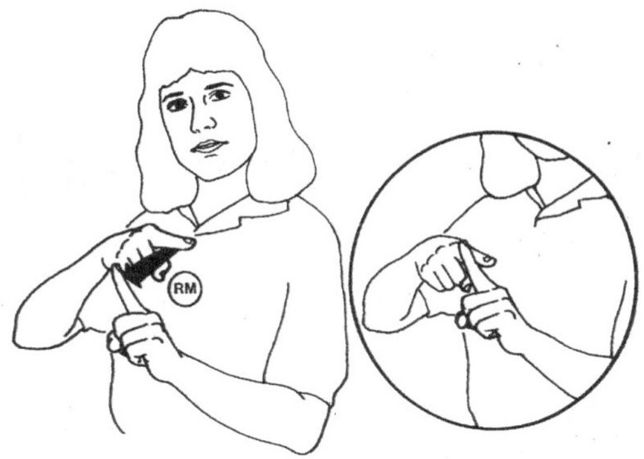

POSITIVE

Your communication journal should include both positive and negative experiences.

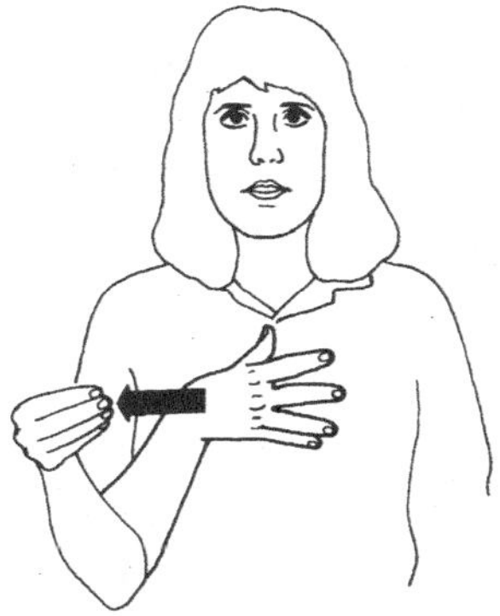

AND

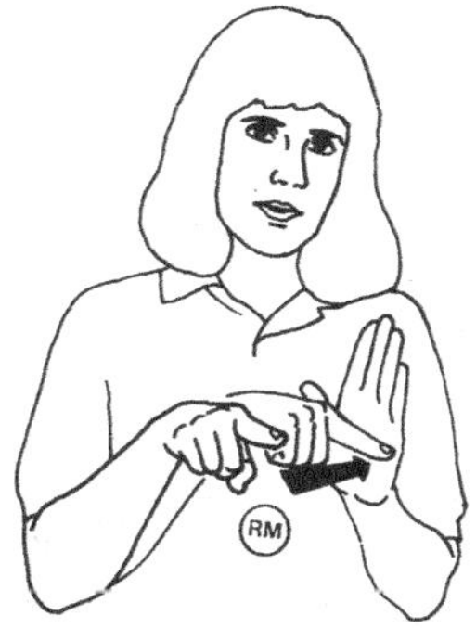

NEGATIVE

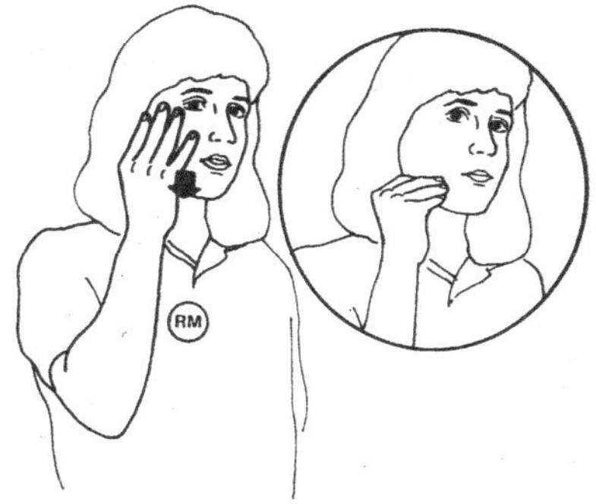

EXPERIENCE.

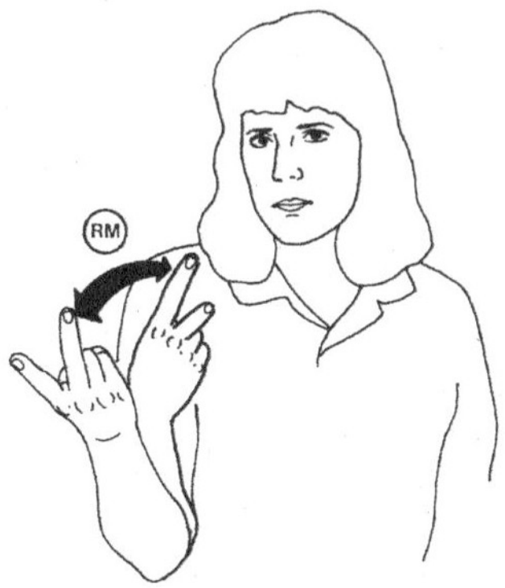

TWO-OF-US

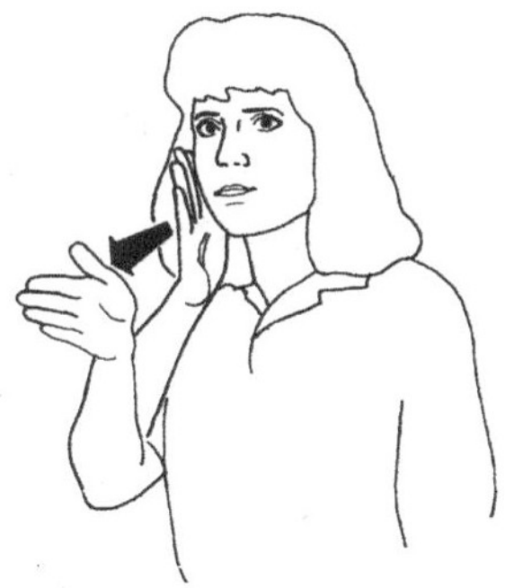

WILL

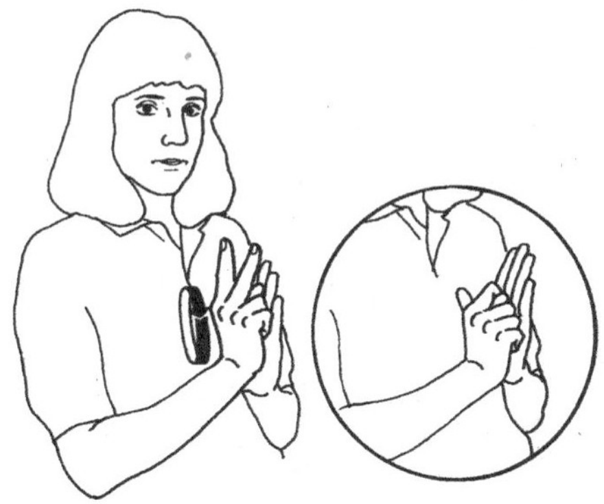

VIDEOTAPE

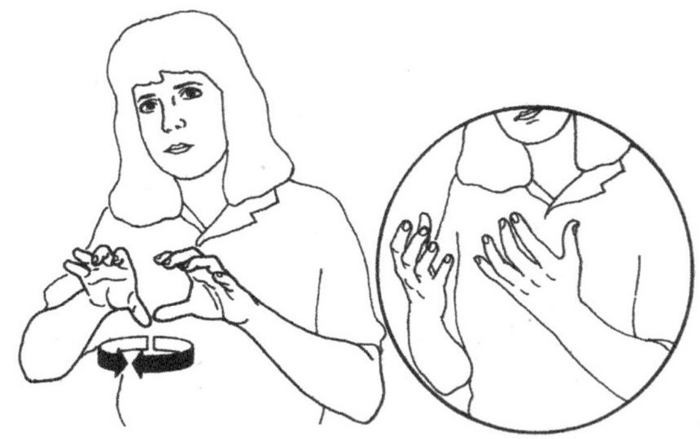

SESSION

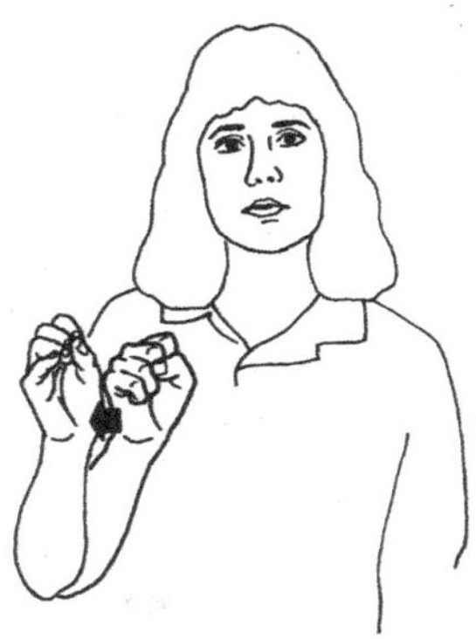

S-O

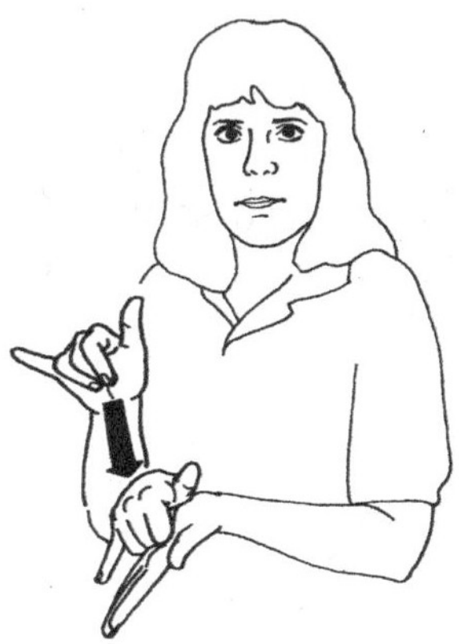

THAT

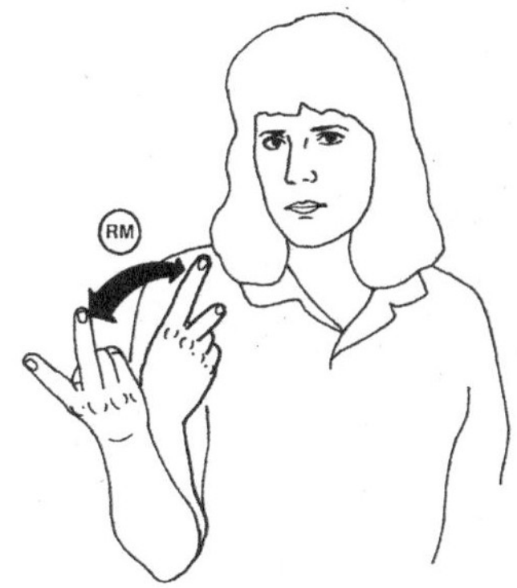

TWO-OF-US

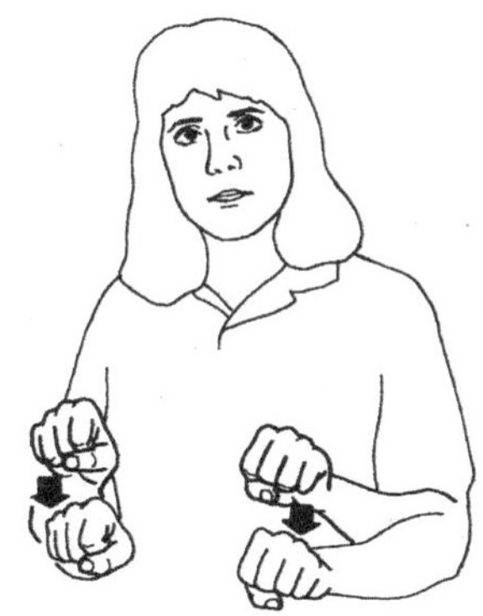

CAN

We will videotape the session so that we can review it later.

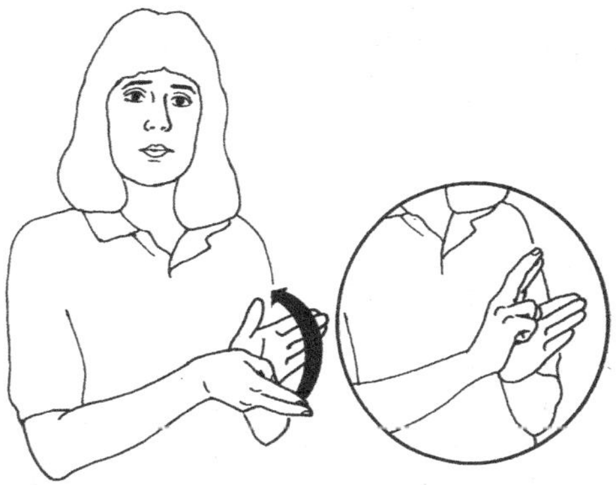

REVIEW

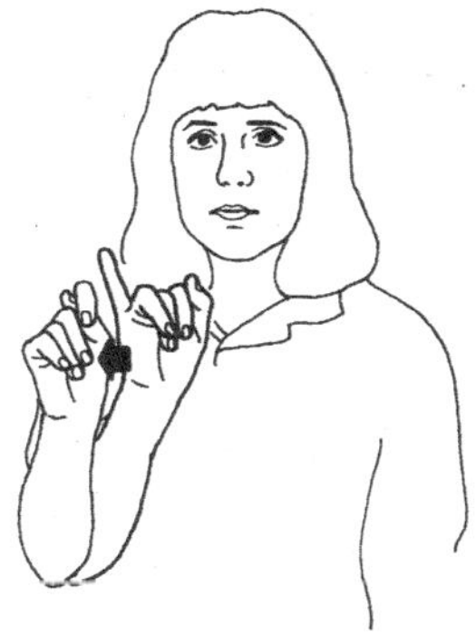

I-T

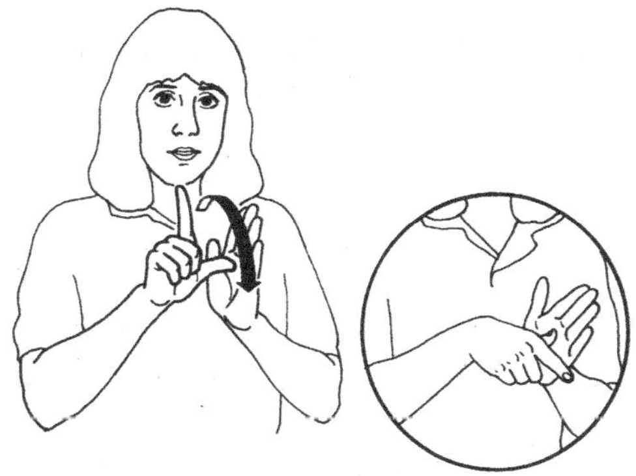

LATER.

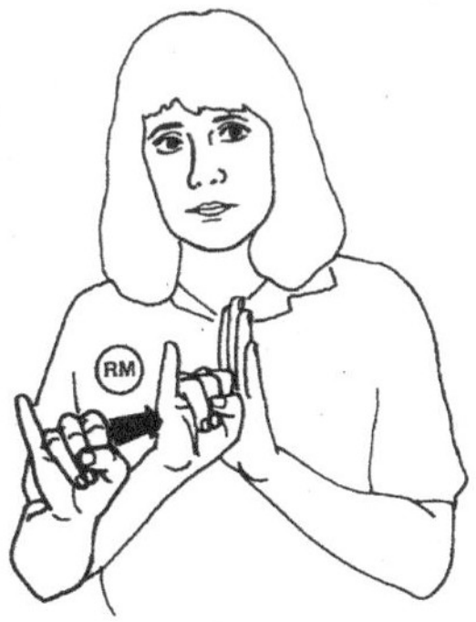

IDENTIFY

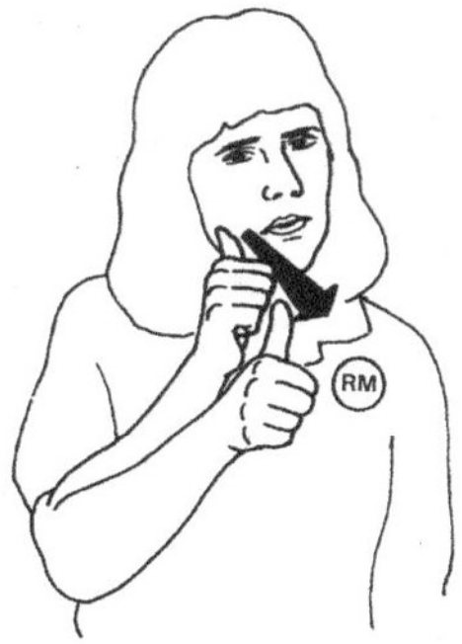

DAILY

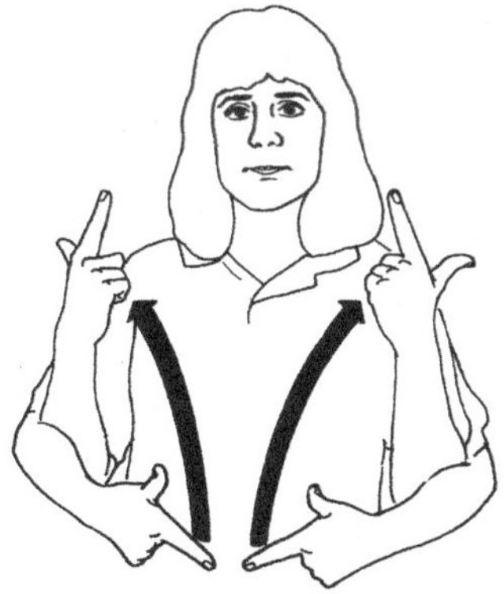

LIFE

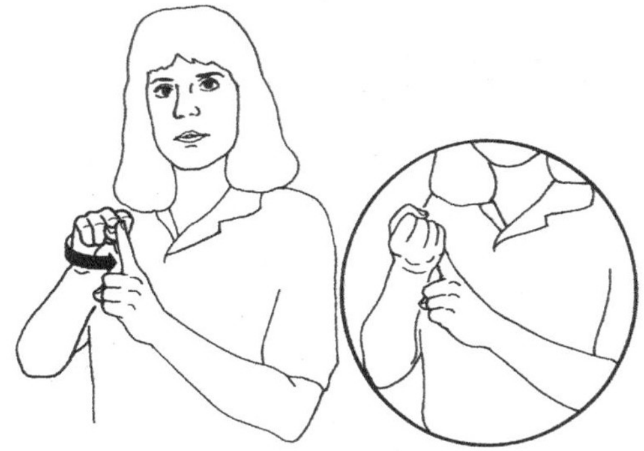

SITUATION

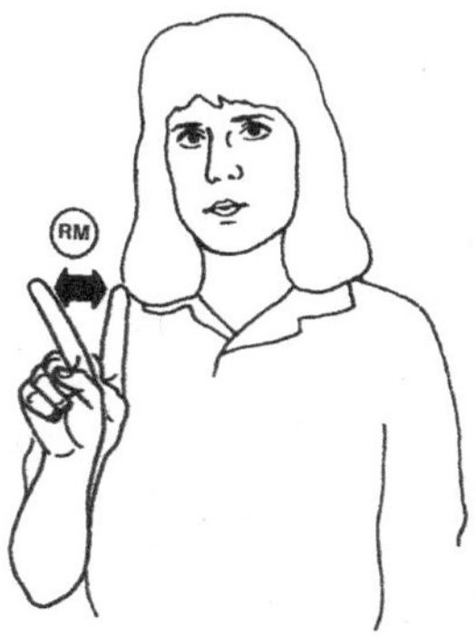

WHERE

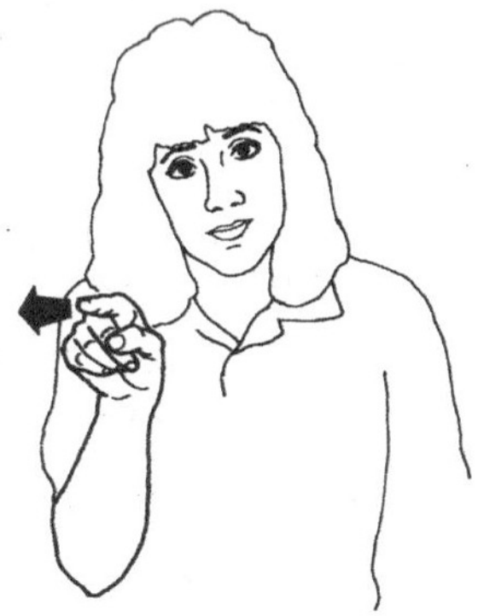

YOU

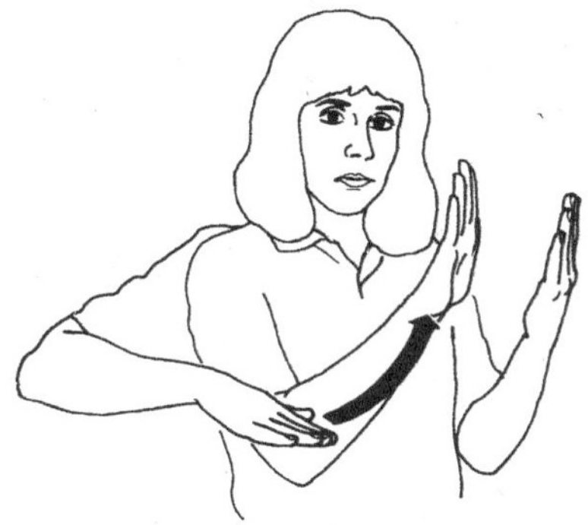

ENCOUNTER

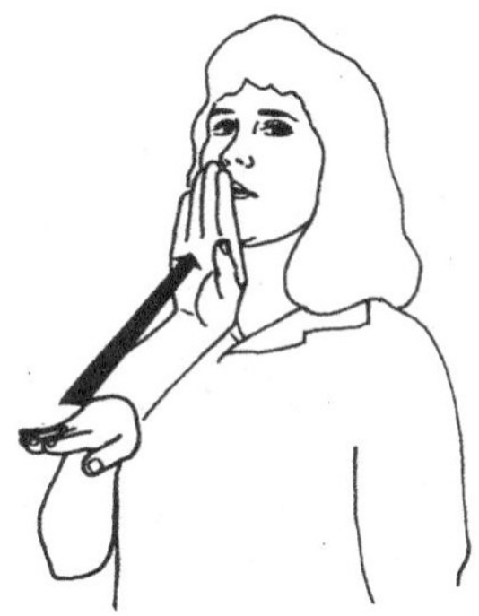

FRUSTRATION

Identify the daily life situations where you encounter frustration related to communication.

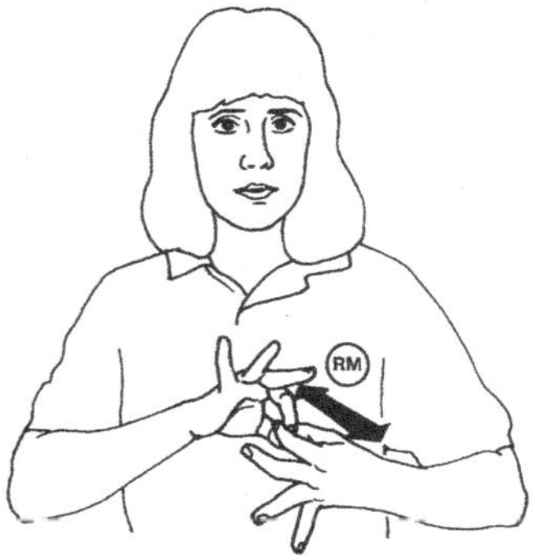

RELATE

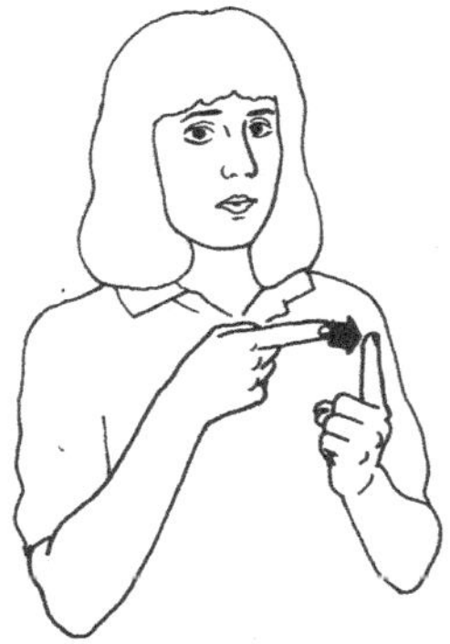

TO

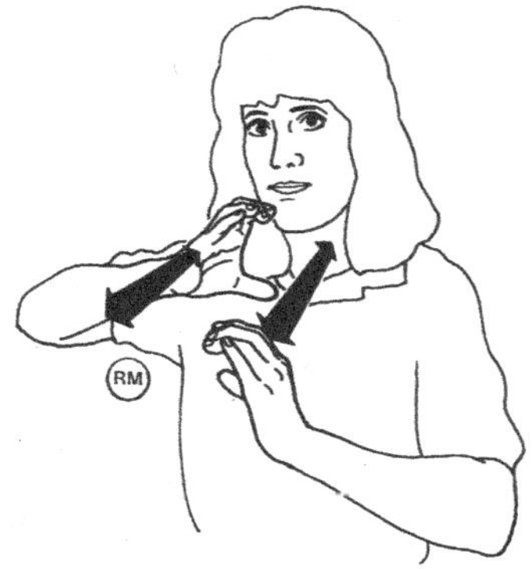

COMMUNICATION.

Chapter 6

Discussion of Test Results and Related Comments

Audiology

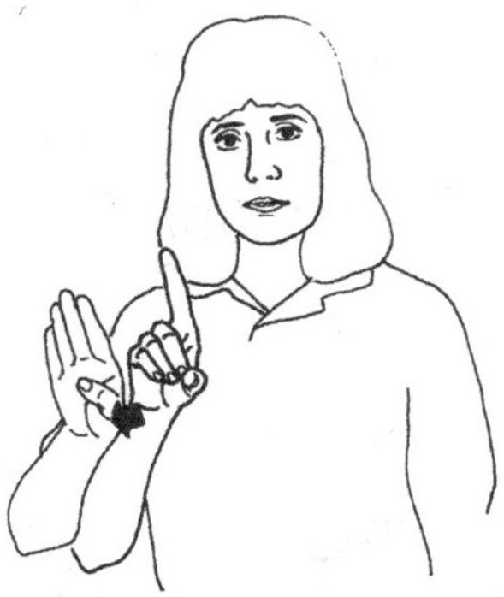

D-B

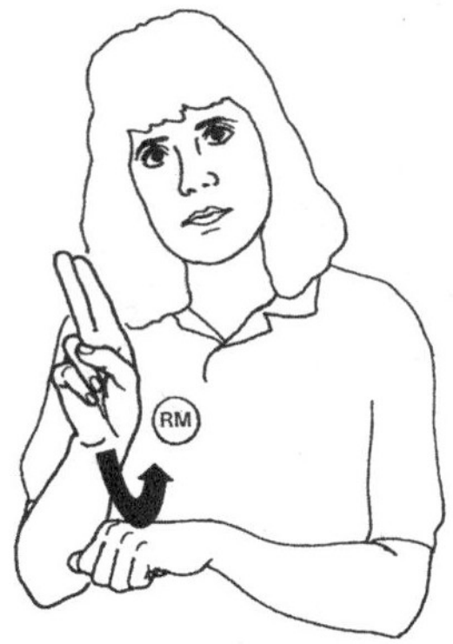

USE

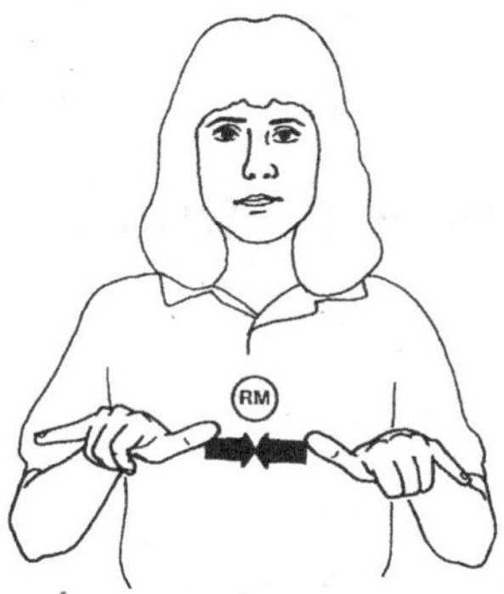

MEASURE

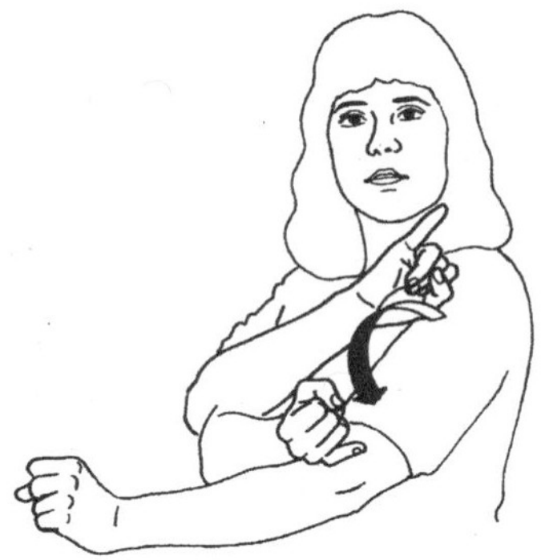

INTENSITY.

DB is used to measure intensity.

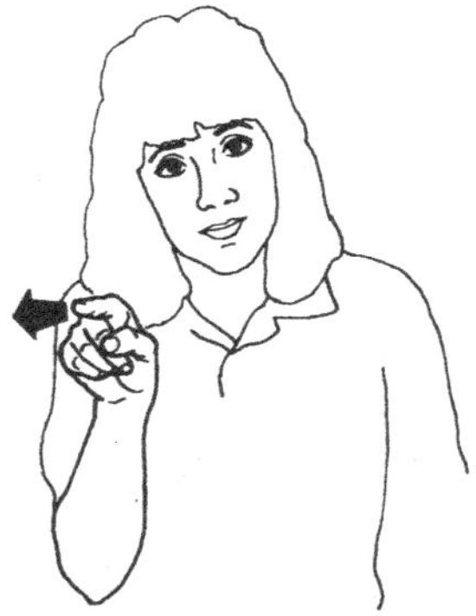

YOU

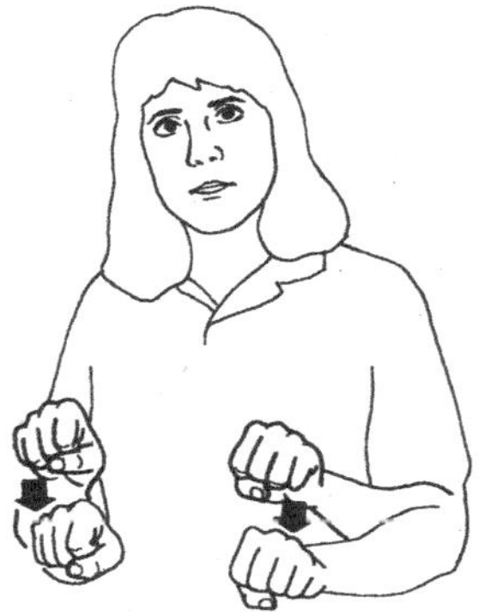

CAN

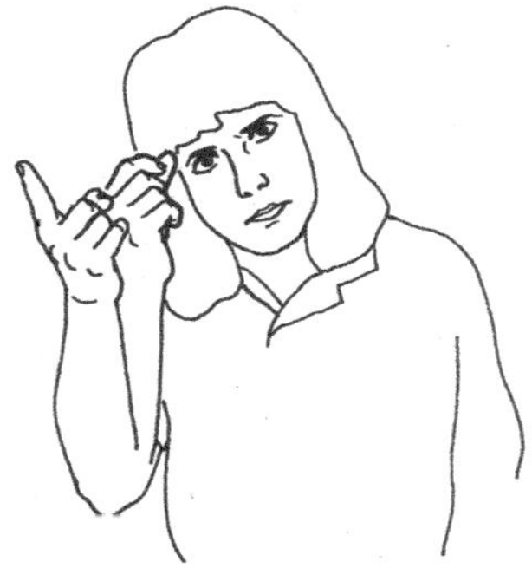

UNDERSTAND

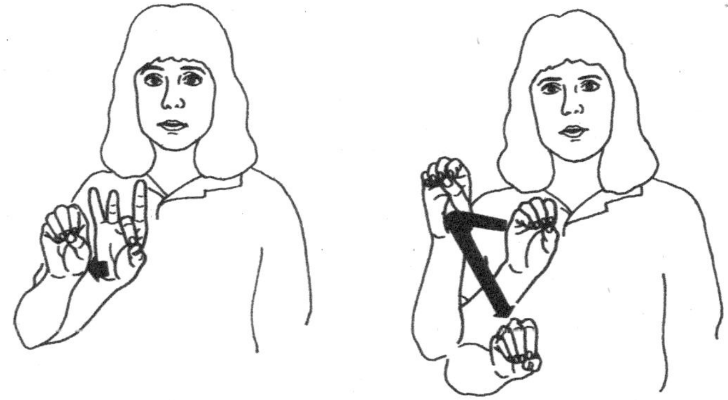

80%

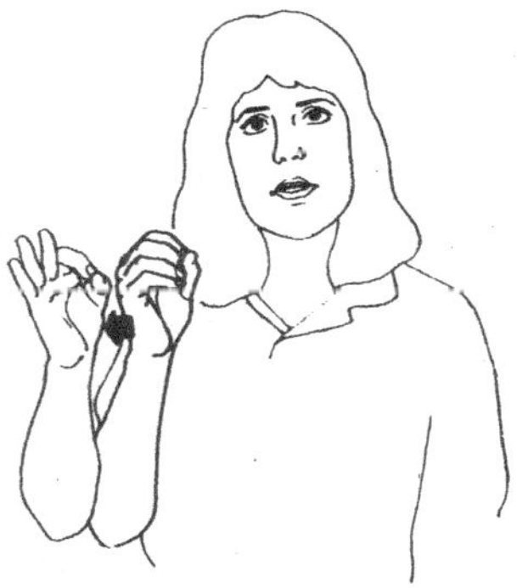

O-F

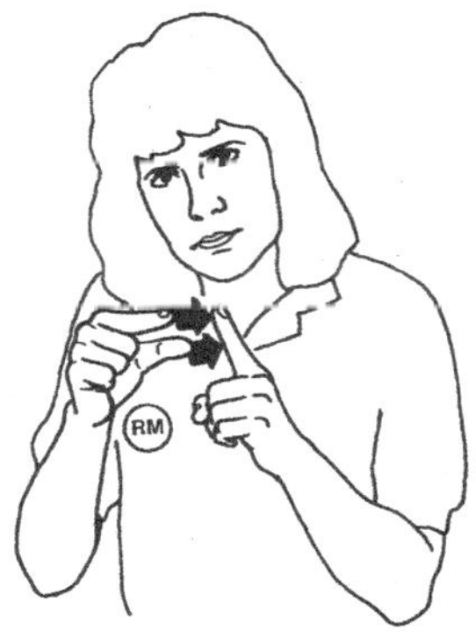

WORD

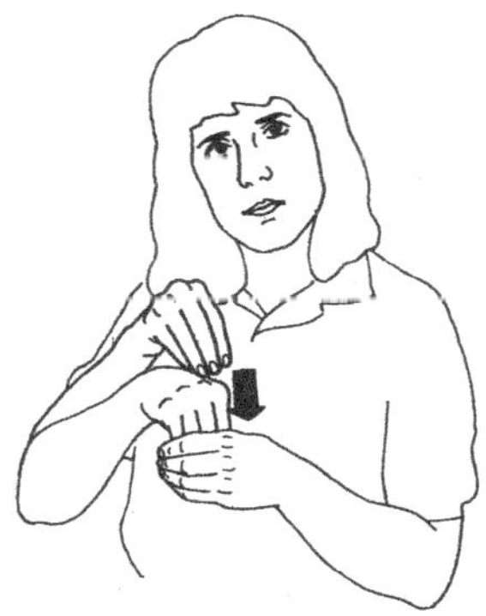

IN

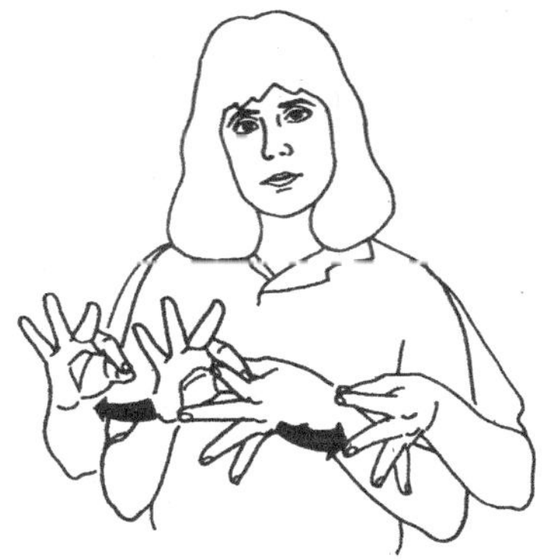

SENTENCE.

You can understand 80% of the words in sentences.

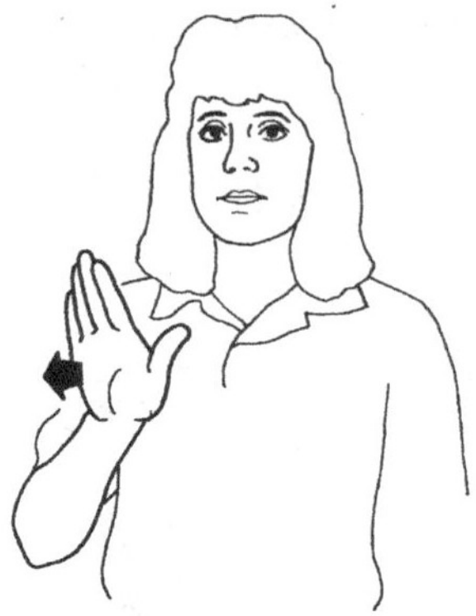

YOUR

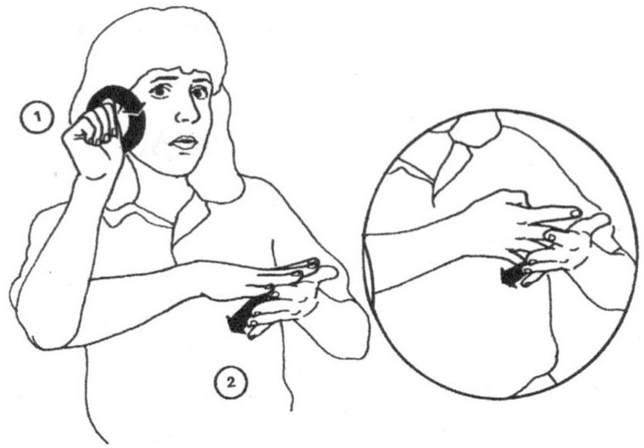

AUDIOGRAM

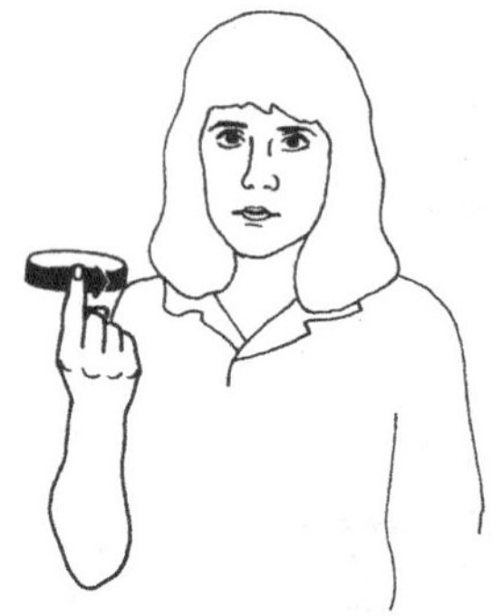

ONLY

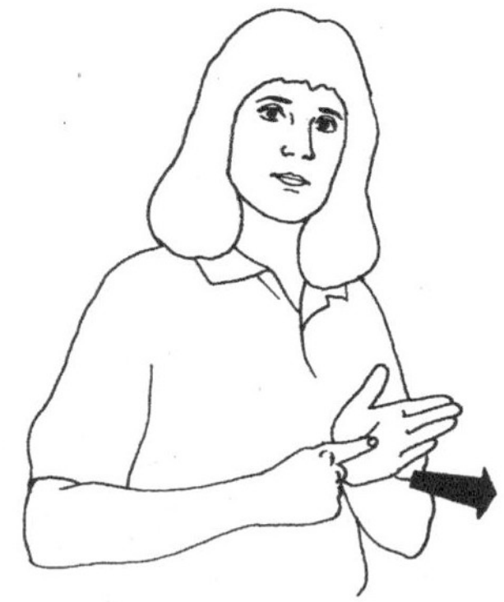

SHOW

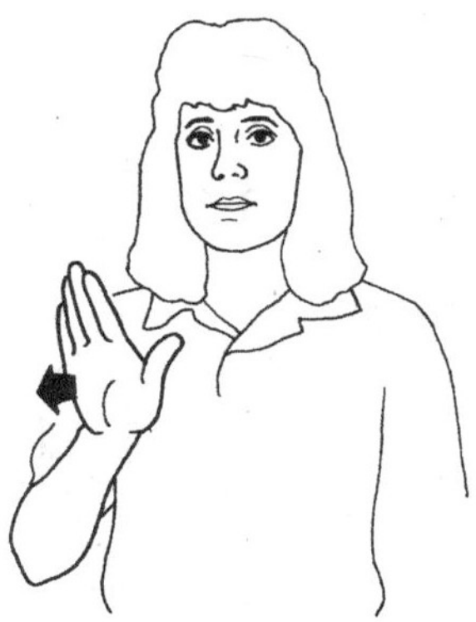

YOUR

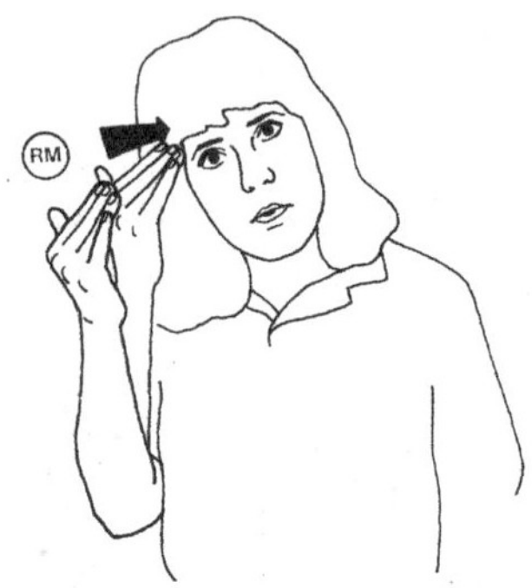

AWARENESS

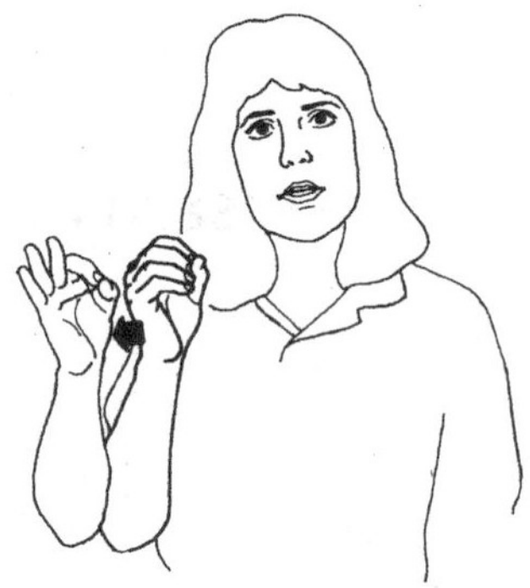

O-F

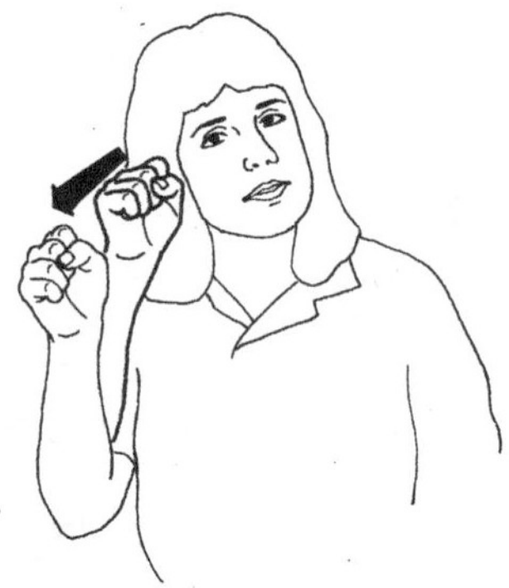

SOUND.

Your audiogram only shows your awareness of sound.

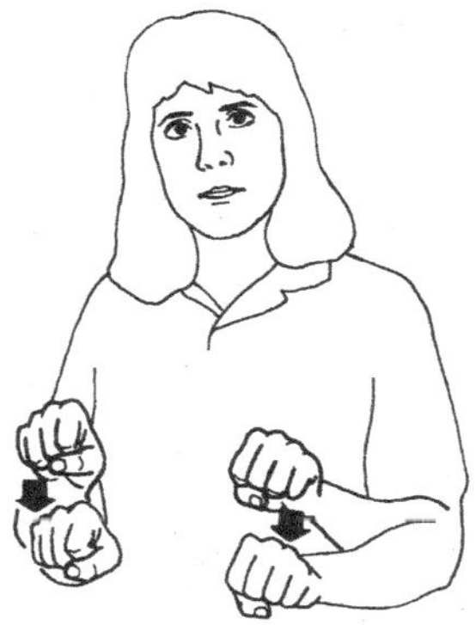

CAN

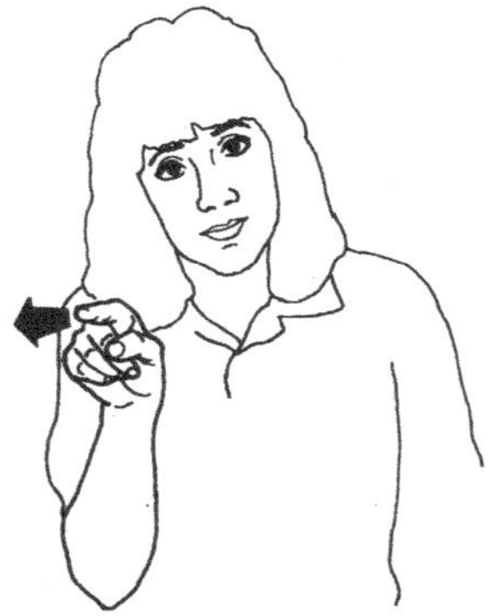

YOU

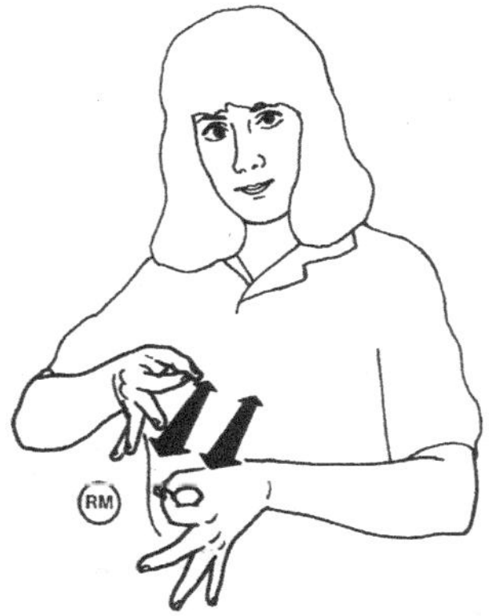

EXPLAIN

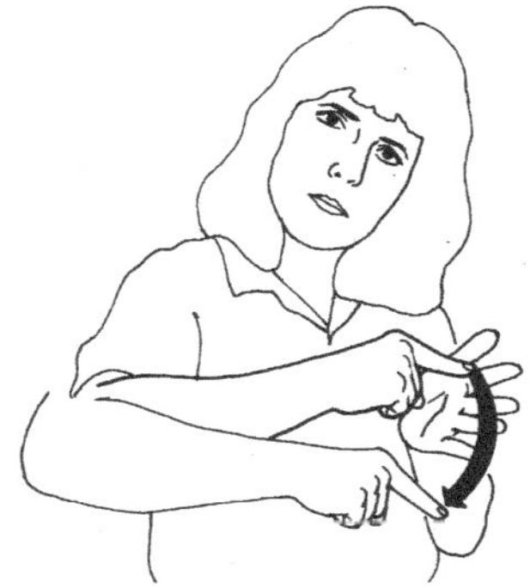

WHAT

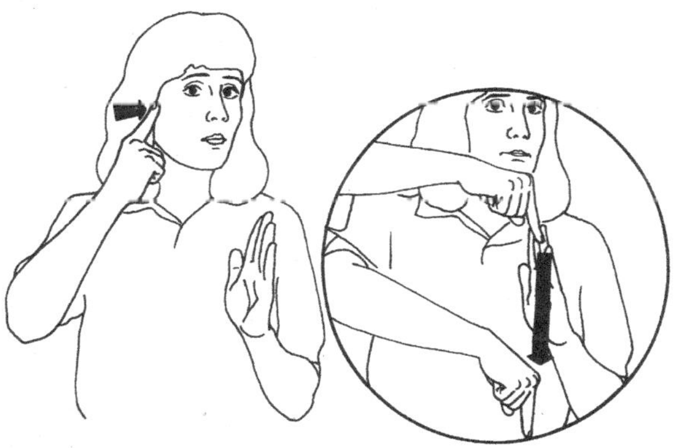

PROFOUND

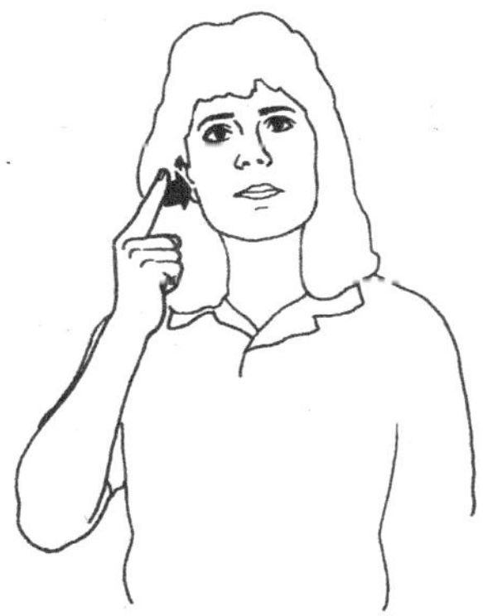

HEARING

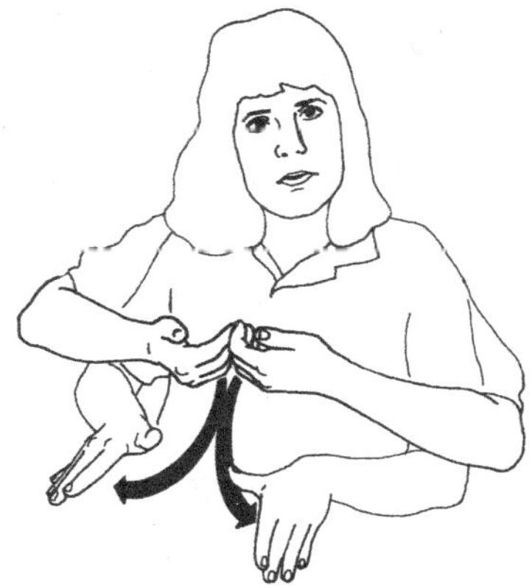

LOSS

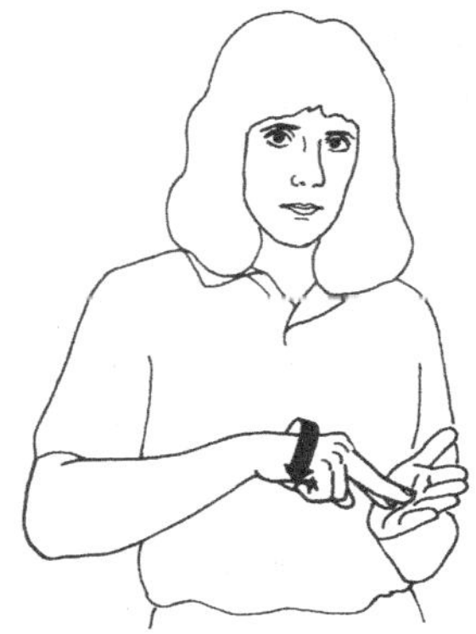

MEAN?

Can you explain what a profound hearing loss means?

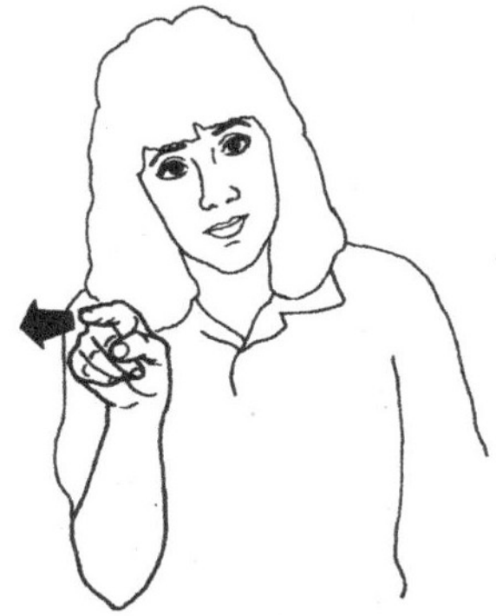

YOU

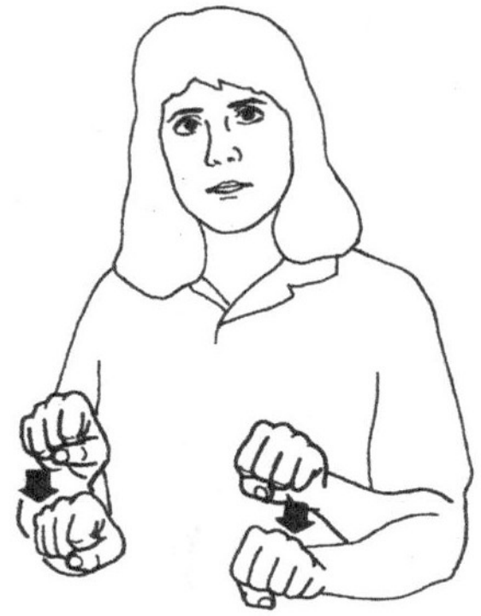

ABLE

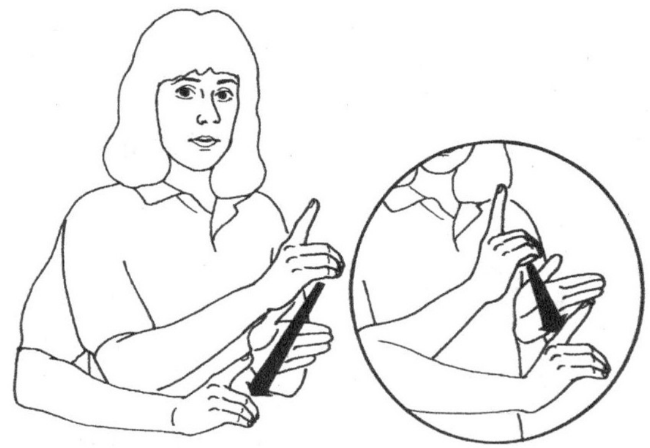

DISCRIMINATE

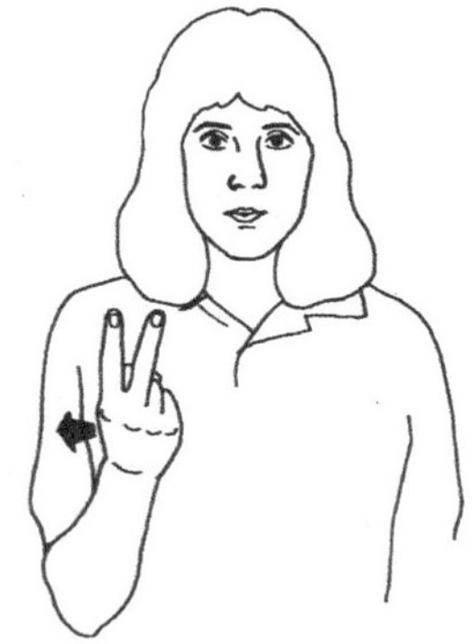

TWO

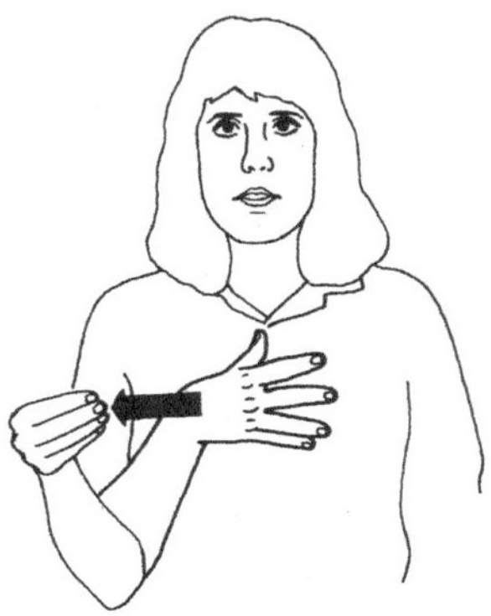

AND

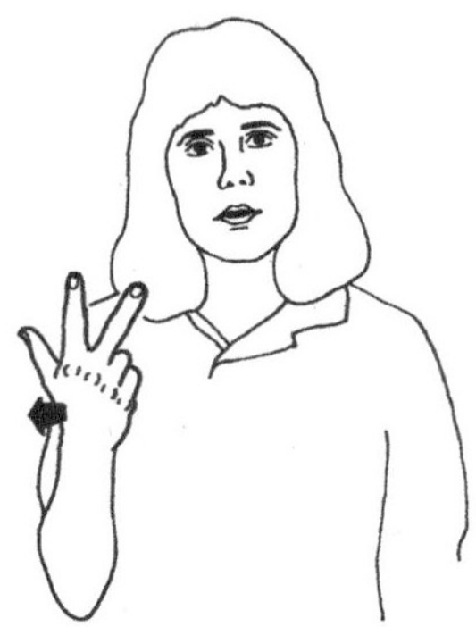

THREE

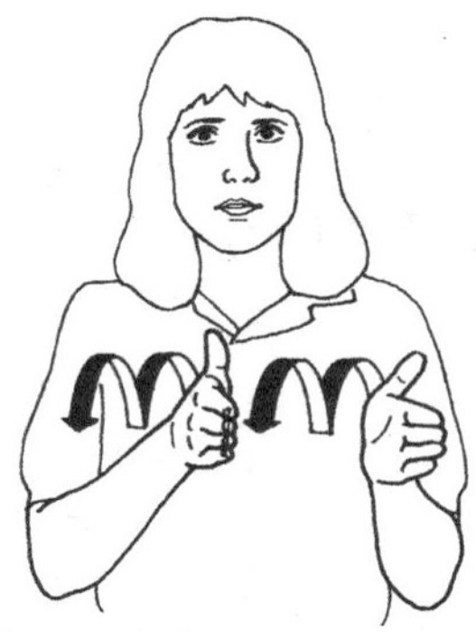

SYLLABLE.

You are able to discriminate two and three syllables.

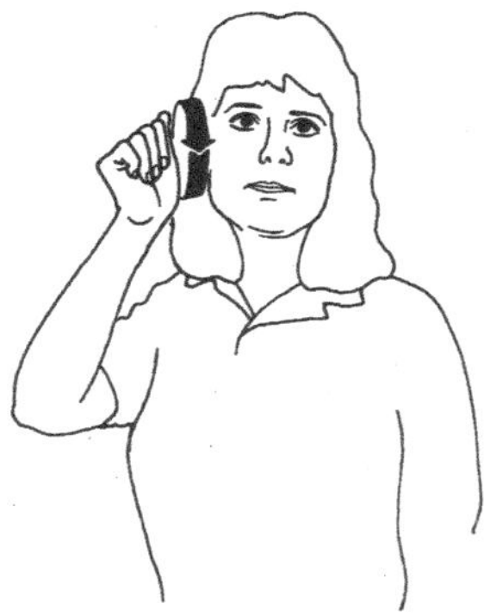

AUDITORY

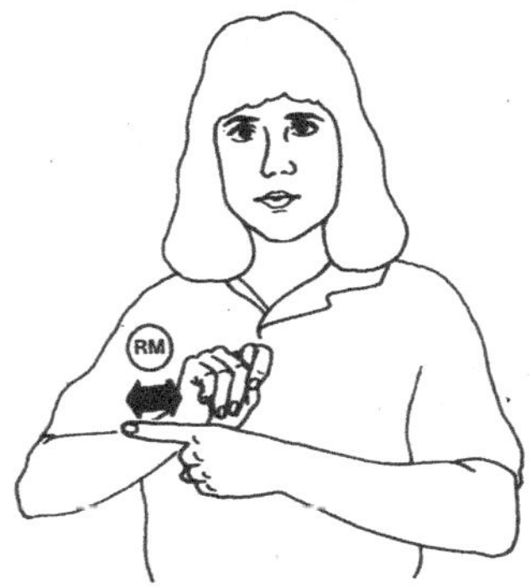

TRAINING

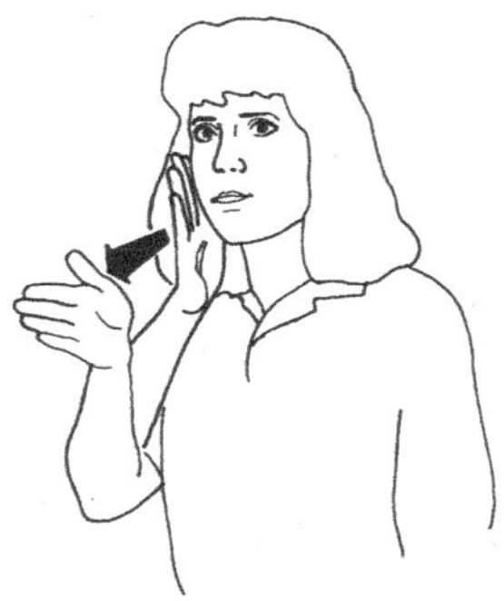

WILL

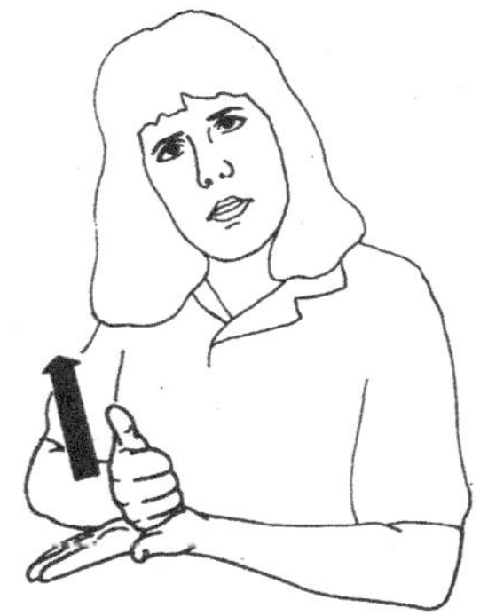

HELP

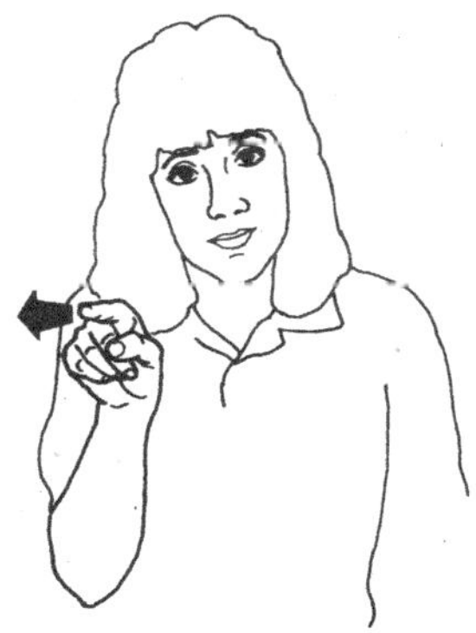

YOU

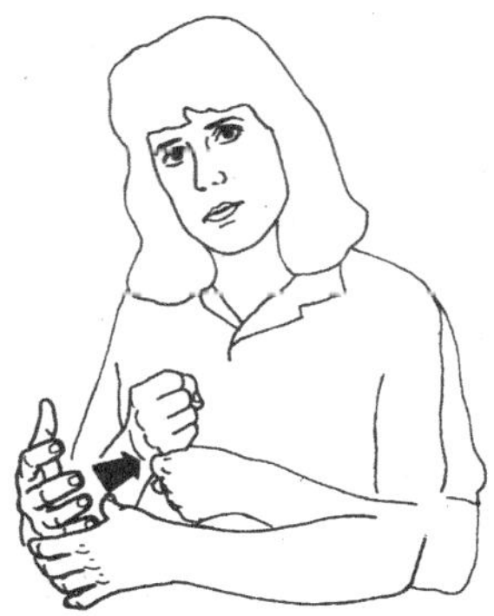

RECEIVE

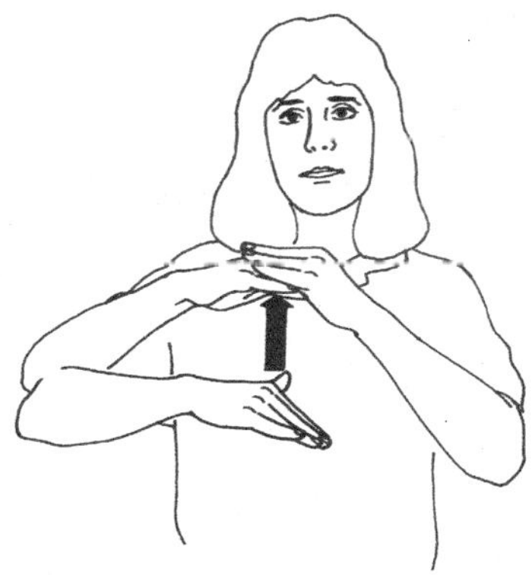

MAXIMUM

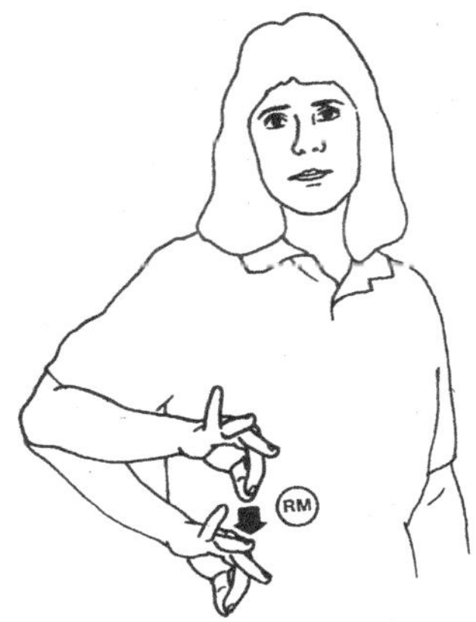

BENEFIT

Auditory training will help you receive maximum benefit from your hearing aid.

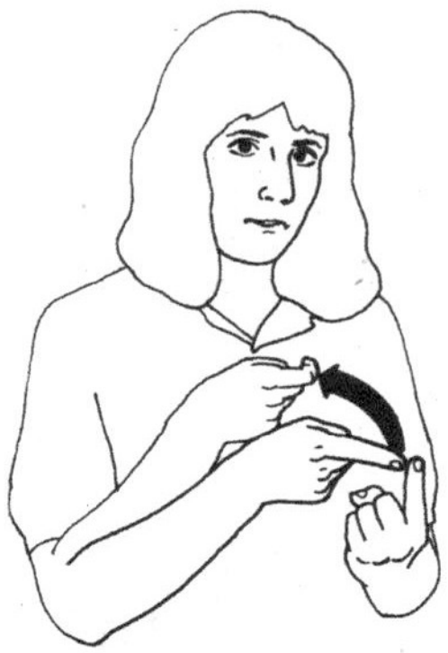

FROM

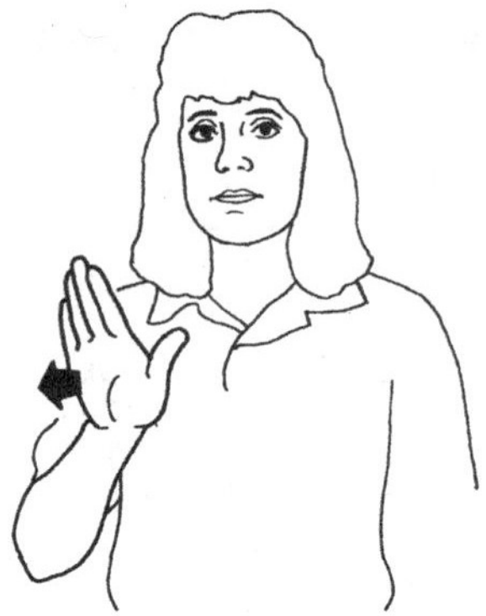

YOUR

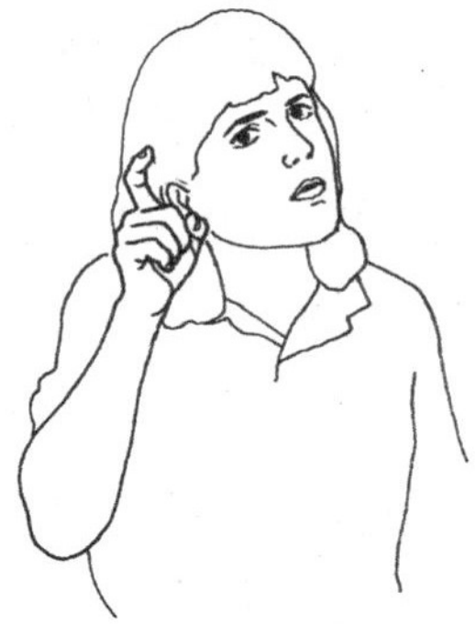

HEARING-AID.

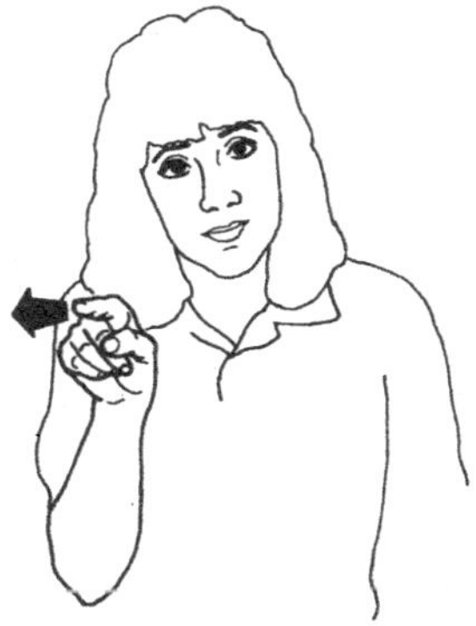

YOU

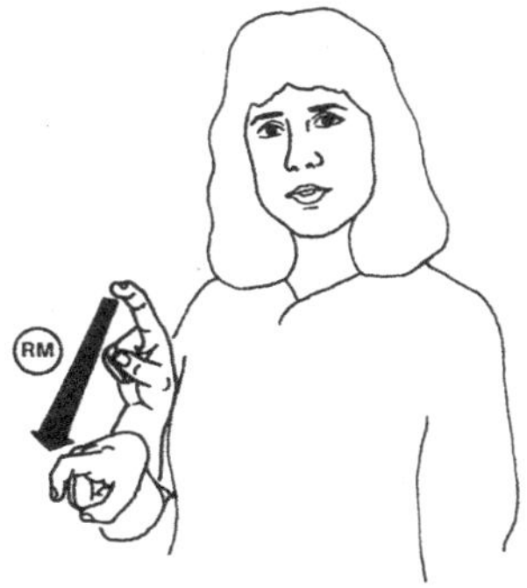

SHOULD

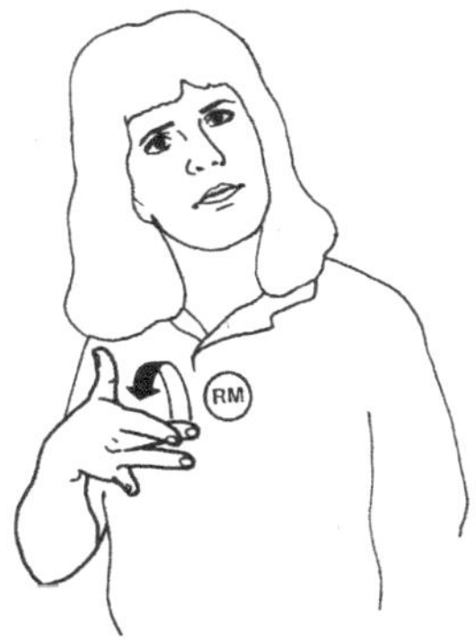

FEEL

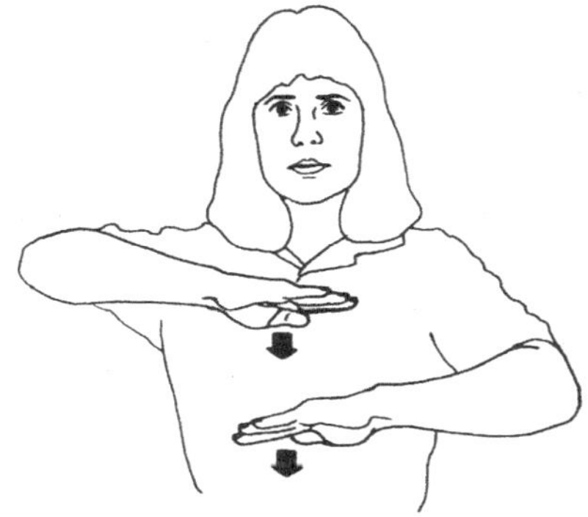

RELIEF

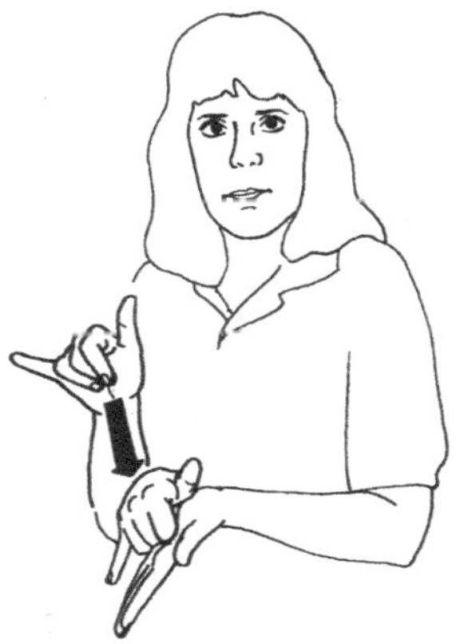

THAT

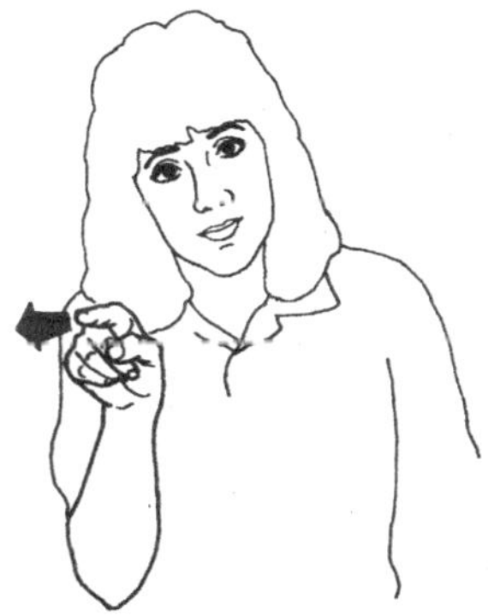

YOU

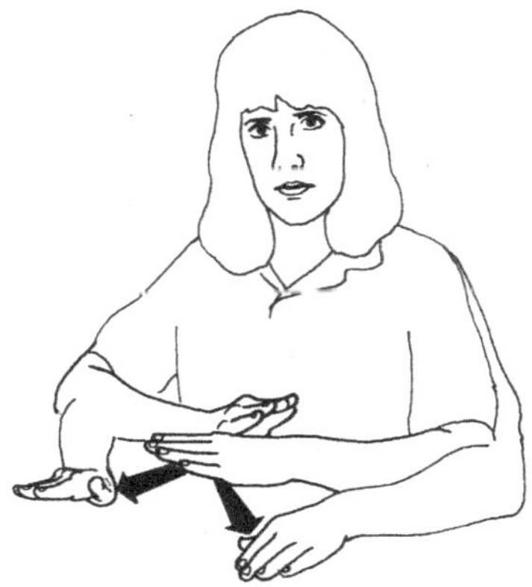

DON'T

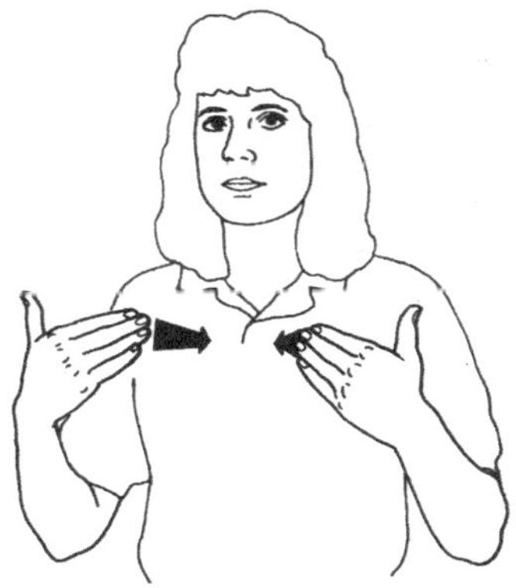

HAVE

You should be relieved that you don't have a middle ear infection.

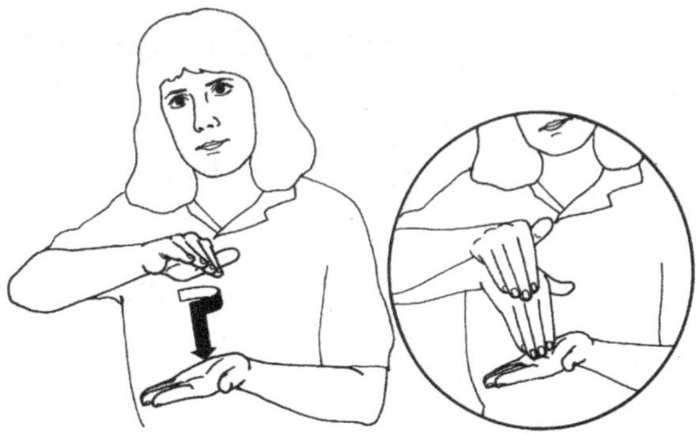

MIDDLE

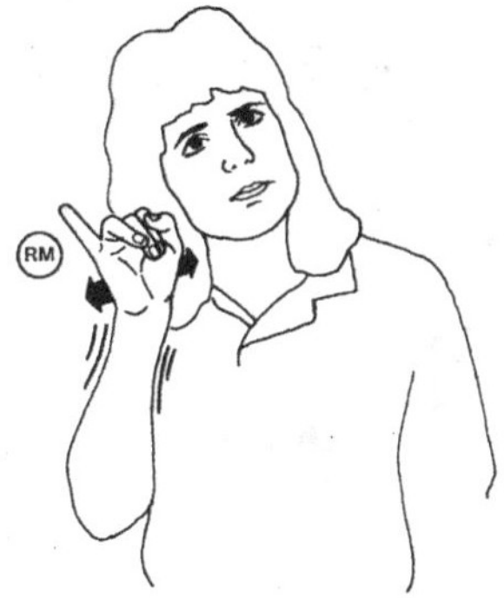

EAR-INFECTION.

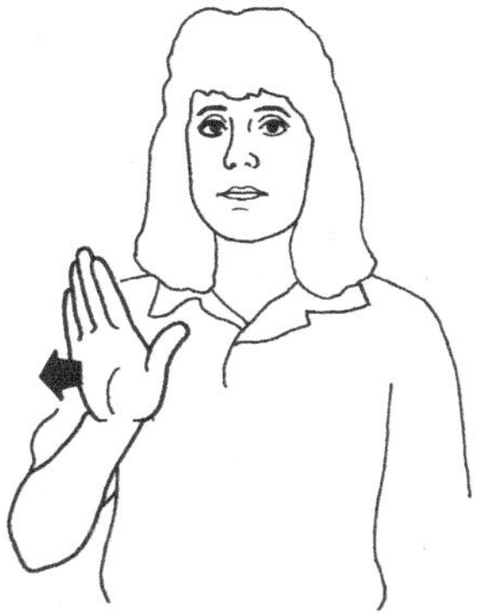

YOUR

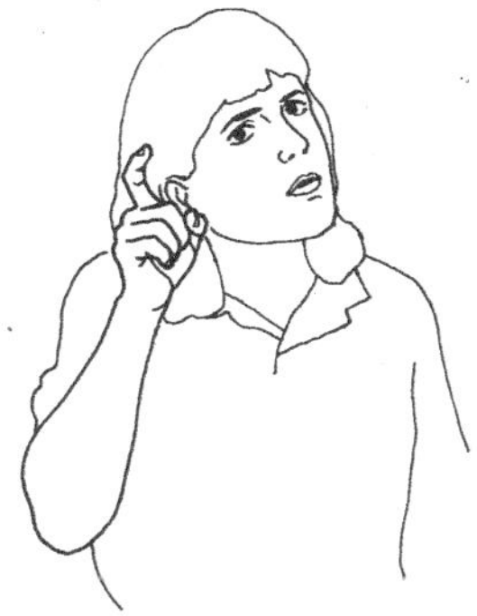

HEARING-AID

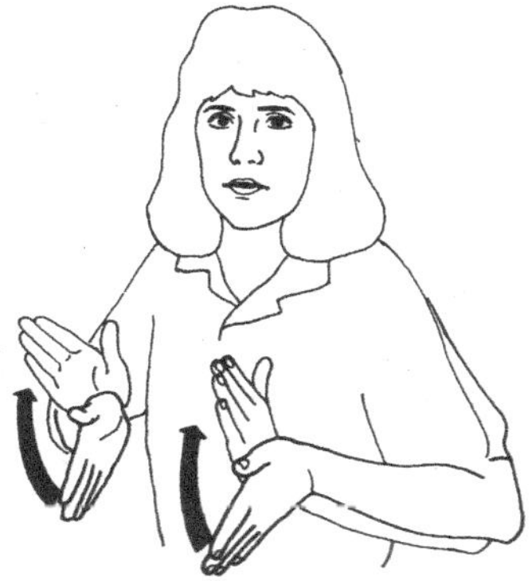

ALLOW

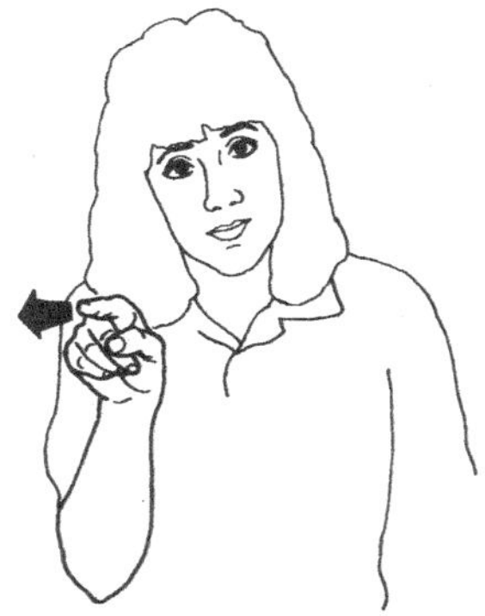

YOU

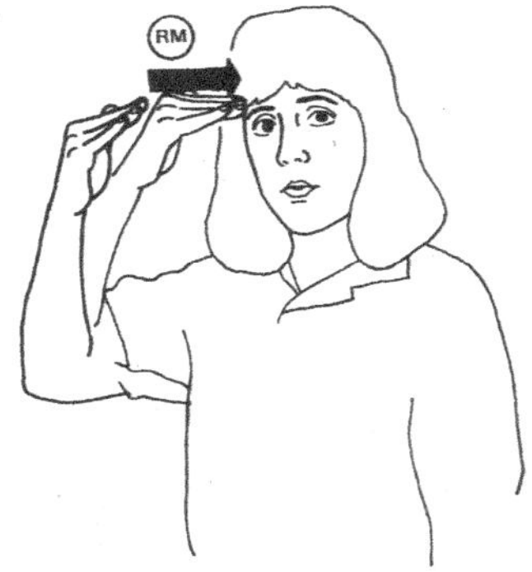

AWARE

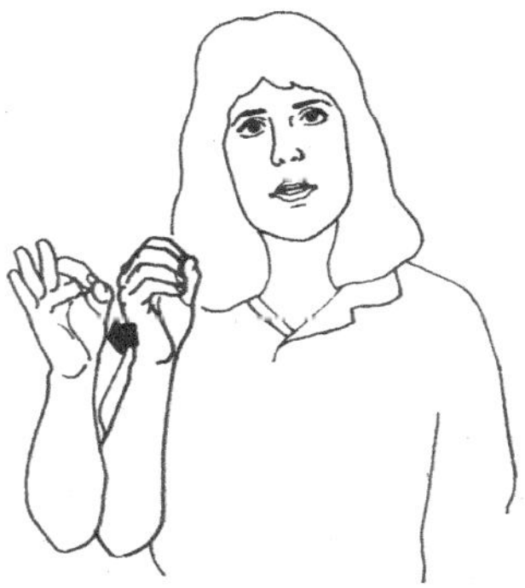

O-F

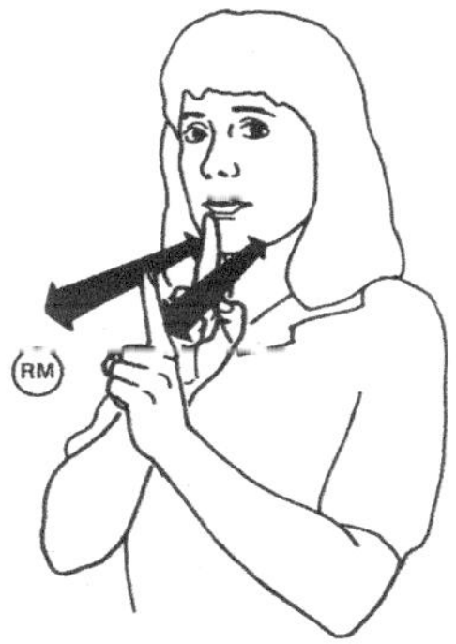

CONVERSATION

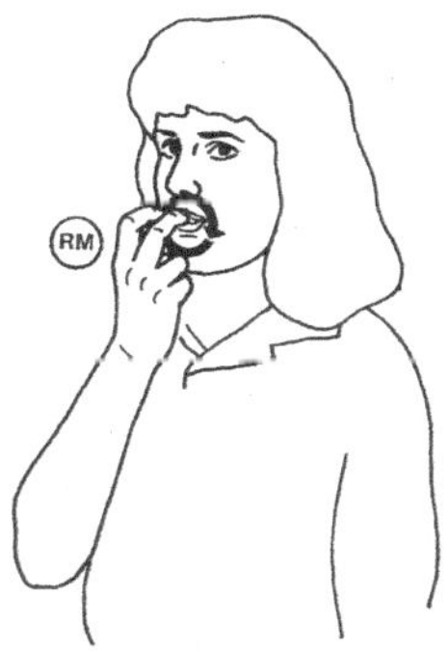

SPEECH.

Your hearing aid allows you to be aware of conversational speech.

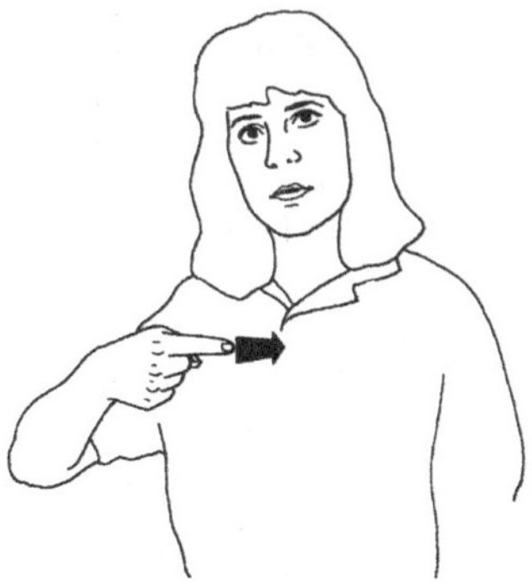

I

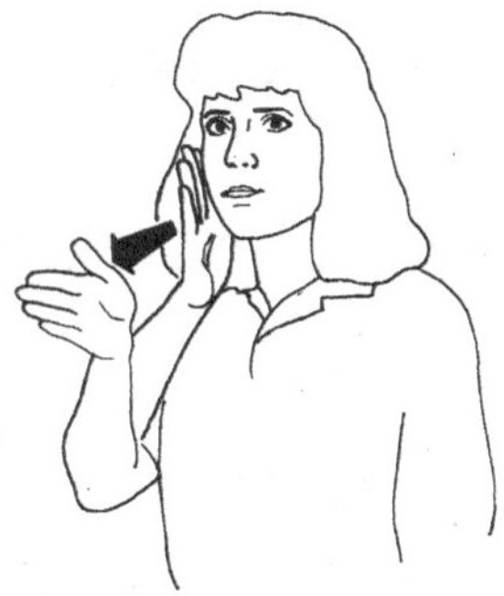

WILL

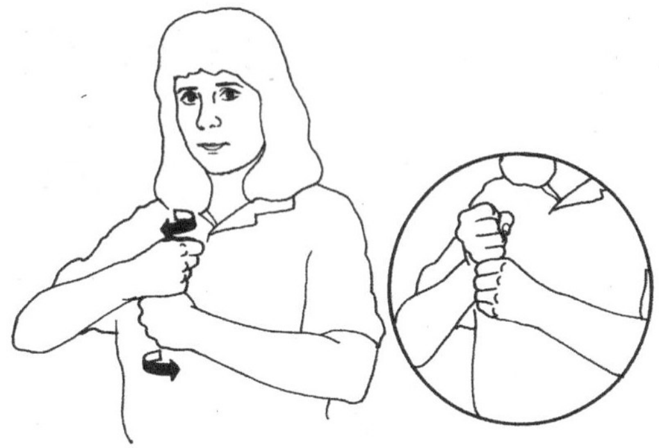

MAKE

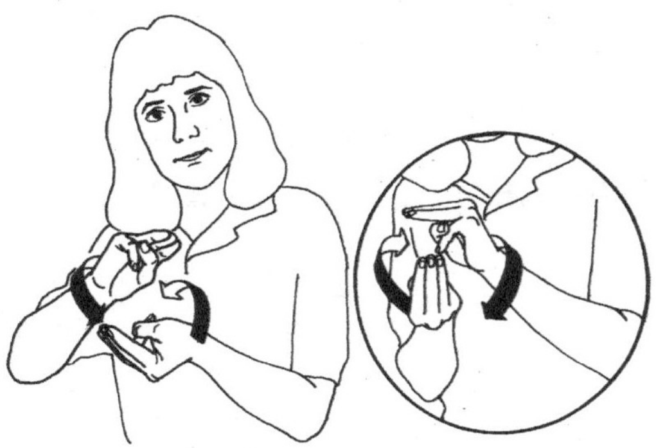

MODIFICATION

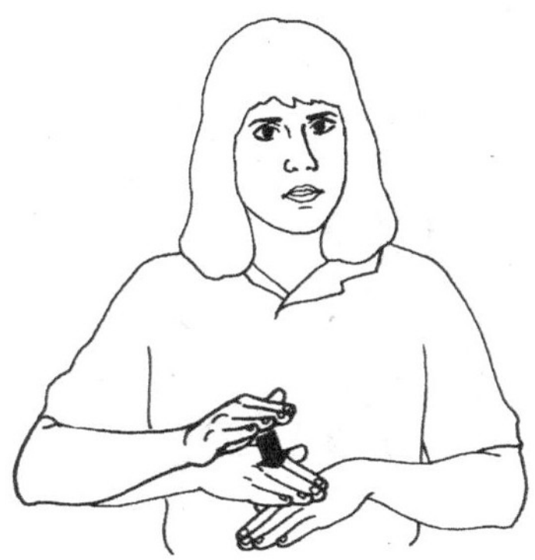

ON

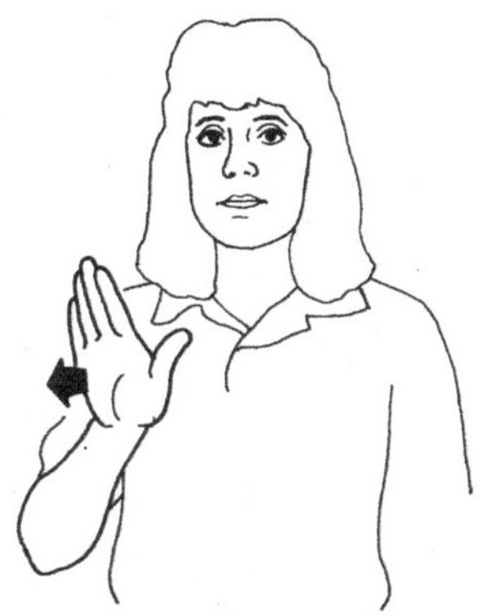

YOUR

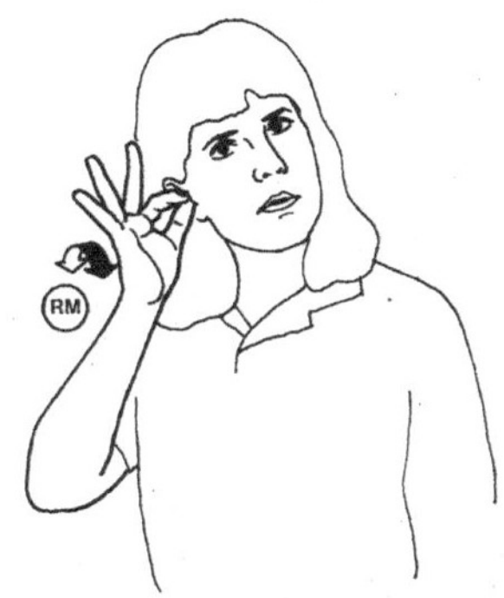

EARMOLD.

I will make modifications on your earmold.

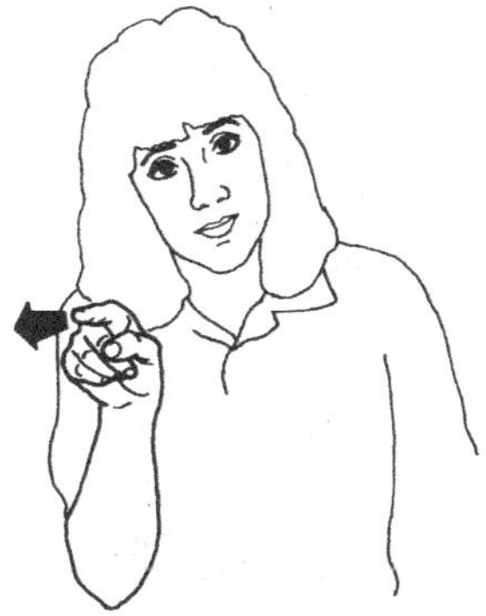

YOU

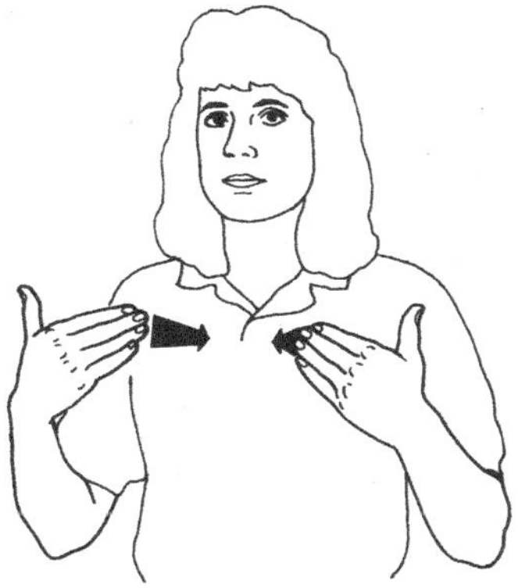

HAVE

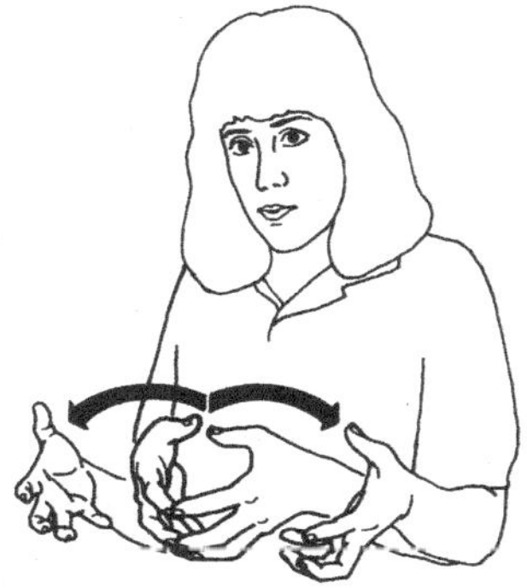

A-LOT

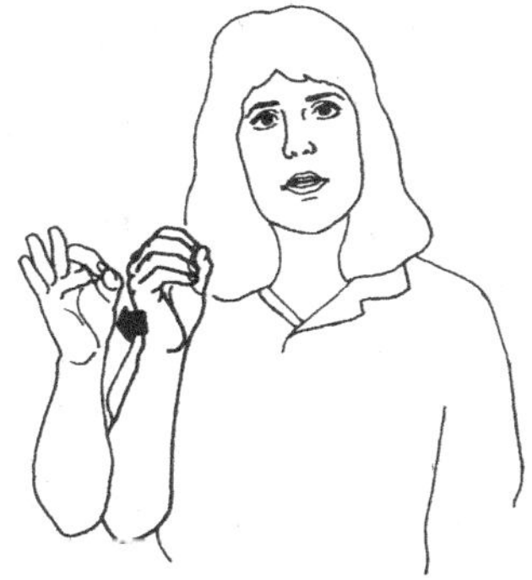

O-F

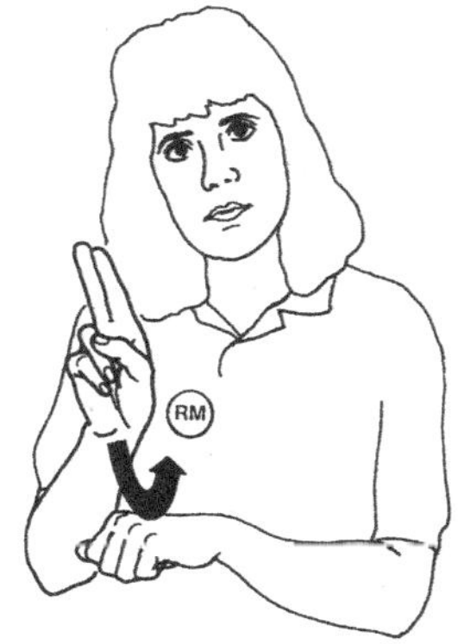

USE

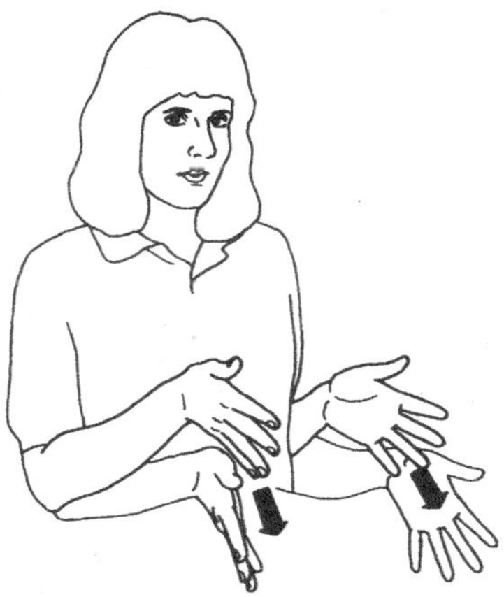

RESIDUAL

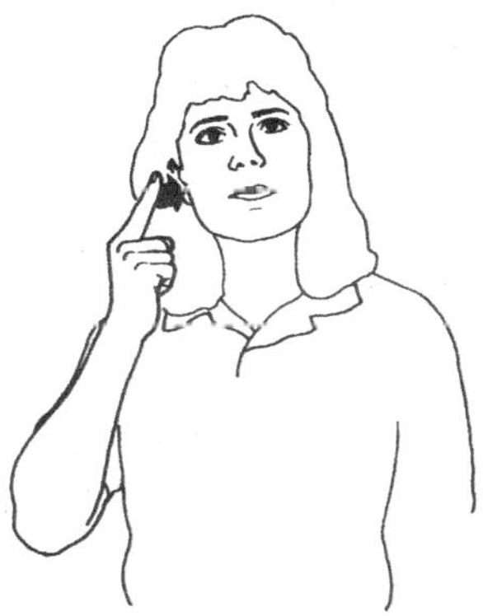

HEARING.

You have a lot of usable residual hearing.

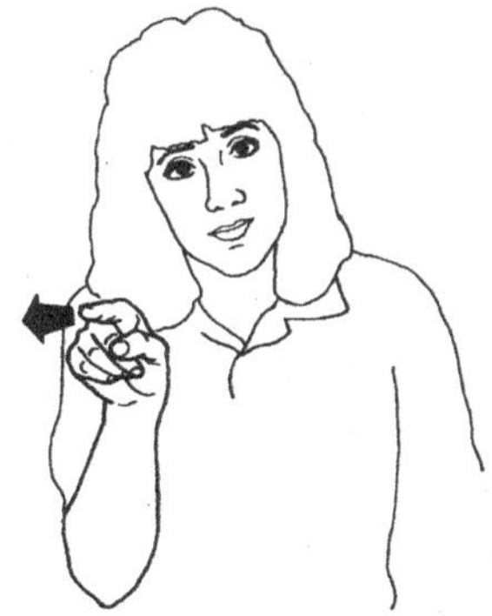

YOU

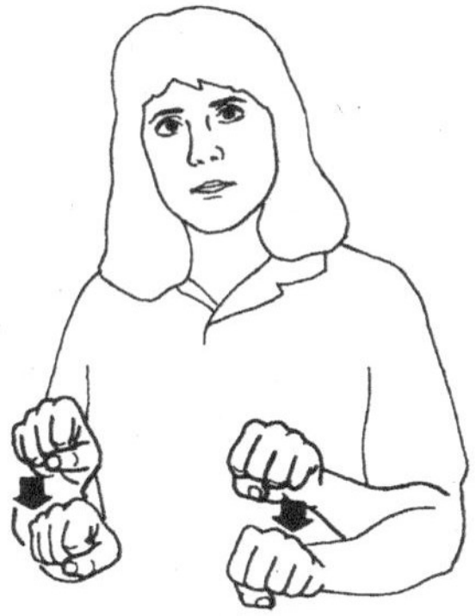

CAN

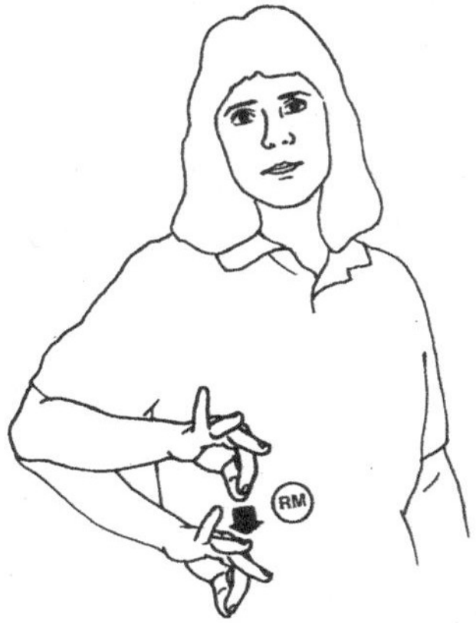

BENEFIT

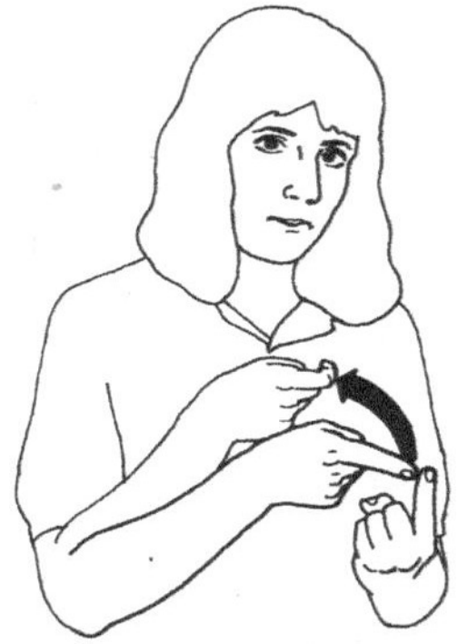

FROM

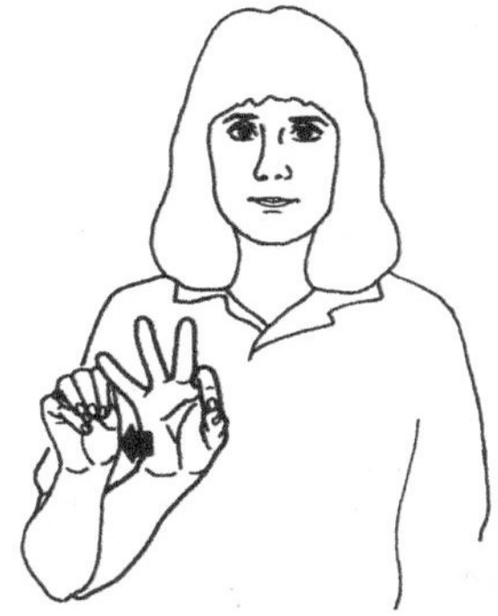

F-M

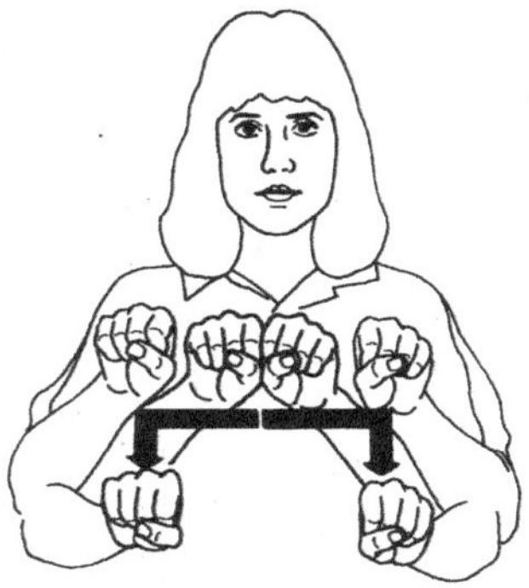

SYSTEM

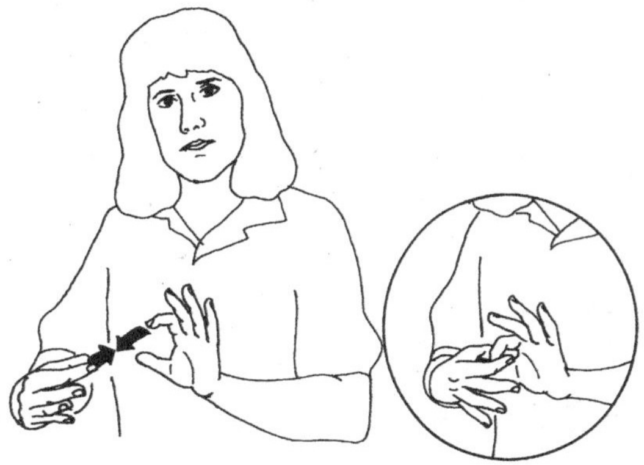

CONNECT

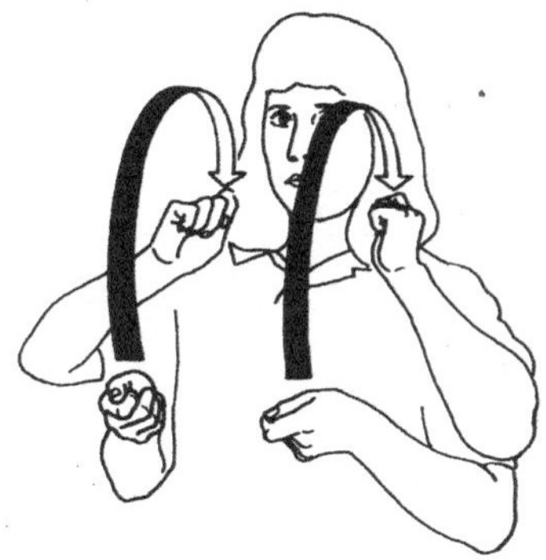

NECK-LOOP.

You can benefit from an FM system connected to a neck loop.

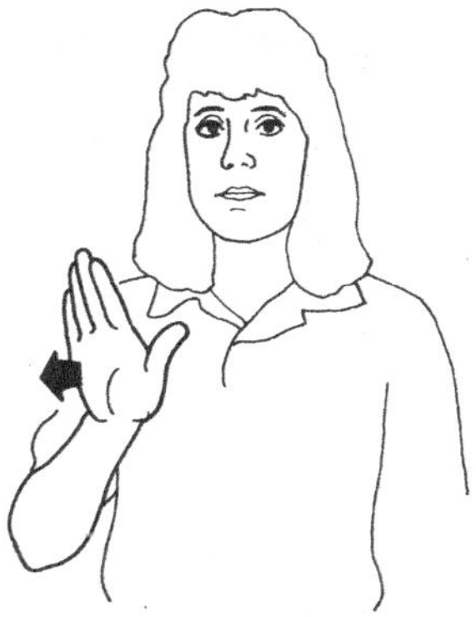

YOUR

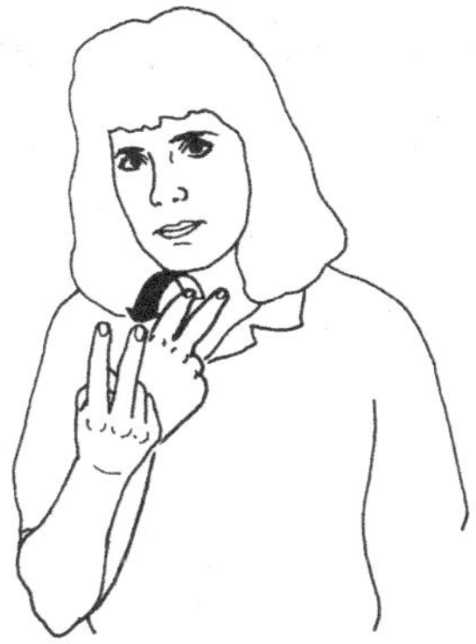

VOICE

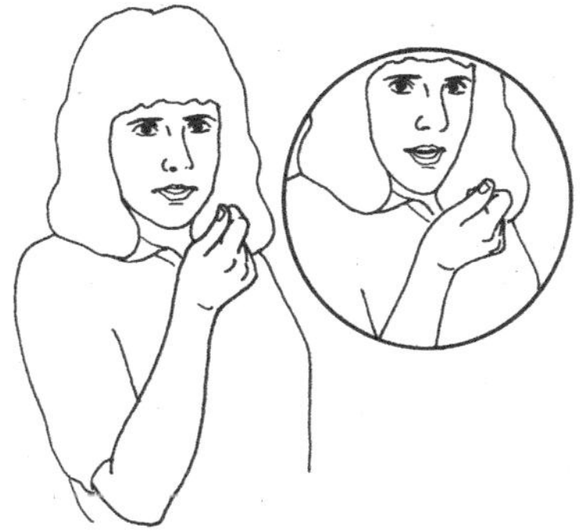

LITTLE-BIT

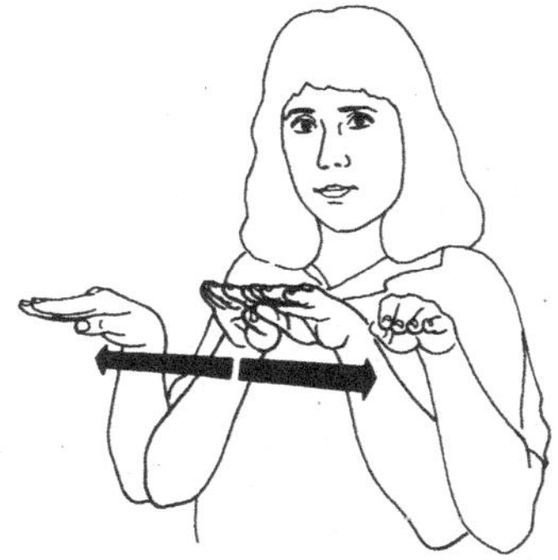

MONOTONE.

Your voice is slightly monotone.

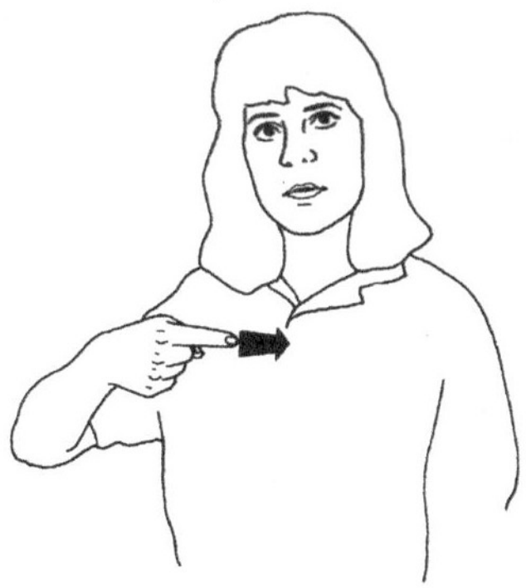

I

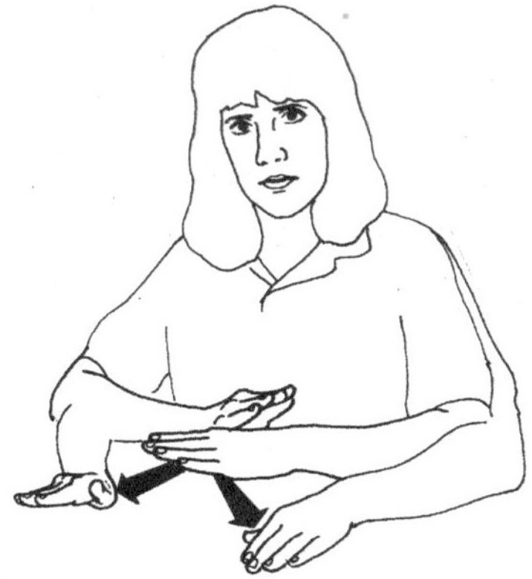

DON'T

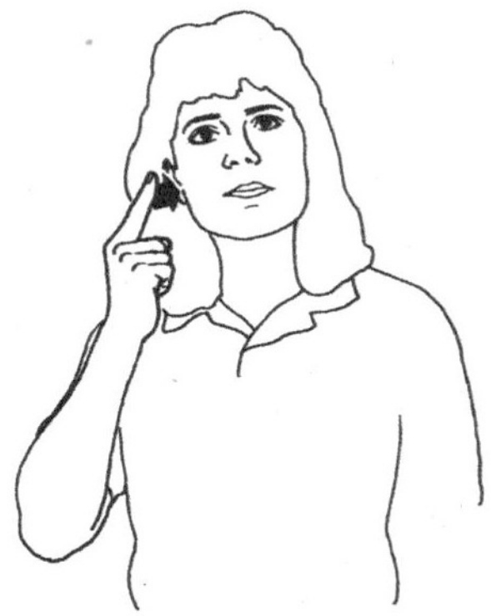

HEAR

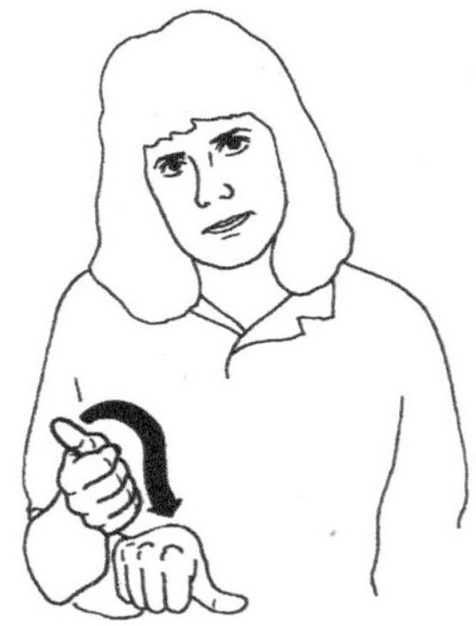

ANY

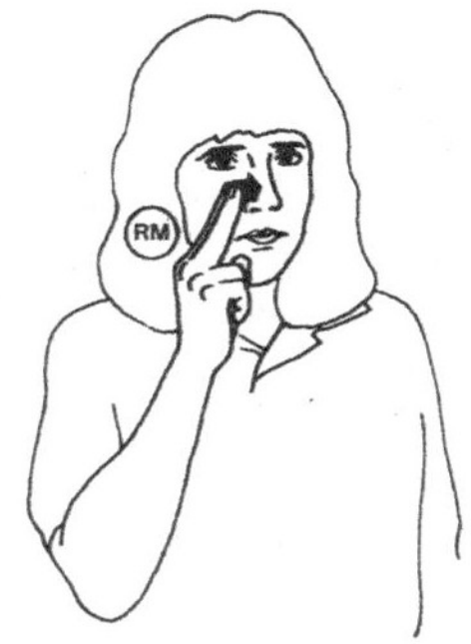

NASAL

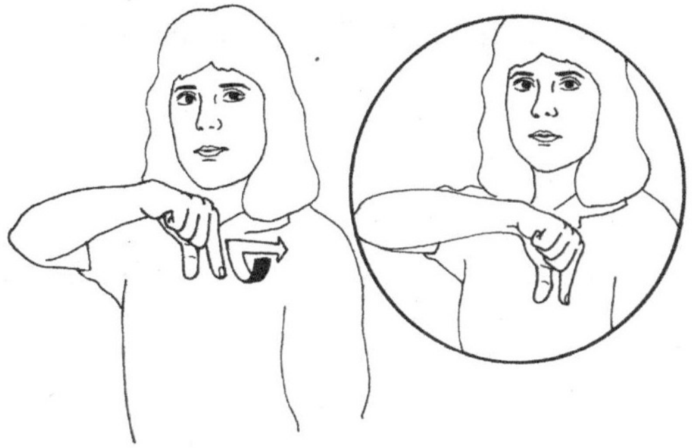

QUALITY

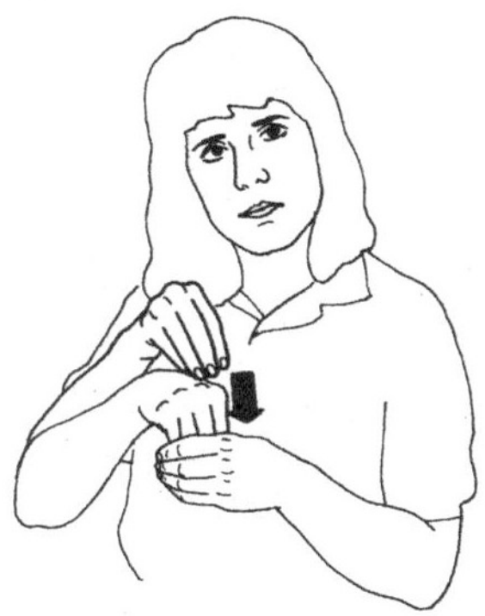

IN

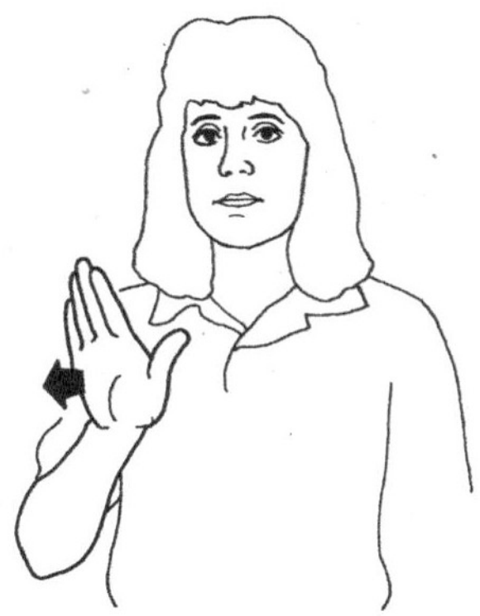

YOUR

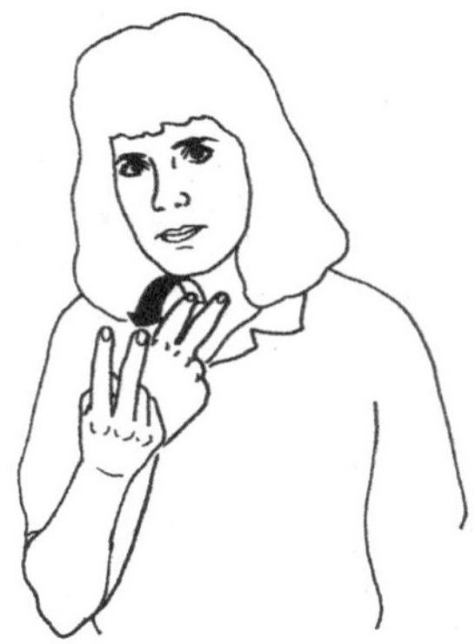

VOICE.

I don't hear any nasal quality in your voice.

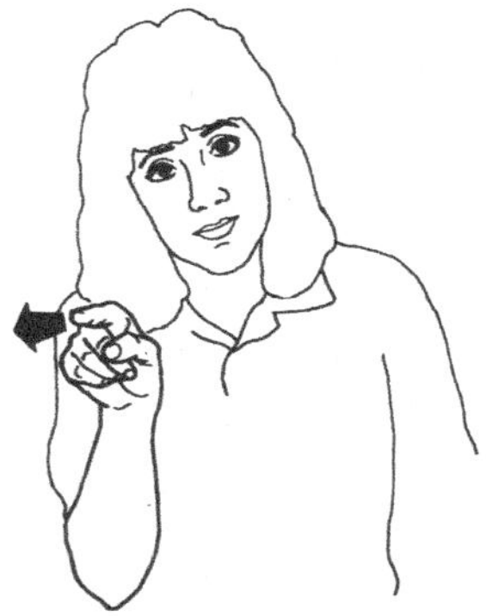

YOU

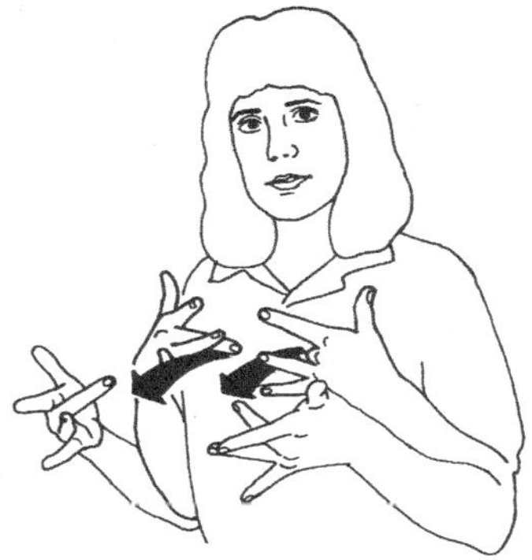

TEND

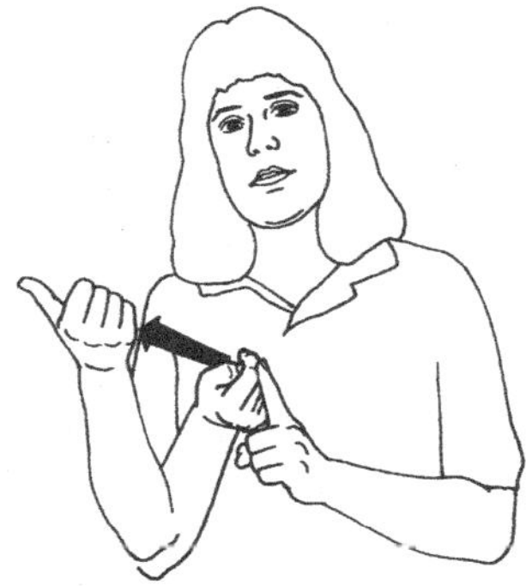

DELETE

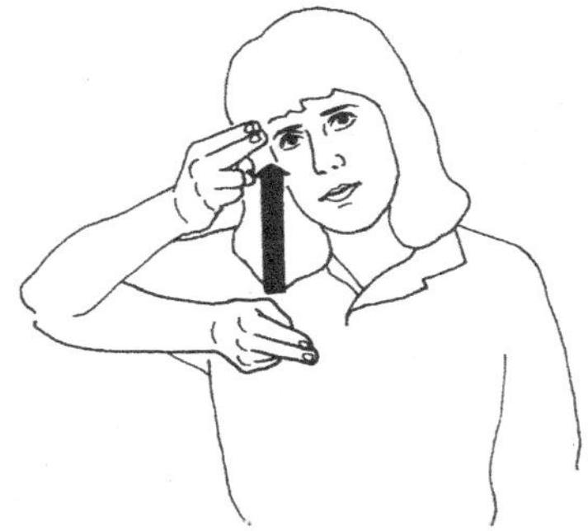

HIGH

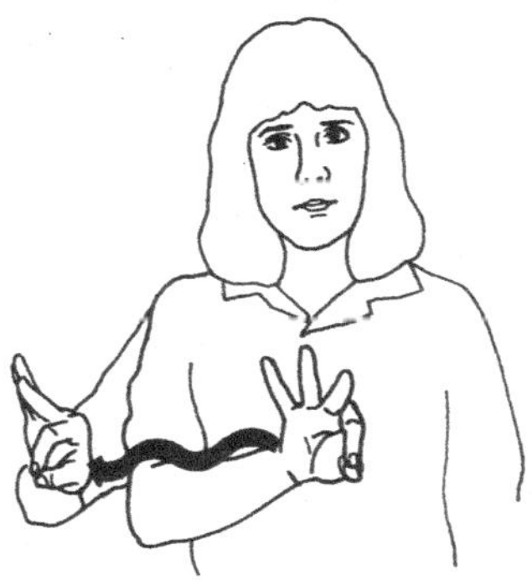

FREQUENCY

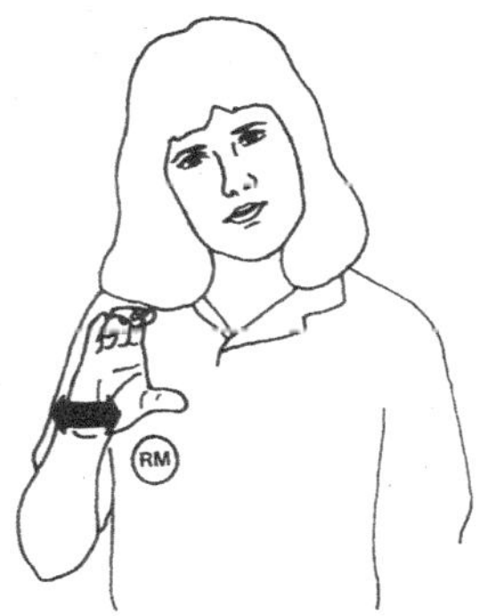

CONSONANT.

You tend to delete high frequency consonants.

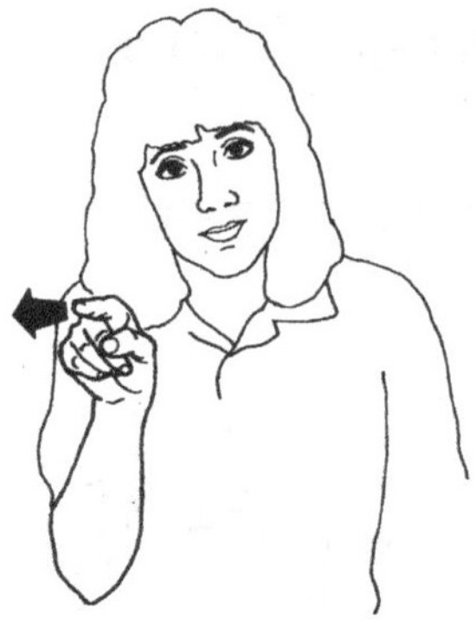

YOU

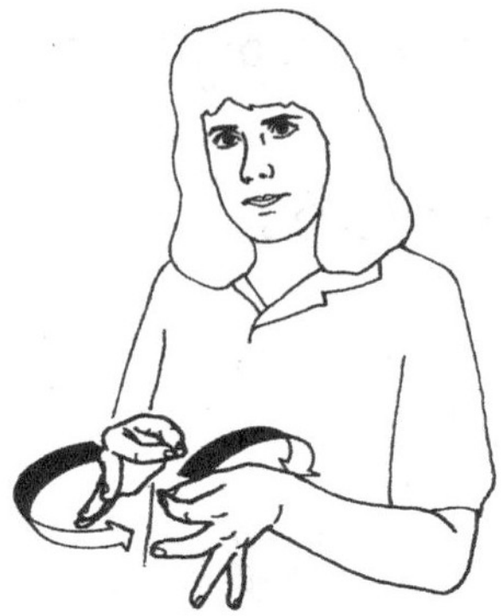

SUBSTITUTE

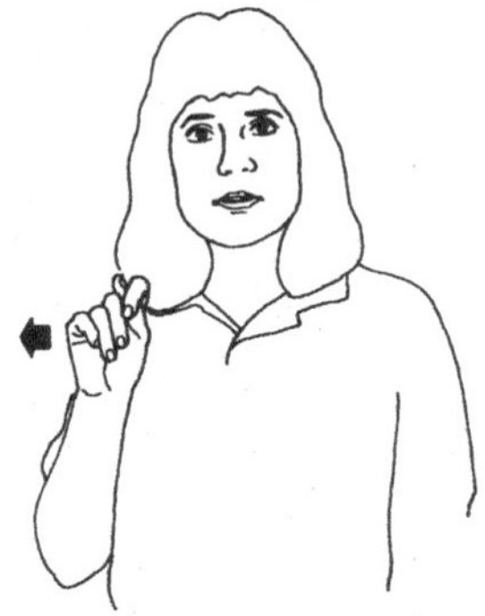

T

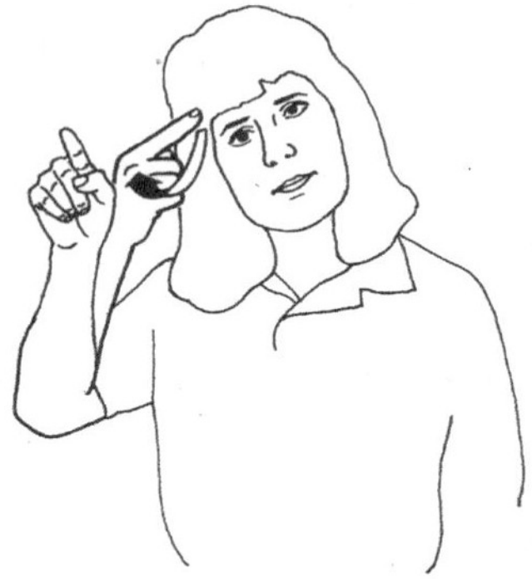

FOR

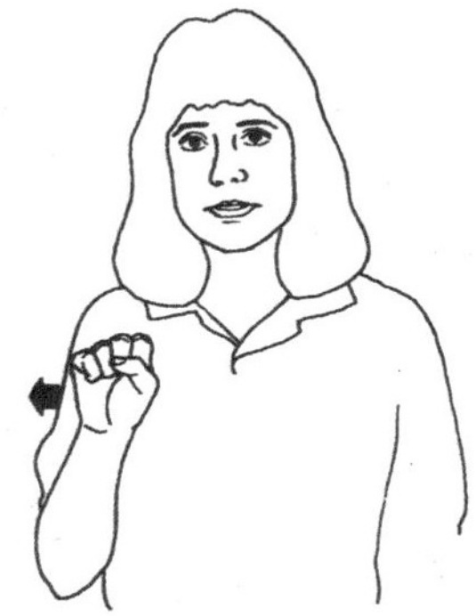

S

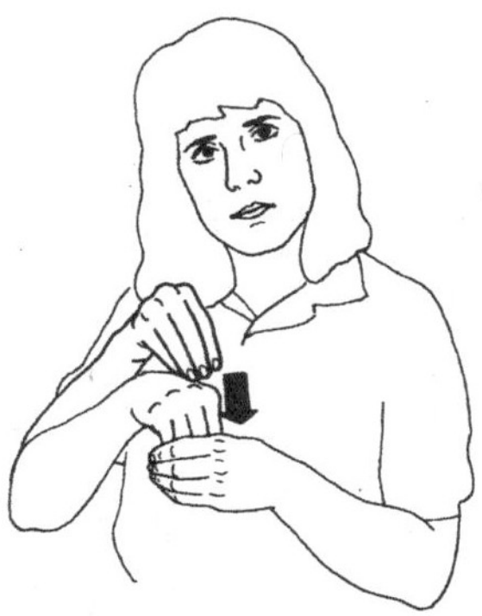

IN

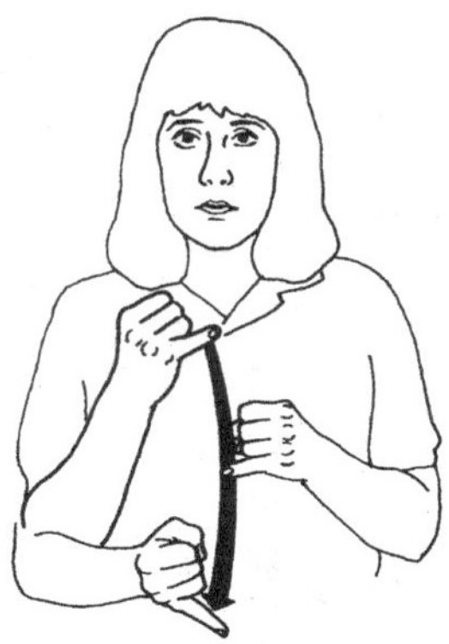

FINAL

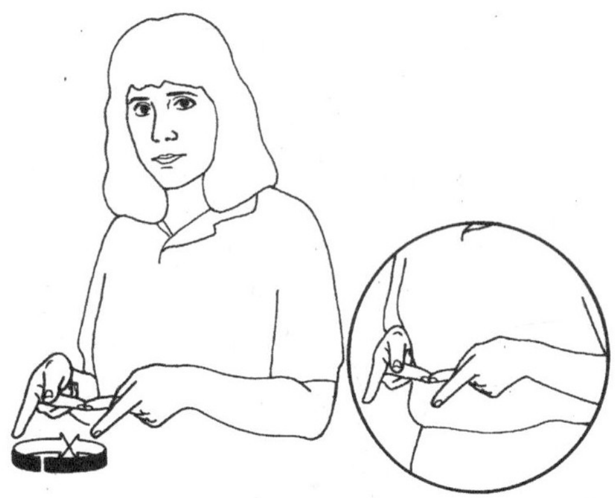

POSITION

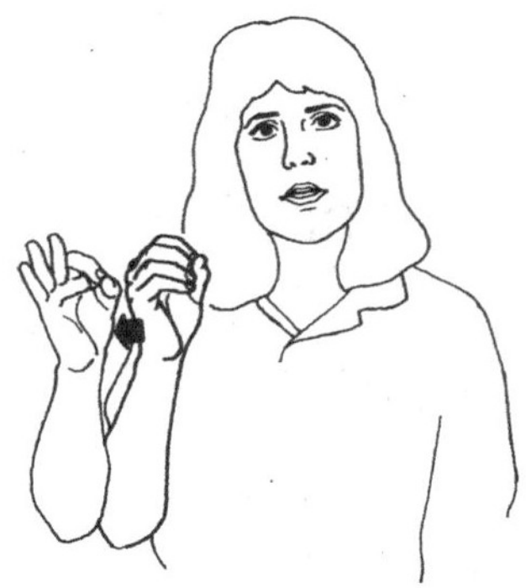

O-F

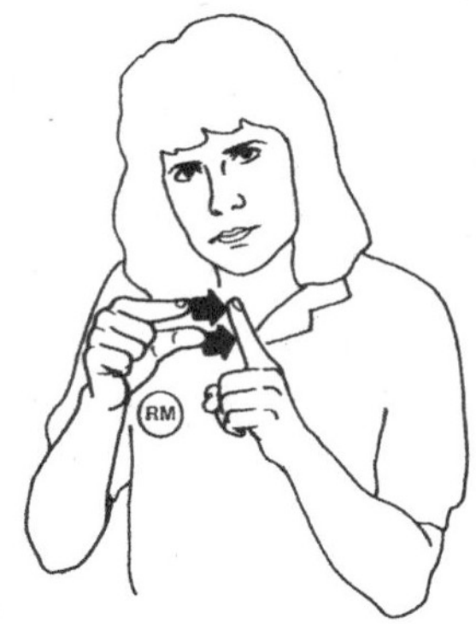

WORD.

You substitute *T* for *S* in the final position of words.

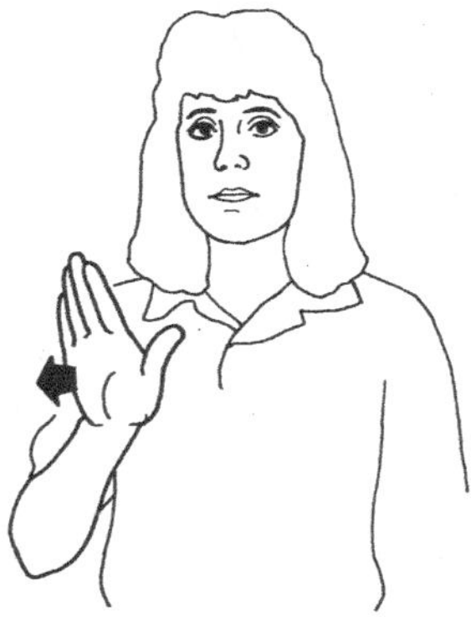

YOUR

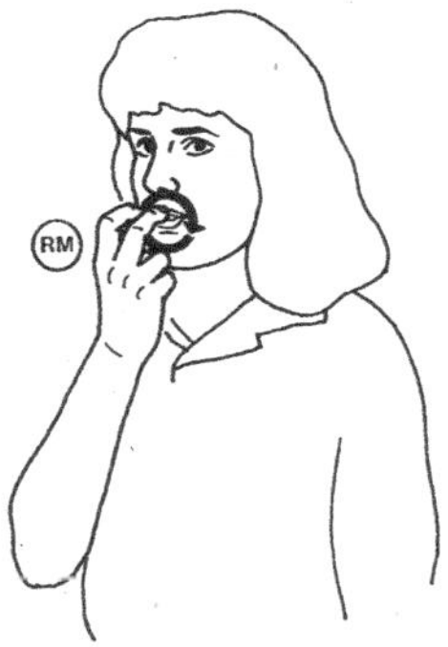

SPEECH

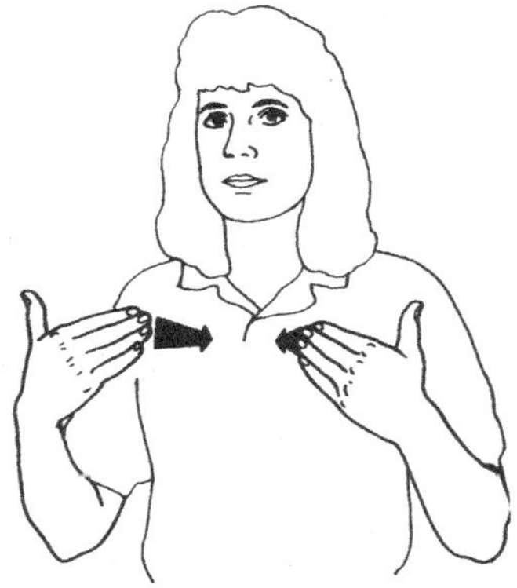

HAS

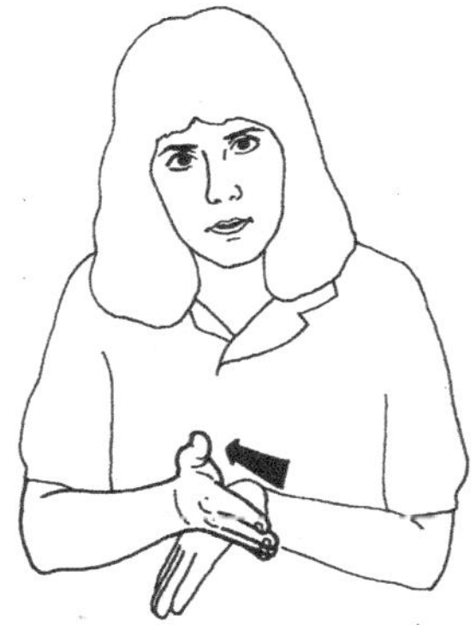

SOME

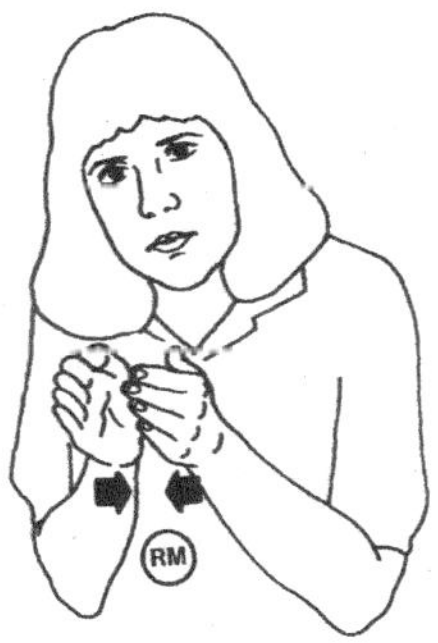

MINOR

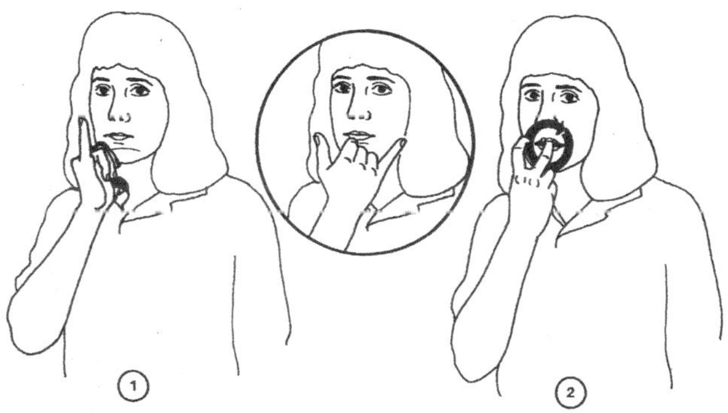

MISARTICULATE.

Your speech has some minor misarticulations.

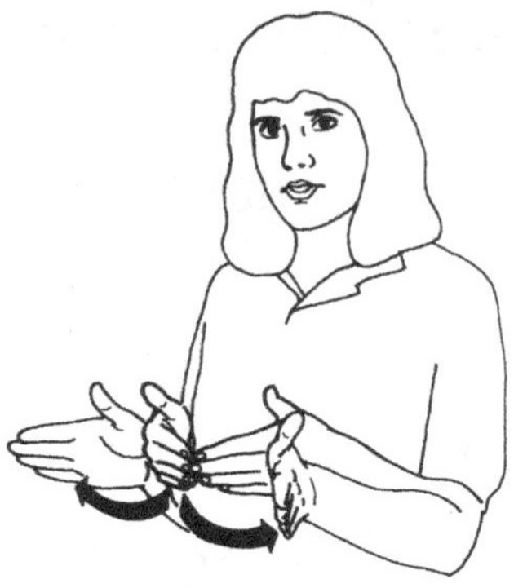

GENERAL

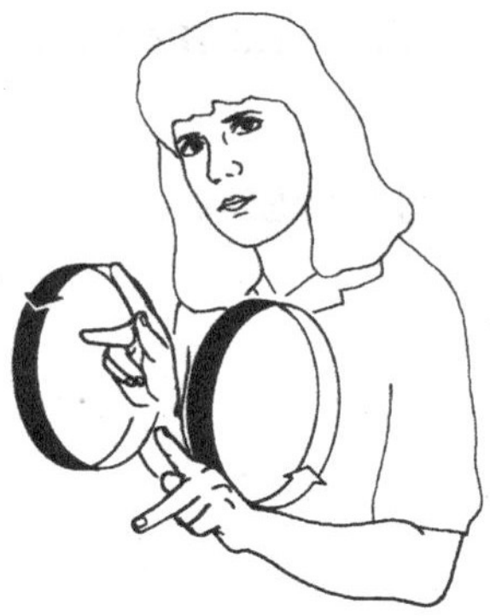

PUBLIC

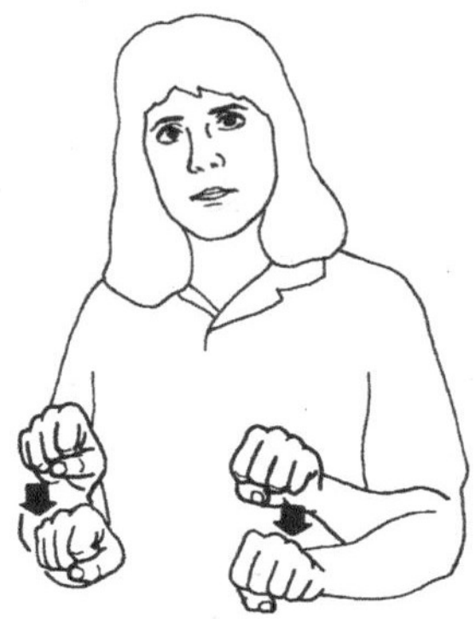

CAN

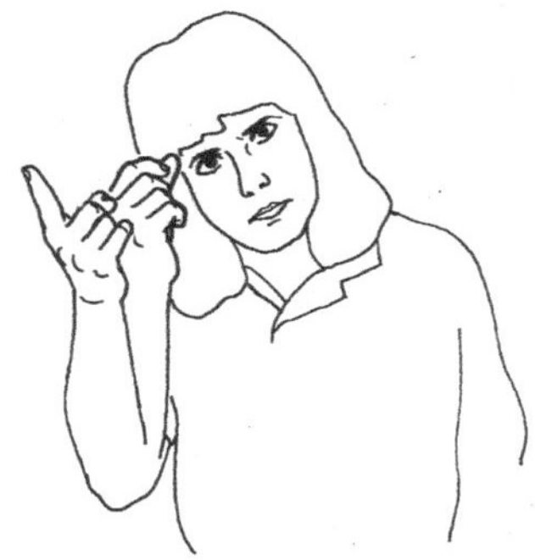

UNDERSTAND

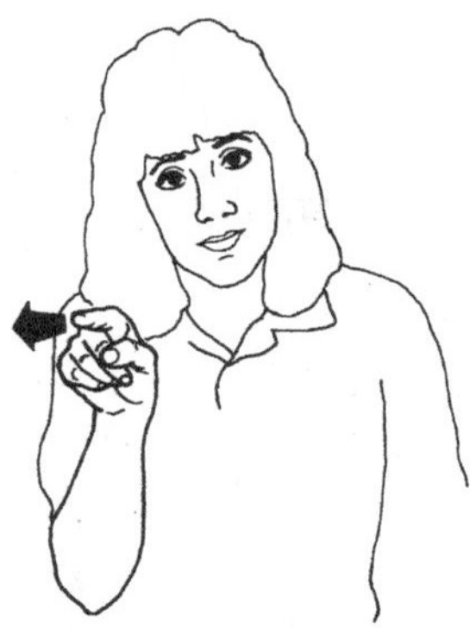

YOU

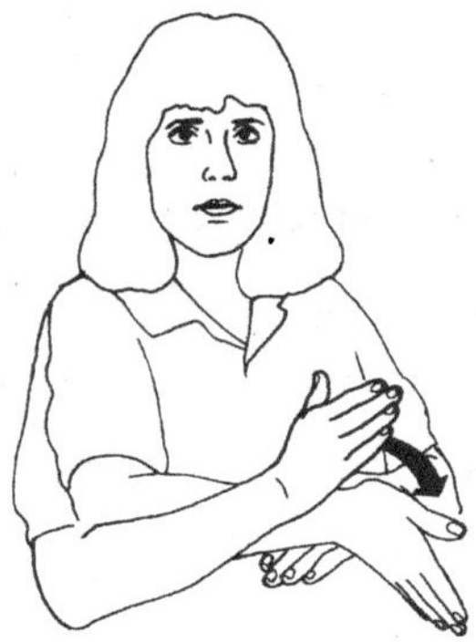

AFTER

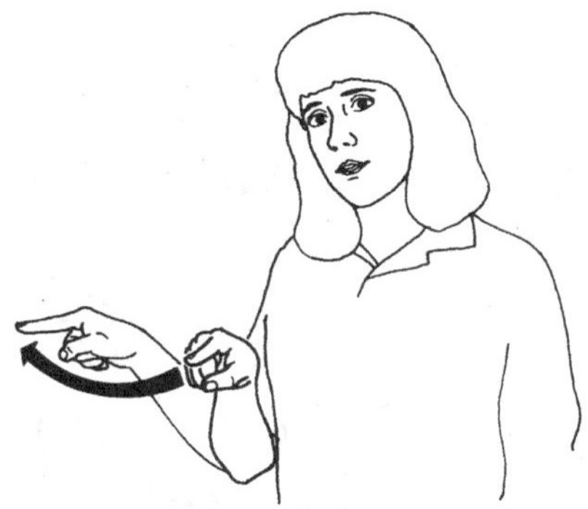

THEY

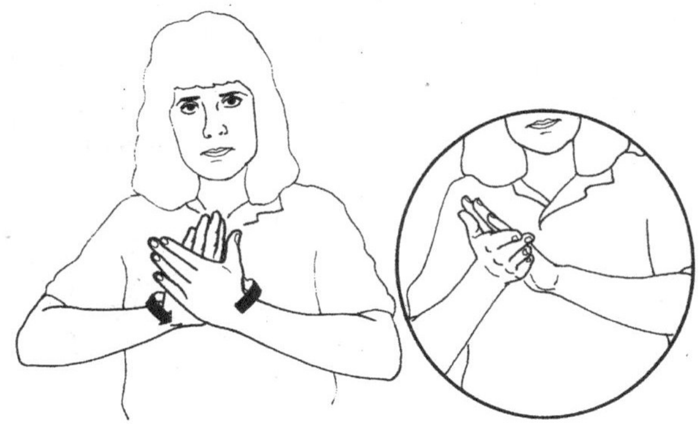

BECOME

The general public can understand you after they become used to your speech.

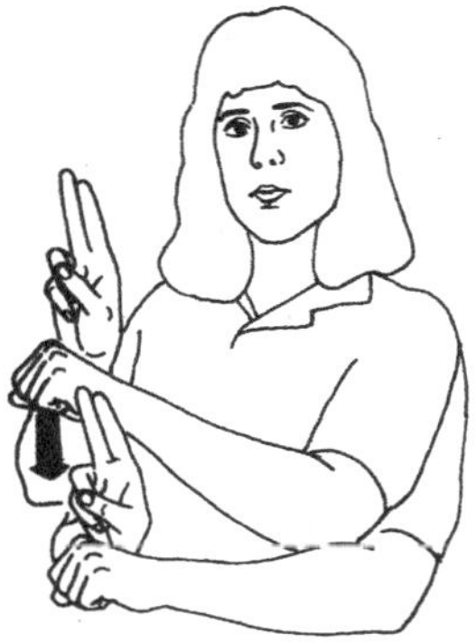

USED-TO

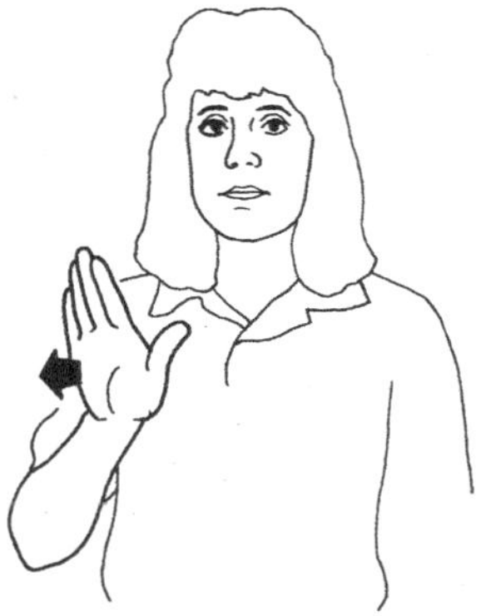

YOUR

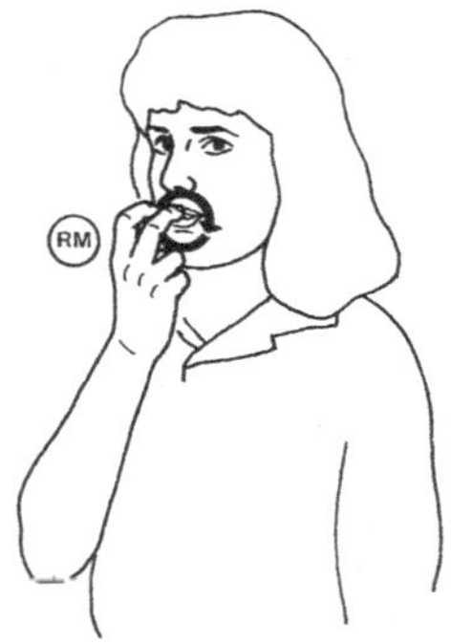

SPEECH.

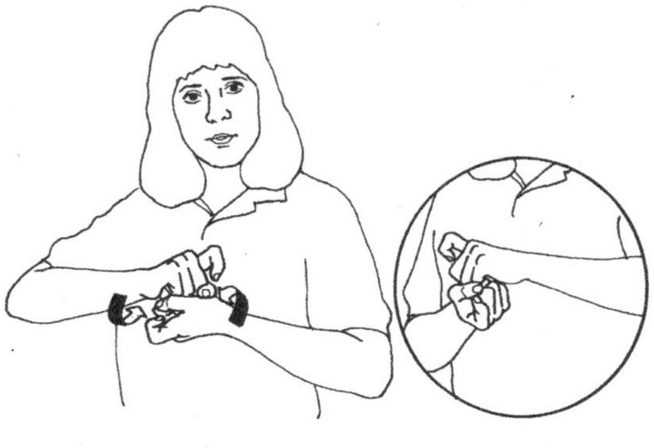

CHANGE

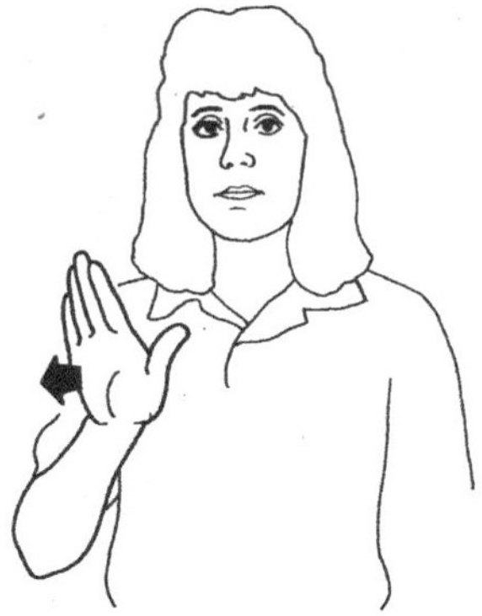

YOUR

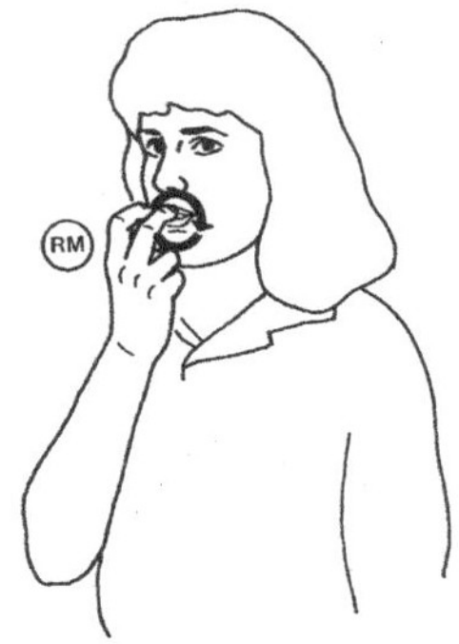

SPEECH

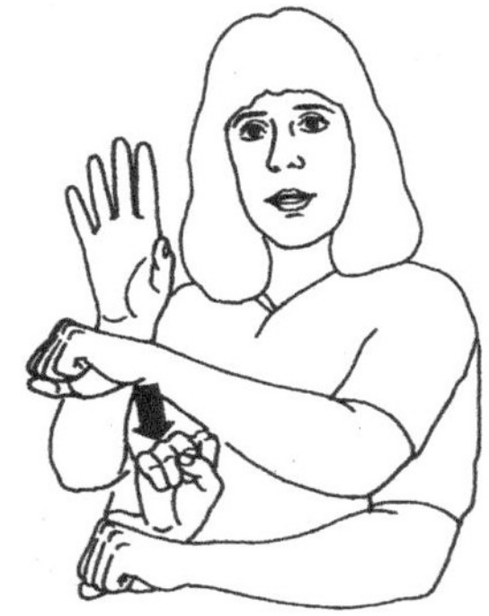

HABIT

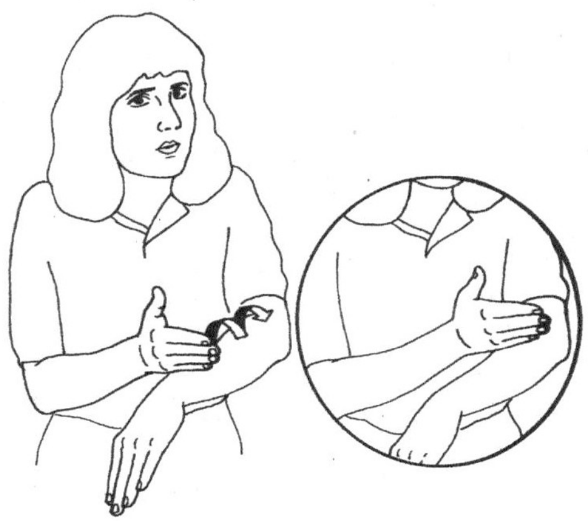

GRADUAL

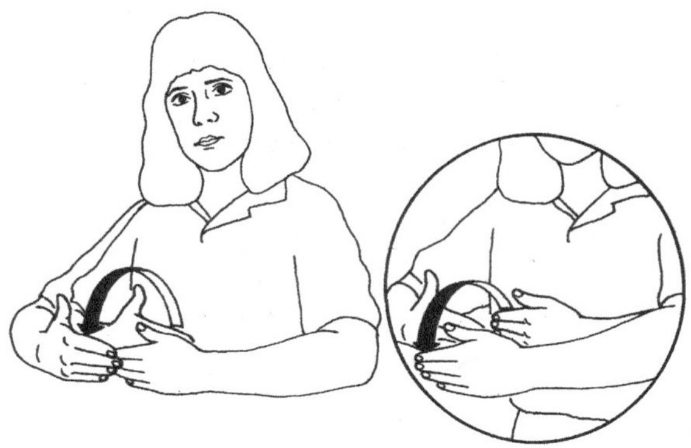

PROCESS.

Changing your speech habits is a gradual process.

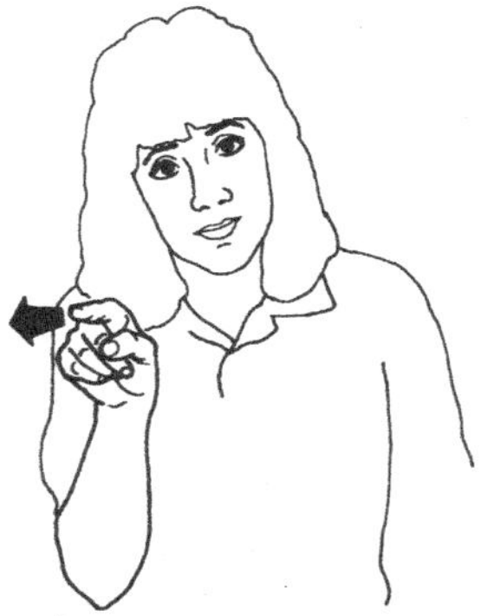

YOU

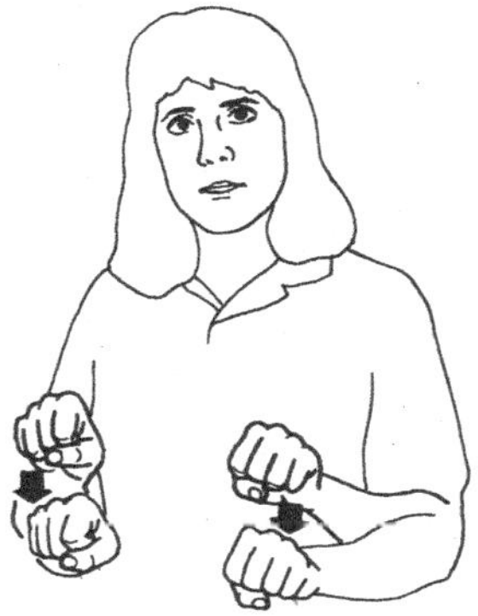

CAN

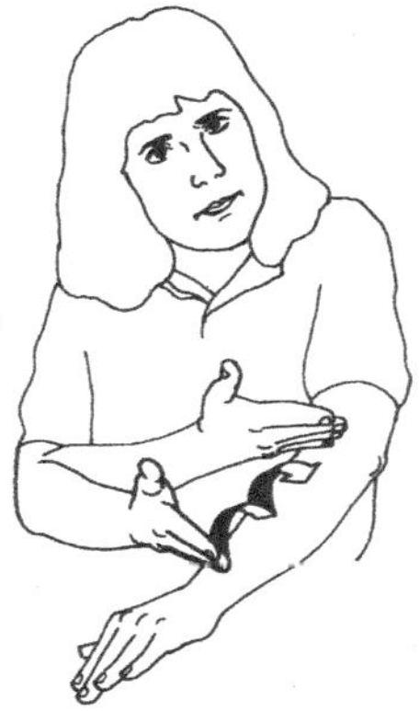

IMPROVE

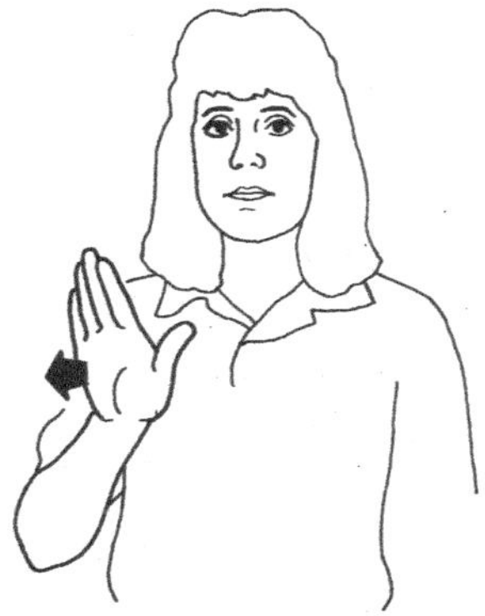

YOUR

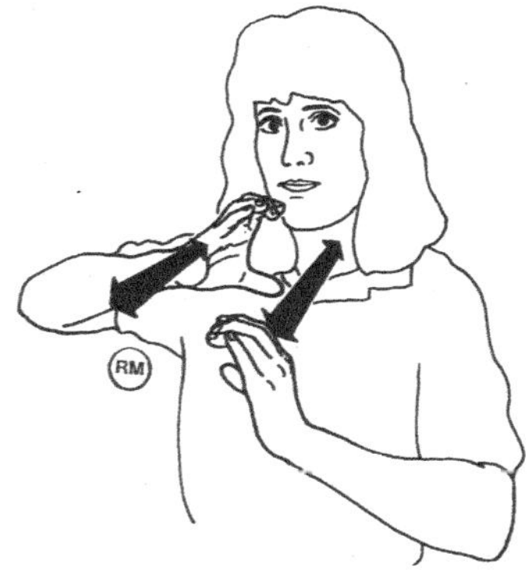

COMMUNICATION

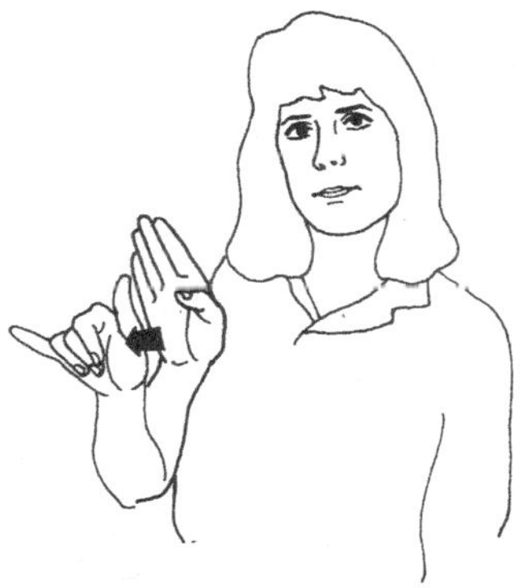

B-Y

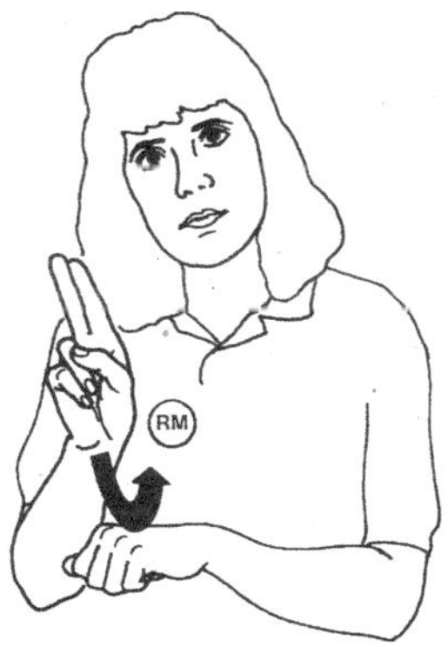

USE

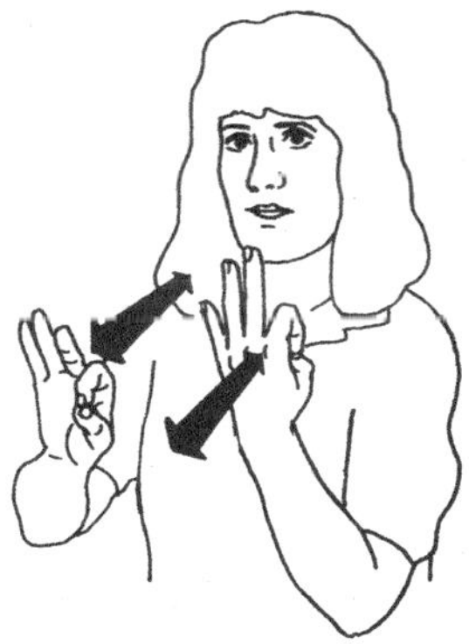

FEEDBACK.

You can improve your communication by using feedback.

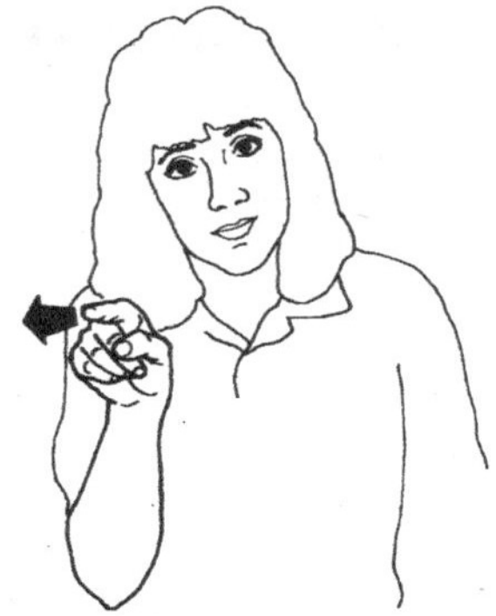

YOU

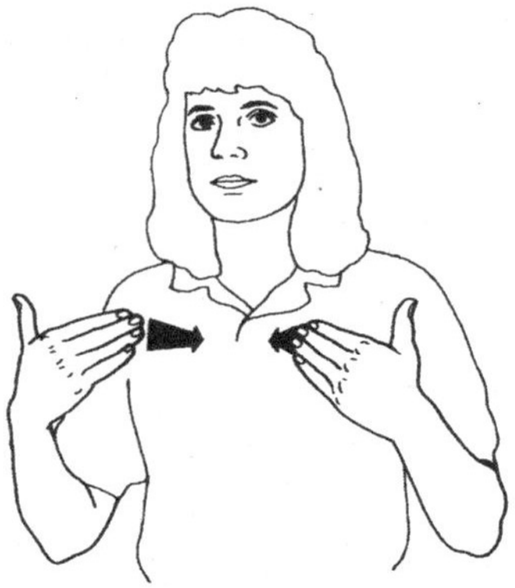

HAVE

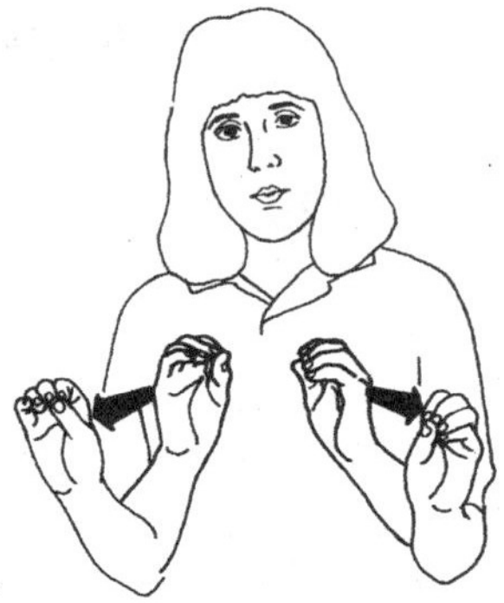

NONE

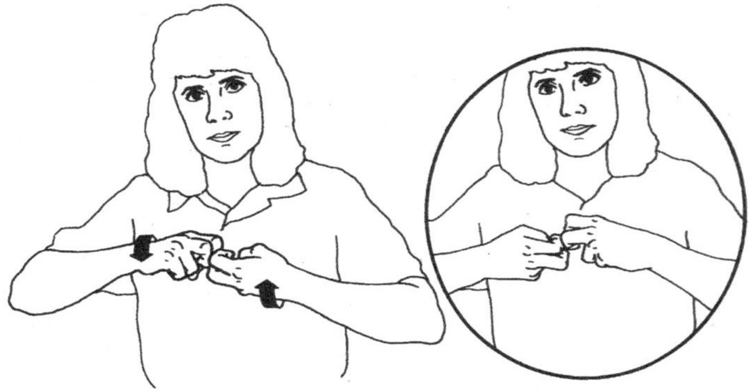

DIFFICULTY

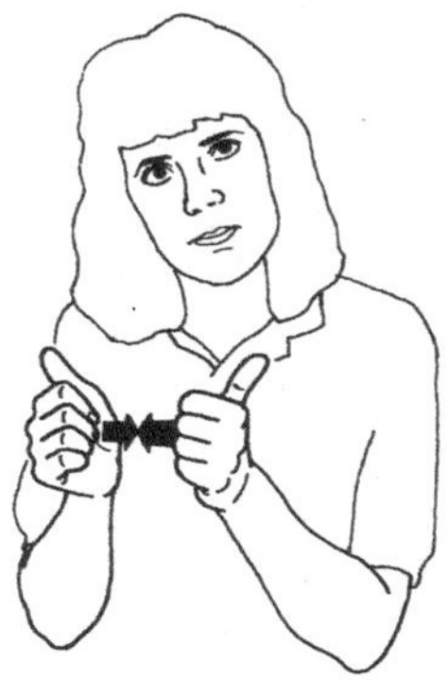

WITH

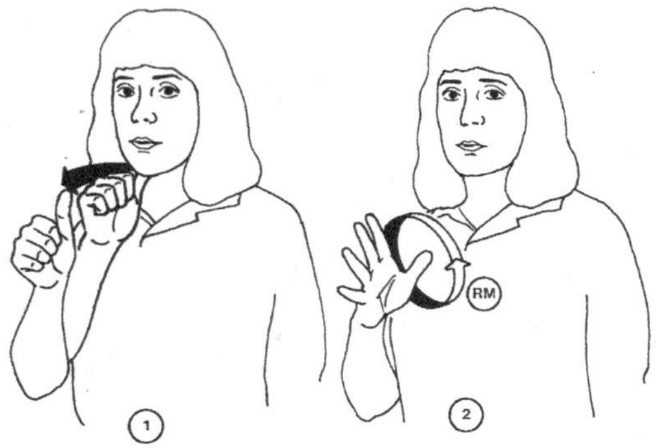

INFORMAL

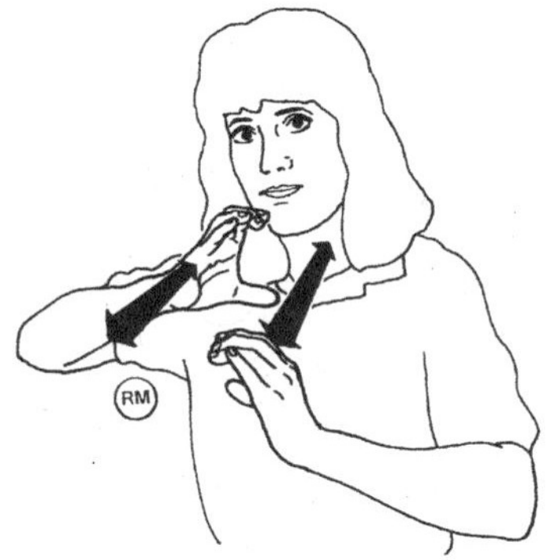

COMMUNICATION

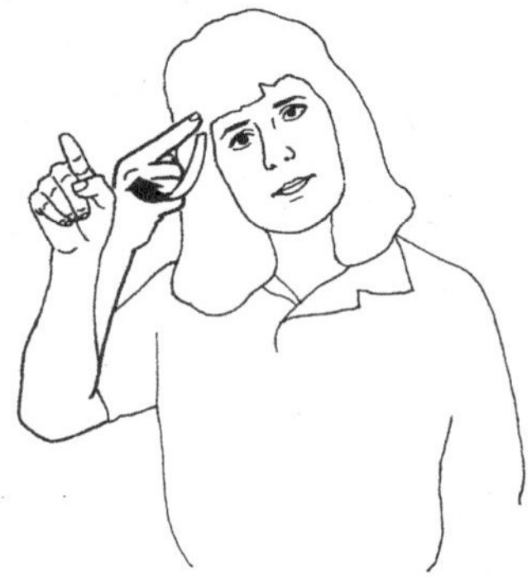

FOR

You have no difficulty with informal communication; for example, socializing with friends.

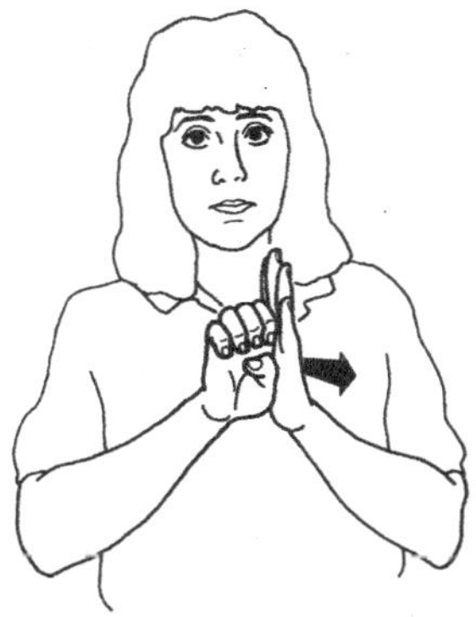

EXAMPLE

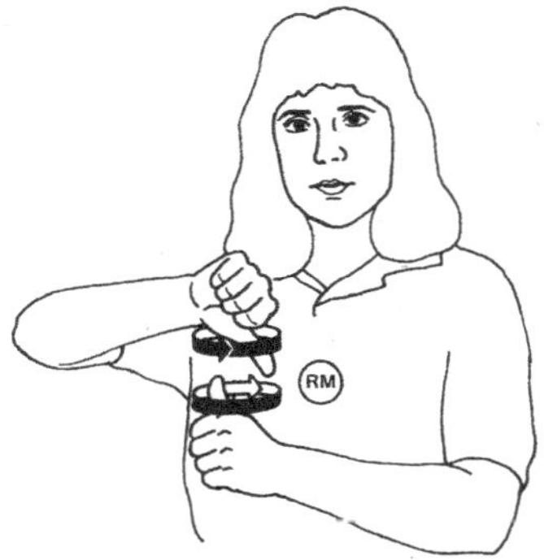

SOCIALIZE

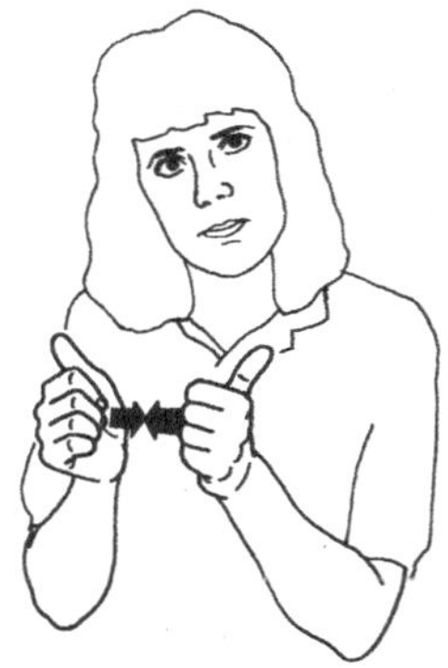

WITH

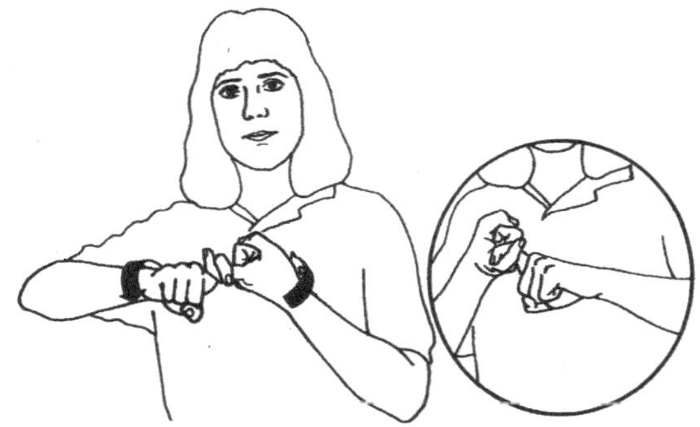

FRIEND.

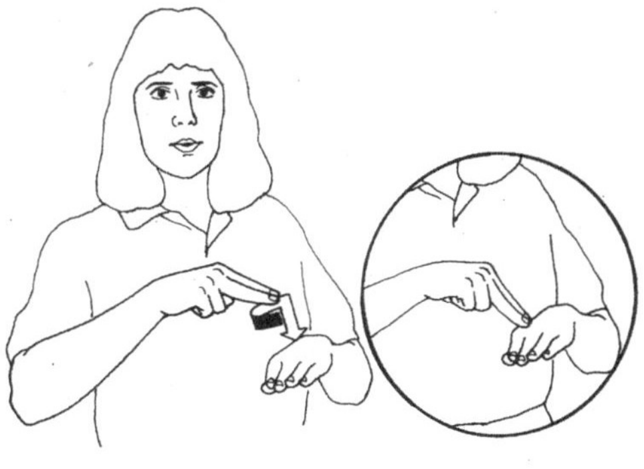

NORMAL

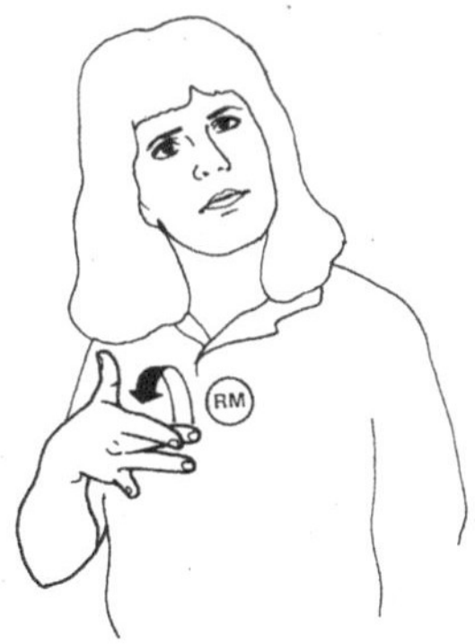

FEEL

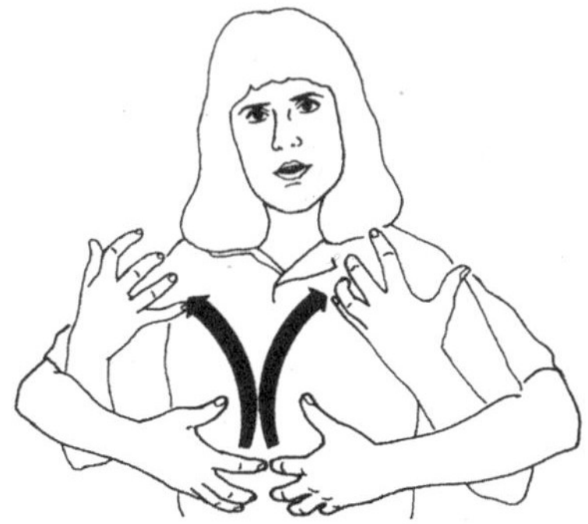

ANGRY

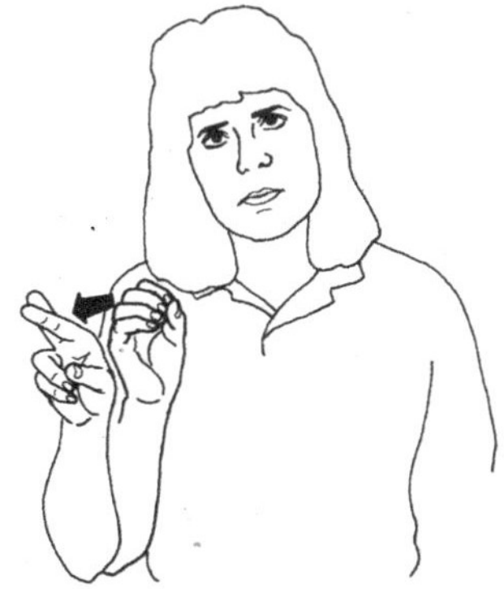

O-R

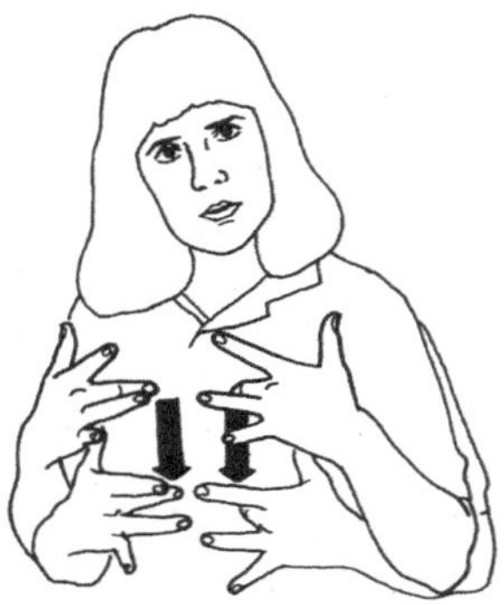

DEPRESSED

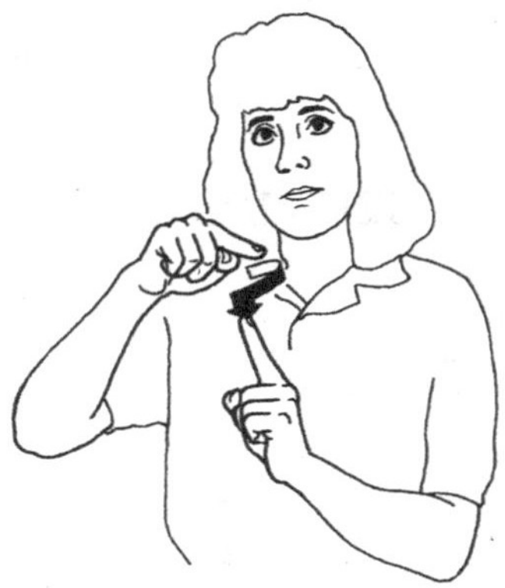

WHEN

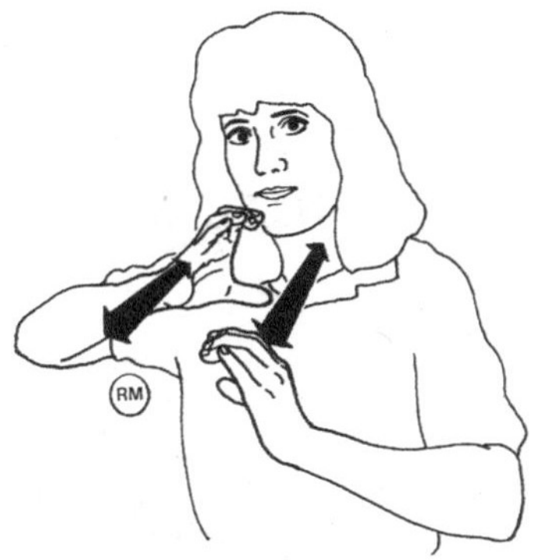

COMMUNICATION

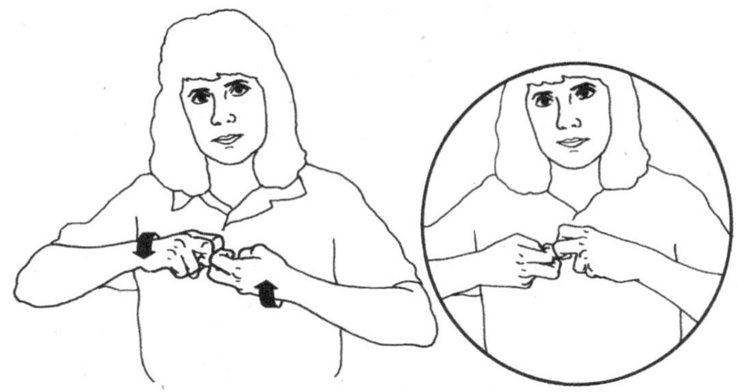

DIFFICULT.

It's normal to feel angry or depressed when communication is difficult.

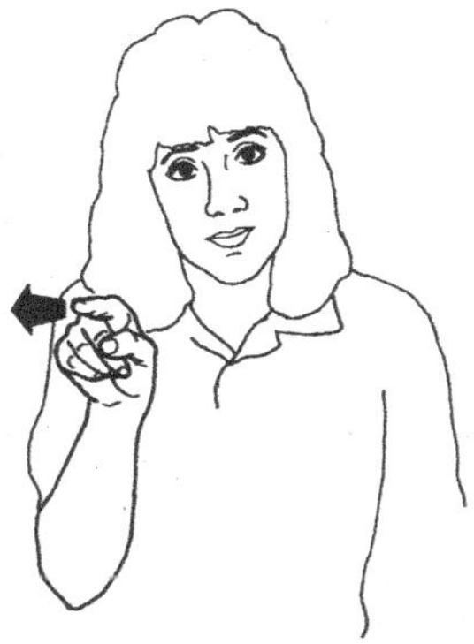

YOU

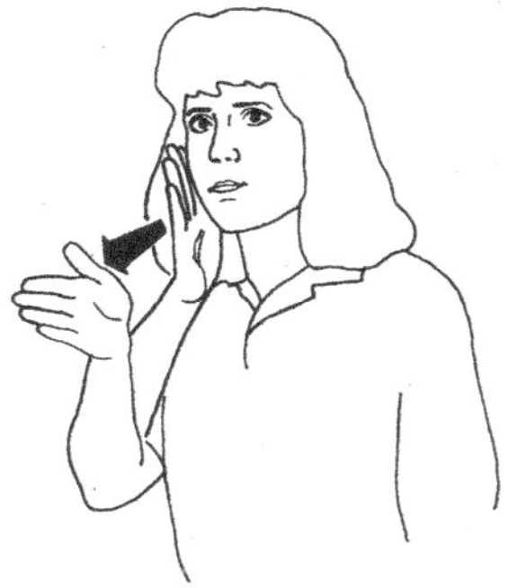

WILL

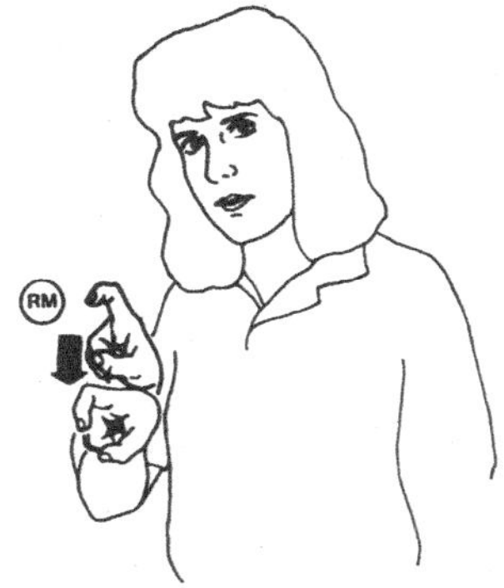

NEED

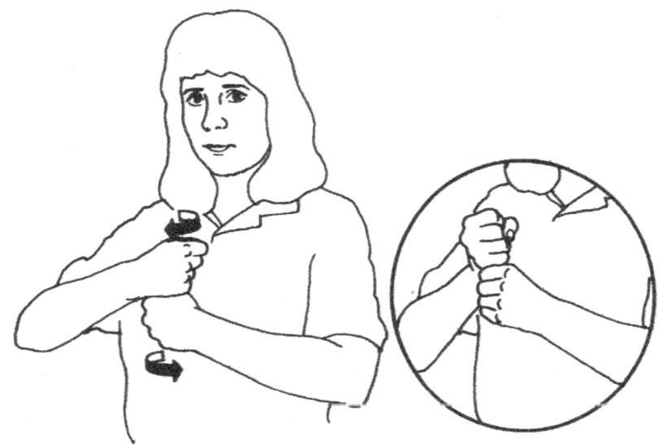

MAKE

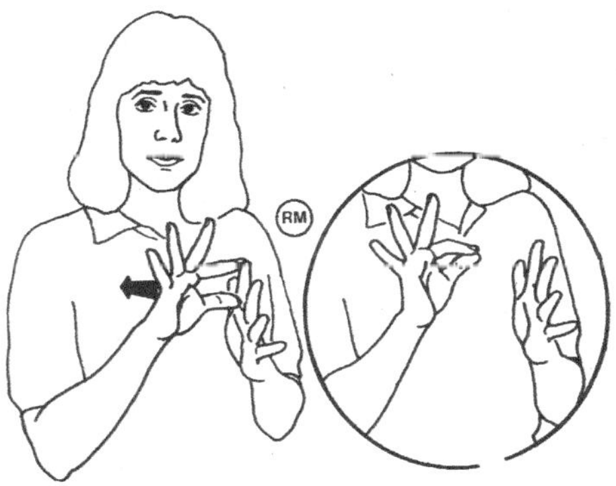

CHOICE

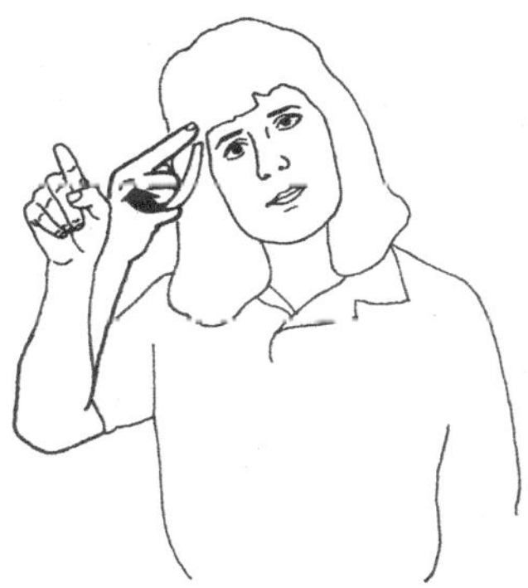

ENSURE

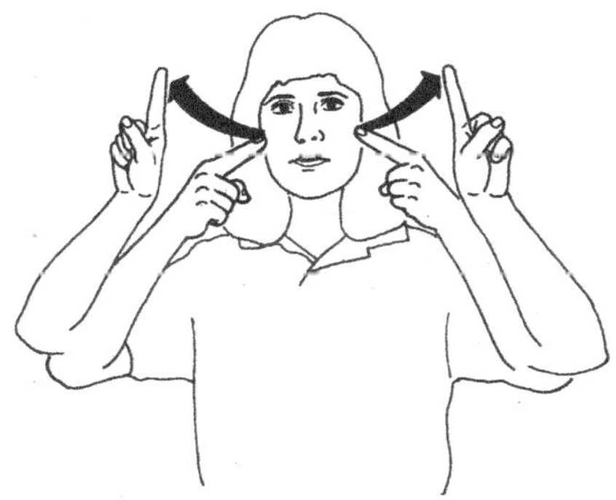

EFFECTIVE

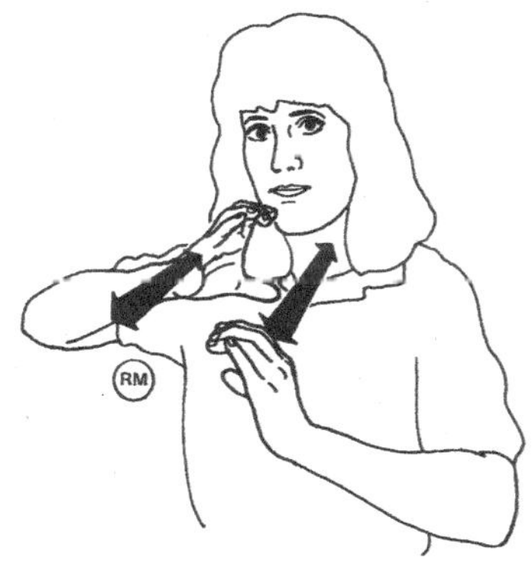

COMMUNICATION.

You will need to make choices to ensure effective communication.

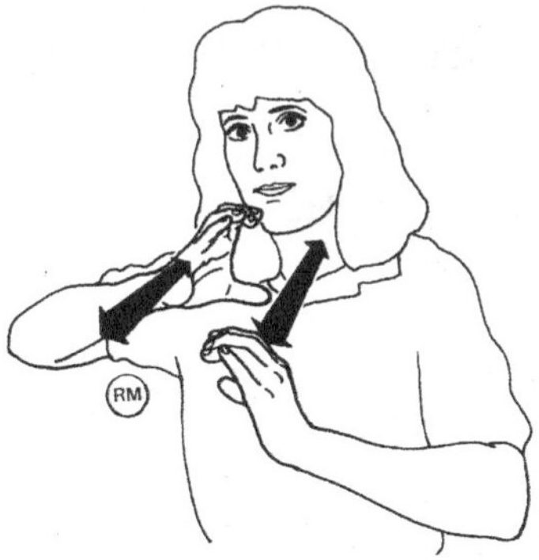

CONVERSE

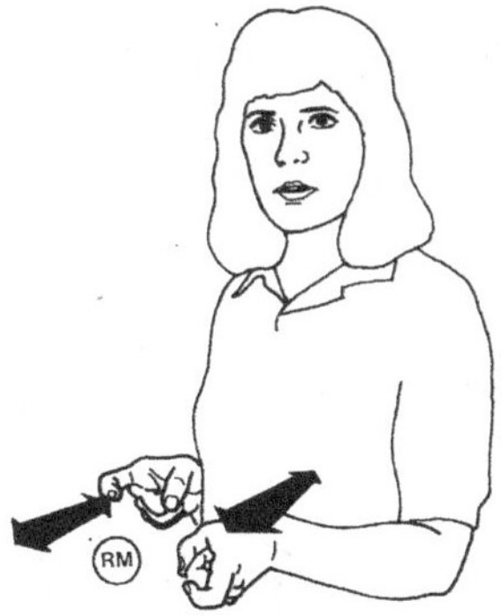

CONTROL

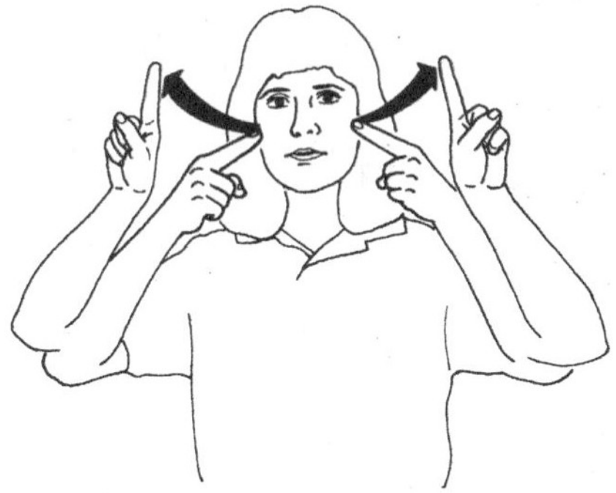

ACHIEVE

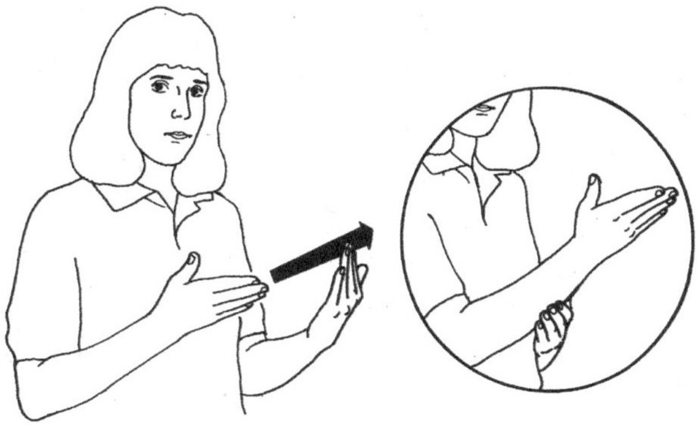

THROUGH

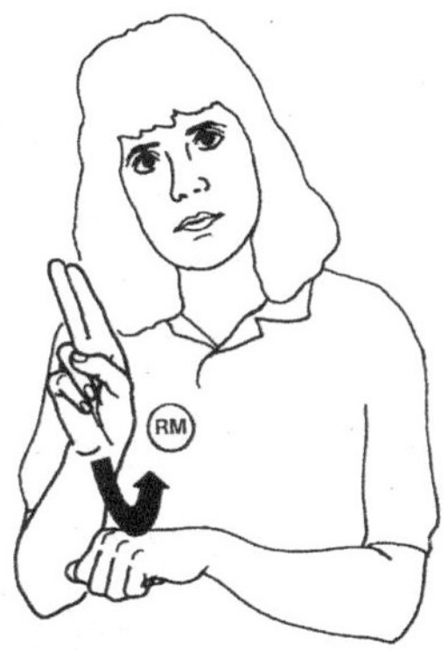

USE

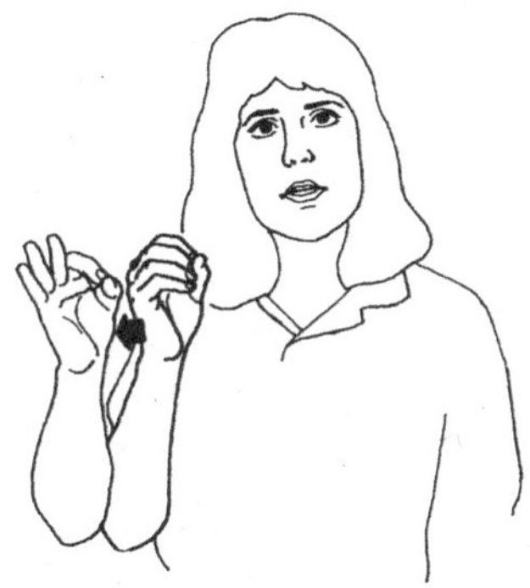

O-F

Conversation control is achieved through the use of yes-no questions.

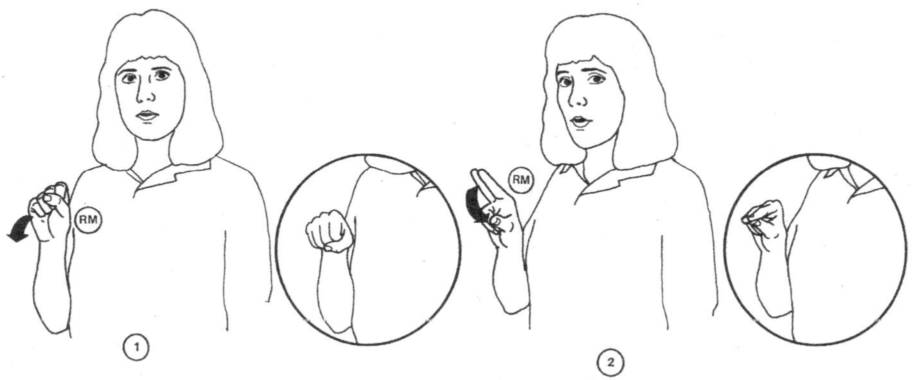

YES-NO

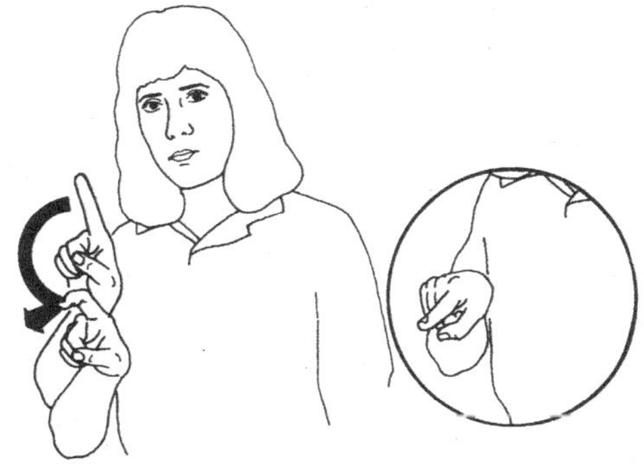

QUESTION.

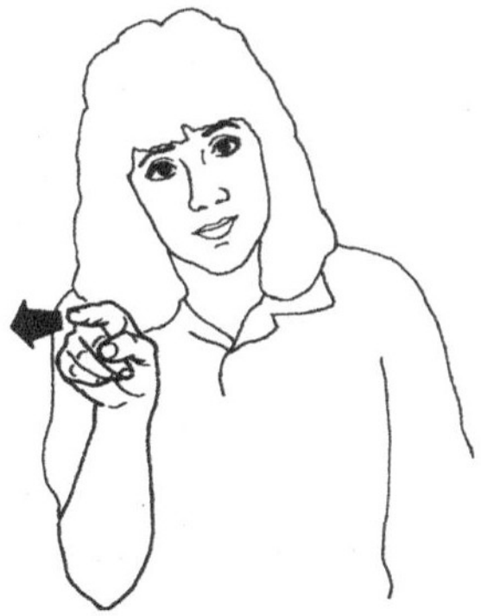

YOU

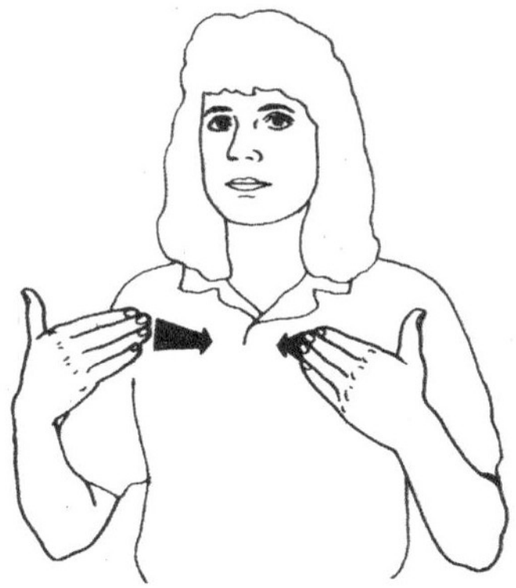

HAVE

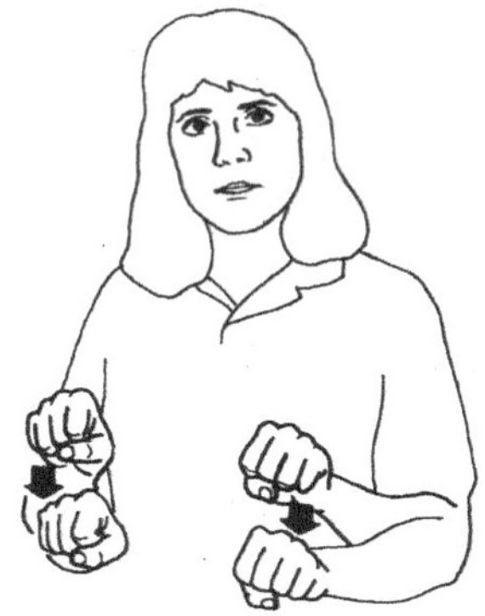

ABILITY

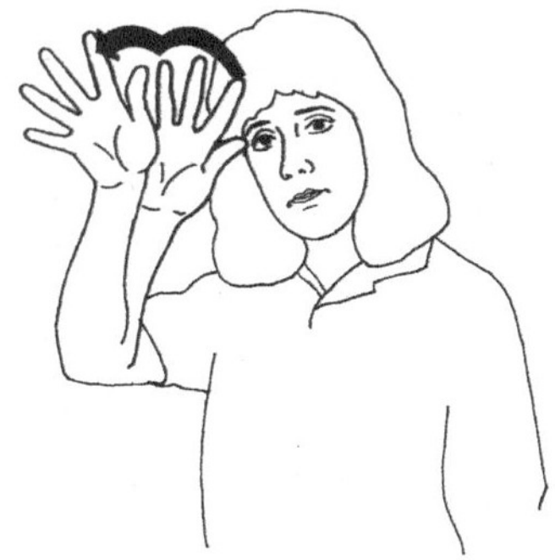

CREATE

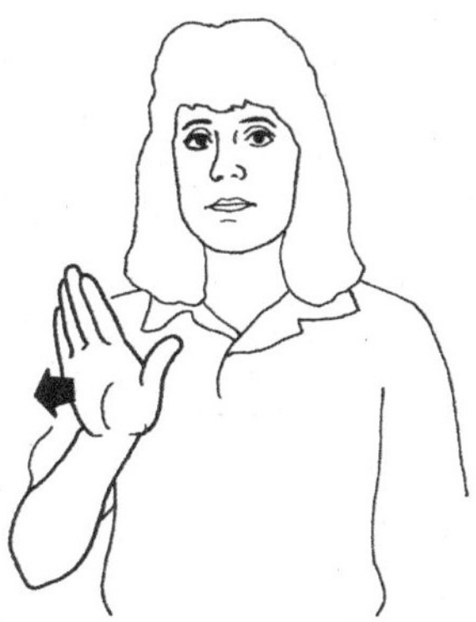

YOUR

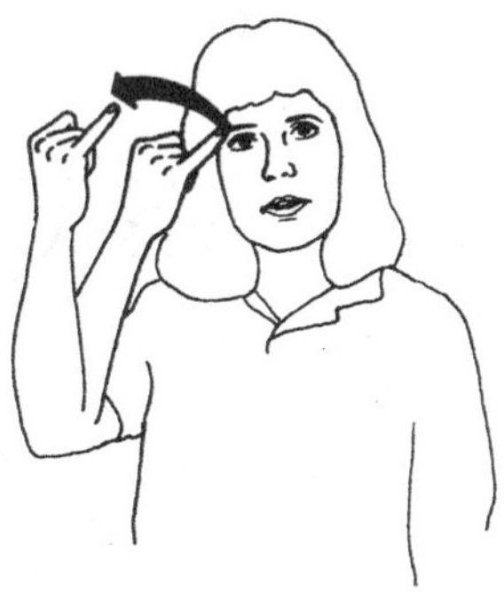

IDEA

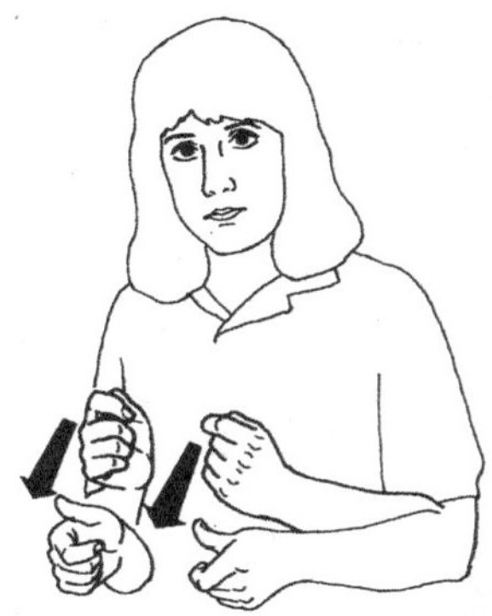

FAST

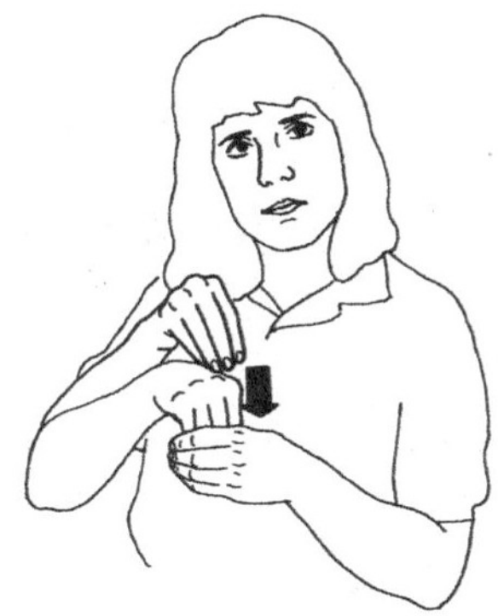

IN

You have the ability to formulate your ideas quickly in various situations.

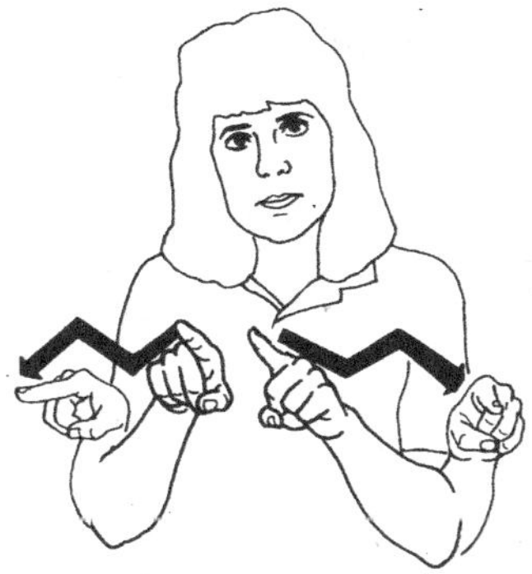

VARIOUS

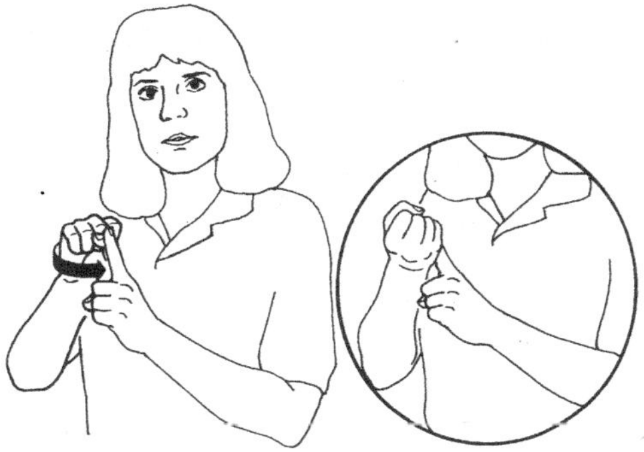

SITUATION.

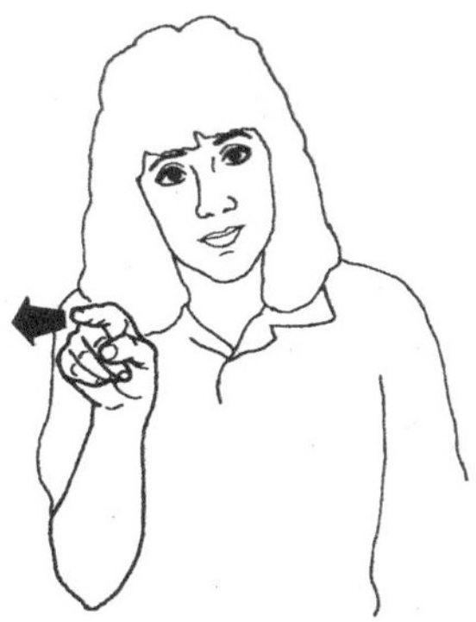

YOU

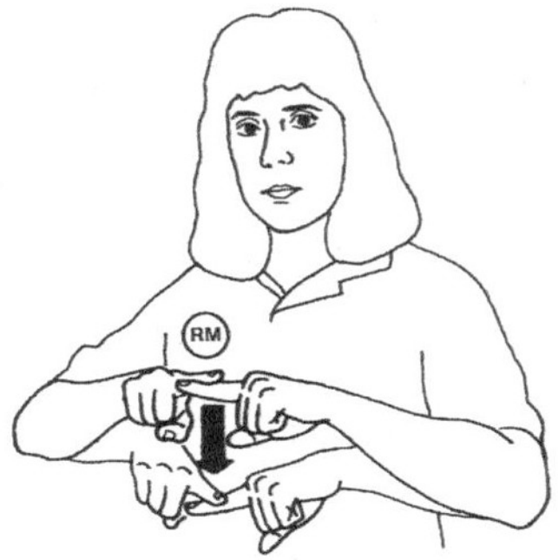

RELY

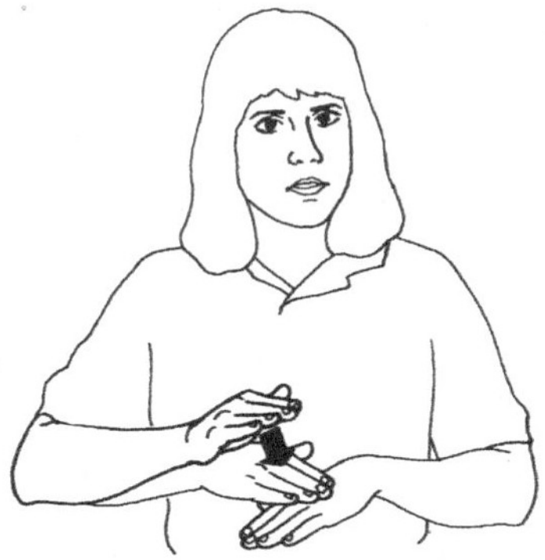

ON

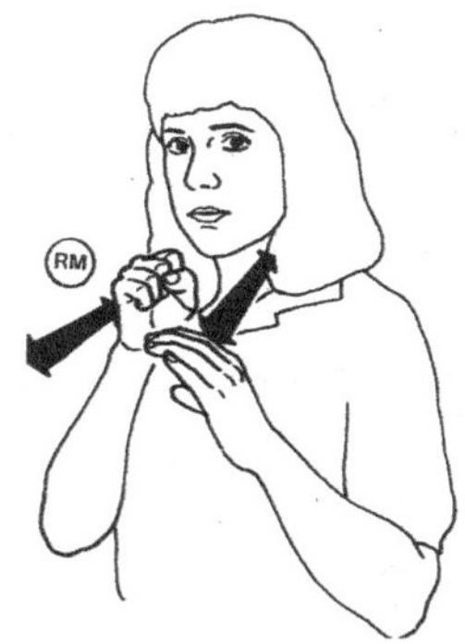

SIMULTANEOUS COMMUNICATION

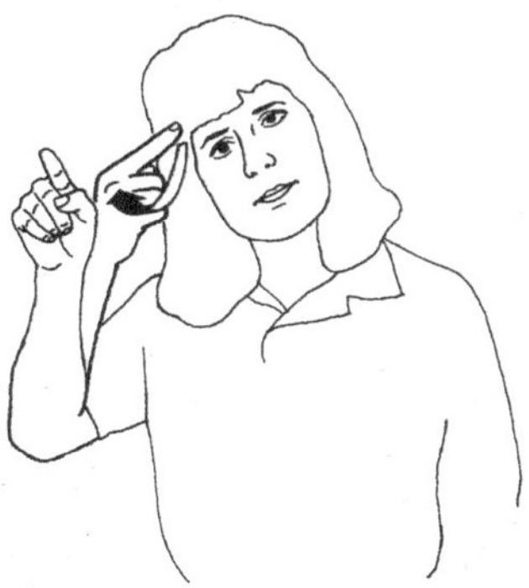

FOR

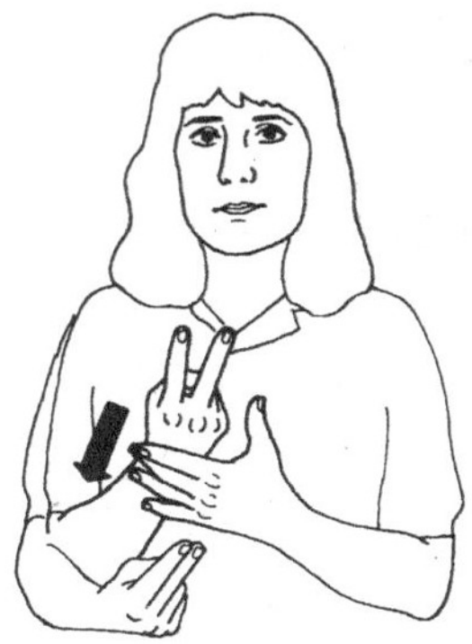

BOTH

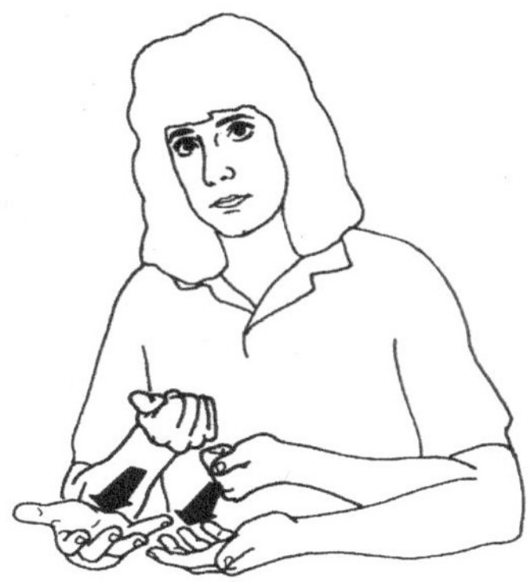

EXPRESSIVE

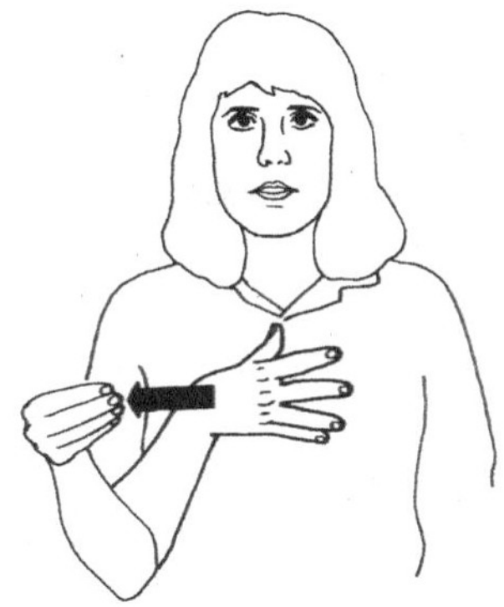

AND

You rely on simultaneous communication for both expressive and receptive communication.

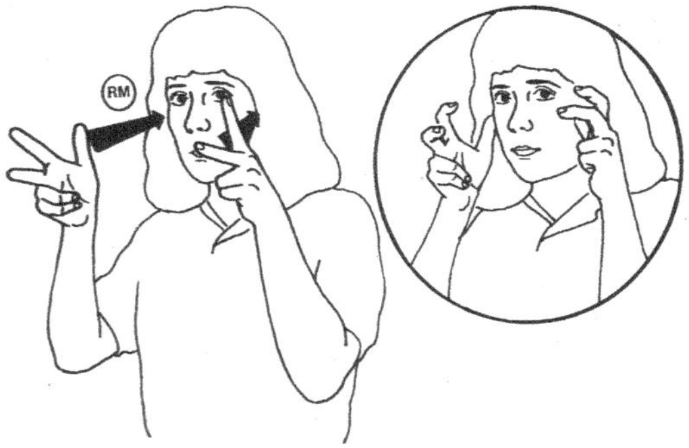

RECEPTIVE

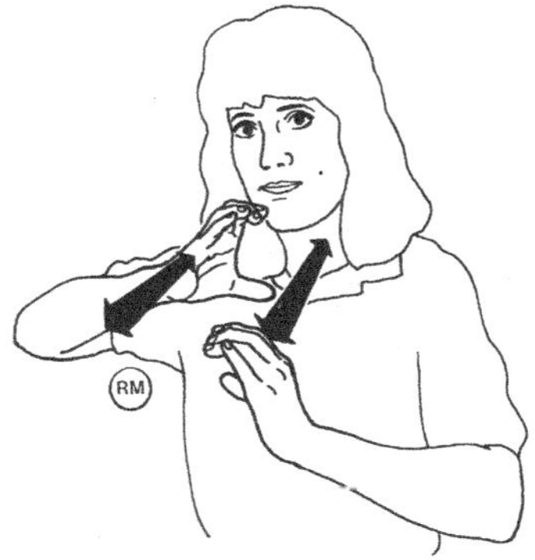

COMMUNICATION.

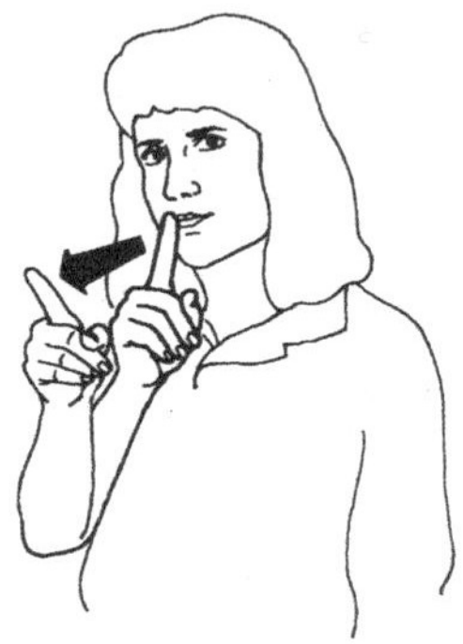

ARE

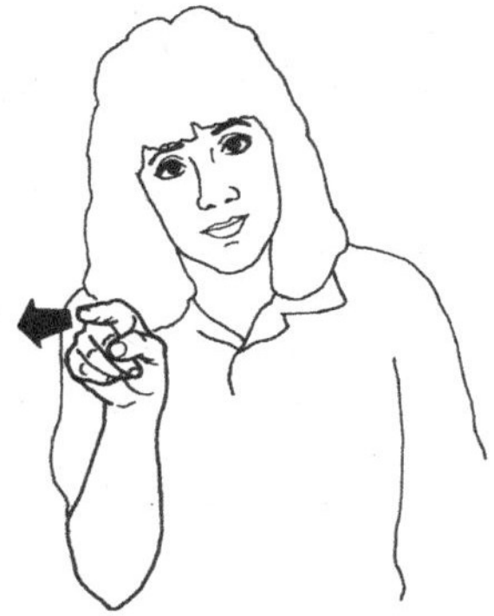

YOU

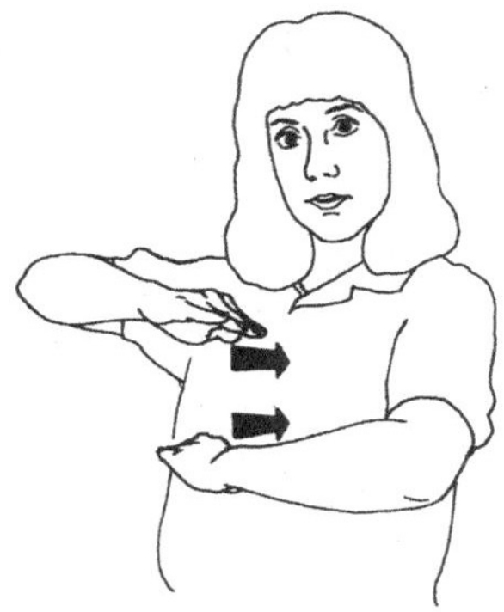

SATISFY

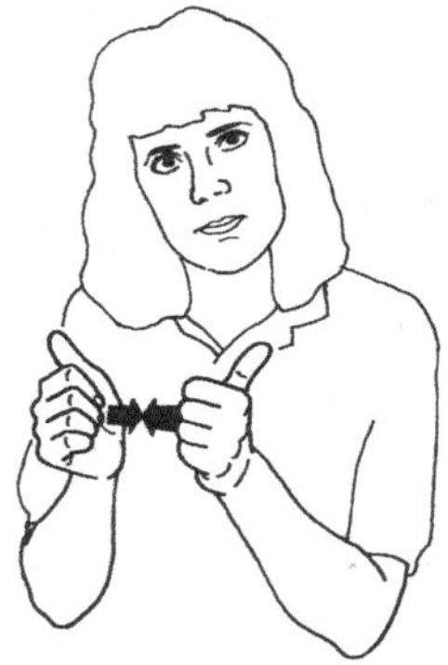

WITH

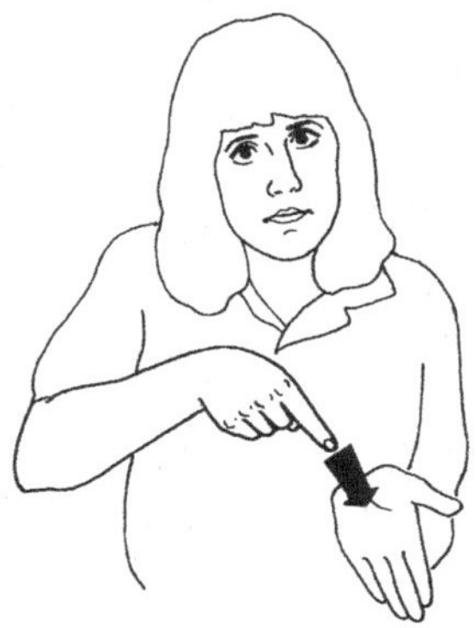

THIS

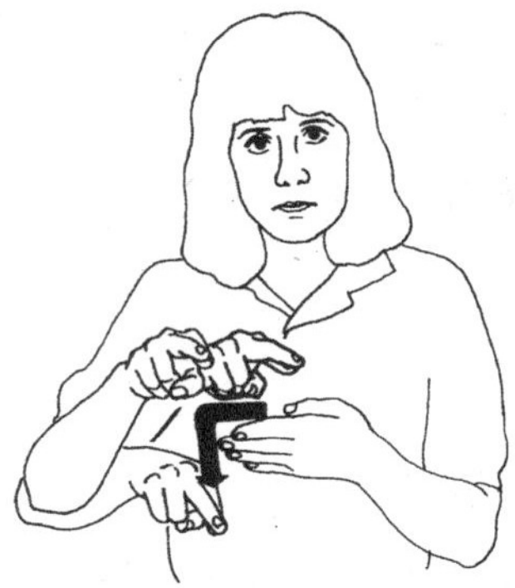

RESULT?

Are you satisfied with these results?

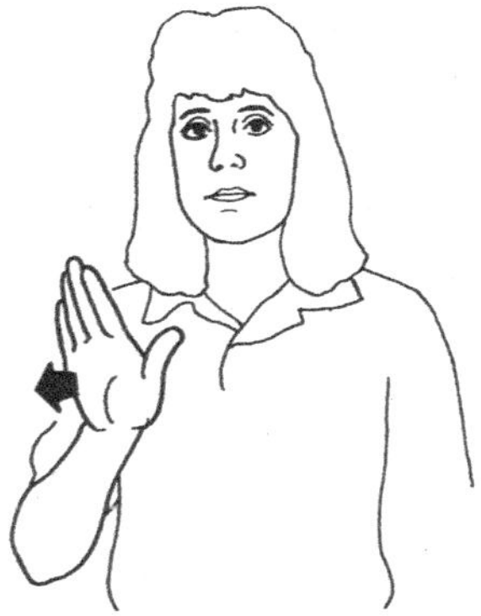

YOUR

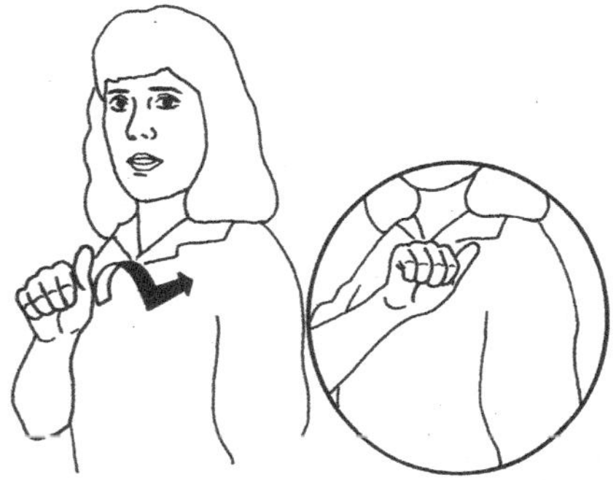

ATTITUDE

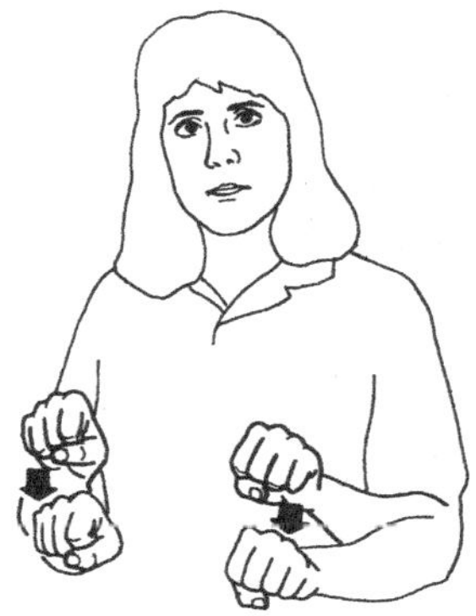

CAN

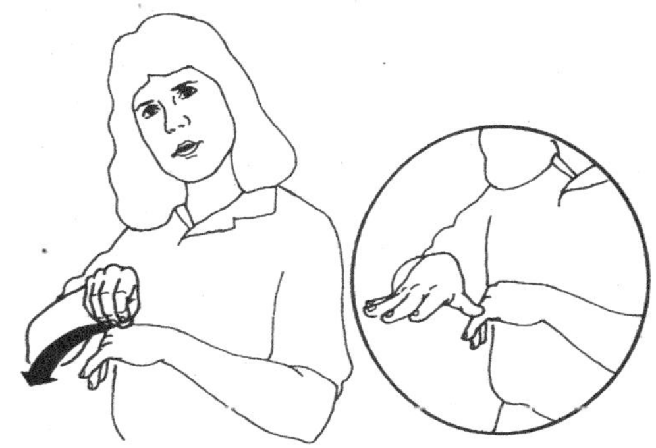

INFLUENCE

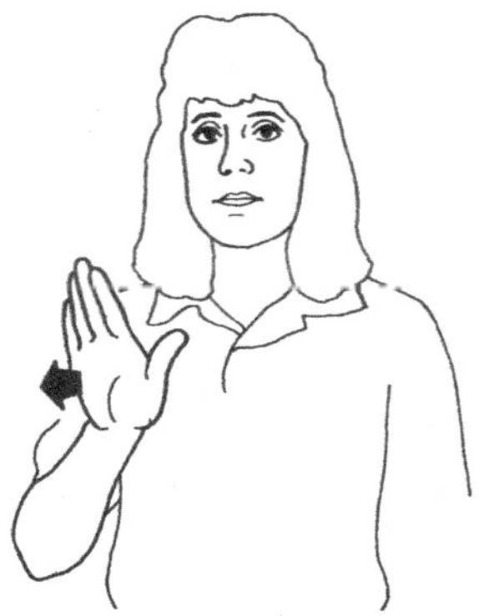

YOUR

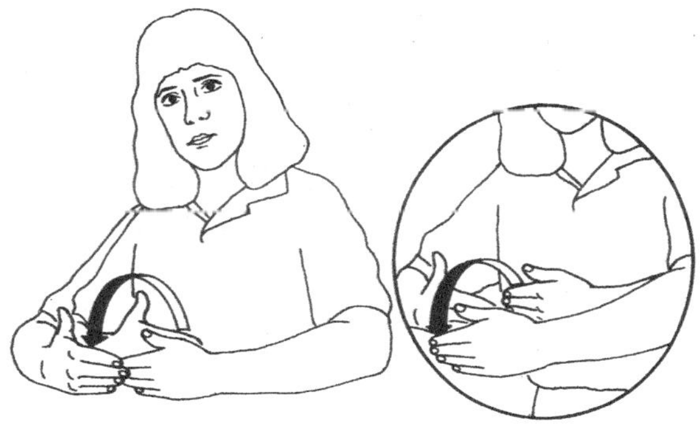

PROGRESS.

Your attitude can influence your progress.

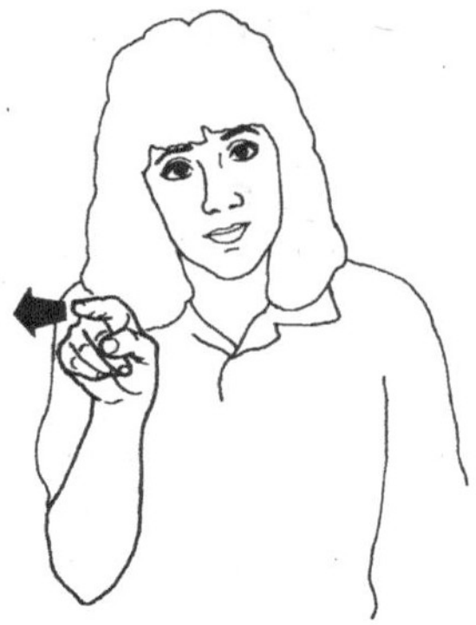

YOU

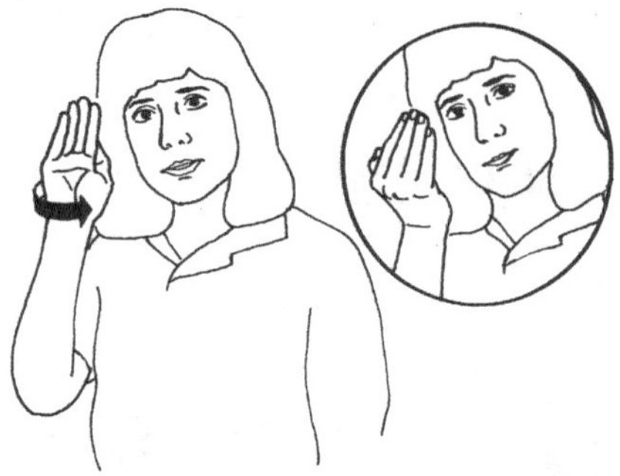

SEEM

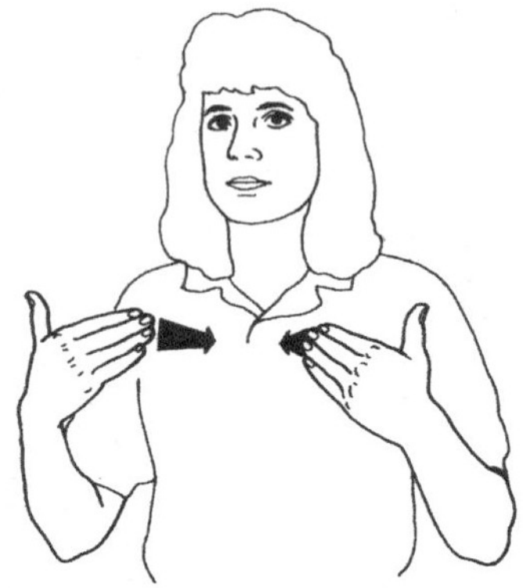

HAVE

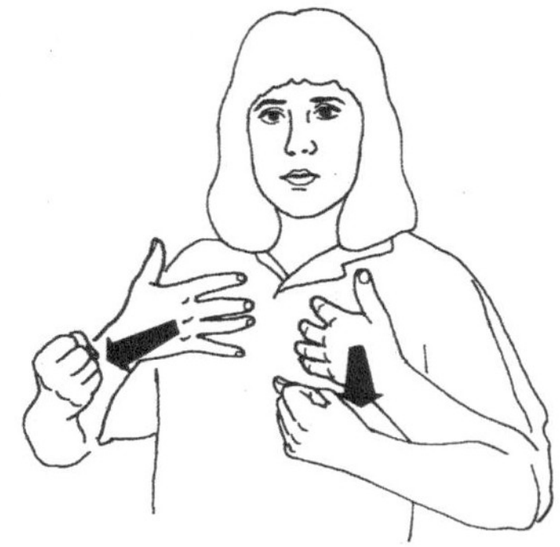

COURAGE

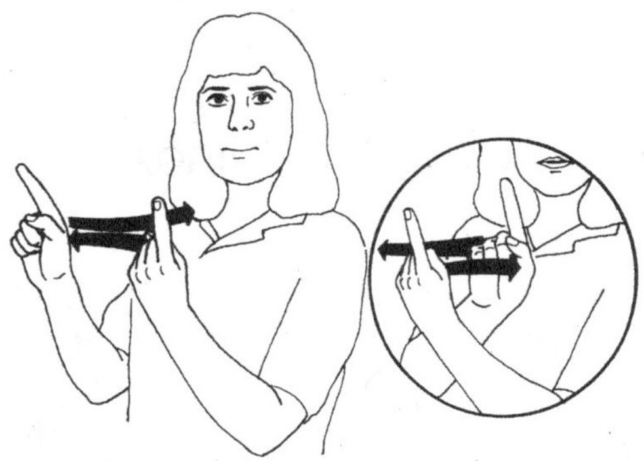

MEET

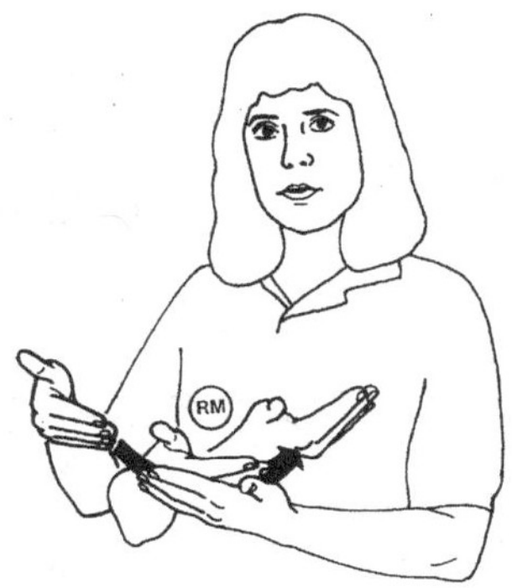

NEW

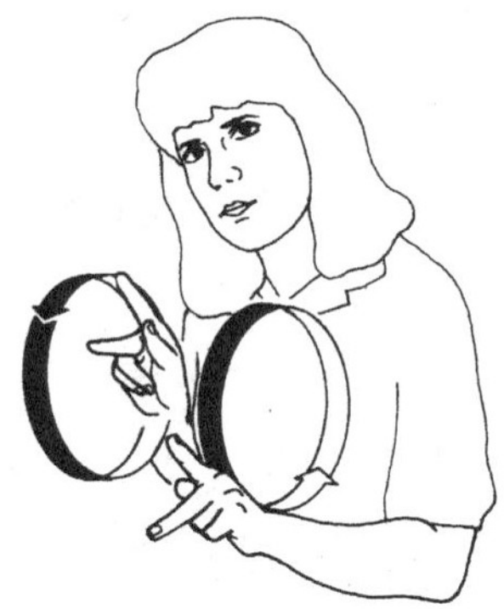

PEOPLE.

You seem to have courage to meet new people.

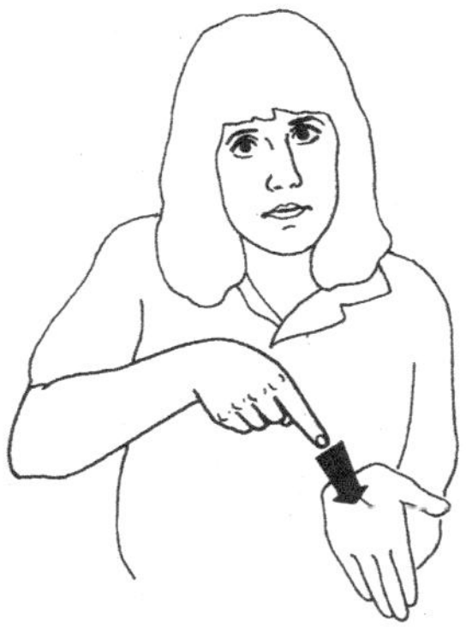

THIS

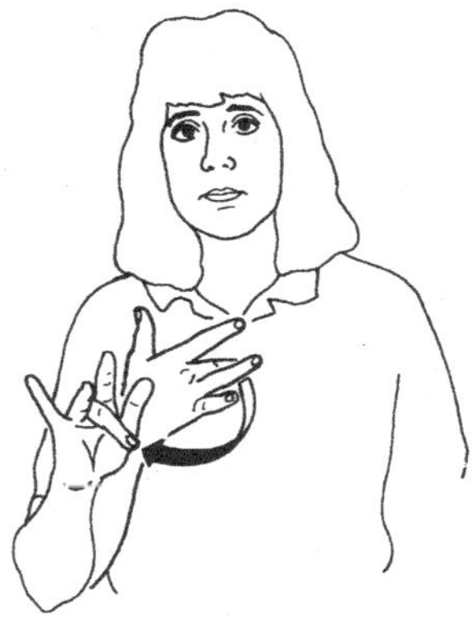

SENSITIVE

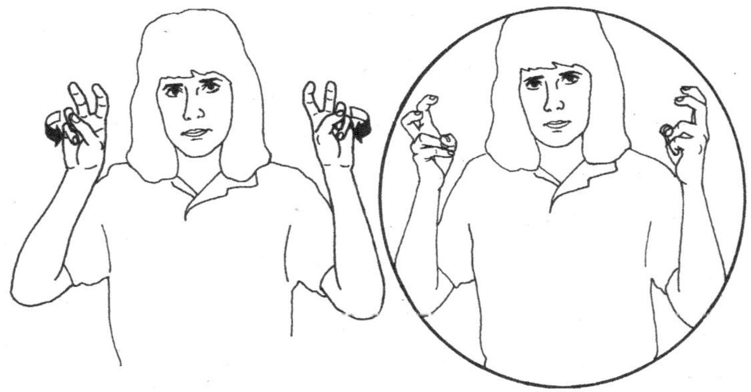

ISSUE.

This is a sensitive issue.

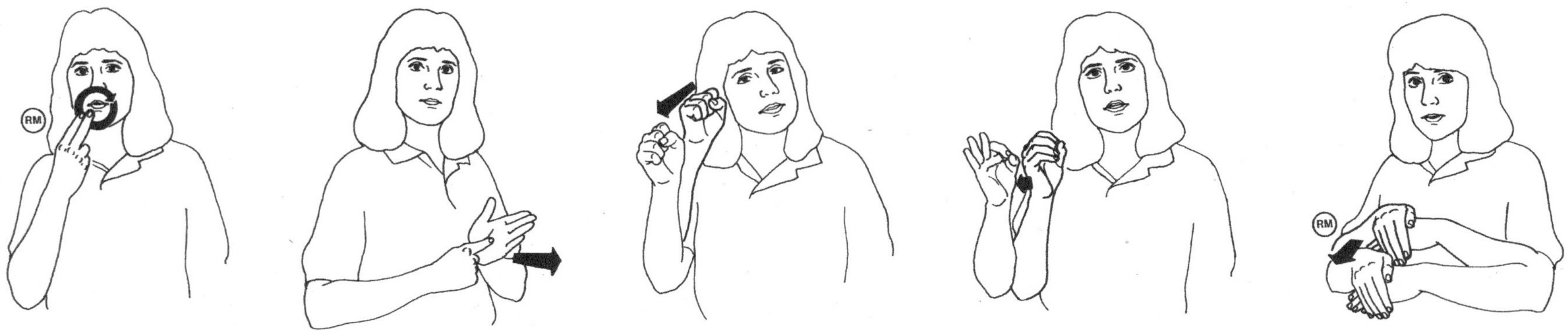

CUED-SPEECH SHOW SOUND O-F ENGLISH

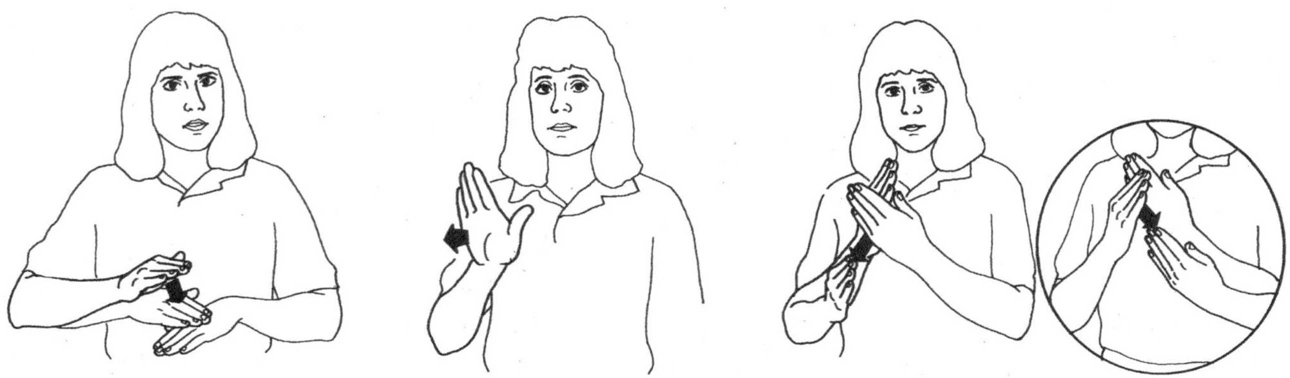

ON YOUR HANDS.

Cued Speech shows the sounds of English on your hands.

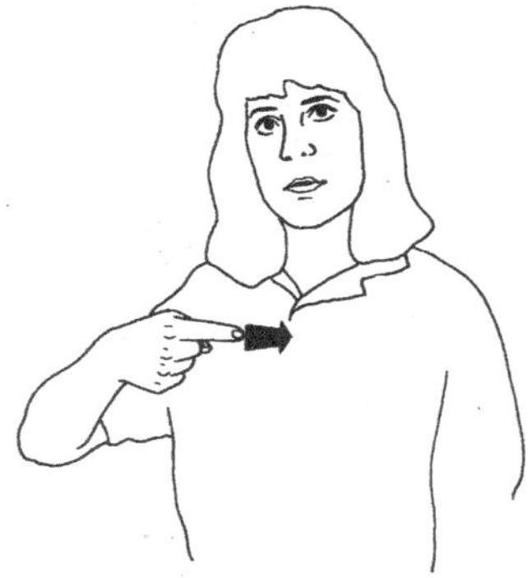

I

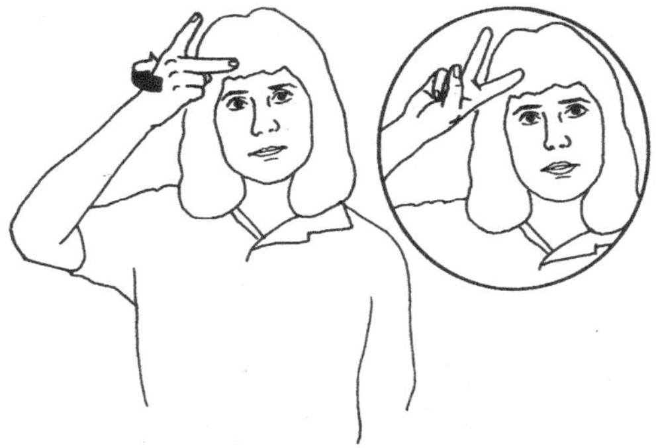

MISUNDERSTAND

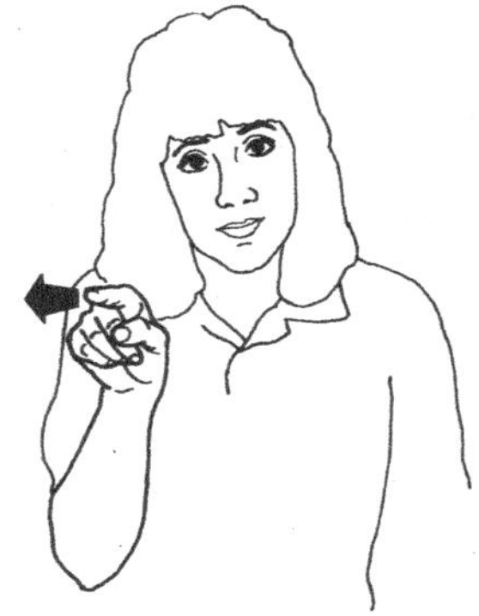

YOU.

I misunderstood you.

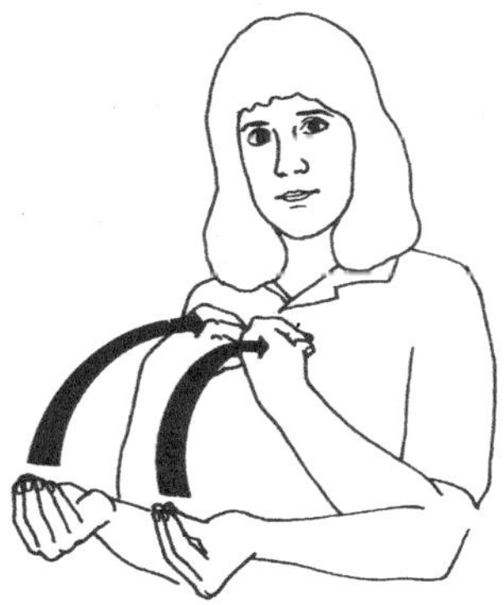

GIVE-ME

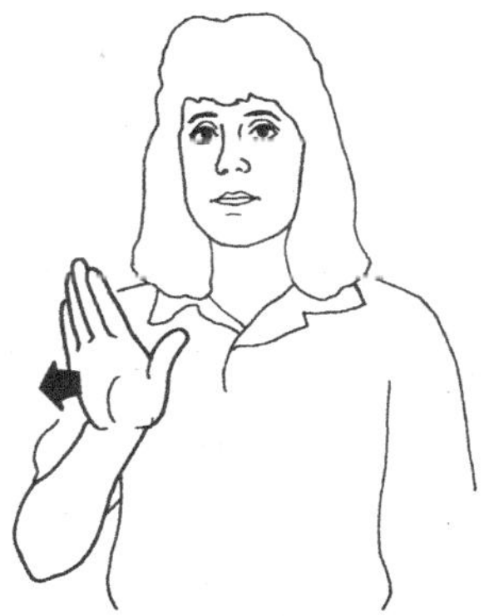

YOUR

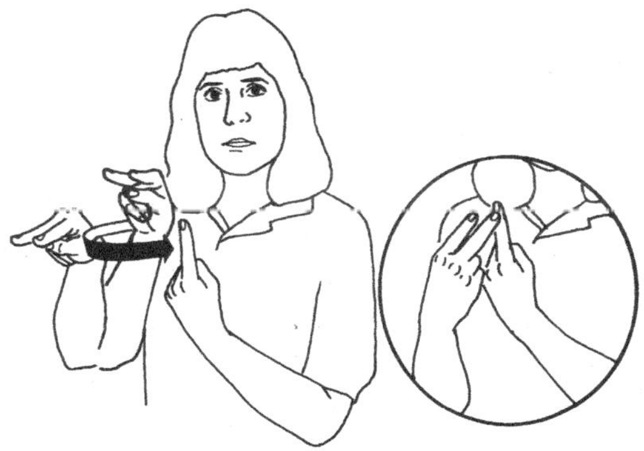

PERSPECTIVE.

Give me your perspective.

Glossary

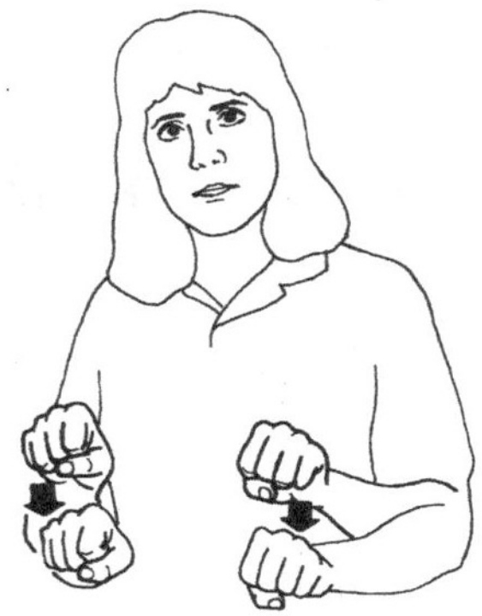

ABILITY/CAN
S hands, chest level, palms down. Simultaneously bring hands down to waist level.

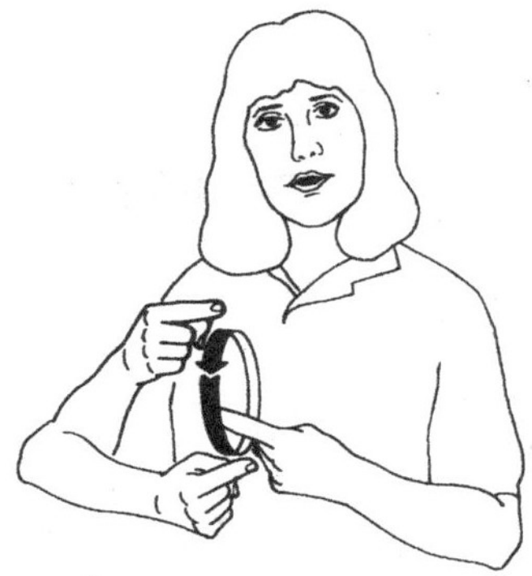

ABOUT
1 hands, palms in, waist level. Circle right hand around left index finger, in a clockwise direction.

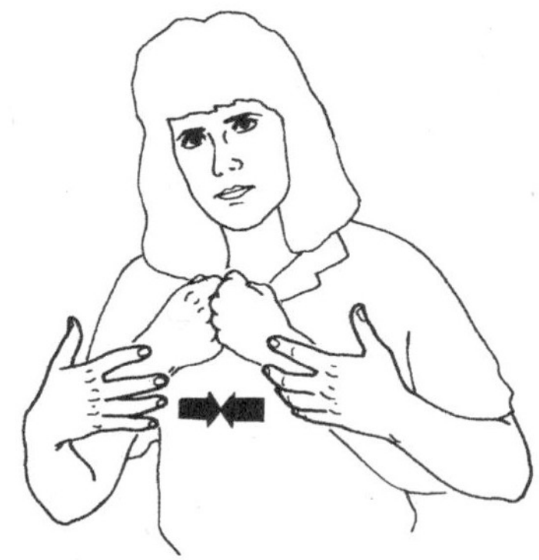

ACCIDENT
5 hands, chest level, palms in. Bring hands together closing to S hands.
Clue: two objects colliding.

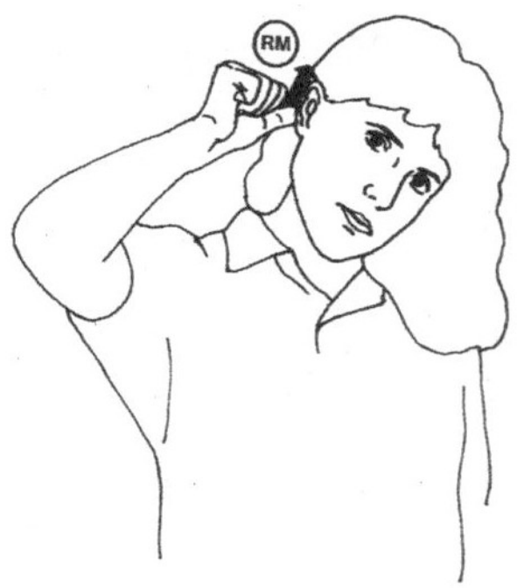

ADJUST THE VOLUME
Right A hand, thumb extended, palm left, behind right ear. Move A slightly upward. Repeat.
Clue: simulates adjusting the volume dial on the hearing aid.

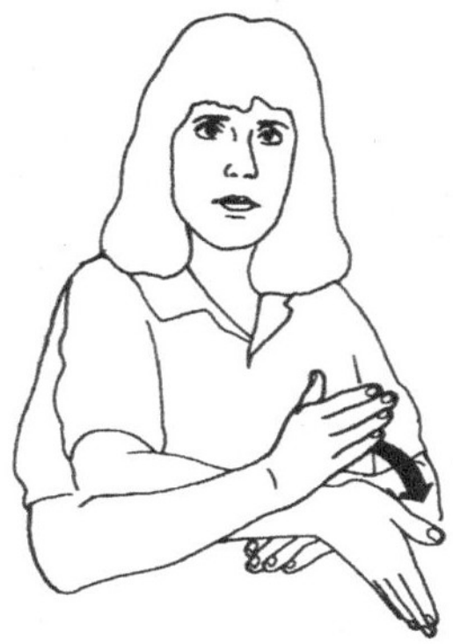

AFTER
Right flat hand, palm left, on left flat hand, palm down, chest level. Move right hand across left hand.

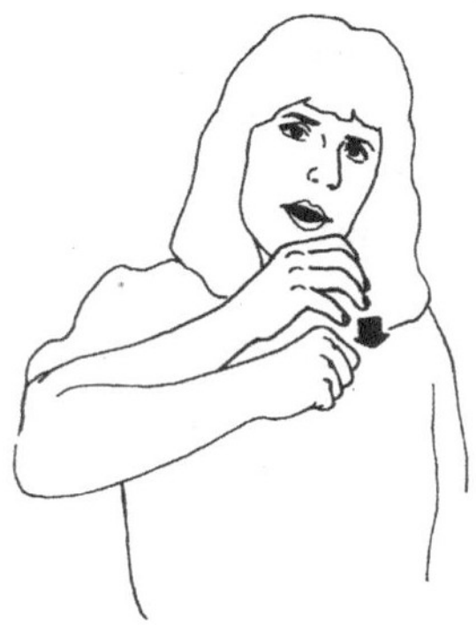

AGE
Right rounded 5 hand at chin, palm in. Move hand down to chest level, closing to S hand.

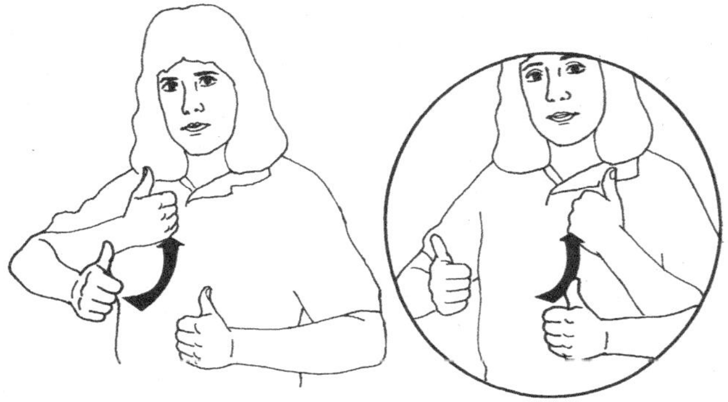

AGGRESSIVE
10 hands, palms in, chest level. Alternately brush hands on chest in circular motions.

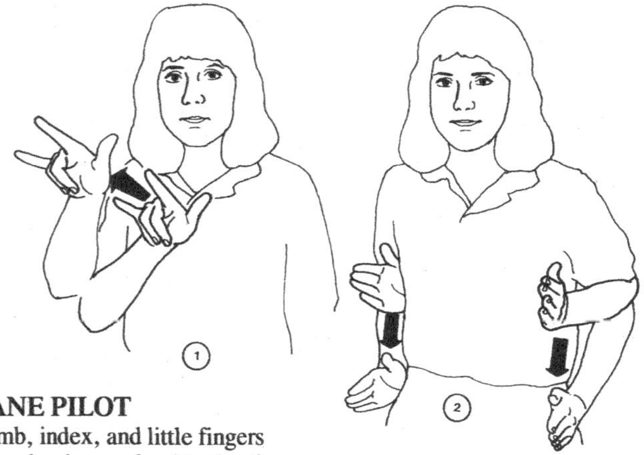

AIRPLANE PILOT
Right thumb, index, and little fingers extended, palm down, shoulder level. Hand points upward, moves slightly. Then change to flat hands, chest level, palms facing, and move down sides of body.

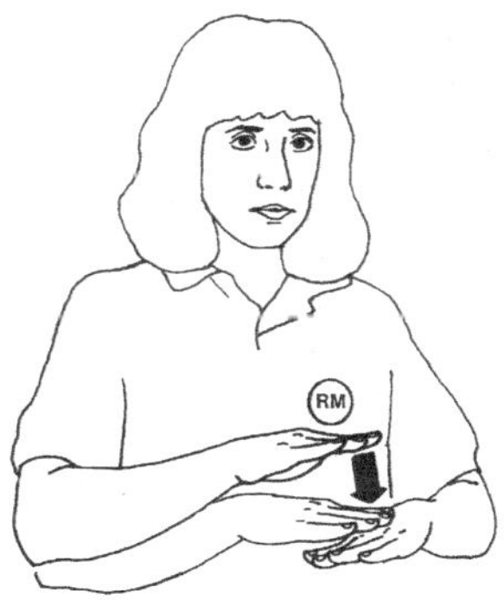

ALERT/WARN
Flat hands, palms down, chest level. Bring right hand down on top of left hand repeatedly.

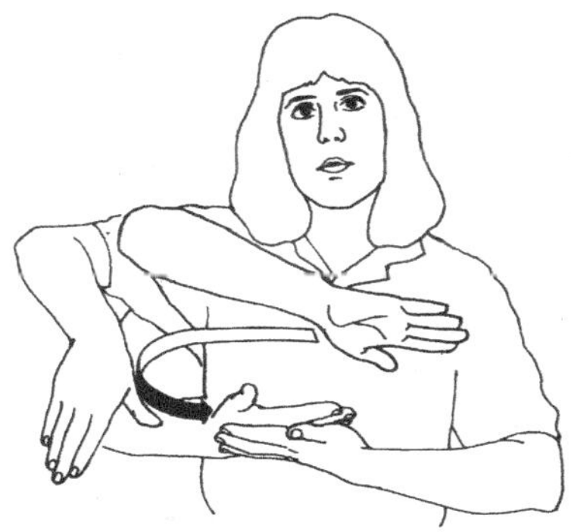

ALL
Flat hands, right palm down, left palm up, chest level. Circle right hand under left hand, ending with right hand on left, palm up.

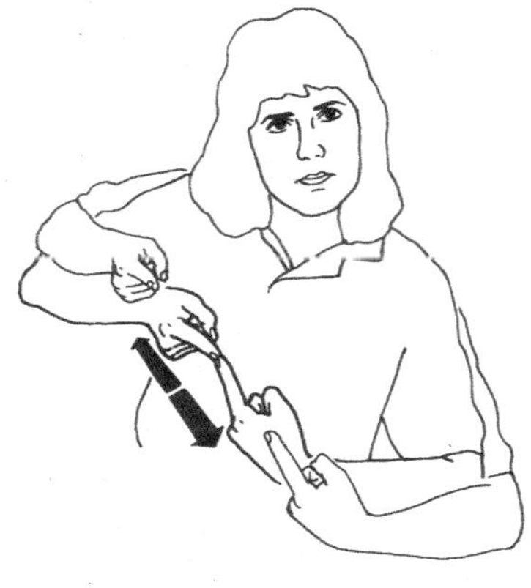

ALLERGIES
1 hands touching, chest level, palms in. Move hands apart with a sharp motion.

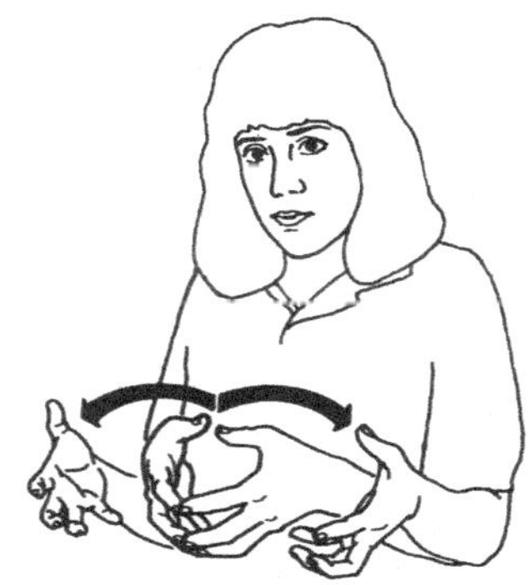

A LOT/MUCH
Rounded 5 hands, palms facing each other, fingertips touching, chest level. Bring hands out to sides.

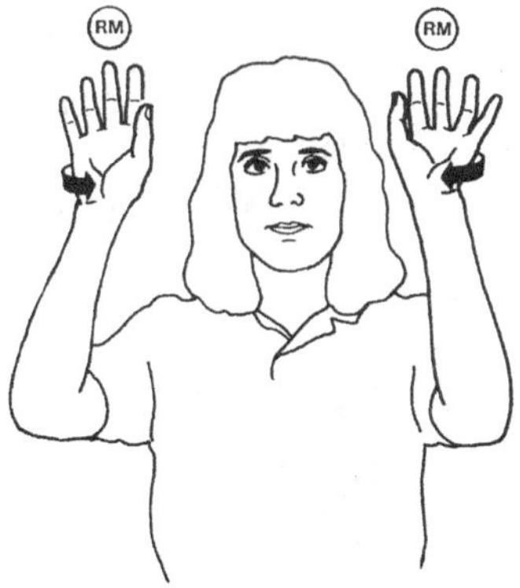

AMBULANCE
Rounded 5 hands, eye level, palms up. Twist slightly back and forth.
Clue: flashing light on an emergency vehicle.

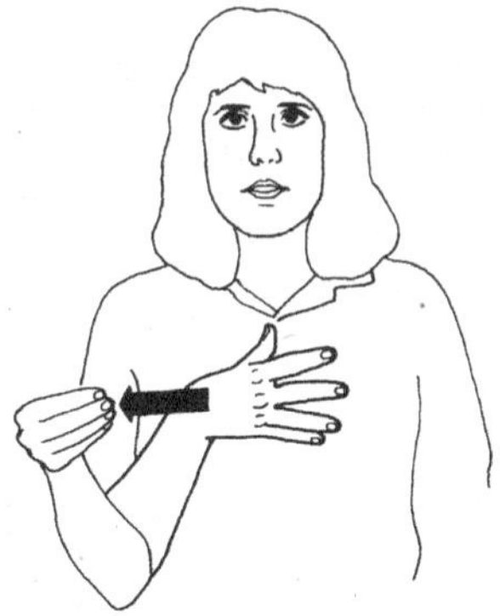

AND
Right 5 hand, chest level, palm in. Bring hand across body while closing to O hand.

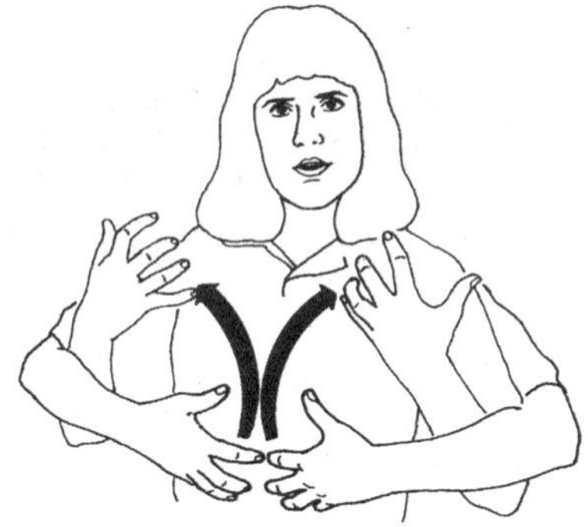

ANGRY
Claw hands, waist level, palms in. Raise to shoulder level in a quick movement.
Clue: anger coming from the inside out.

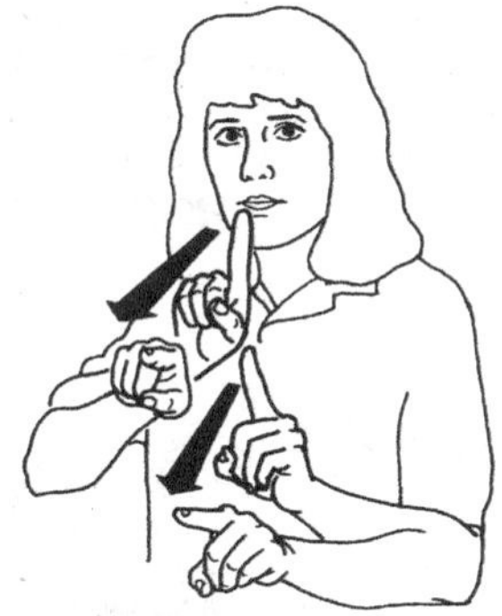

ANSWER
1 hands, right hand at chin, left hand slightly forward, palms out. Move hands simultaneously to palms down.

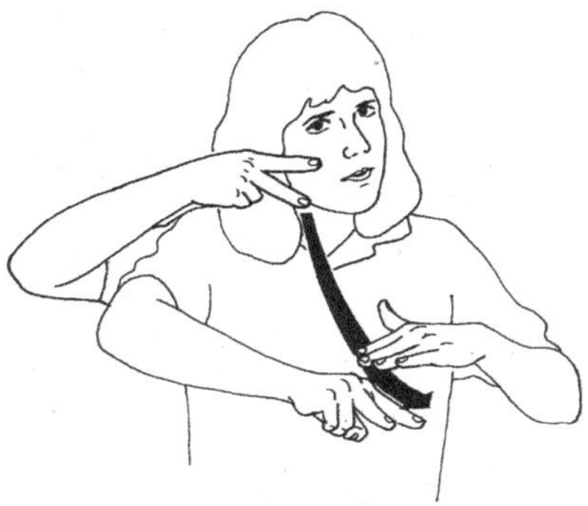

ANTICIPATORY
Left palm down, chest level, right V hand at cheek, palm in. Pass right hand under left.
Clue: seeing into the future.

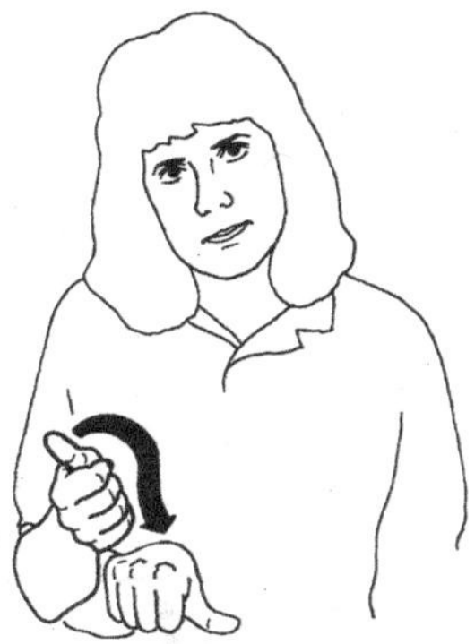

ANY
Right A hand, shoulder level, palm left. Move to waist level in a counterclockwise direction to palm down.

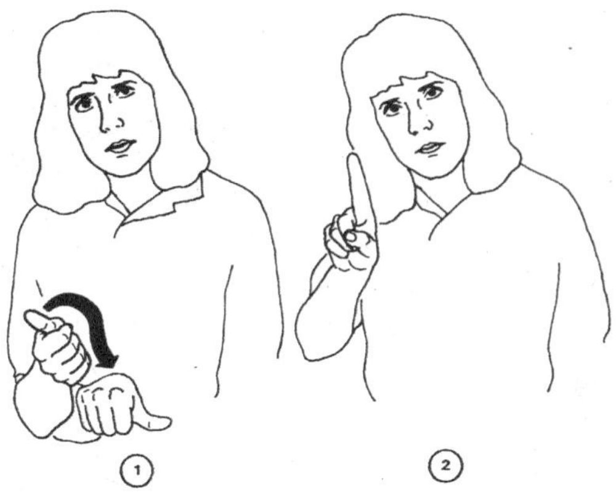

ANYONE
Right A hand, shoulder level, palm left. Move to waist level in a counterclockwise direction to palm down. Change A to 1 hand, shoulder level, palm out.

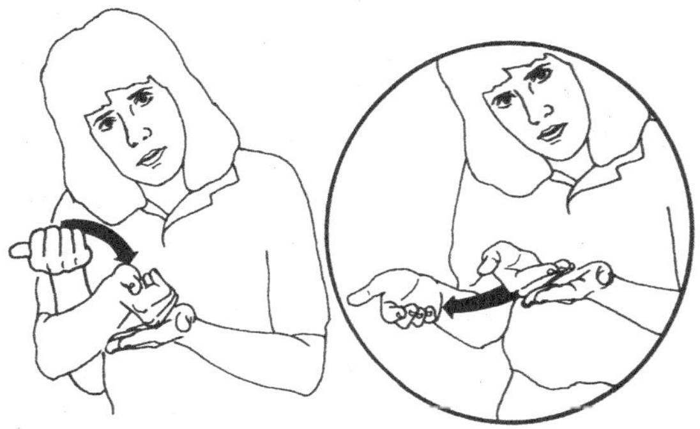

ANYTHING
Right A hand, shoulder level, palm up. Left flat hand, palm up, waist level. Move A down to left palm in counter-clockwise direction. Flatten hand to palm up when reaching waist level. Move from left to right.
Clue: any + thing.

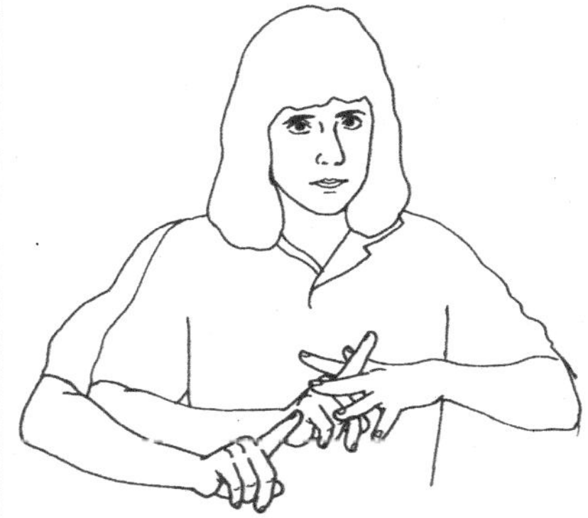

APPEAR/ARISE/POP UP
Left 5 hand, palm down, chest level. Right 1 hand, palm out, waist level. Bring right hand up, ending with right 1 between left index and middle fingers.

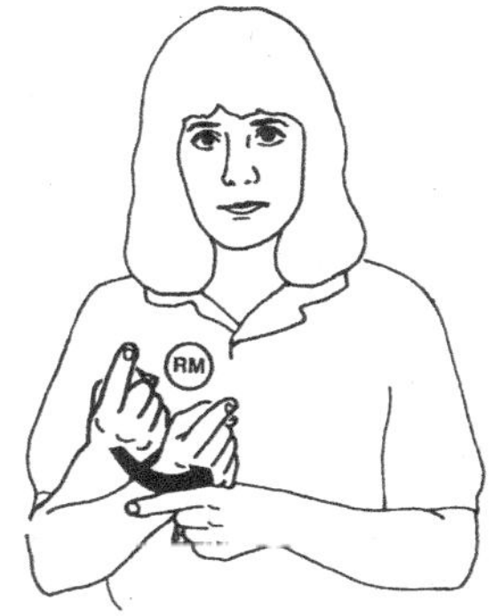

APPROPRIATE/PROPER
1 hands, waist level, palms facing each other. Bounce right hand repeatedly on left hand.

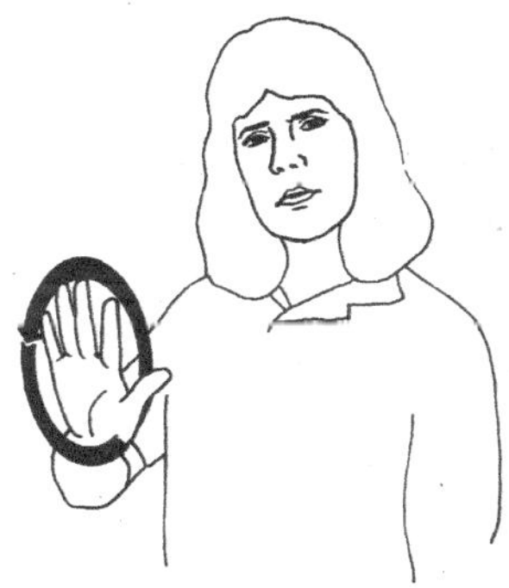

APPROXIMATE
Right 5 hand, chest level, palm out. Circle in a counter-clockwise direction.

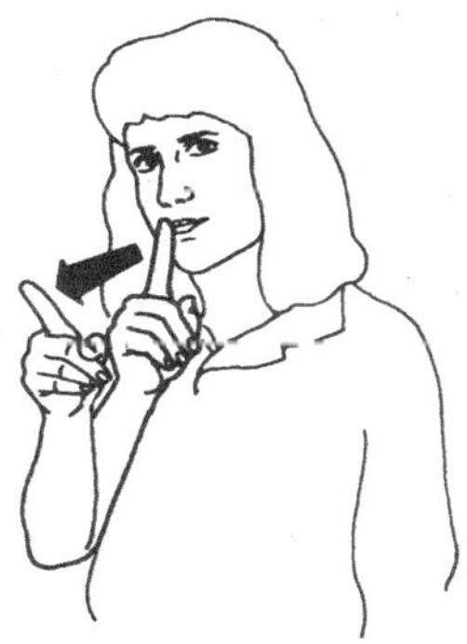

ARE/AM/IS/TO BE
Right 1 hand at mouth, palm left. Move hand directly out from mouth.

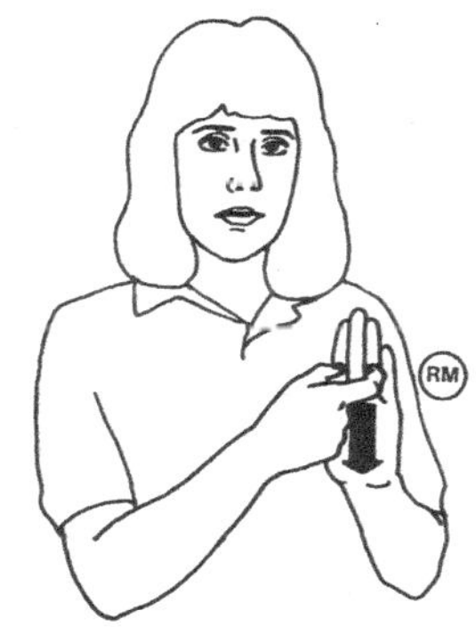

ARTICLE
Left flat hand, palm right, chest level. Right bent index and thumb, palm right, fingertips resting on left palm. Bring right hand down left palm.

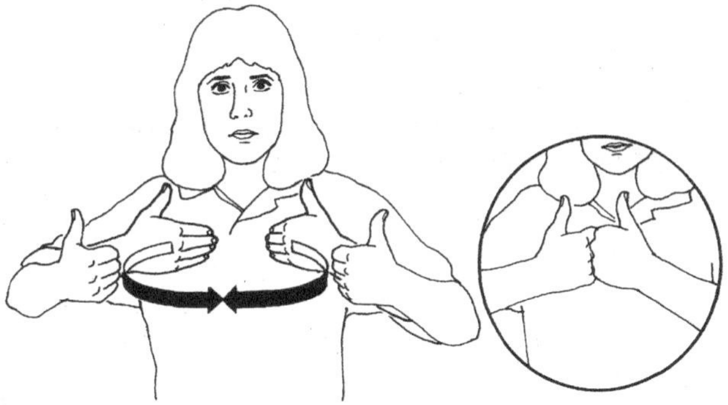

ASSERTIVE
Flat hands, chest level, palms in. Move to 10 hands away from body. Bring 10 hands together, knuckles touching.

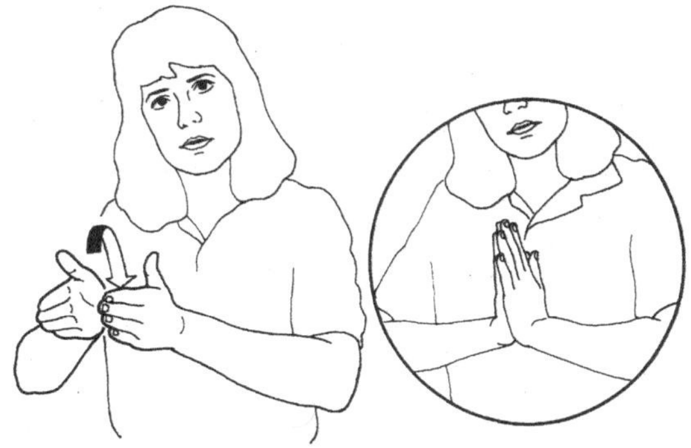

ASK
Flat hands, fingertips forward, palms facing each other, waist level. Move hands simultaneously so fingertips are up and palms are together at chest level.

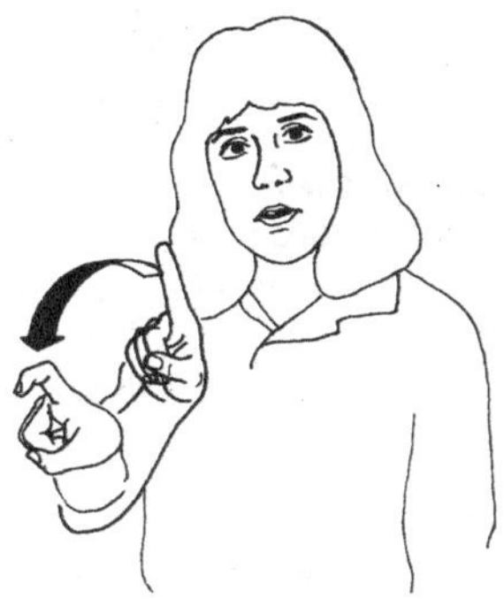

ASK
Right 1 hand at shoulder level, palm out. Move hand forward to X handshape.

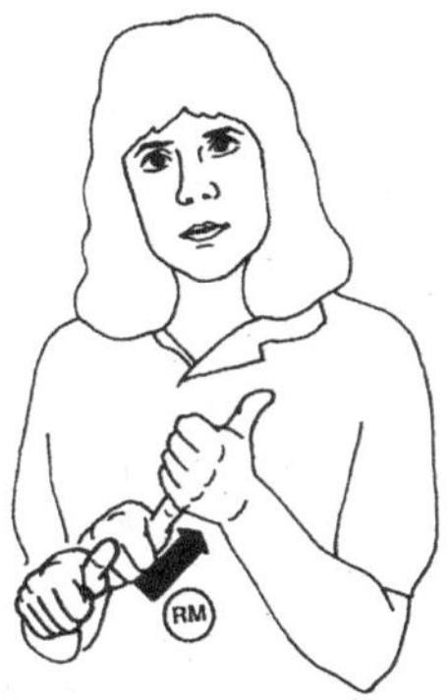

ASSIST/AID
A hands, palms facing, chest level. Place right A directly below left A. Move thumb of right A up to base of left A repeatedly.

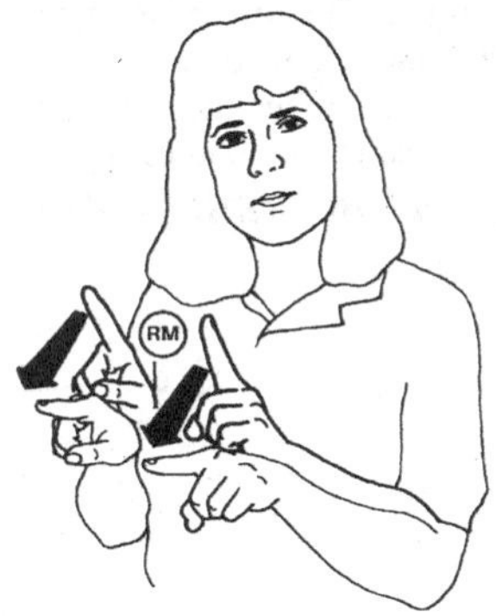

ATTEND/GO TO
1 hands, shoulder level, palms out. Move hands simultaneously down and up. Repeat.

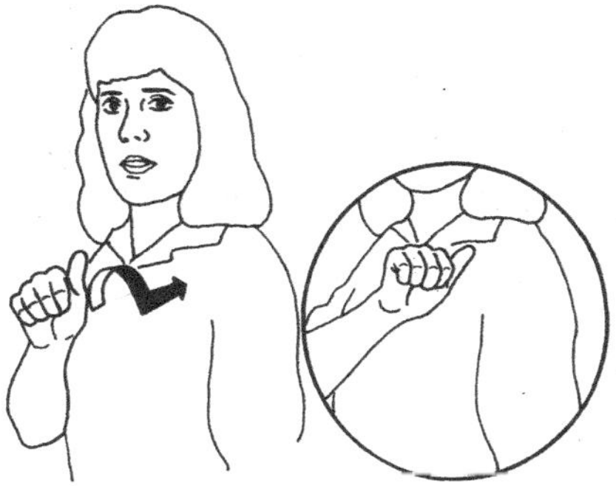

ATTITUDE
Right A hand, shoulder level, moves in a clockwise direction and come to rest on the left side of chest.

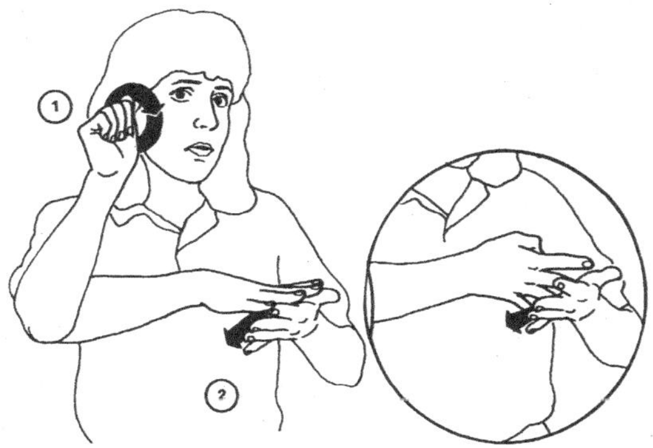

AUDIOGRAM
Right A hand, ear level, palm out. Circle clockwise once. Right 4 hand, palm down, left 5 hand, palm up, waist level. Move right hand down and then across left palm.
Clue: audiology + graph.

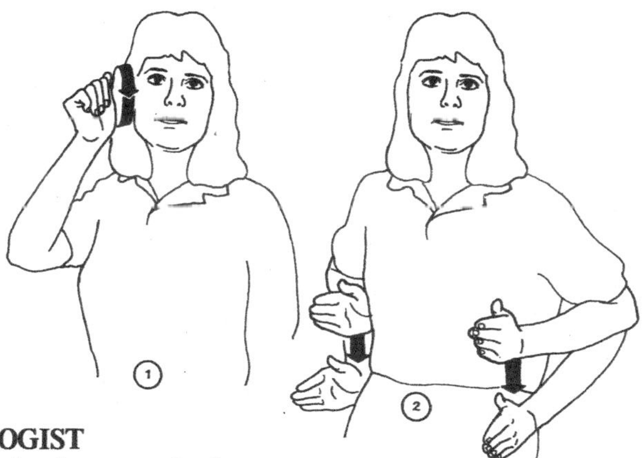

AUDIOLOGIST
Right A hand, palm out, ear level. Circle hand in clockwise direction, opening to flat hand while bringing hand down side of body. Left flat hand also moves down side of body.

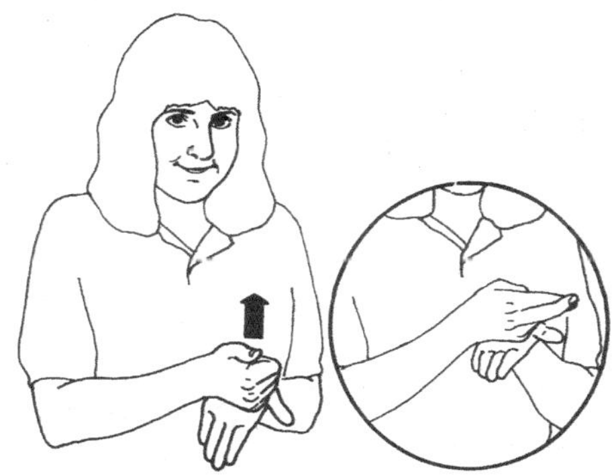

AURAL REHABILITATION
Right A hand, palm left. Left flat hand, palm up, waist level. Rest A on left palm. Raise left palm while changing right A to R handshape.
Clue: initialized sign—same sign motion for help and therapy.

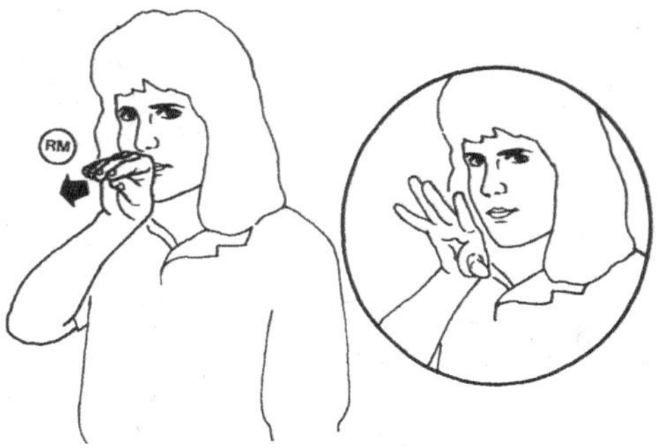

BABBLE
Right O hand in front of mouth, fingertips out. Open to 5 hand and close to O hand. Repeat movement.

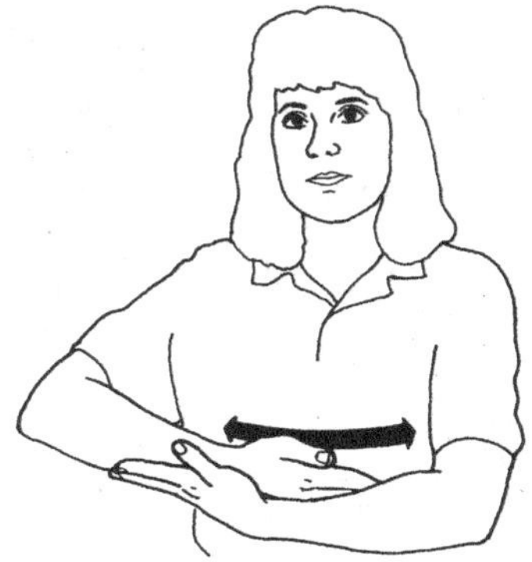

BABY
Flat hands, palms up, chest level, right hand on top of left hand. Rock arms back and forth.
Clue: motion of rocking a baby.

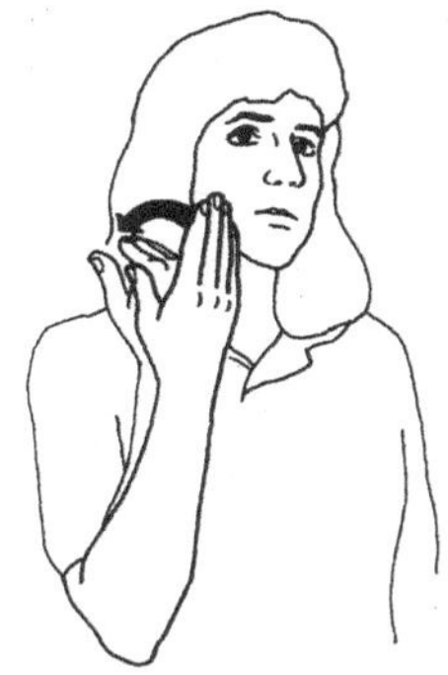

BACK OF MOUTH
Right flat hand, fingertips up, palm back, right cheek level. Flick fingertips down to point back.

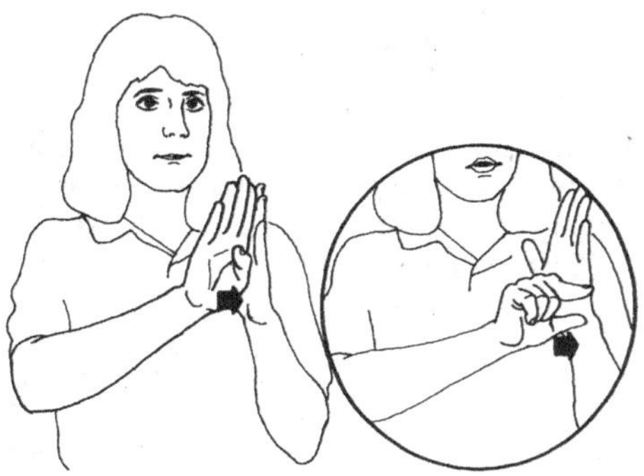

BACKGROUND
Left flat hand, chest level, palm right. Right B hand on left flat hand. Move B down left hand, changing to G.

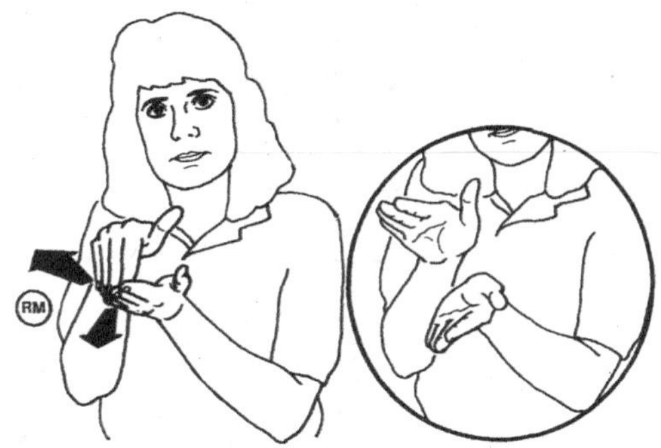

BARKING
Right flat hand on top of left flat hand, fingertips touching. Move fingers apart and back together. Repeat movement.
Clue: jaws of a dog when barking.

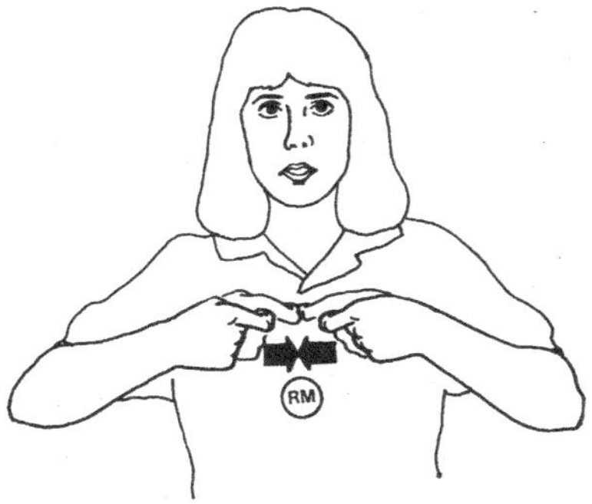

BATTERY
X hands, chest level, palms in. Tap index fingers together. Repeat movement.

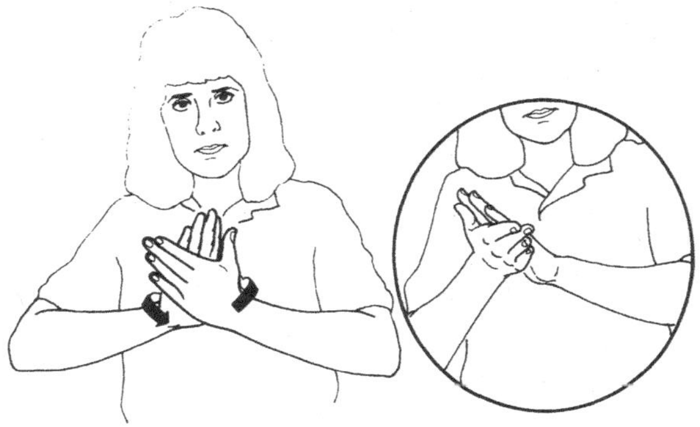

BECOME
Flat hands, right palm on top of left palm, chest level. Rotate hands 180 degrees in opposite directions.

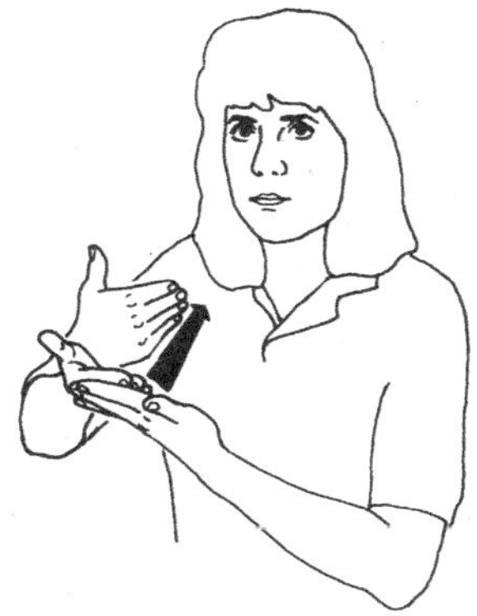

BEFORE
Flat hands, chest level, palms in, right hand in left palm. Bring right hand back to shoulder.

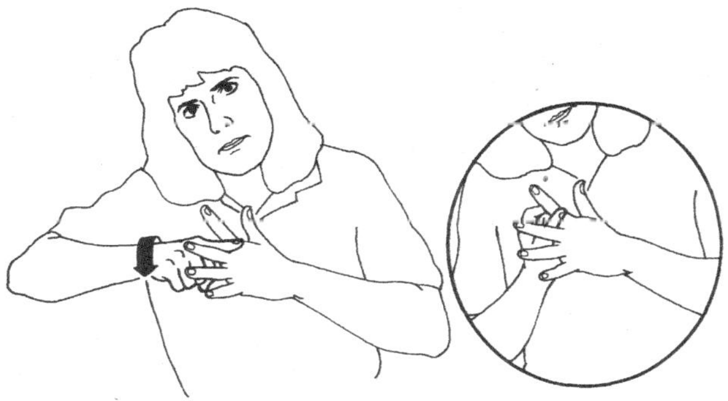

BEGIN/START
Left 5 hand, chest level, palm facing side. Right 1 hand, index finger inserted into left hand, between the index and middle fingers. Rotate right hand 180 degrees in a clockwise direction.
Clue: inserting key in ignition to start car.

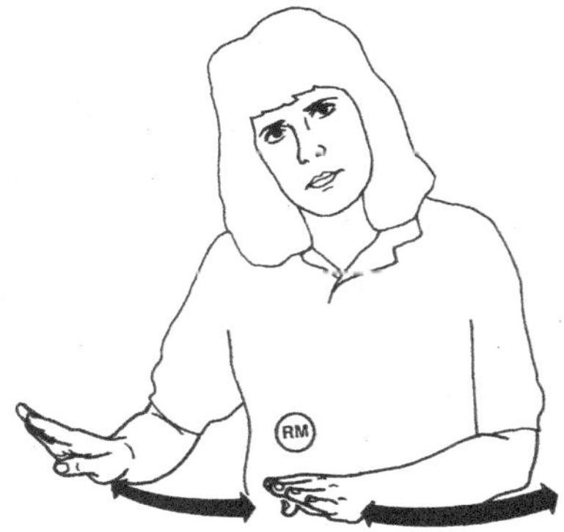

BEHAVIOR
B hands, waist level, palms down. Move hands side to side simultaneously. Repeat movement.

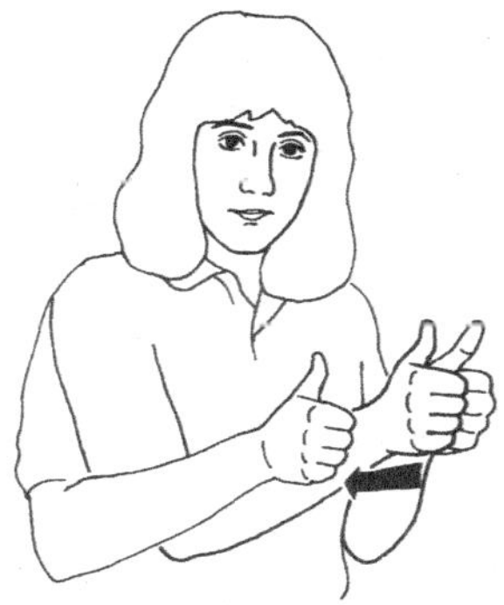

BEHIND
A hands, chest level, knuckles touching. Move right hand directly behind left hand.
Clue: putting one object behind another.

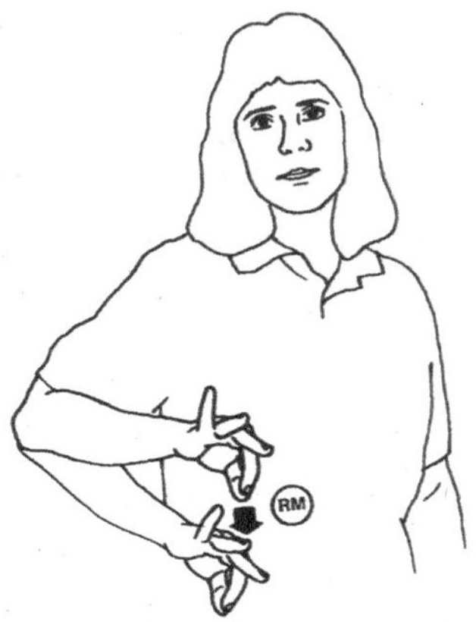

BENEFIT
Right F hand, chest level, palm down. Move down right side of body. Repeat movement.
Clue: putting something in your pocket.

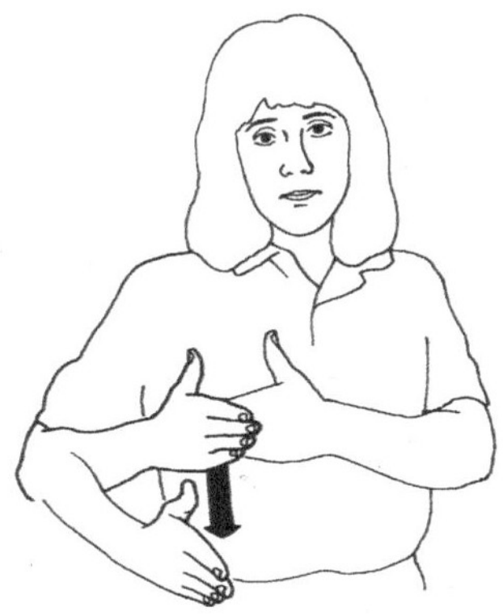

BESIDE
Flat hands, palms in, right fingers on back of left hand, chest level. Bounce right hand to the right.

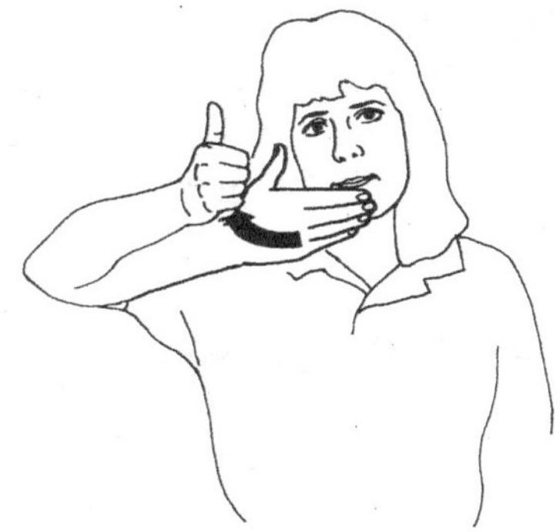

BETTER
Right flat hand, at chin, palm in. Move to right side of face, closing to A hand.

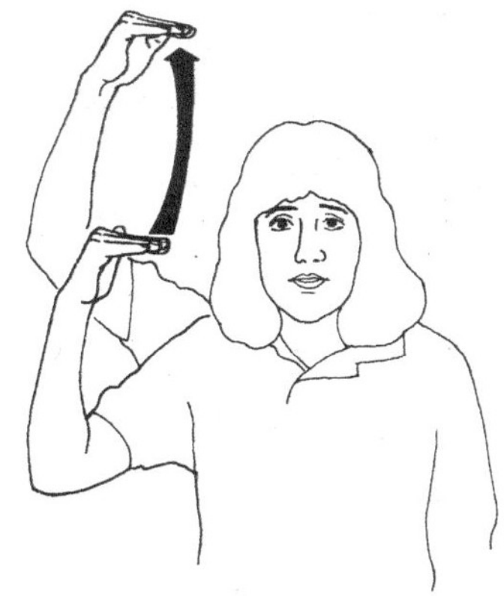

BIG/TALL
Right bent flat hand, palm left, eye level. Move hand up, above head.
Clue: showing the height of something.

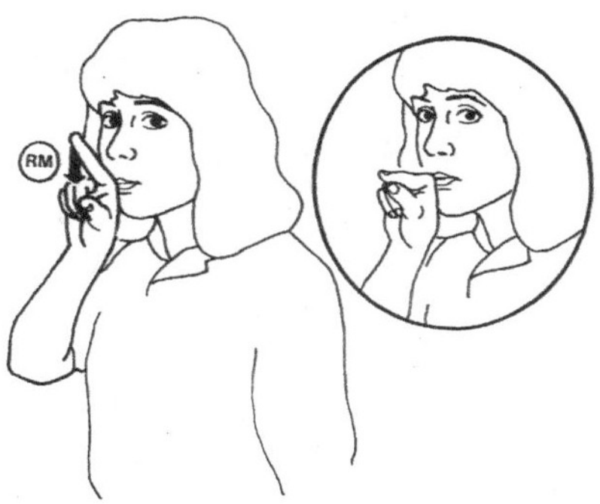

BIRD
Right G hand, fingers pointing out, in front of mouth. Close and open index finger and thumb repeatedly.
Clue: the beak of a bird.

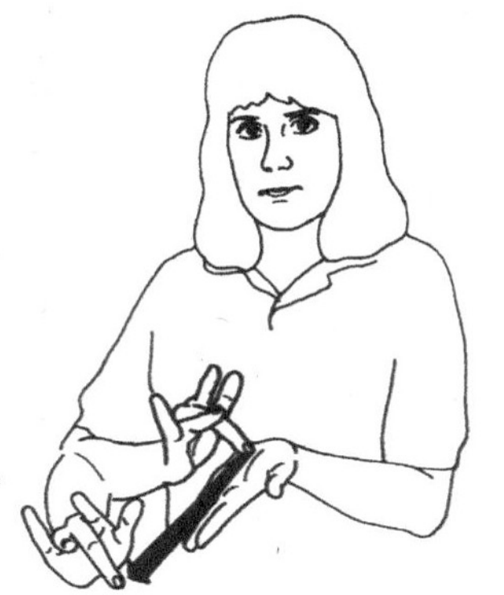

BLANK
Left flat hand, palm up, waist level. Right hand, palm down, middle finger touching left flat hand. Move right hand across left hand.

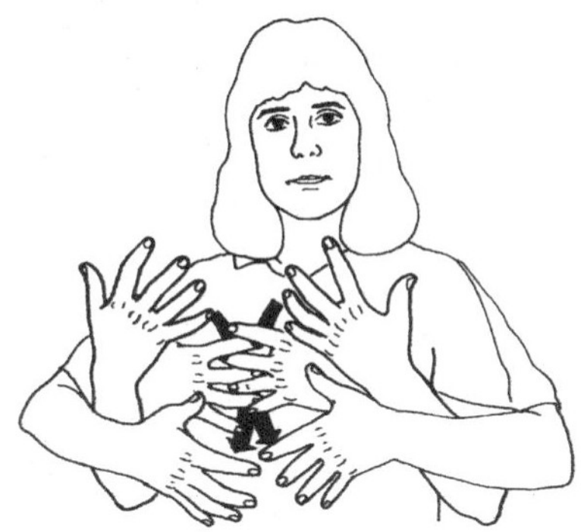

BLEND
Rounded 5 hands, chest level, palms in. Bring hands down as fingertips lightly interlock.
Clue: two things coming together.

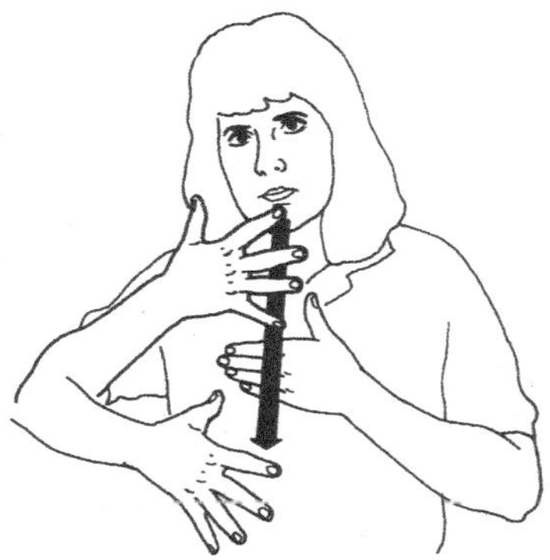

BLOOD
Left flat hand, at chest, palm in. Right 5 hand at chin, palm in. Move right hand down while fingers wiggle.
Clue: a cut that is bleeding.

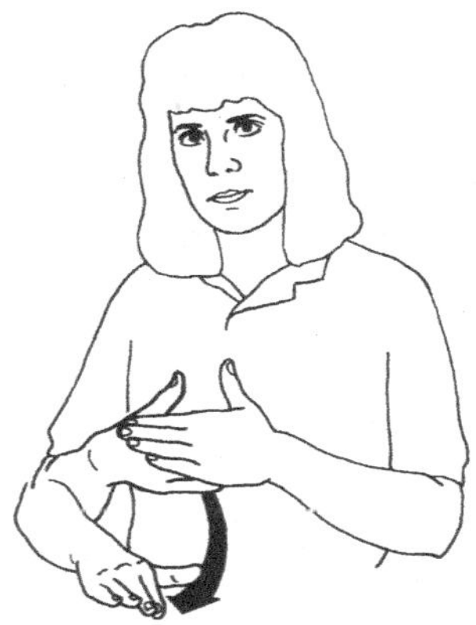

BORN/BIRTH
Flat hands, palms in, chest level, right hand inside left. Move right hand under and out from left.
Clue: baby being born.

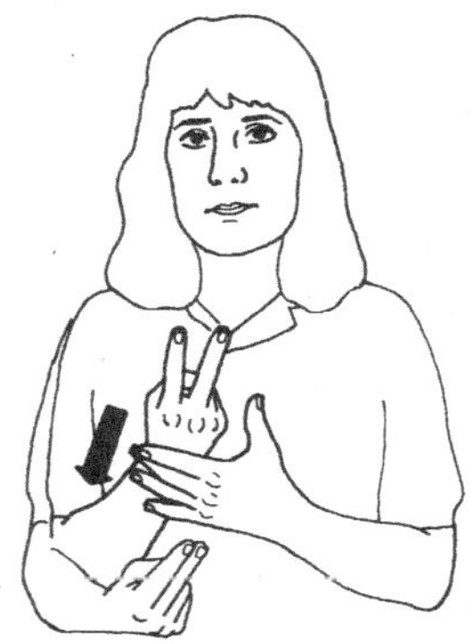

BOTH
Cupped left hand, chest level, palm in. Right V hand, palm in, in left hand. Pull right V down left hand. Right hand becomes U hand.

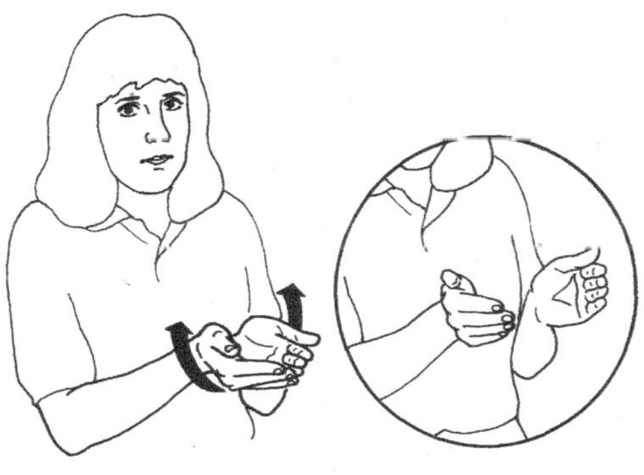

BOWL
Curved hands, chest level, palms up, hands touching. Move hands up slightly.
Clue: resembles the shape of a bowl.

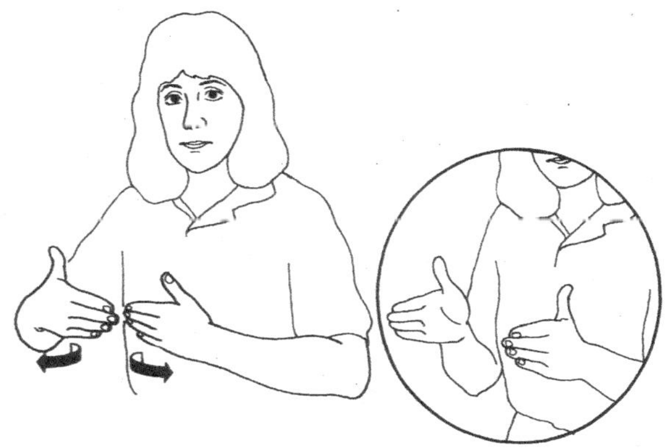

BOX
Flat hands, palms in, chest level. Move right and left hands at wrist simultaneously so palms face each other.

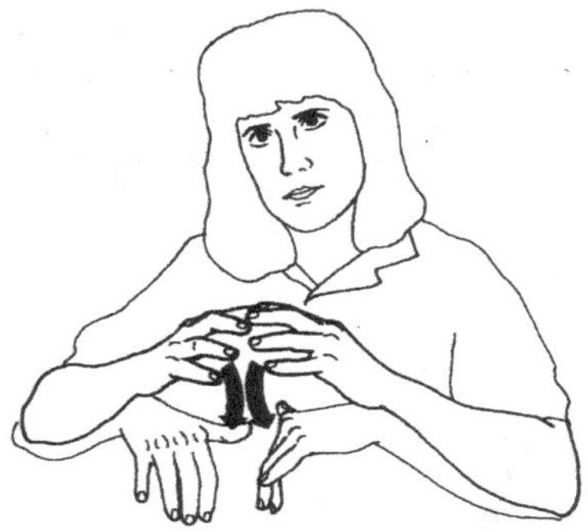

BREAKDOWN
5 hands, slightly clawed, at shoulder level, palms facing. Slightly interlace fingers. Move hands to palms down simultaneously.
Clue: something collapsing.

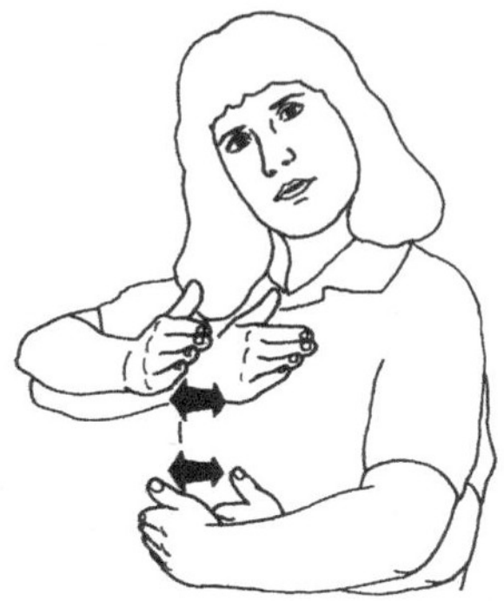

BREATHE
Flat hands, palms in, chest level, right hand above left. Simultaneously move both hands in and out from body, keeping palms flat.
Clue: lungs and chest filling and emptying of air.

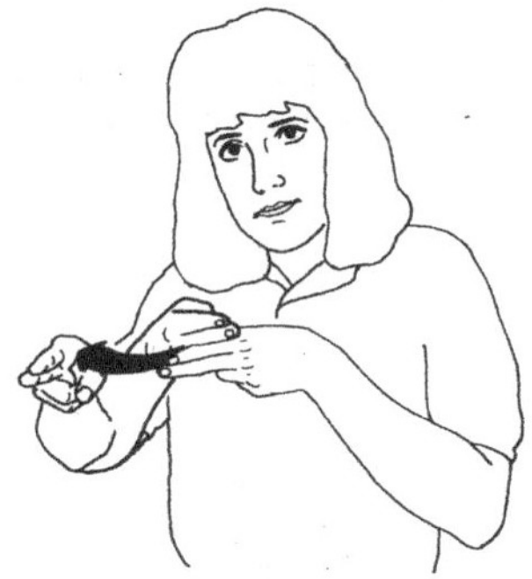

BRIEF/SHORT
U hands, chest level. Rest right U on left U. Move right U across left U using wrist.

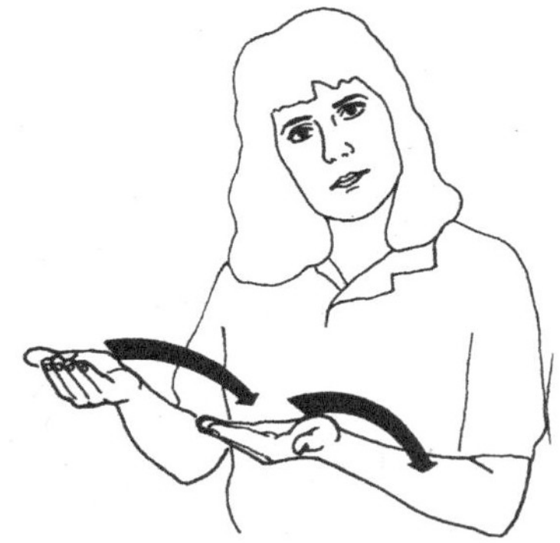

BRING
Flat hands, palms up, chest level, slightly to right side. Right hand in front of left hand. Move simultaneously to front of chest.

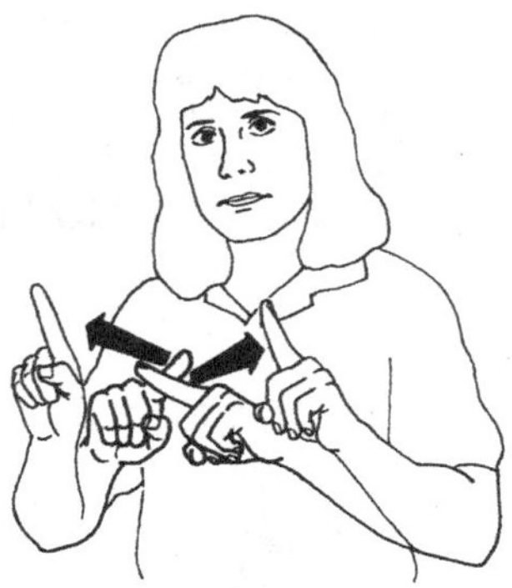

BUT
1 hands, chest level, palms out. 1 hands cross. Move hands apart.

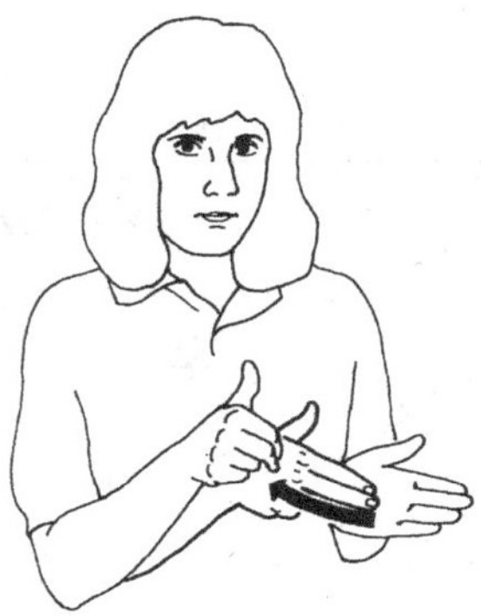

BUTTER
Left flat hand, waist level, palm up. Right U hand, palm down. Brush right U down left palm. Repeat movement.
Clue: spreading butter on bread.

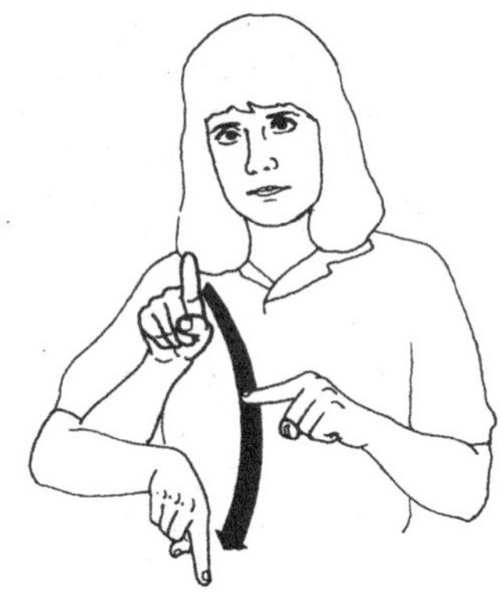

CAN'T
1 hands, palms down, left hand waist level, right hand at shoulder level. Right hand moves down, striking left fingertips. Shake head from side to side while signing.

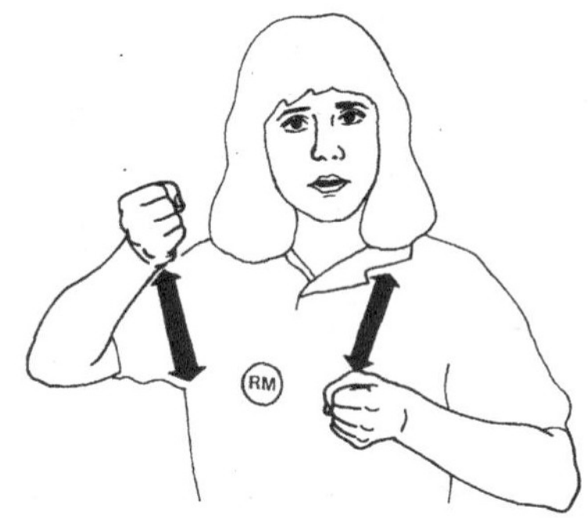

CAR
S handshapes move as in steering a car.

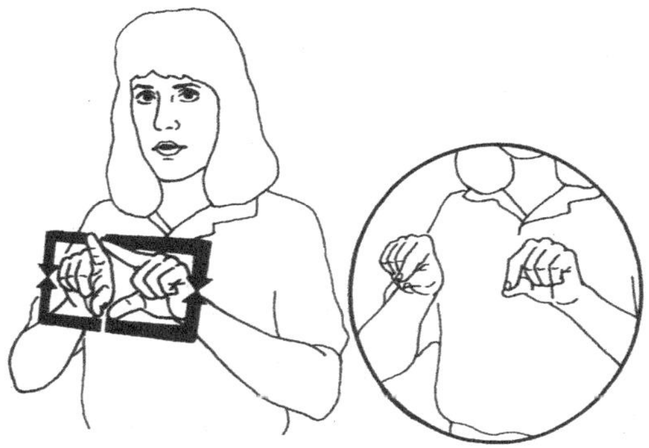

CARD
L hands, palms out, thumbs touching at chest level. Move hands apart, ending with index fingers touching thumbs.

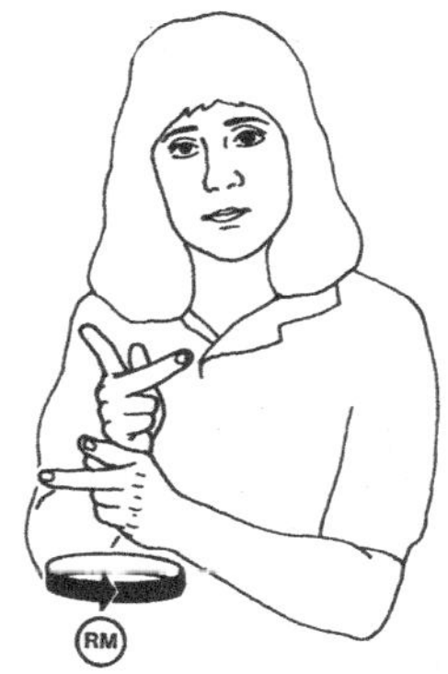

CARE/SUPERVISE
V hands, waist level, palms to sides, right hand on top of left. Circle hands together in a clockwise direction. Repeat movement.

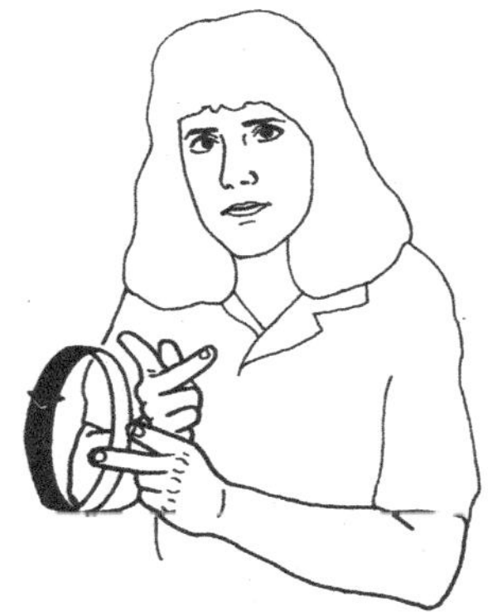

CAREFUL
V hands, chest level, palms to sides, right hand on top of left. Simultaneously move hands in a circular direction, away from body. Repeat movement.

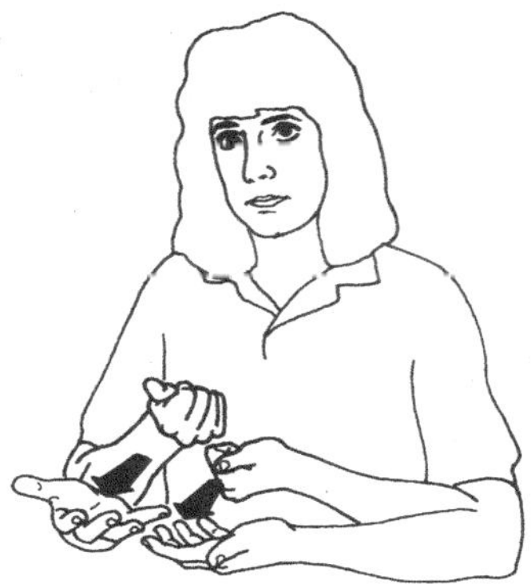

CAUSE
A hands, chest level, palms up. Move both hands away from body, opening to 5 hands.

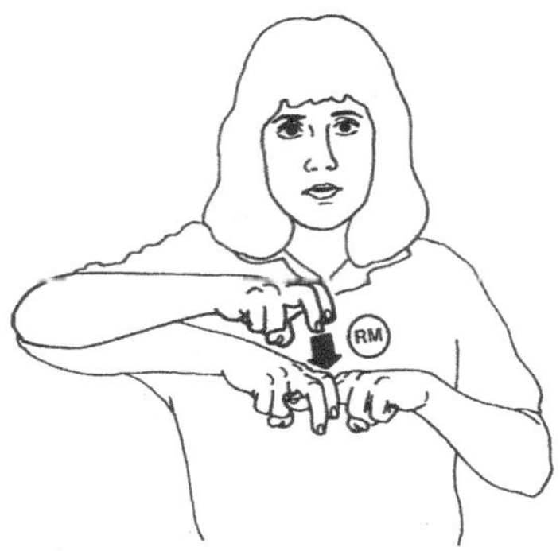

CHAIR
H hands, palms down, chest level. Bring right hand down on top of left and bounce several times.

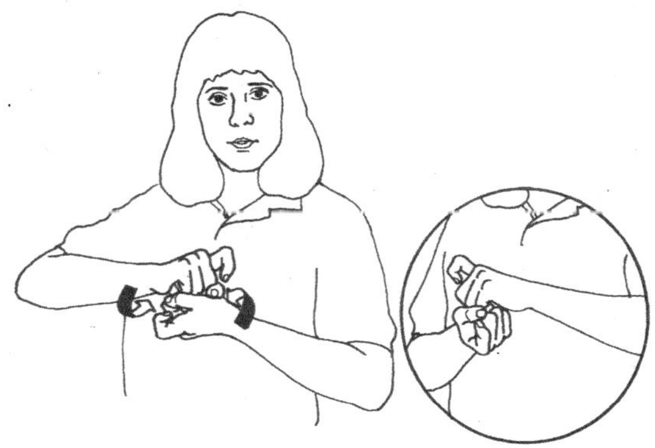

CHANGE
X hands, chest level, right palm on left palm. Rotate hands 180 degrees, ending with left palm on right palm.

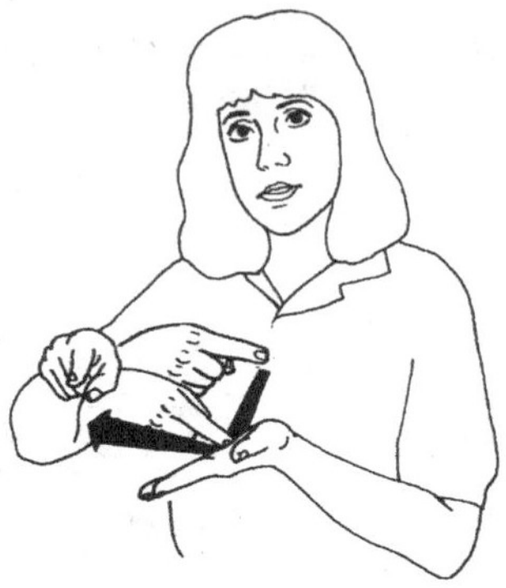

CHECK (verb)
Left flat hand, chest level, palm up. Right 1 hand, chest level, palm down. In open left palm, make a checking motion with right 1 hand.

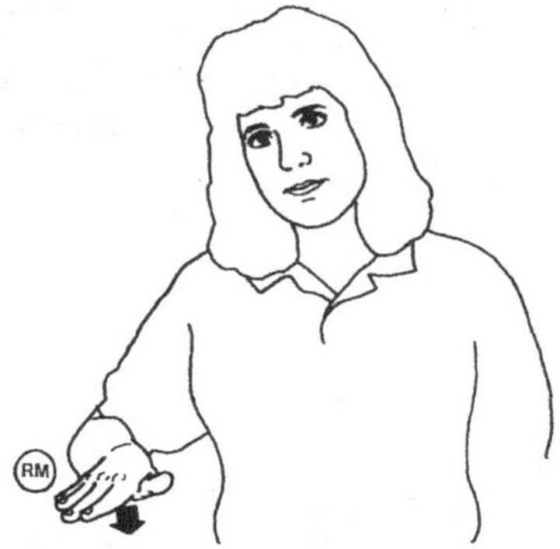

CHILD
Right 5 hand, palm down, waist level. Move hand up and down slightly.
Clue: patting a child's head.

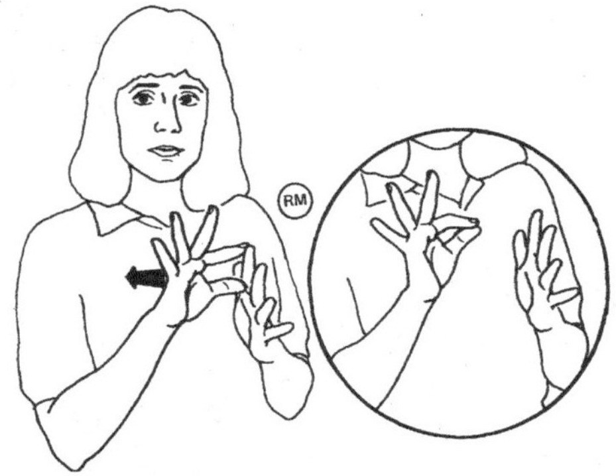

CHOICES
Right F hand, palm left. Left 5 hand, palm right, chest level. Move F to left index finger. Separate F at thumb and index finger while touching left index fingertip. Move back to F quickly. Repeat at middle finger.

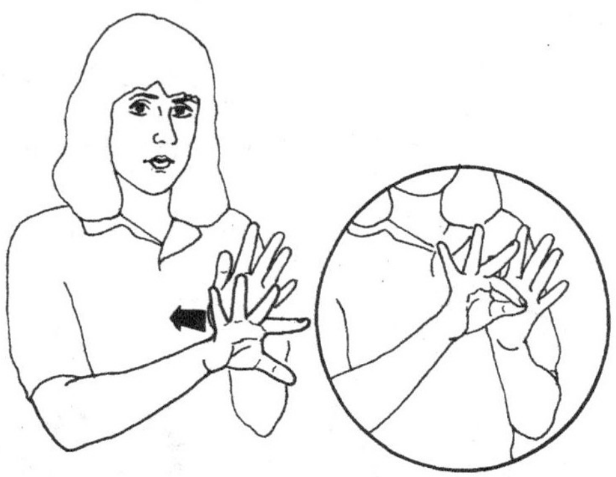

CHOOSE
Right 5 hand, chest level, palm out. Left 5 hand, chest level, palm right. Brush right 5 against left palm, changing to an F hand.
Clue: picking out your choice of something.

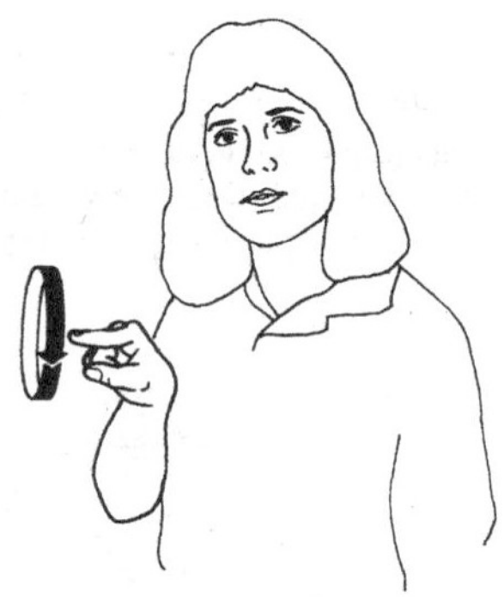

CIRCLE
Right 1 hand, palm out, moves in clockwise direction.
Clue: drawing a circle on a piece of paper.

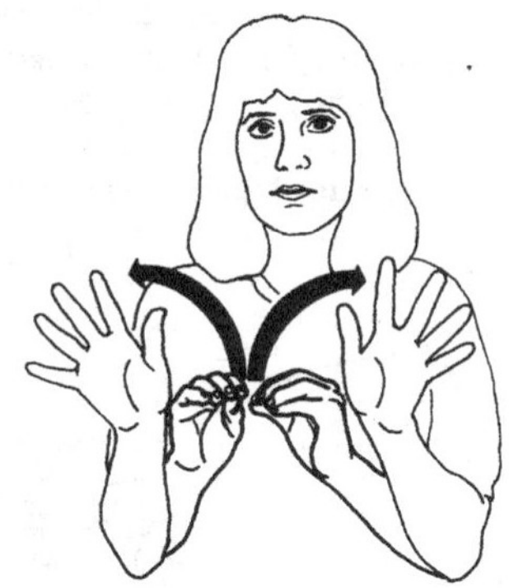

CLARITY
O hands, chest level, palms out. Simultaneously move to 5 hands, palms out.

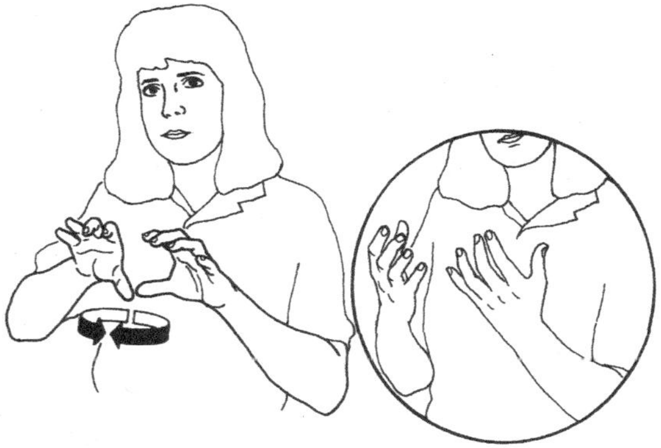

CLASSES
C hands, chest level, palms out, thumbs touching. Bring hands out in a circle until little fingers almost touch.

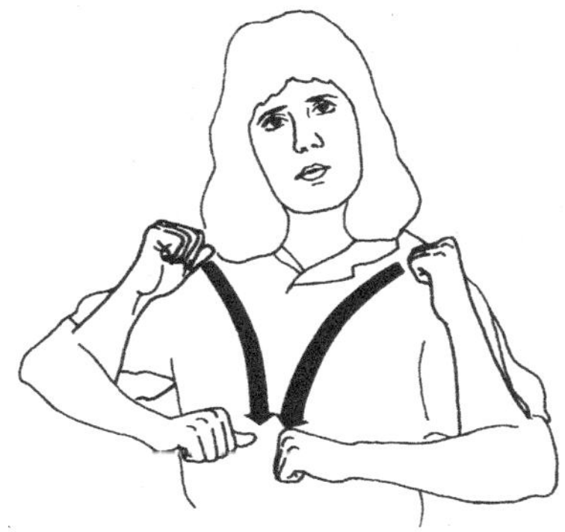

COAT
A hands, thumbs touching shoulders. Bring hands out and down to waist.

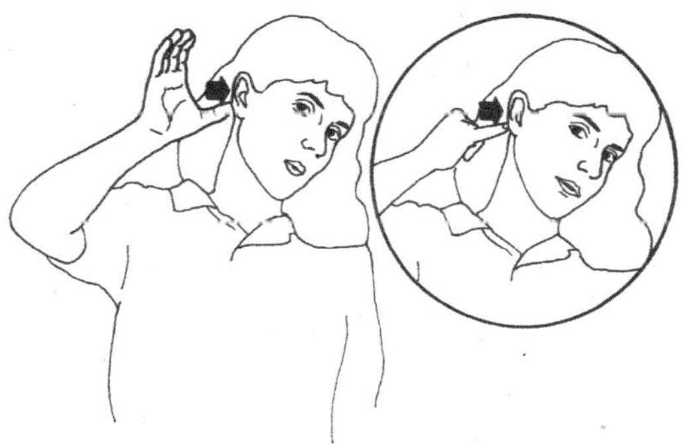

COCHLEAR IMPLANT
Right C hand, palm out, thumb behind right ear. Move down behind right ear changing C to I hand.

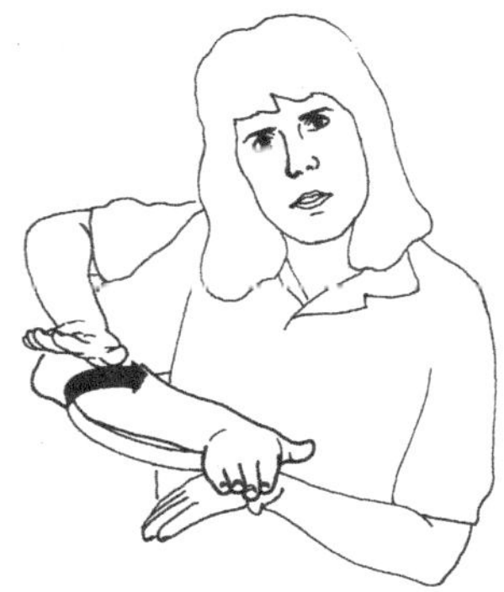

COLLEGE
Flat hands, waist level, palms together. Move right hand in a curving motion out and up from left hand.

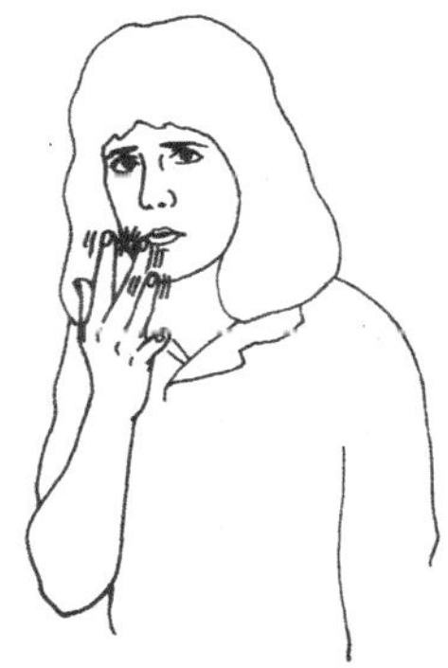

COLORS
Right 5 hand, palm facing in, at chin. Middle fingertips alternately touch chin.

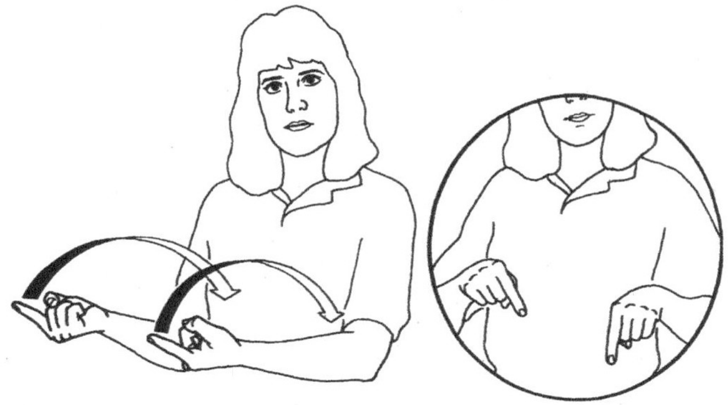

COME BACK
1 hands, chest level, palms up, right hand in front of left. Bring hands up and in to body, ending with fingers pointing down.

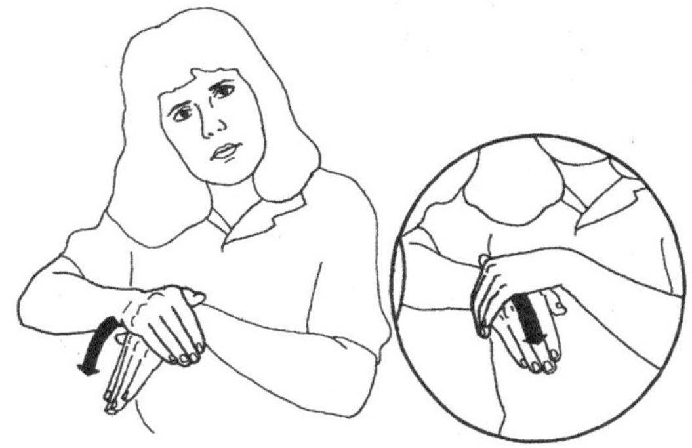

COMFORTABLE
Flat hands, chest level, palms down. Place right hand on top of left hand, pull left hand up and out to top of right hand. Repeat alternating hands.

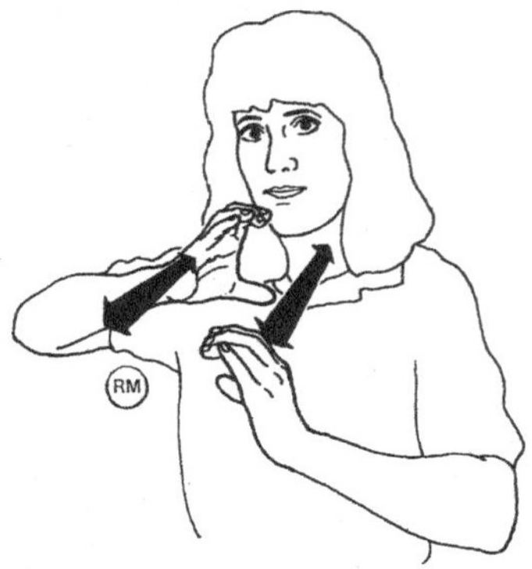

COMMUNICATION
C hands, chin level, palms face each other. Move hands alternately away from face.

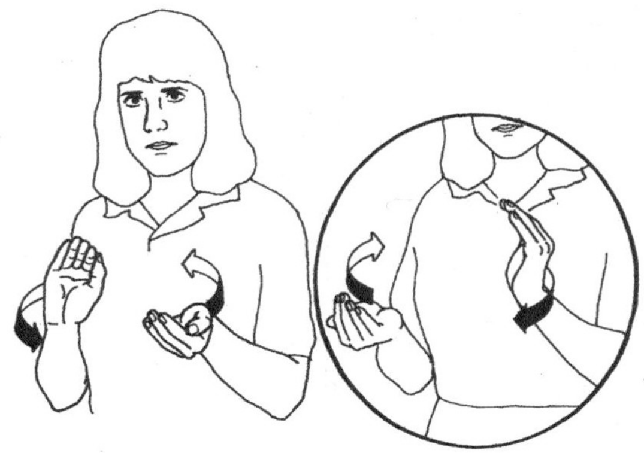

COMPARISON
Slightly curved hands, shoulder level, palms facing each other. Alternate hands toward and away from body. *Clue: examining two items in your hand.*

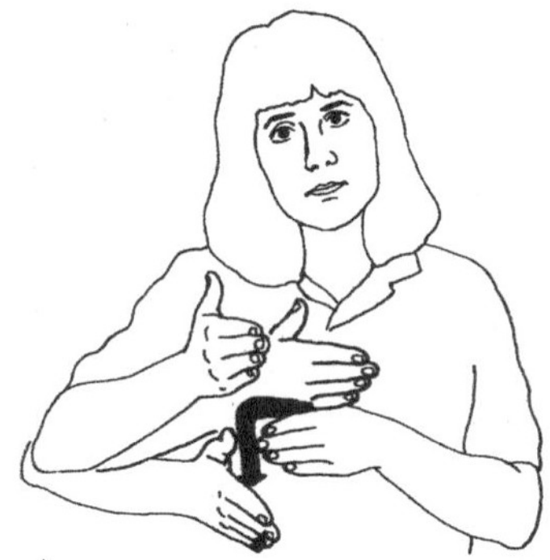

COMPLETE
Flat hands, chest level, right hand across left hand. Move right hand along left index finger, then straight down.

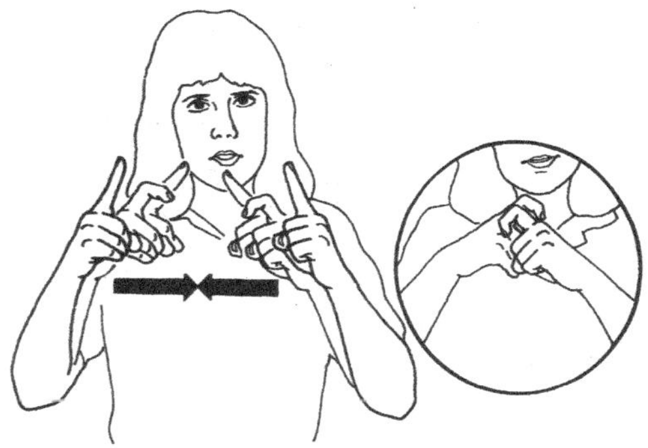

COMPLEX
1 hands, palms facing, shoulder level. As hands cross each other in front of face, fingers change from 1 to X hands repeatedly.

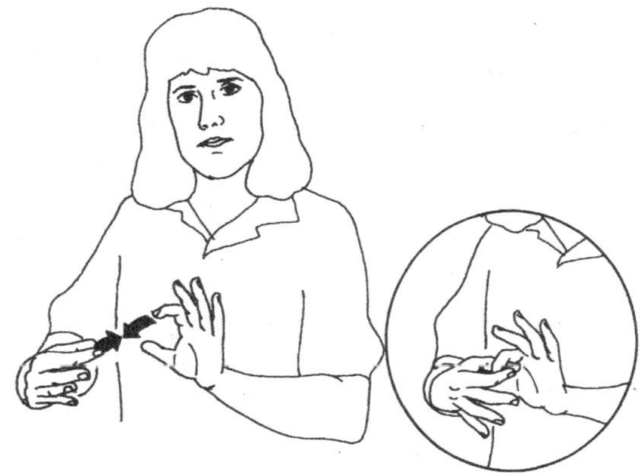

CONNECT
Rounded 5 hands, palms facing, chest level. Bring hands together, ending with thumbs and index fingers interlocked.

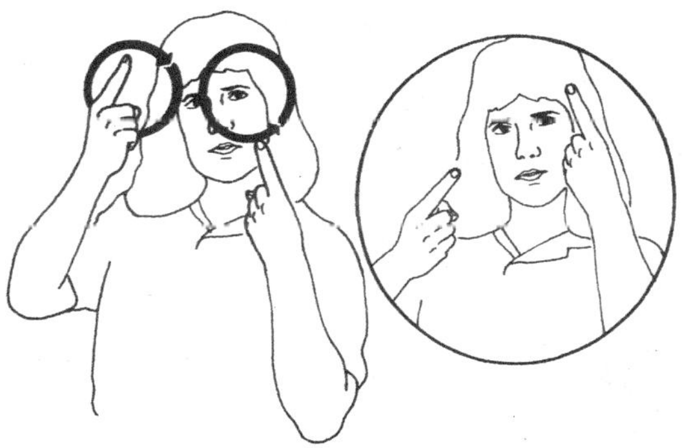

CONSIDER
1 hands, head level, palms in. Circle alternately in front of face.

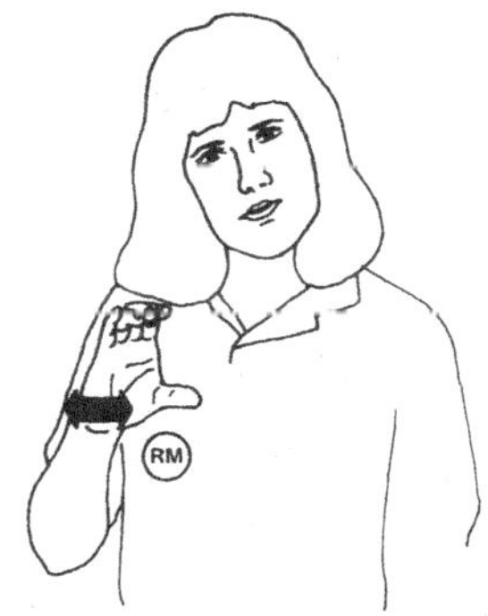

CONSONANT
Right C hand, palm out, chest level. Shake slightly, side-to-side.

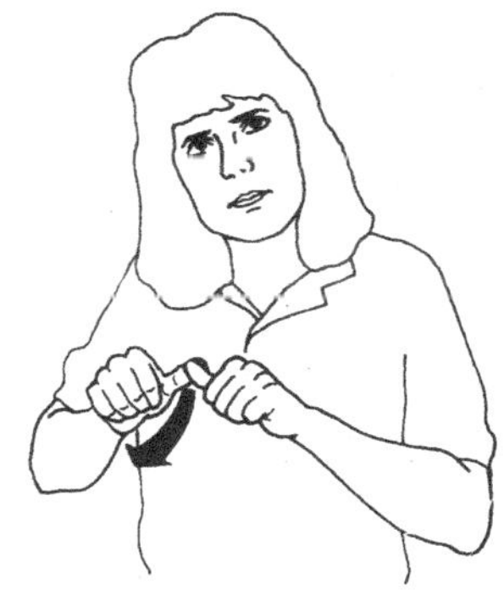

CONSTANT
A hands, chest level, palms down, thumbs touching. Move out from body twice.

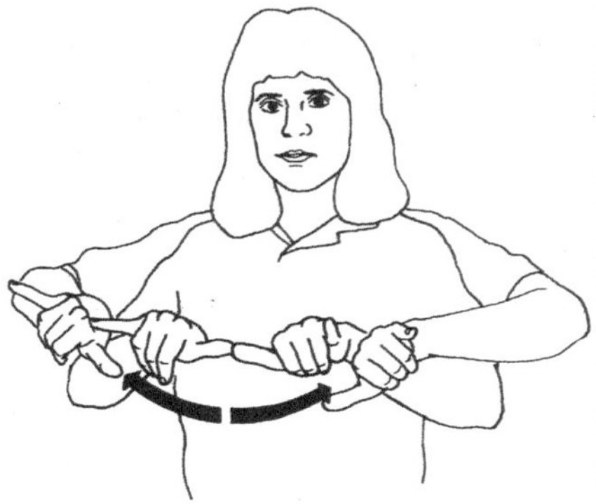

CONTINUUM
Y hands, palms down, thumbs touching, waist level. Bring hands apart and swing up to sides.

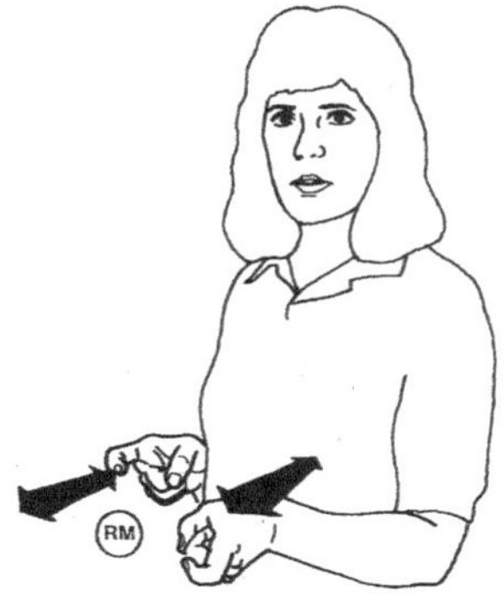

CONTROL
X hands, palms facing each other, chest level. (X index fingers pointing out.) Alternately move hands back and forth, away from body. Repeat.

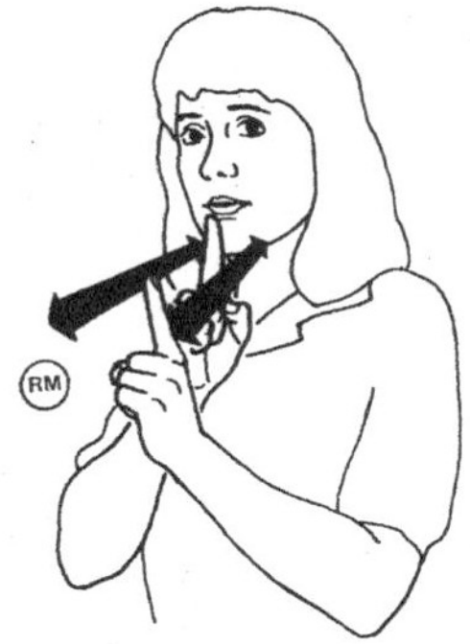

CONVERSE/TALK
1 hands, chin level, palms facing each other slightly. Alternately move hands back and forth to chin.

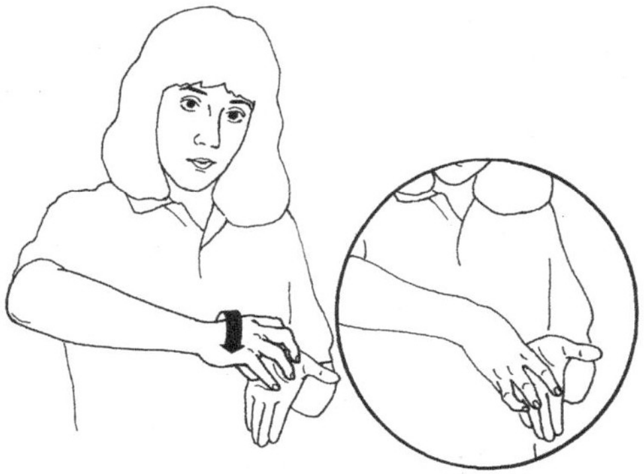

COOKIE
Left flat hand, palm up, chest level. Right claw hand, palm down, fingertips resting on left palm. Turn right hand from side-to-side.
Clue: using a cookie cutter.

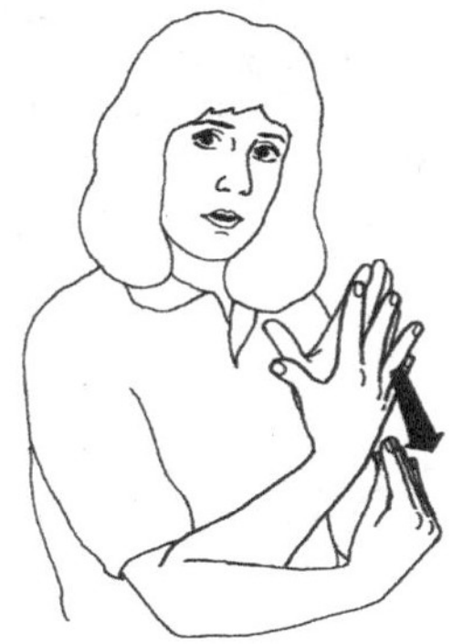

COPY
Left 5 hand, palm out, shoulder level. Right 5 hand fingers on left hand. Bring right hand out and close hand so fingertips touch.
Clue: your right (dominant) hand is making a copy of your left hand.

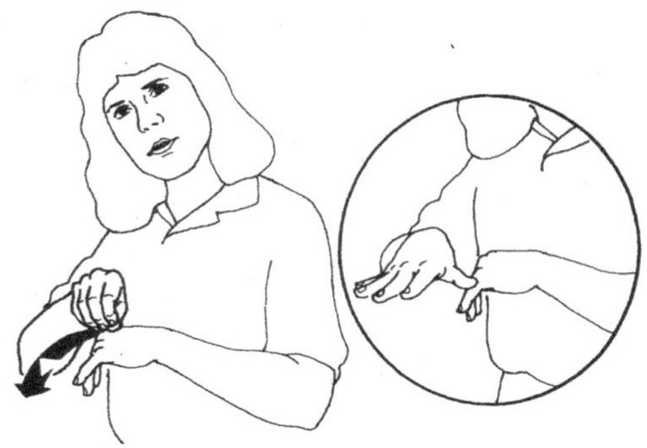

COUNSELING/INFLUENCE
Right O hand on back of left flat hand, at chest level, palms down. Move right hand away from body, opening to 5 handshape, palm down. Repeat.

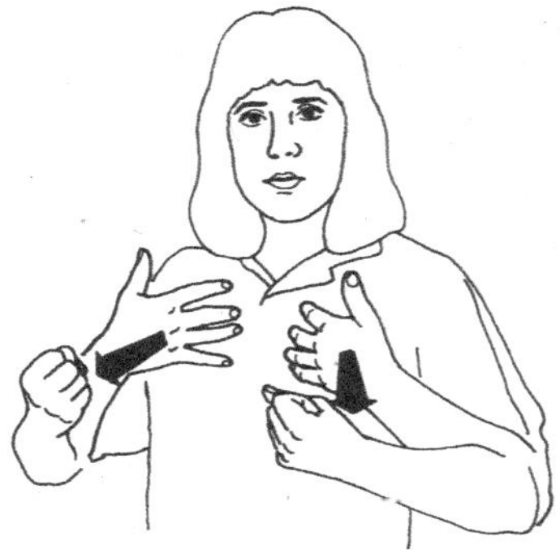

COURAGE
5 hands fingertips touching shoulders. Move forward into S handshapes.

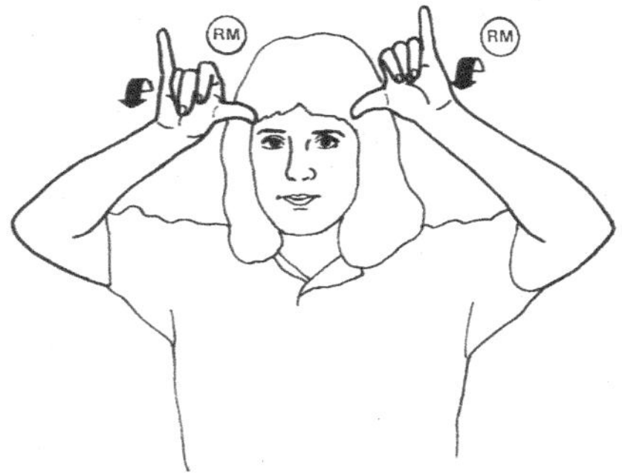

COW
Y hands, thumbs on side of head near temples. Rotate hands down.
Clue: resembles the horns on a male steer.

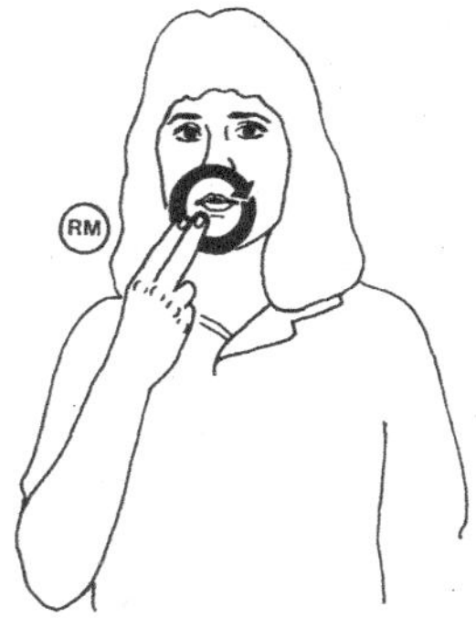

CUED SPEECH
Right H hand, palm in, at mouth level. Move in small counterclockwise circle.

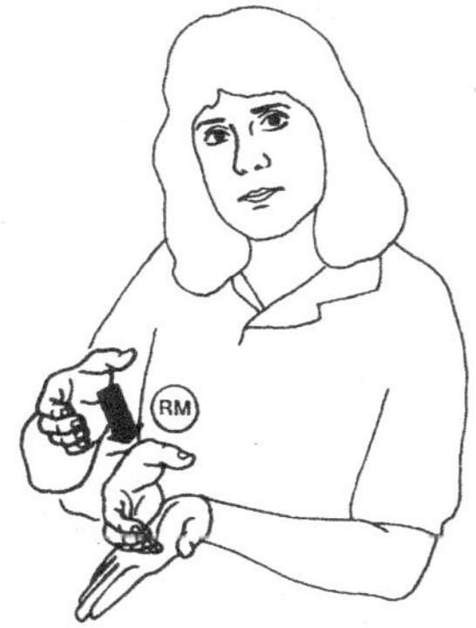

CUP
Right C hand, palm facing left. Move up and down on left flat palm.
Clue: the movement shape is similar to a cup in your hand.

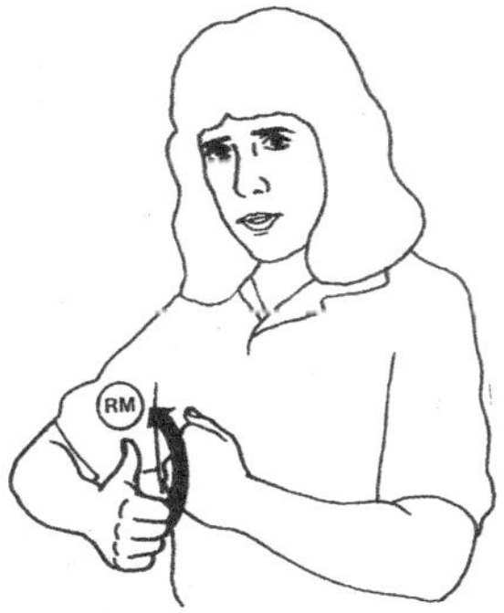

DANGEROUS
Right A hand, thumb up, palm in. Left S hand, palm in, chest level. Right hand in front of left. Brush A against left hand. Repeat.

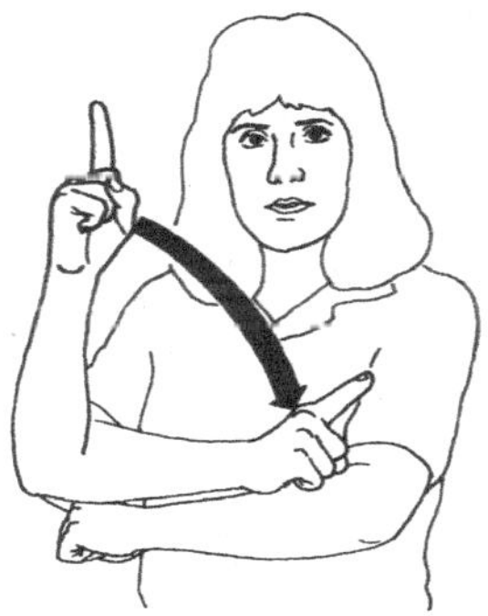

DAY
Left arm folded at waist, palm down. Right 1 hand, palm left, arm straight up, elbow on back of left hand. Bring right arm down in front of body to rest on top of left arm.

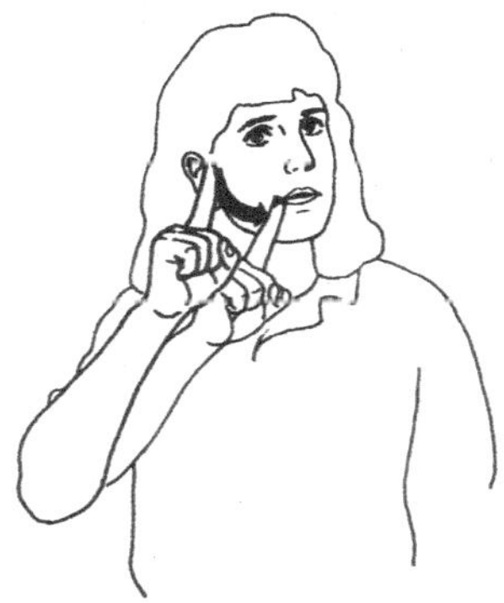

DEAF
Right 1 hand points to right ear, then side of mouth.

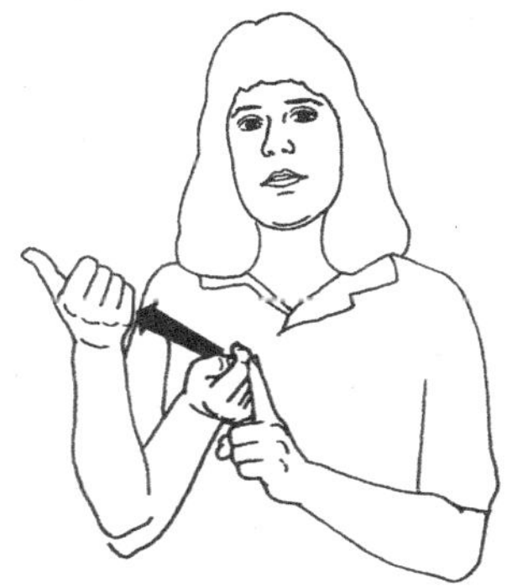

DELETE/ELIMINATE
Left 1 hand, chest level, palm right. Right closed hand, thumb touching index finger, palm in, touching left index finger. Quickly flick right thumb against index finger.

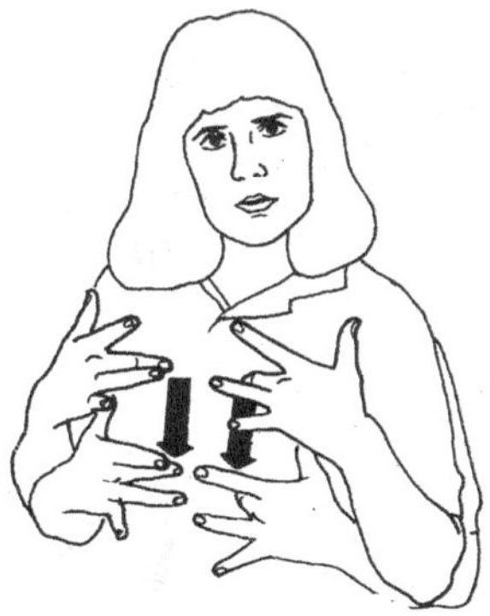

DEPRESSED
5 hands, palms in, middle fingers touching chest. Move hands down.

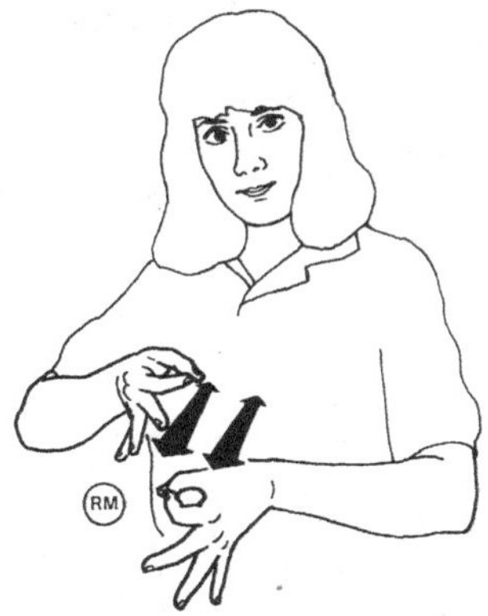

DESCRIBE/EXPLAIN
F hands, palms facing each other, waist level. Alternately move hands back and forth.

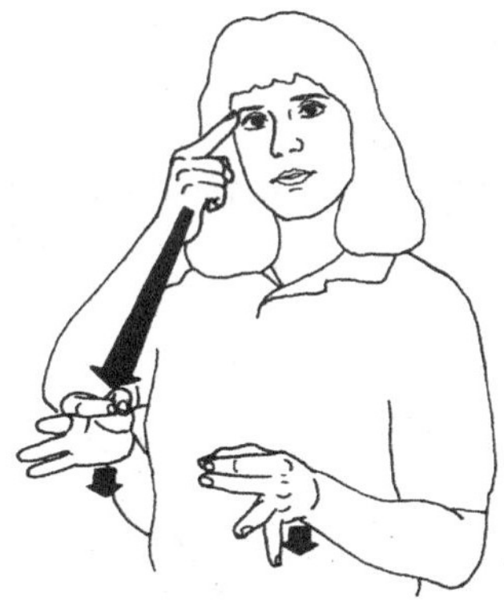

DETERMINE
Right 1 hand, palm in, touching right temple. Left F hand, palm right, chest level. Move right hand down, changing to F handshape, palm facing left palm.

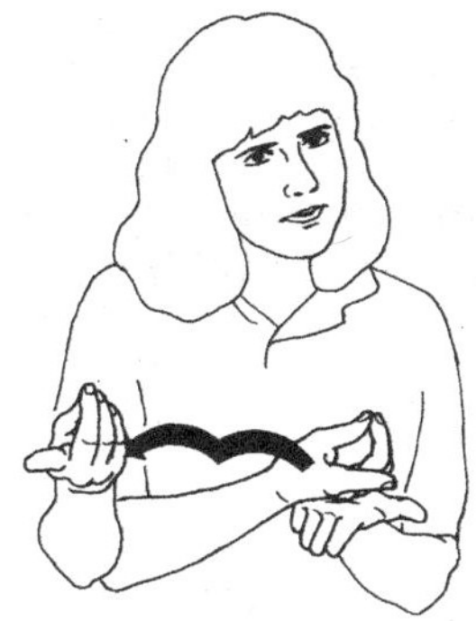

DEVICES
Right D hand, palm up. Left flat hand, palm up, chest level. D hits left palm, then moves to the right, bouncing two times.

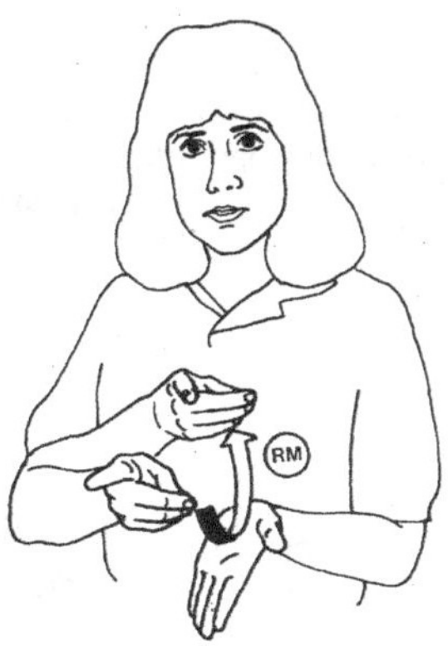

DICTIONARY
Left flat hand, palm up, chest level. Right D hand, palm left, on left palm. Circle right hand in a clockwise direction on left palm.
Clue: flipping through pages in a book.

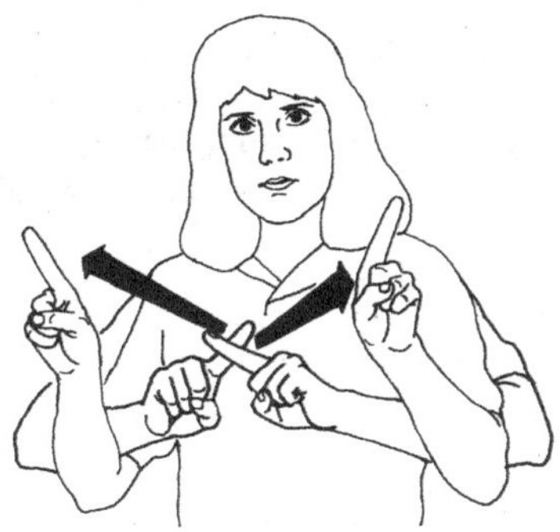

DIFFERENT
1 hands, chest level, palms out, fingers crossed. Move hands apart.

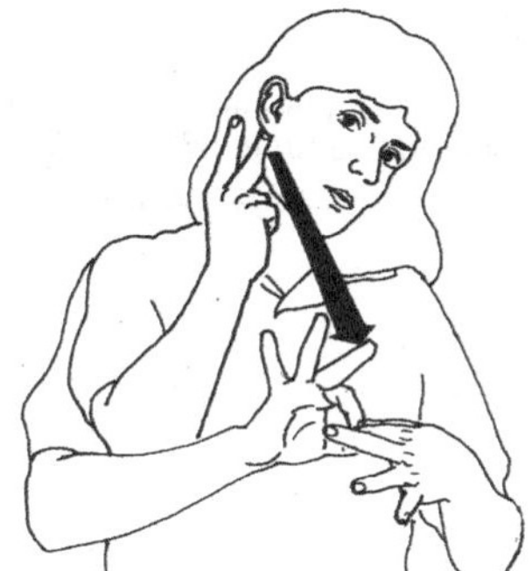

DIRECT AUDIO INPUT
Right V hand behind right ear. Move hand down, changing to F handshape. Interlock thumb and index finger with left F hand.

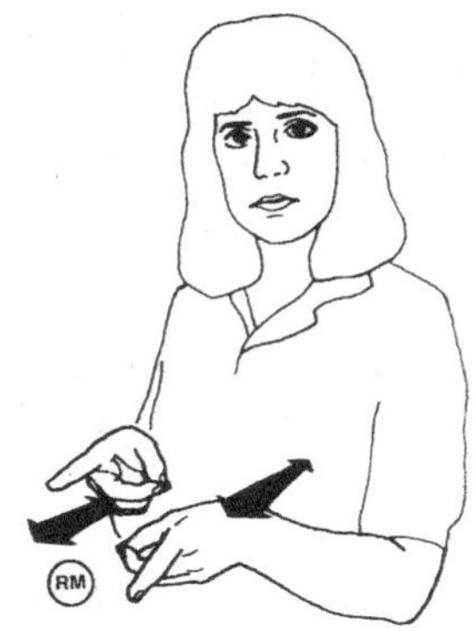

DIRECTIONS
D hands, palms facing each other, waist level. Move alternately back and forth.

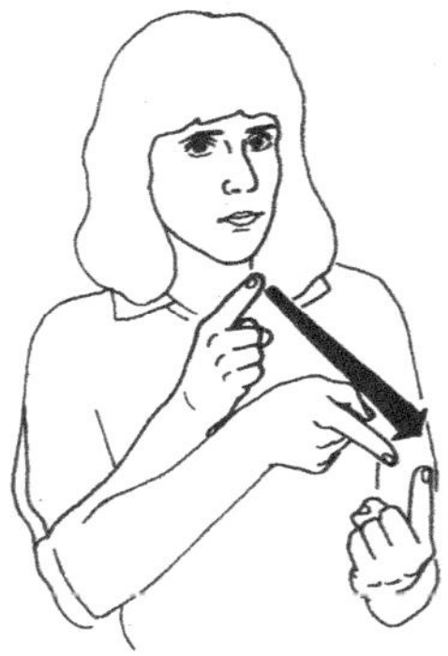

DIRECTLY
Right 1 hand, finger up, palm in, chest level. Left 1 hand, finger up, palm right, chest level. Move right hand at wrist until index fingers touch.

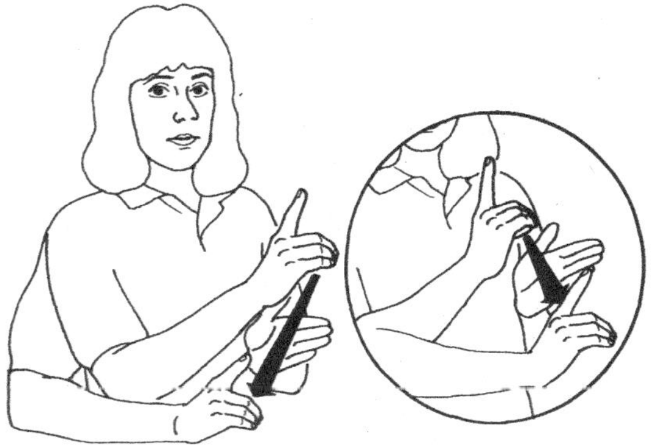

DISCRIMINATE
Left flat hand, palm right, chest level. Right D hand, palm left, on left palm. Right hand crisscrosses left palm.

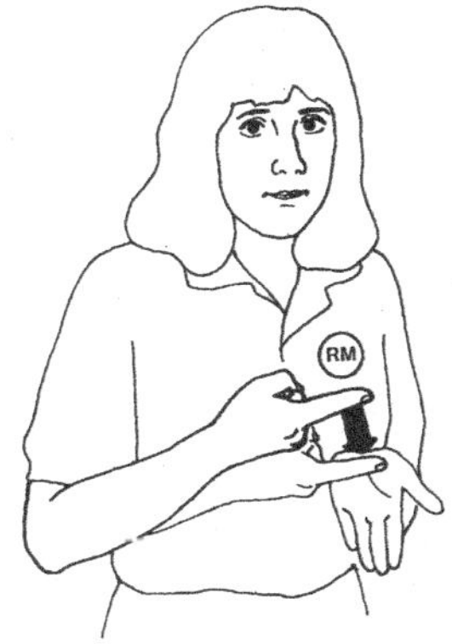

DISCUSS
Right 1 hand, palm in, chest level. Left flat hand, palm up, chest level. Right 1 taps left palm repeatedly.

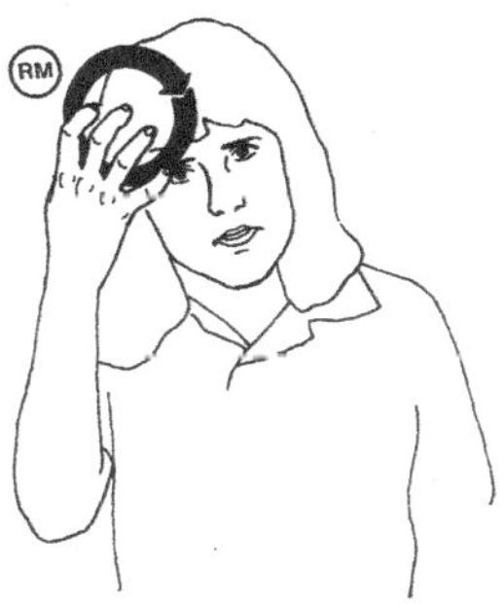

DIZZINESS/DIZZY
Claw hand, head level, palm in. Move hand in a counterclockwise direction.

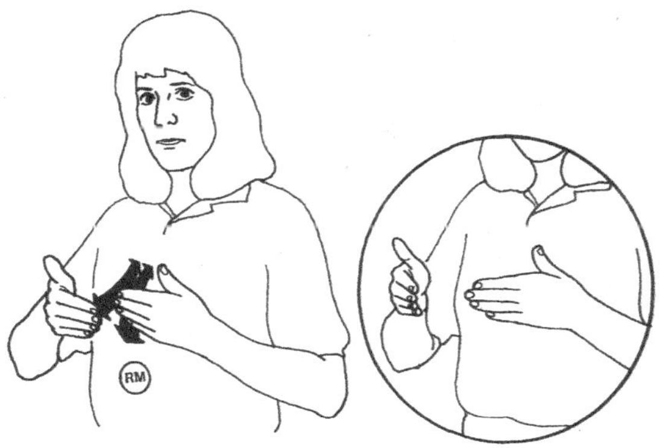

DOESN'T MATTER
Flat hands, palms in, chest level, right hand slightly in front of left. Flap right hand back and forth across left hand fingertips. Repeat. Shake head while producing this sign.

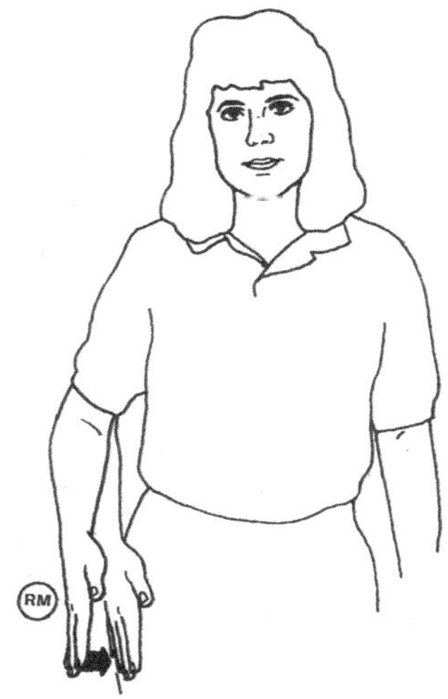

DOG
Right flat hand slaps right thigh.
Clue: calling a dog.

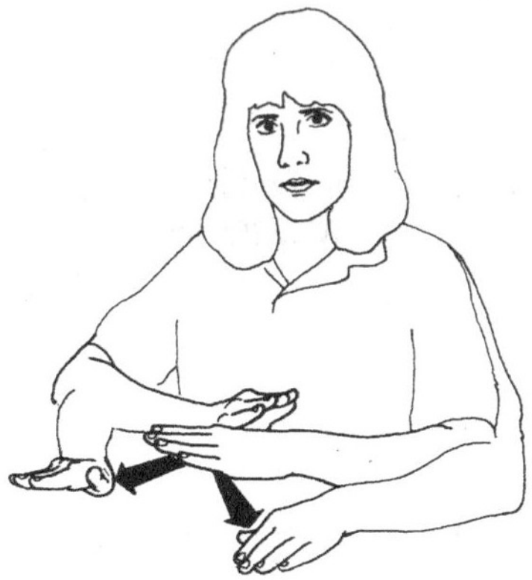

DON'T
Flat hands, waist level, palms down, hands crossed. Uncross hands in a quick movement.

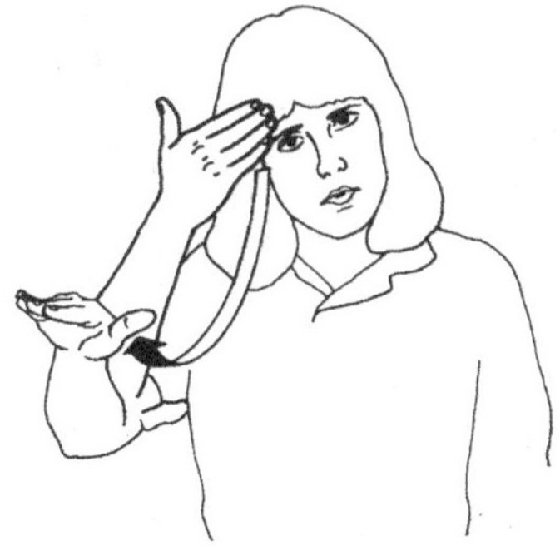

DON'T KNOW
Right flat hand, palm in, fingertips touching right temple. Sweep away from face to palm down.

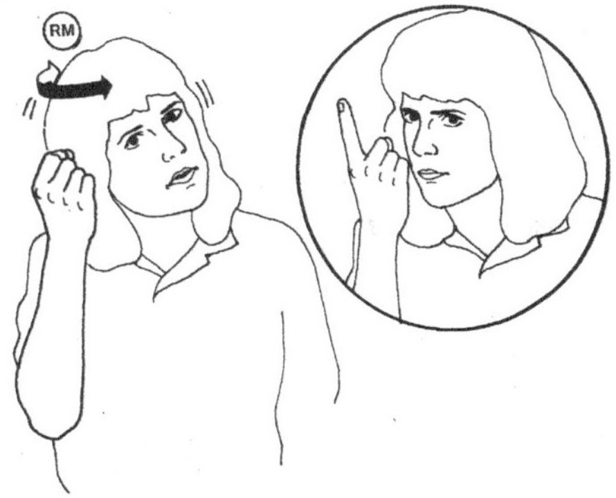

DON'T UNDERSTAND
Right S hand, palm in at right side of forehead. Flick index finger up quickly to 1 handshape. Shake head "no."

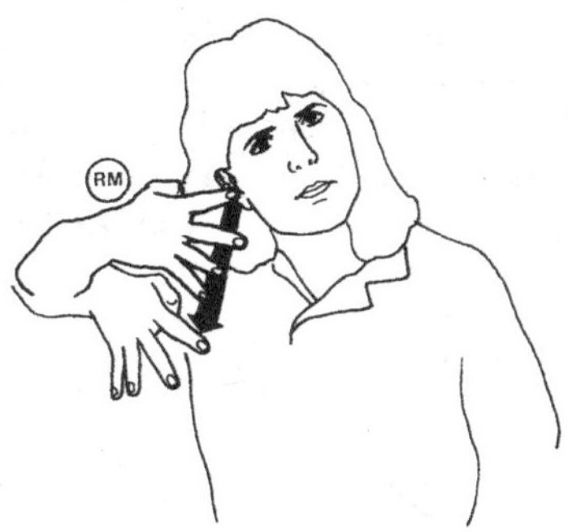

DRAINAGE
Right 4 hand, palm in, at ear. Move hand up and down.
Clue: draining ears.

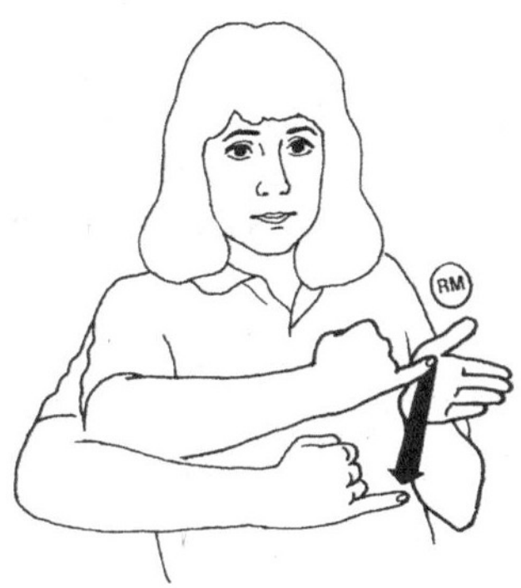

DRAW
Right I hand, palm in. Left flat hand, palm tilted, waist level. Place I at thumb of left hand and move down left palm in a wavy line.

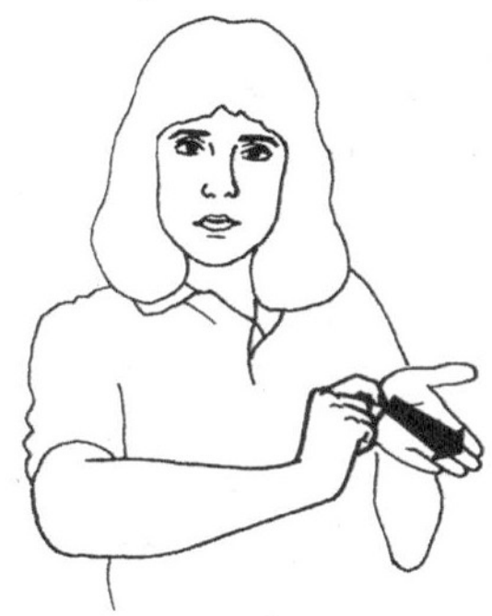

DRAW A LINE
Right hand closed, thumb and index finger touching, palm down. Left flat hand, palm up, chest level. Place right thumb and index finger on heel of left palm and move across palm to fingertips.

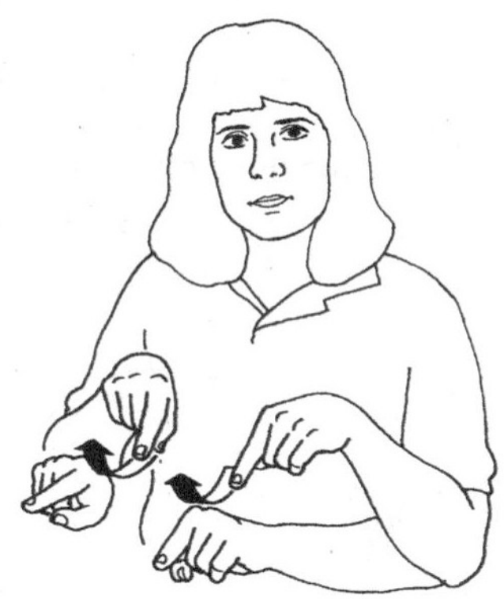

DURING
1 hands, palms down, chest level. Move in a slight curve up and away from body simultaneously.

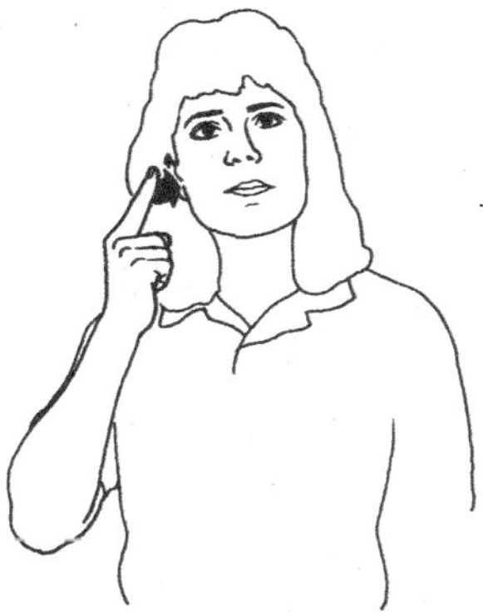

EAR/HEAR/HEARING
Right 1 hand points to one or both ears.

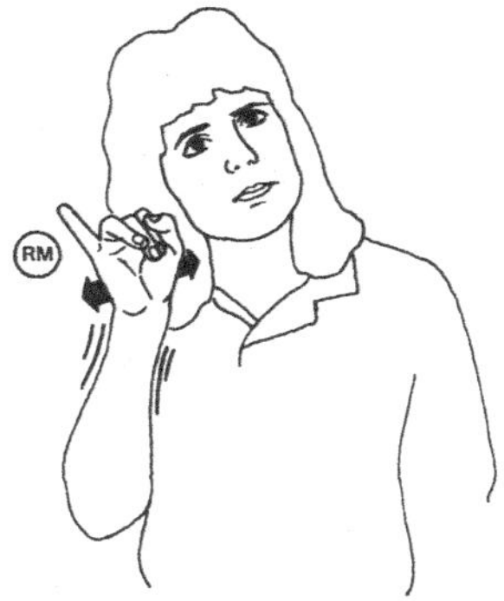

EAR INFECTION
Right I hand, ear level, palm out. Shake hand back and forth.

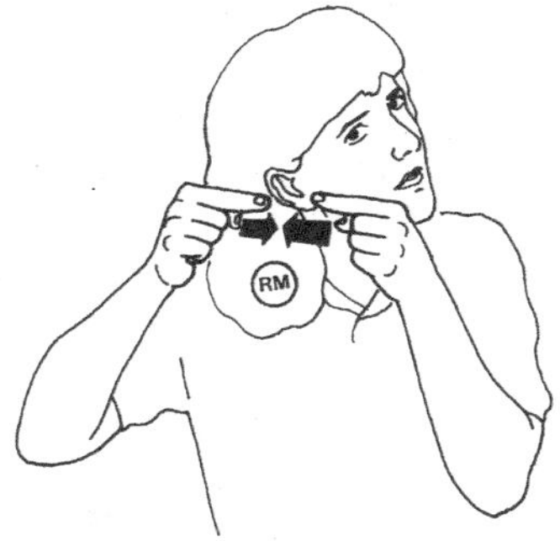

EARACHE
1 hands, palms in, index fingers facing, at right ear. Move index fingers toward and away from each other. Repeat.

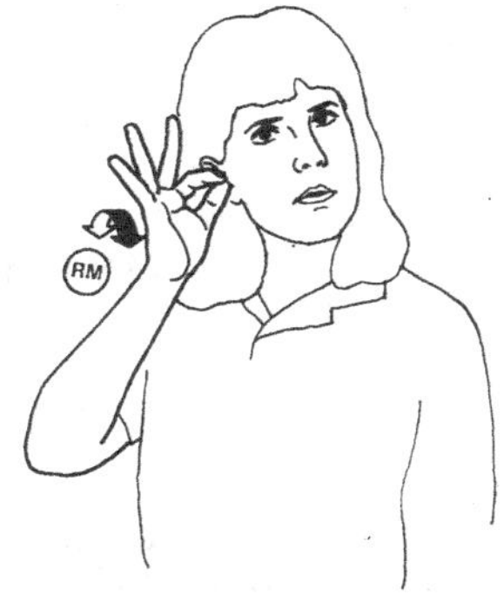

EARMOLD
Right F hand, palm in, at right ear. Twist slightly back and forth.
Clue: the action of inserting an earmold.

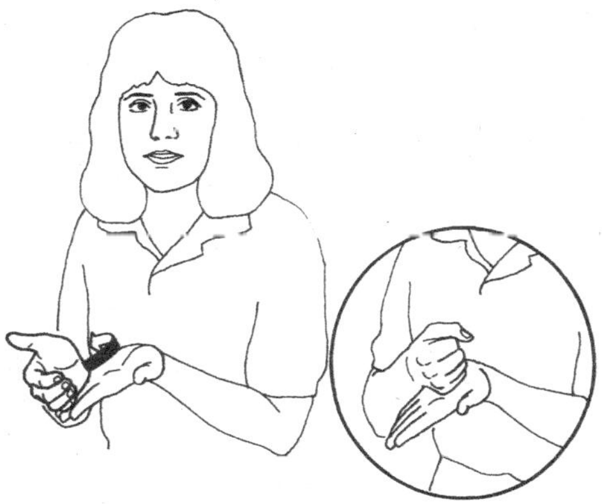

EARN
Left flat hand, palm up, waist level. Right C hand, palm in. Right hand brushes across left palm, closing to A handshape.
Clue: collecting money in the palm of your hand.

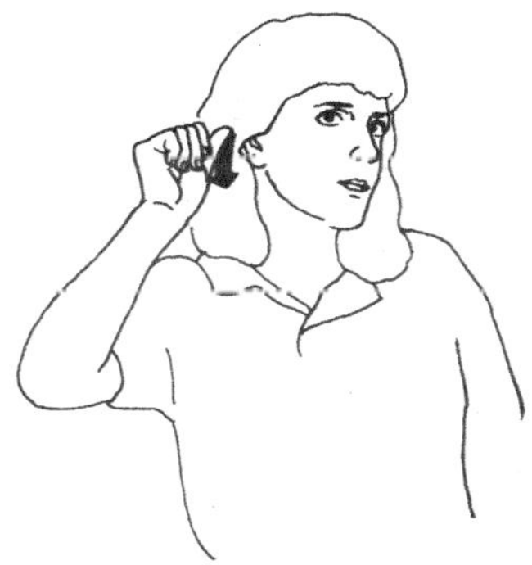

EAR SURGERY
Right A hand, palm out, thumb behind right ear. Move hand down.

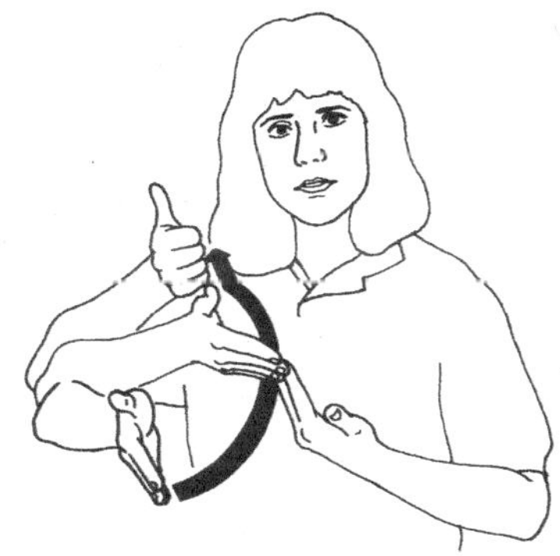

EASIER
Flat hands, palms up, waist level. Left hand on top of right fingers. Bring right hand up, brushing left fingertips, ending in 10 handshape.

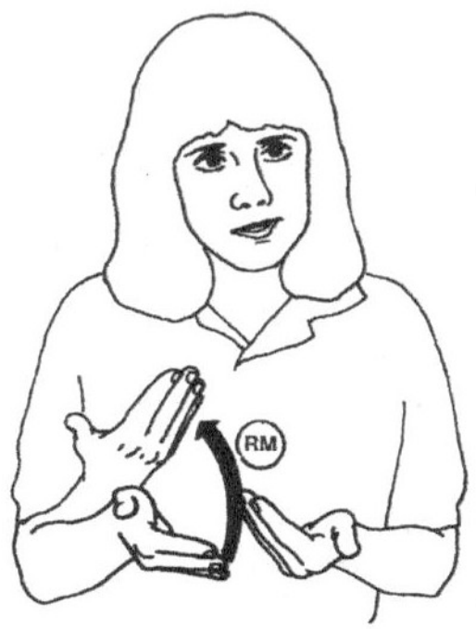

EASY
Flat hands, palms up, waist level. Fingertips of right hand come up from under left hand and brush fingertips of left hand repeatedly.

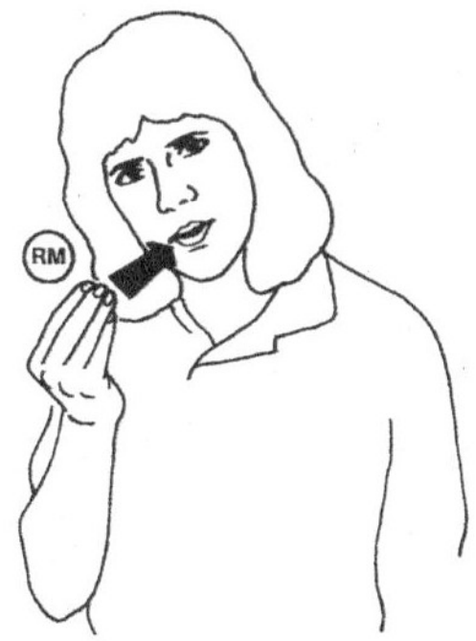

EAT
Right flat O hand, palm in, at mouth. Move repeatedly towards mouth. *Clue: putting food in mouth.*

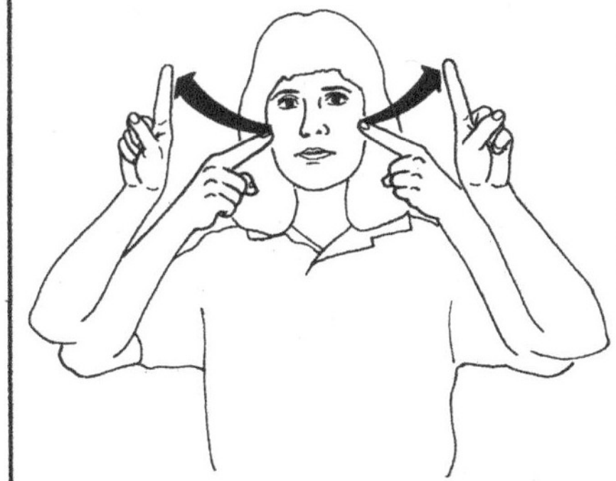

EFFECTIVE/ACHIEVE
1 hands, palms down, touching corners of mouth. Swoop up to palms out, eye level.

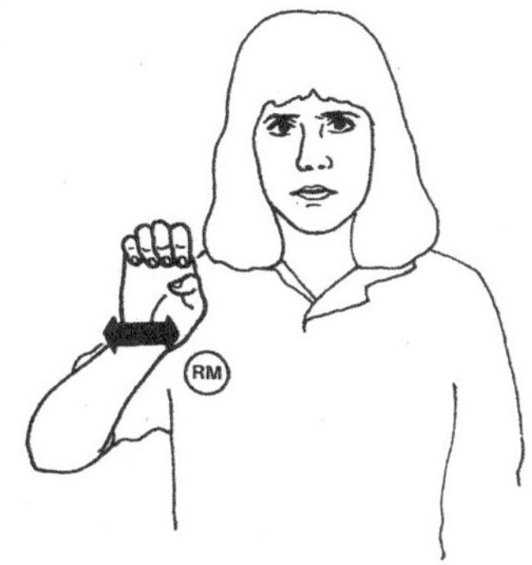

EMERGENCY
Right E hand, palm out, shoulder level. Shake hand left to right repeatedly.

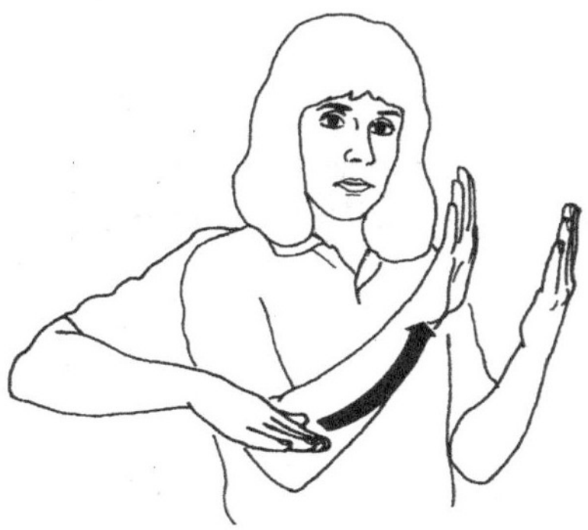

ENCOUNTER
Flat hands, left palm out, chest level. Right hand out from body, palm down, chest level. Right hand sweeps in towards body, until palms face each other.

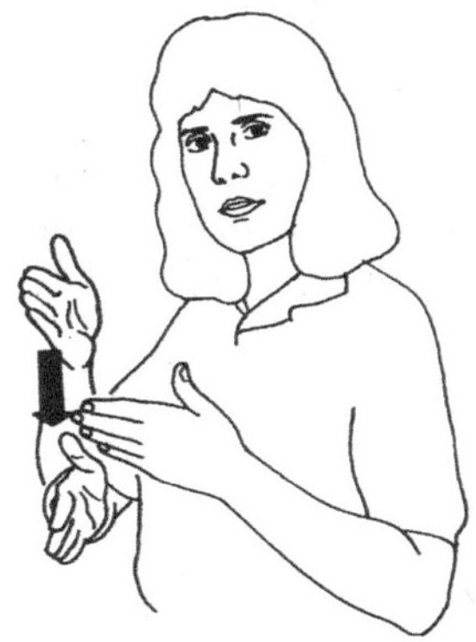

END
Flat hands, chest level, left palm right, right palm in, right hand above left, near fingertips. Bring right hand straight down.

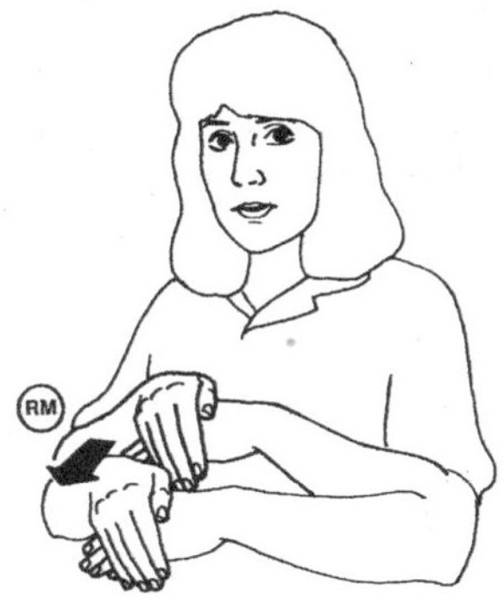

ENGLISH
Left flat hand, palm down, waist level. Right hand, palm down, clutches left hand.

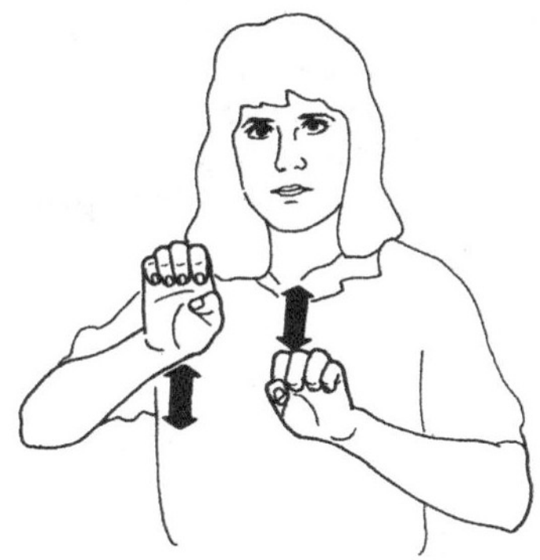

EVALUATE
E hands, chest level, palms out. Alternately move hands up and down.

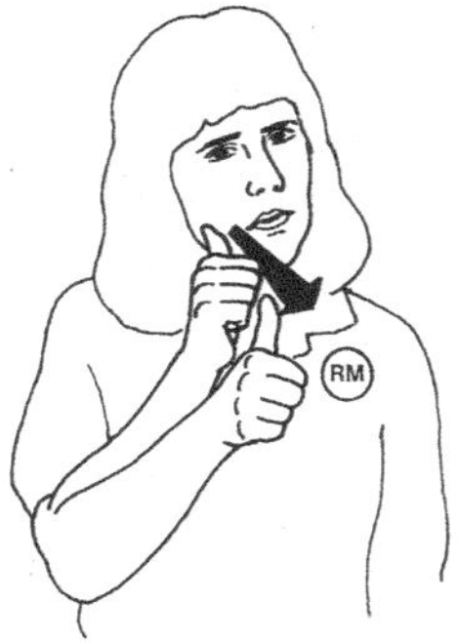

EVERYDAY
Right A hand, thumb extended, palm left, at right cheek. Quickly stroke A out from face slightly. Repeat.

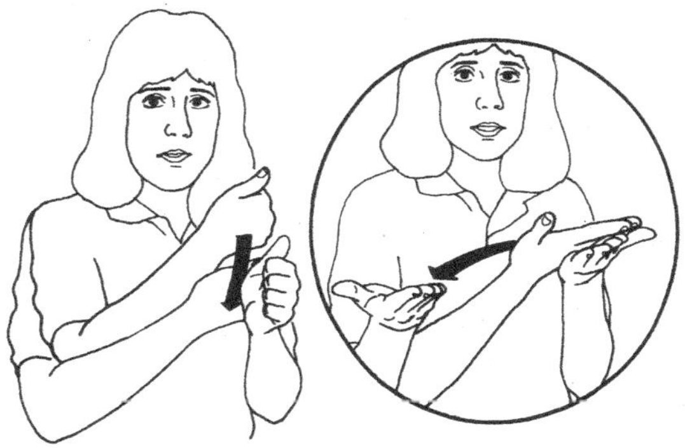

EVERYTHING
A hands, waist level. Left hand, palm right, right hand, palm in. Right hand comes down thumb on left hand and moves to right, opening to 5 hand, palm up.

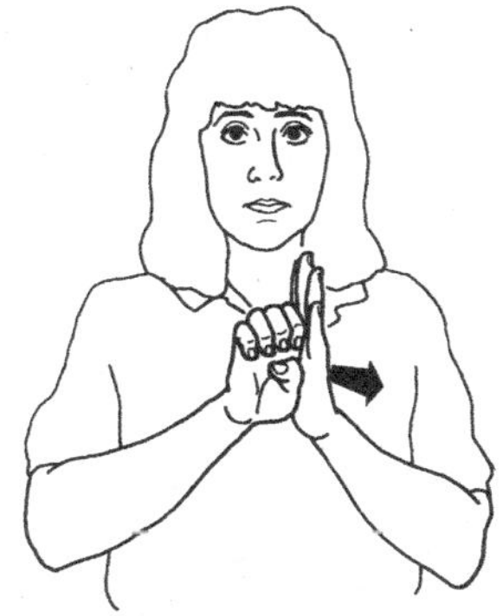

EXAMPLE
Left flat hand, chest level, palm right. Right E hand touching left palm. Move hands forward.

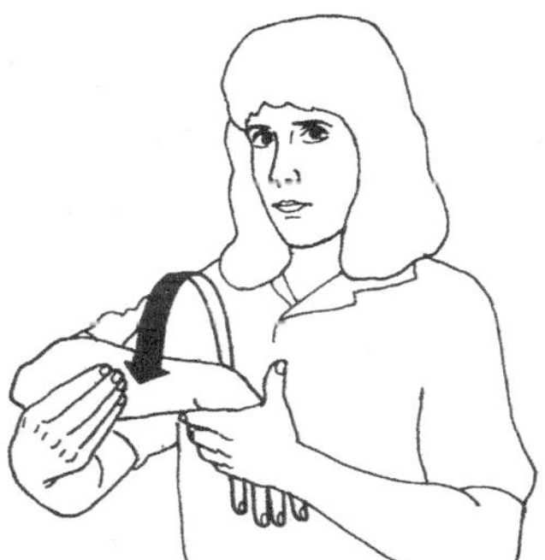

EXHALATION
Left C hand, palm in, chest level. Right O hand in left hand. Bring right hand out of left.
Clue: air coming out of lungs.

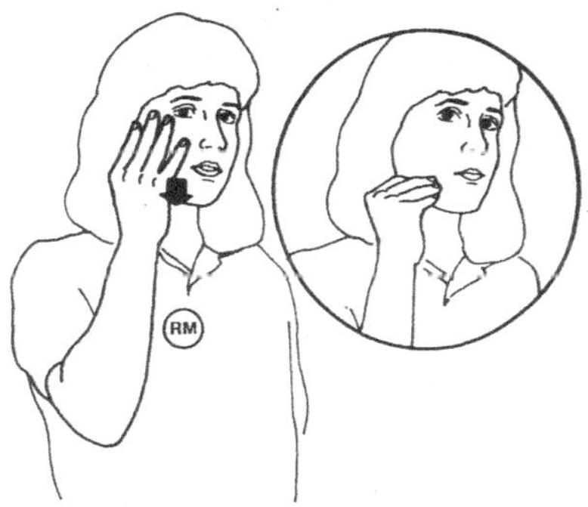

EXPERIENCE
Right 5 hand on right cheek. Bring hand down side of face, closing to O hand. Repeat movement.

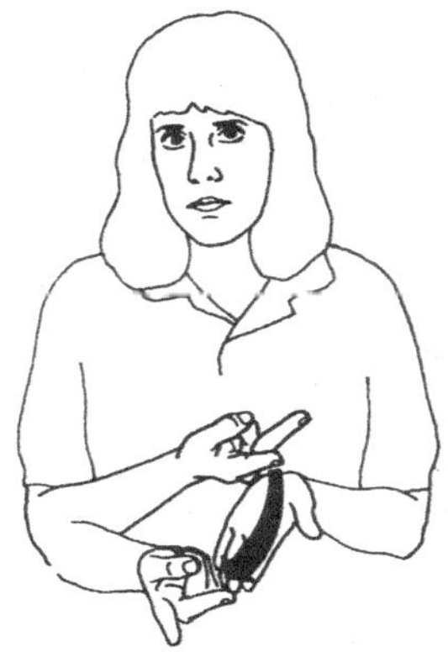

FAIL
Right V hand, palm up. Left flat hand, palm up, waist level. Place V at left wrist and sweep across left palm, slightly beyond fingertips.

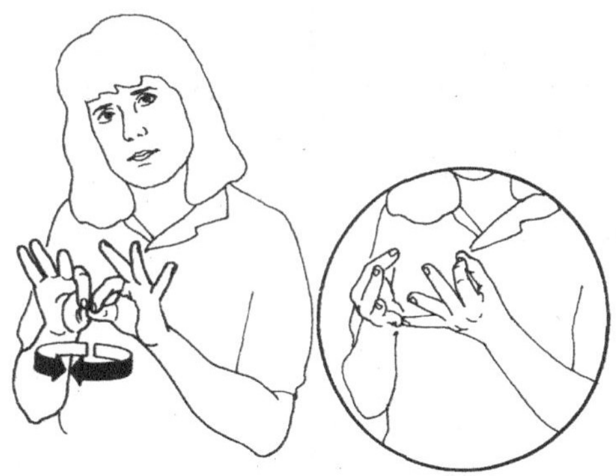

FAMILY
F hands, chest level, palms out, thumbs touching. Bring hands out in a circle until little fingers touch.

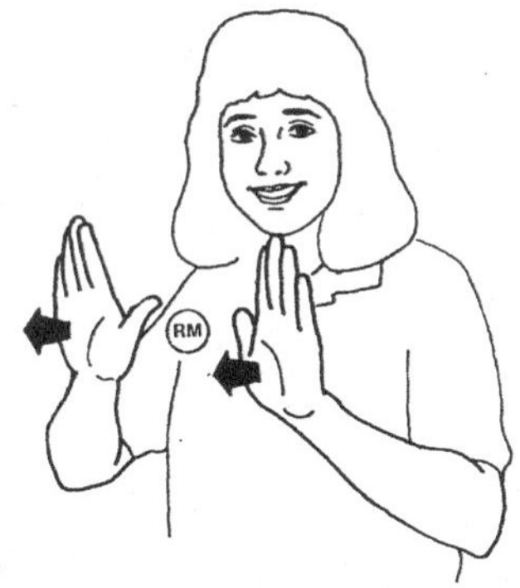

FANTASTIC/WONDERFUL
Flat hands, palms out, chest level. Push hands simultaneously away from body. Repeat.

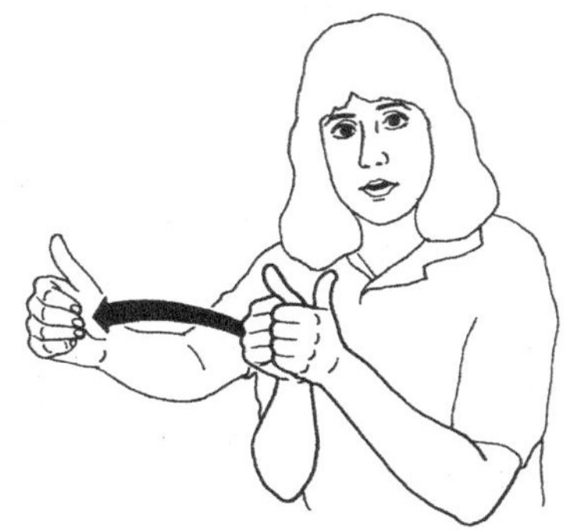

FAR
10 hands, palms facing each other, chest level. Quickly move right 10 away from left, extending right arm.

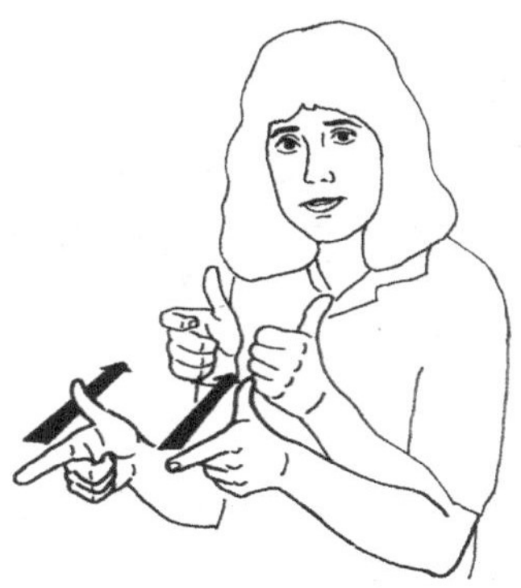

FAST
L hands, palms facing each other, chest level. Simultaneously pull back hands and quickly crook index fingers.

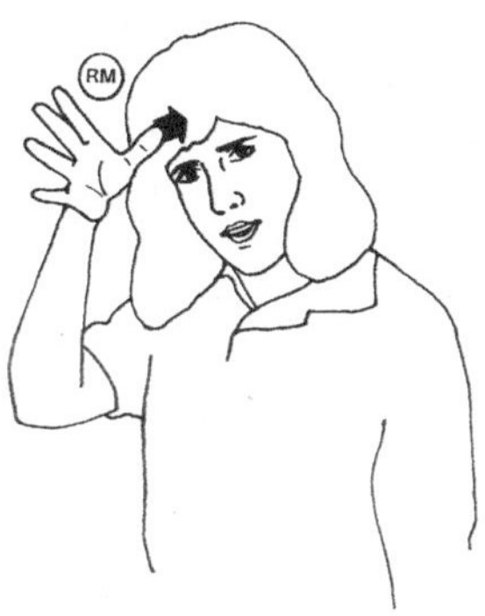

FATHER
Right 5 hand, palm left. Repeatedly tap forehead with thumb.

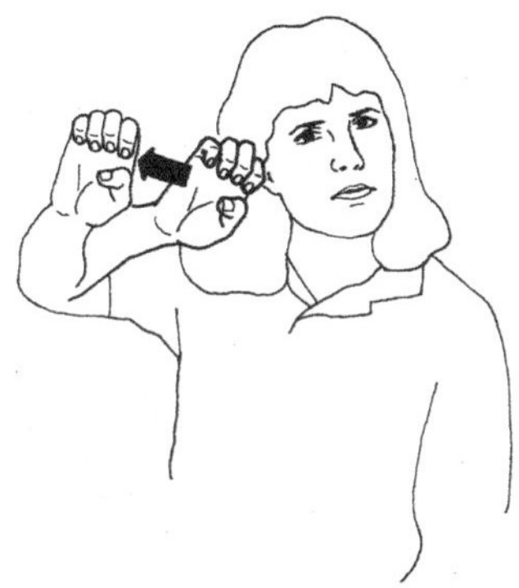

FEEDBACK
Right E hand, palm out, right ear level. Move back and forth from ear repeatedly.
Clue: simulates the EEEEE sound from a hearing aid.

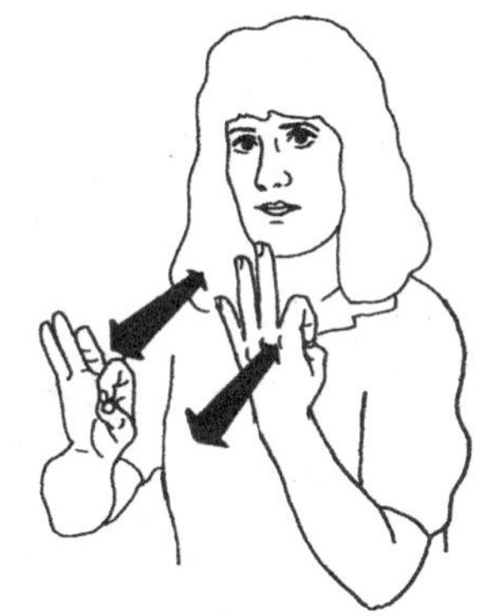

FEEDBACK
F hands, right palm out, left palm in, chin level. Move hands alternately away from and towards face.

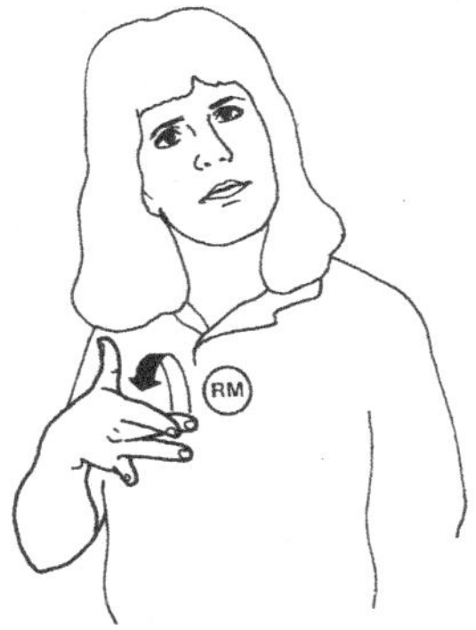

FEEL
Right 5 hand, middle finger bent, palm in, fingertips left, chest level. Touch middle finger to chest and flick up and slightly away from chest.

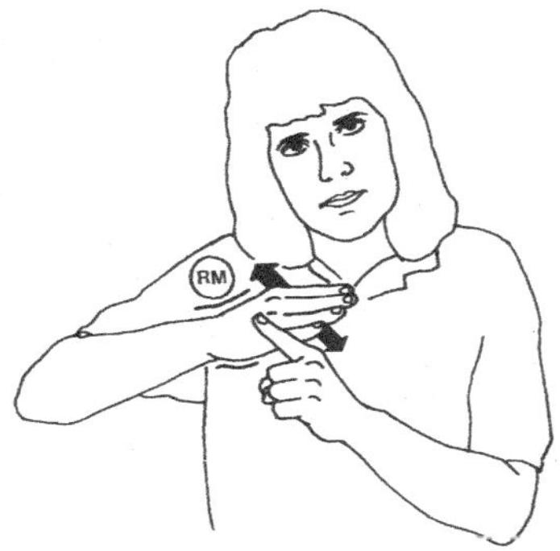

FEVER
Left 1 hand, palm right, chest level. Right B hand, palm down, touching top of left index finger. Right hand slides up and down on left finger.
Clue: the temperature going up and down on thermometer.

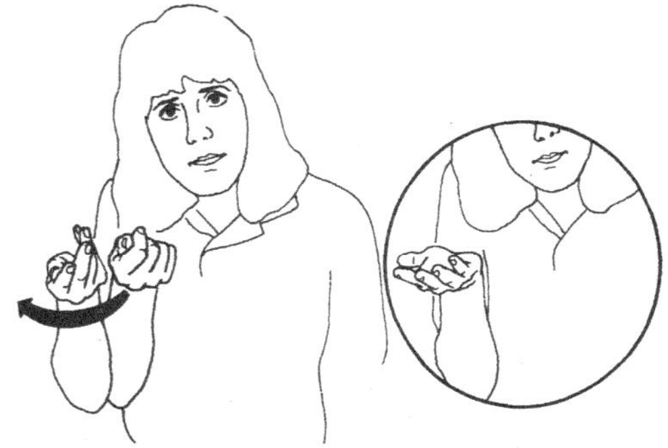

FEW
Right A hand, palm up, chest level. Beginning with index finger, extend each finger slowly while thumb moves across inside base of each.

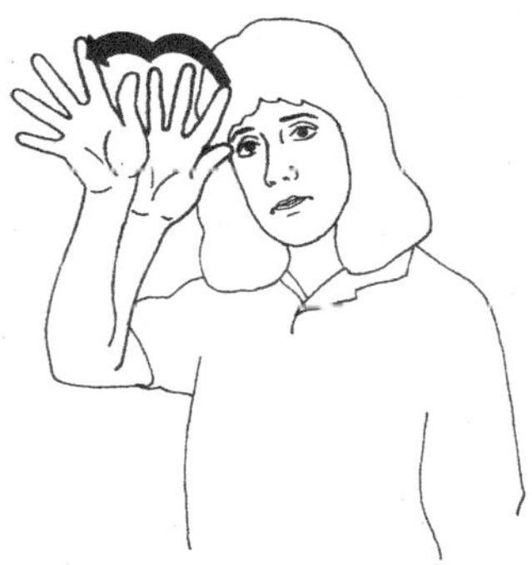

FIGURATIVE
Right 5 hand, palm left, index finger touching forehead. Bring hand out from head in a slightly choppy movement.

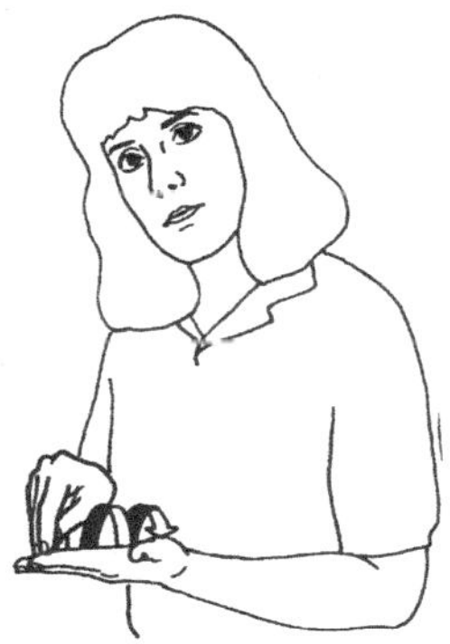

FILL IN
Left flat hand, waist level, palm up. Right O hand, palm down, on left fingertips. Bounce right O down left palm.

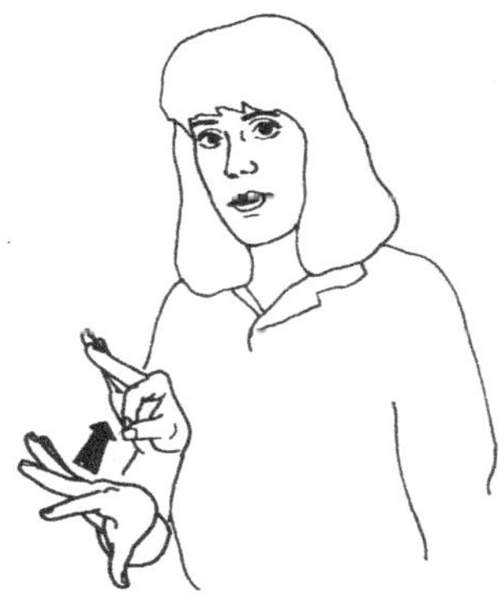

FIND
Right 5 hand, palm down, waist level. Move to chest level while changing to F hand.

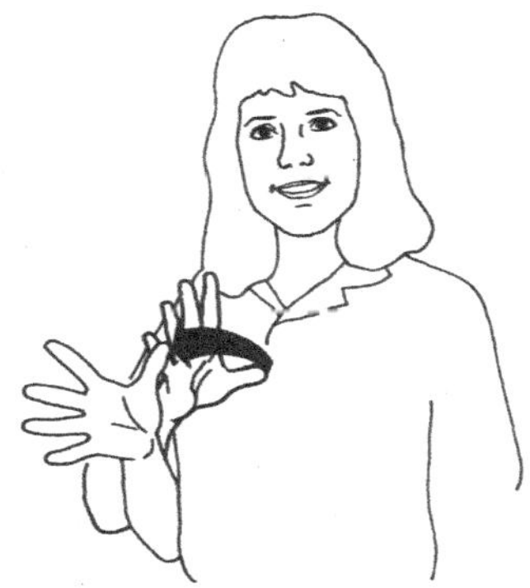

FINE
Right 5 hand, palm left, thumb touching center of chest. Move hand away from chest.

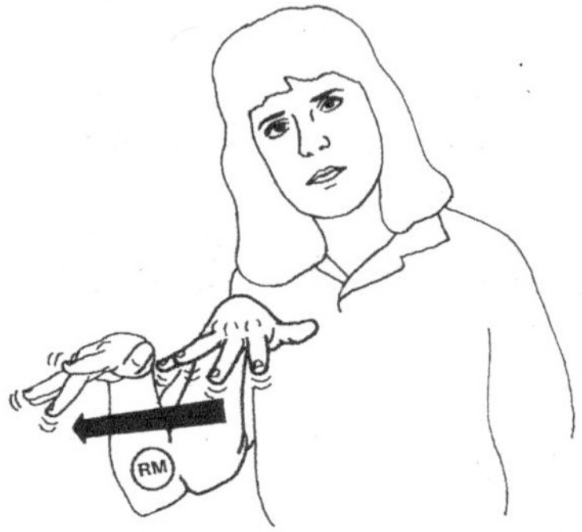

FINGERSPELLING
Right 5 hand, palm down, waist level. Wiggle fingers while moving hand to the right.
Clue: representing the finger forming various letters.

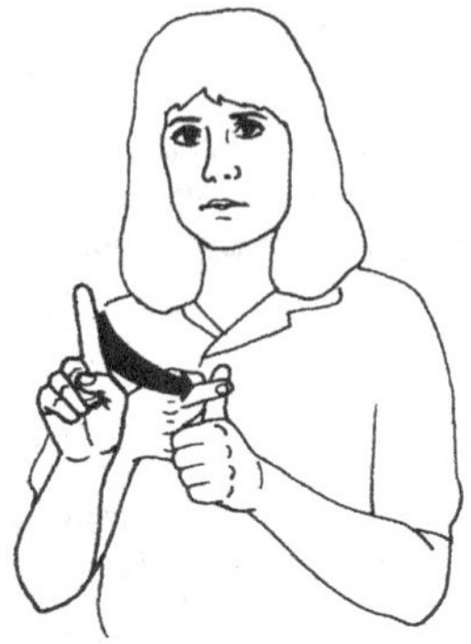

FIRST
Right 1 hand, palm out, shoulder level. Left 10 hand, palm right, chest level. Twist right wrist around so index finger touches left thumb.

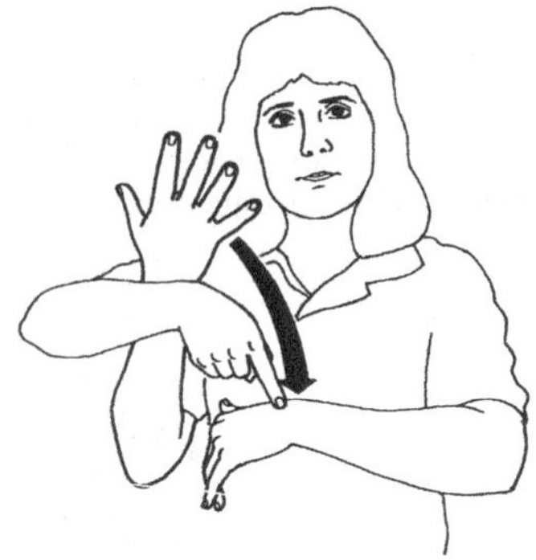

FIVE TIMES
Right 5 hand, palm in, near shoulders. Left flat hand, palm down, arm extended across waist. Bring right hand down, ending with 1 hand tapping left wrist.

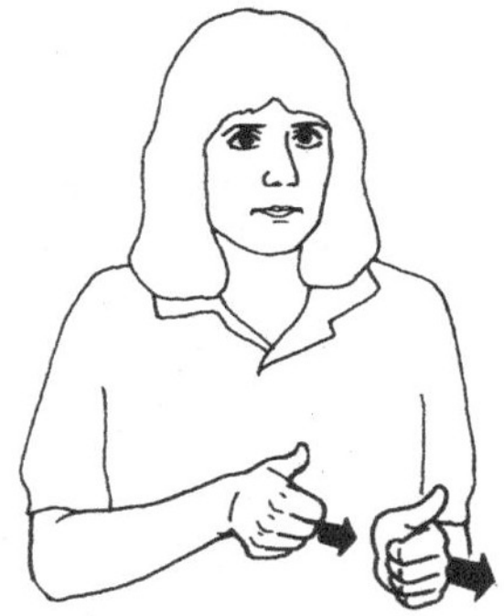

FOLLOW
A hands, palms face sides, chest level. Right A behind left A. Move both forward simultaneously.

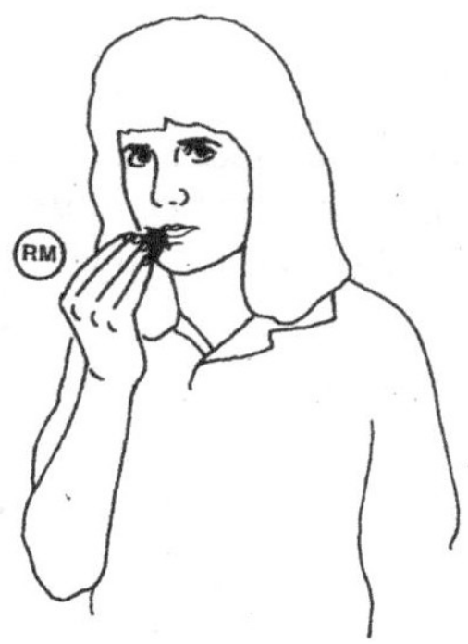

FOOD
Right O hand, palm in, at mouth. Move hand to and from mouth.
Clue: the action of eating.

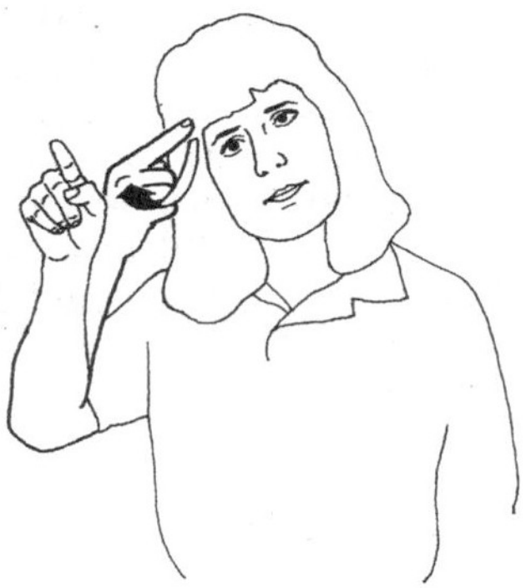

FOR
Right 1 hand, palm in, fingertip on right temple. Move away from face to palm out.

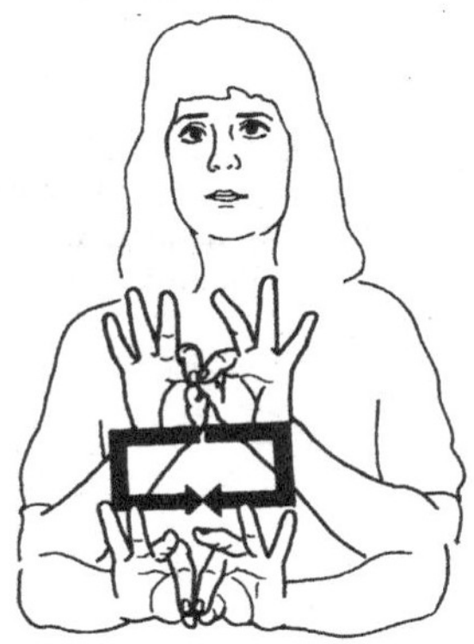

FORM
F hands, palms out, chest level, thumbs touching. Move hands in outline of a square.

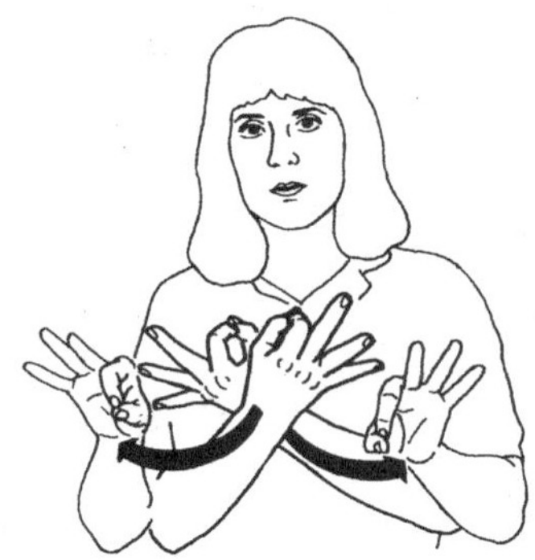

FREE
F hands, palms in, crossed at wrists, chest level. Move F hands to palms out.

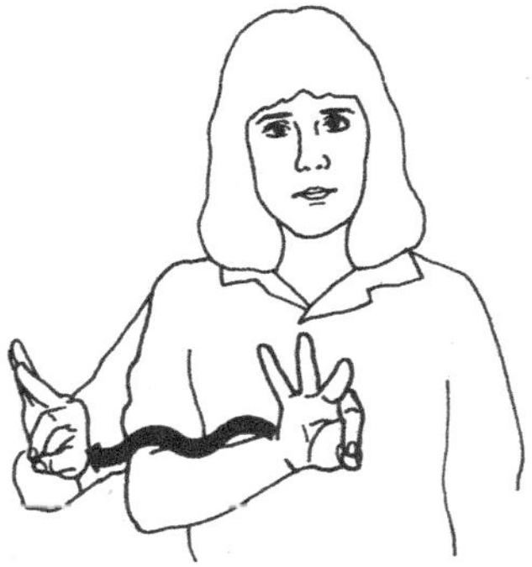

FREQUENCIES
Right F hand, palm out, chest level. Bounce down at wrist and arc to the right. Repeat.

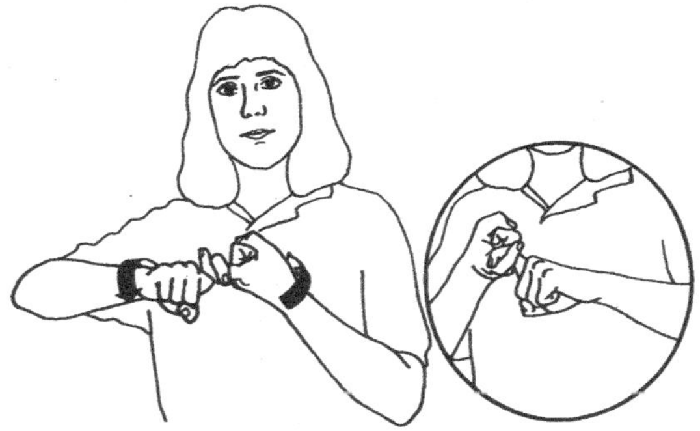

FRIENDS
X hands, right palm down, left palm up, chest level. Link X hands. Move to right palm up, left palm down, linking X hands.

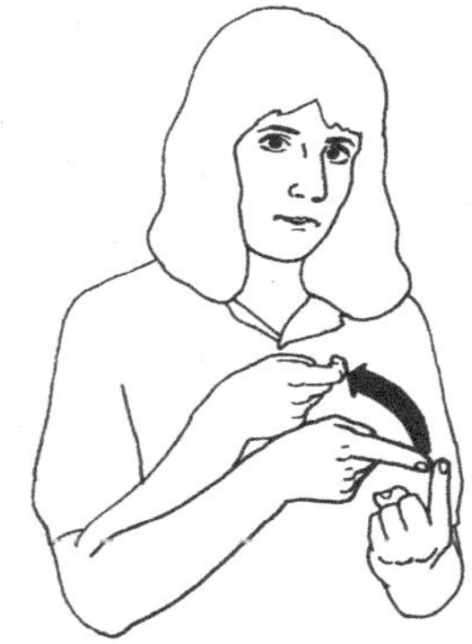

FROM
1 hands, right palm left, left palm right, chest level. Right index finger touches left index finger, then moves away, changing to X hand.

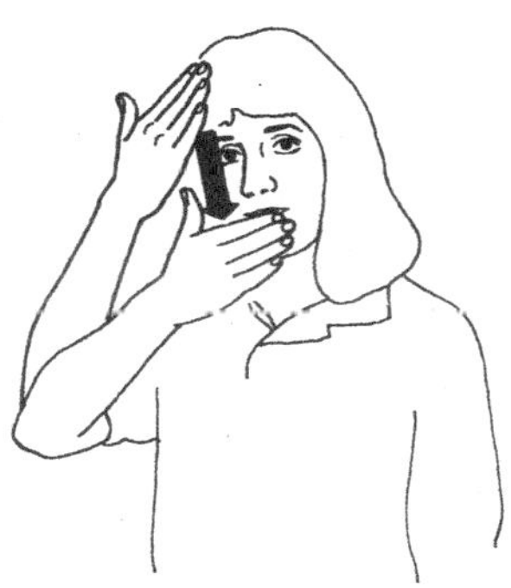

FRONT
Right flat hand, fingertips left, palm in, forehead level. Quickly move down to chin level.

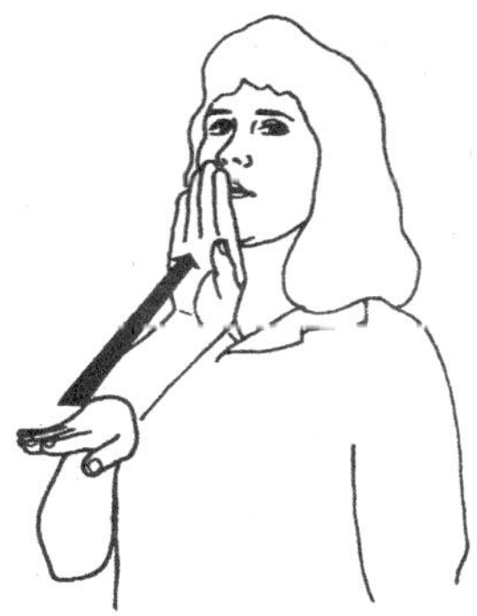

FRUSTRATION
Right B hand, palm down, chest level. Swiftly bring hand towards body, tapping on chin.

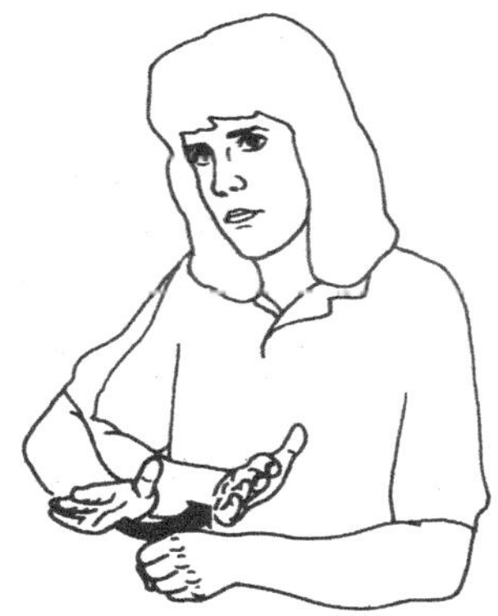

FULL
Right flat hand, palm down, waist level. Left S hand, palm towards body, waist level. Move right hand across left S.

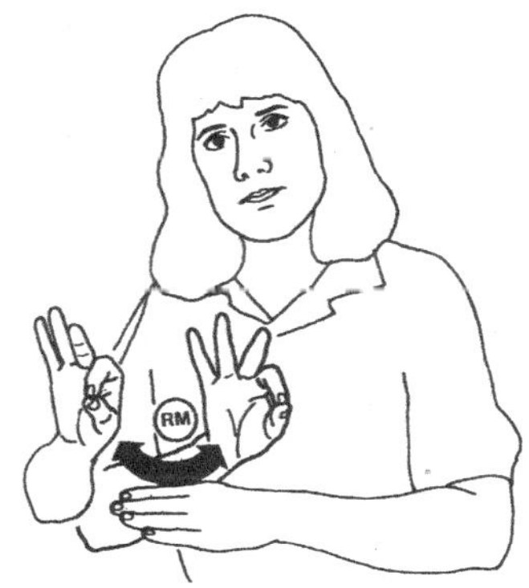

FUNCTION
Right F hand, palm out. Left B hand, palm down, waist level. Base of F sweeps back and forth across left index finger.

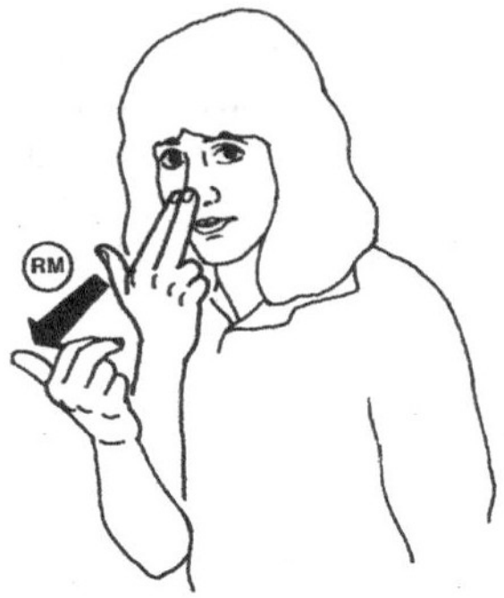

FUNNY
Right U hand, thumb extended, palm in, fingertips on tip of nose. Move right hand away from face while retracting U. Repeat.

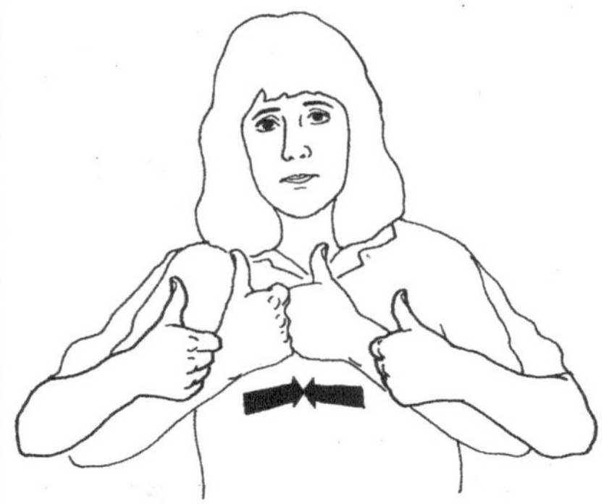

GAME
10 hands, chest level, palms in. Move hands together, knuckles touching.

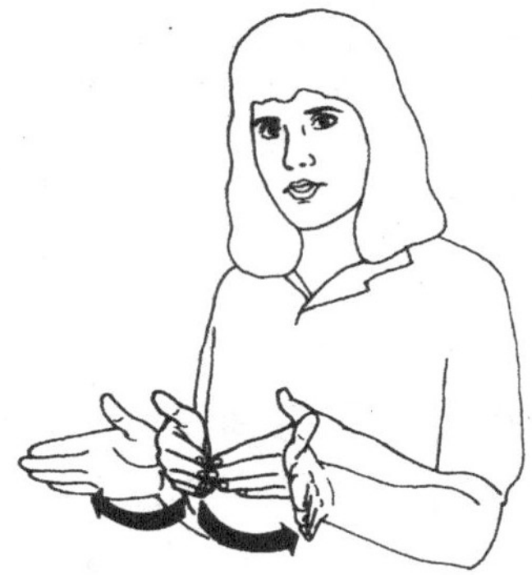

GENERAL
Flat hands, palms in, fingertips touching, chest level. Move hands apart.

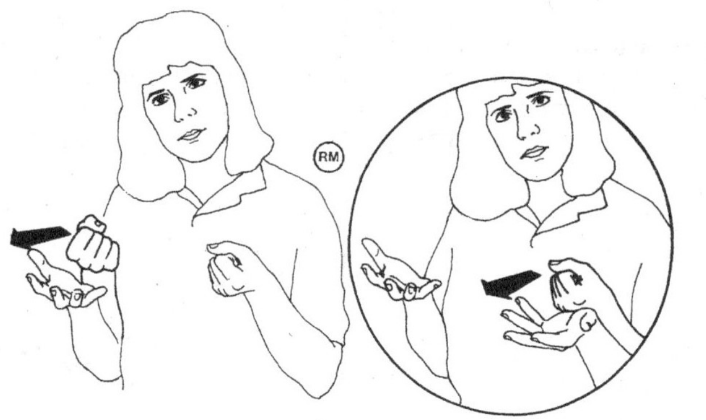

GESTURE
S hands, chest level, palms up. Alternately move hands out, opening to 5 hands. Repeat movement.

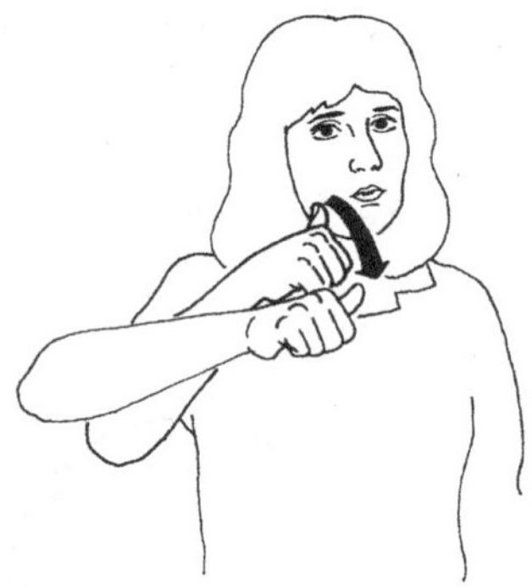

GIRL
Right A hand, thumb on lower right cheek. Move thumb down along face and slightly beyond. Repeat.
Clue: string from a girl's bonnet.

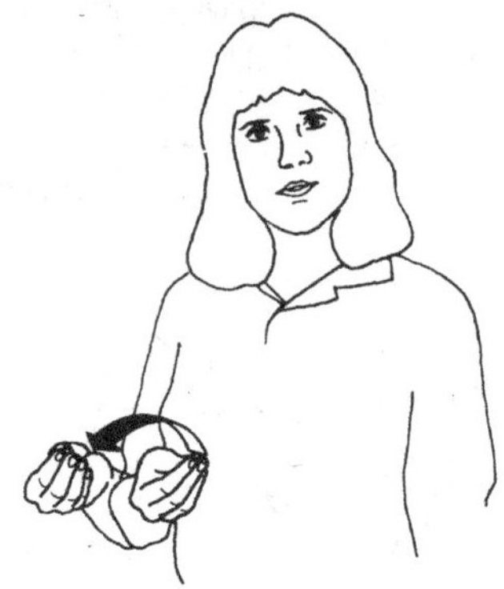

GIVE
Right O hand, palm in, below shoulder. Bring out from body ending with palm up.

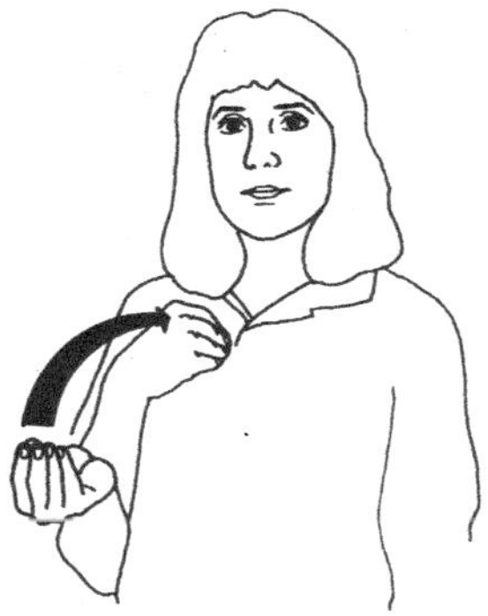

GIVE-ME
Right O hand, palm up, chest level. Bring hand back toward body, ending with fingertips on chest.

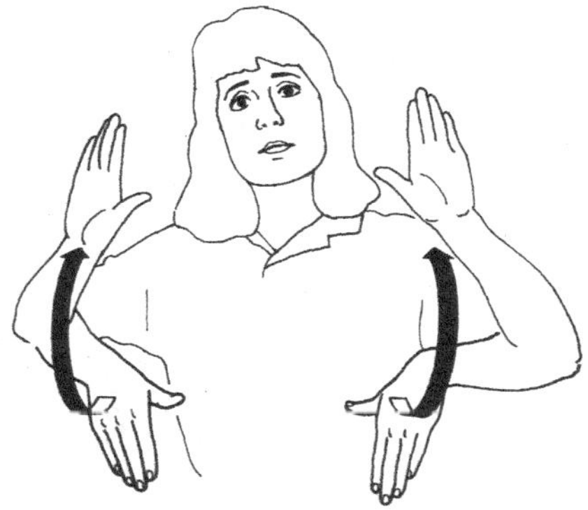

GIVE UP
Flat hands, waist level, palms down. Quickly bring hands up, palm facing out.

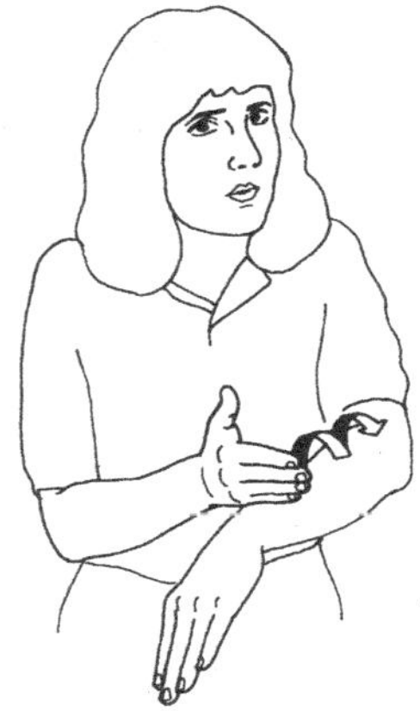

GRADUAL
Right flat hand, palm left, rests on left arm (fingertips at wrist). Slide right hand slowly up left arm to elbow.

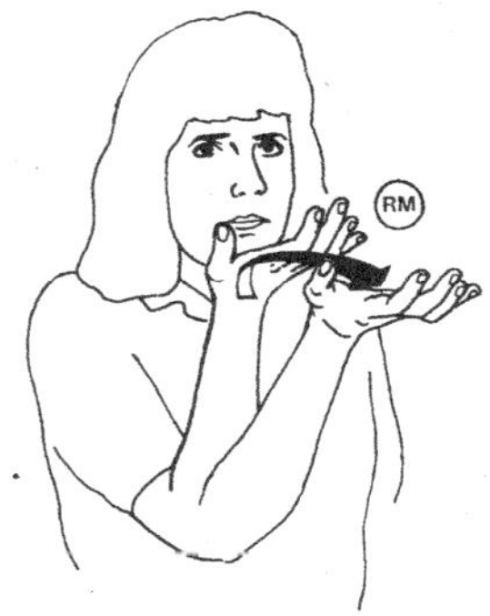

GRASS
Right 5 hand, at chin, palm up. Repeatedly bring hand up and out from chin.

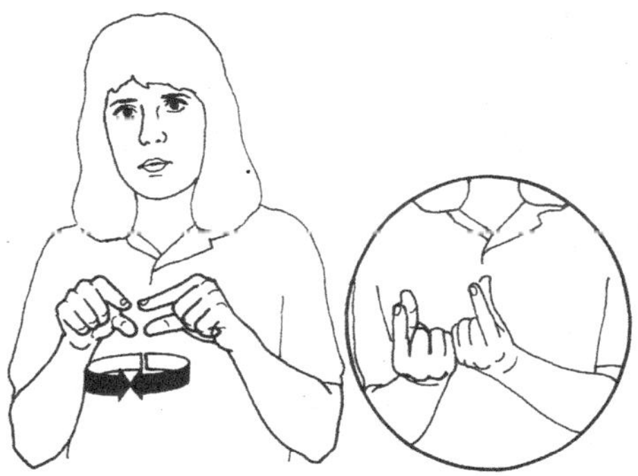

GROUP
G hands, chest level, palms out, thumbs almost touching. Bring hands out in circle until hands touch.

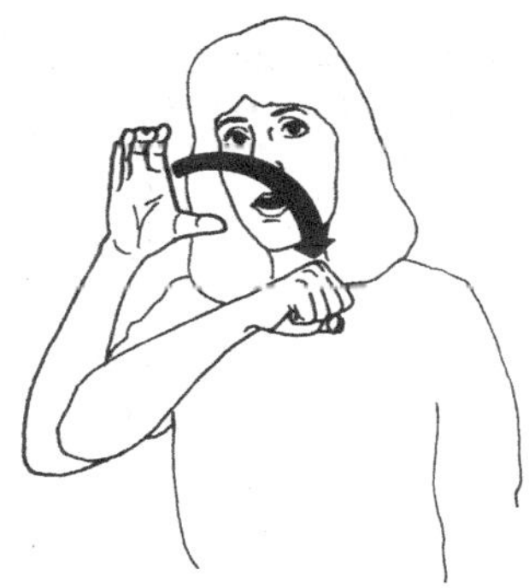

GUESS
Right C hand, palm left, face level. Move across face, changing to S hand, palm down.

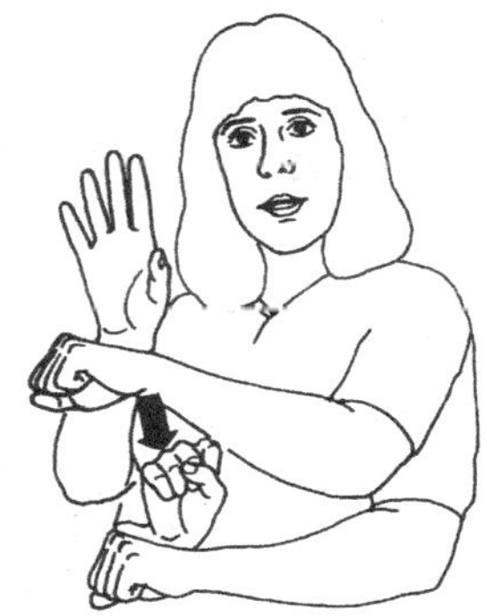

HABIT
Right 5 hand, palm out. Left S hand, palm down. At chest level, cross wrists, right behind left. Simultaneously move hands down and change right 5 to S hand.

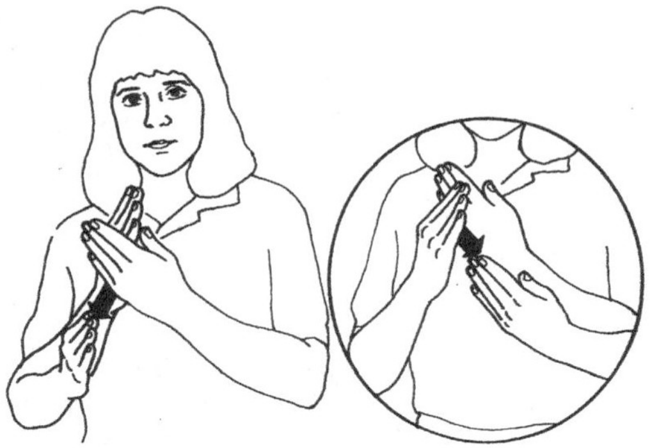

HANDS
Flat hands, chest level. Brush right hand across left palm, then brush left hand across right palm.

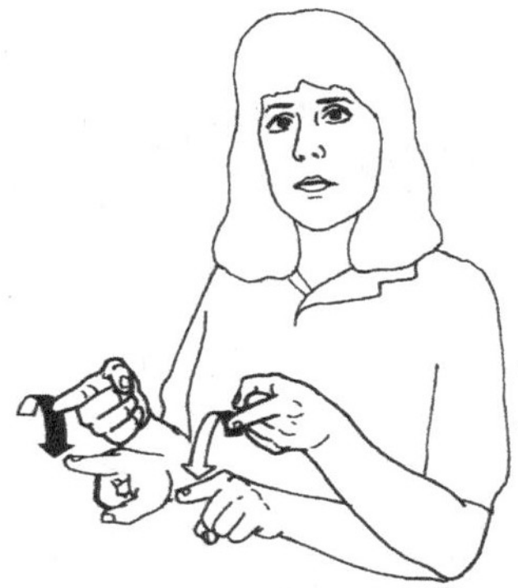

HAPPEN/EVENT/OCCUR
1 hands, waist level, palms up. Simultaneously turn hands over, palms down.

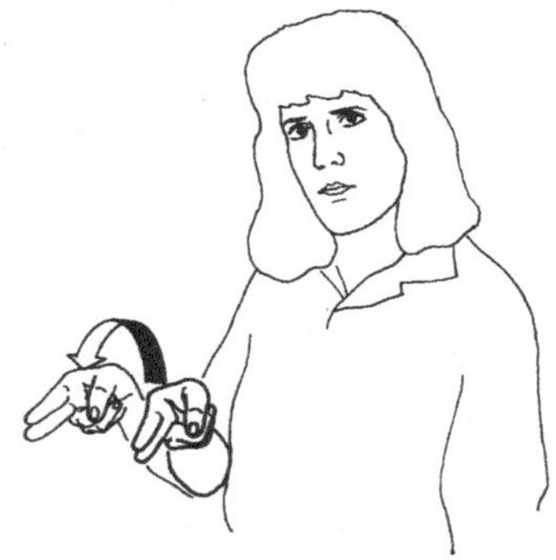

HARD OF HEARING
Right H hand, palm in, chest level. Bounce hand twice, while moving hand to the right slightly.

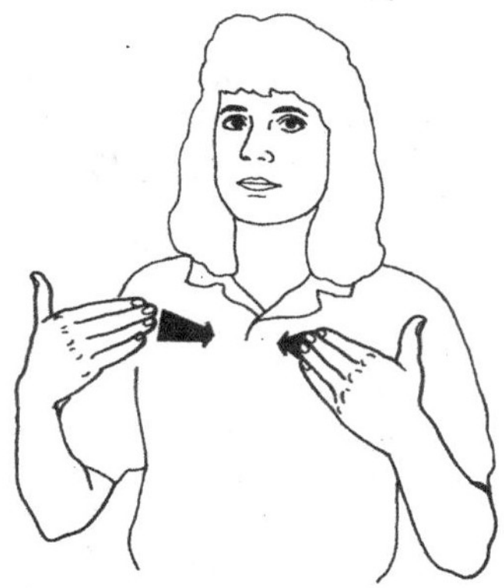

HAS/HAVE
5 hands, chest level, palms in. Simultaneously bring hands into chest until fingertips touch chest.

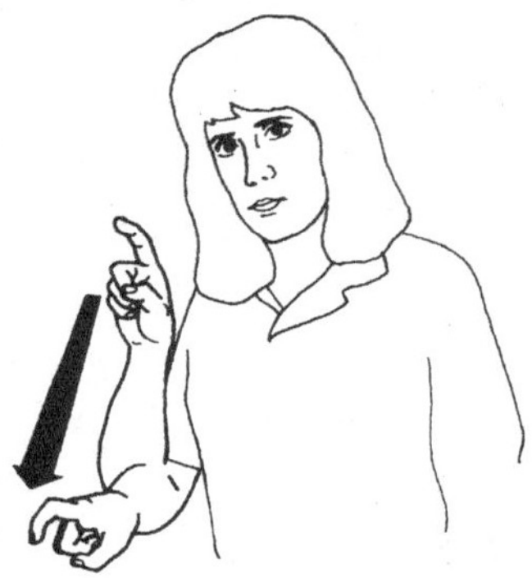

HAVE TO/MUST
Right X hand, chest level, palm out. Move hand down in a short, strong movement.

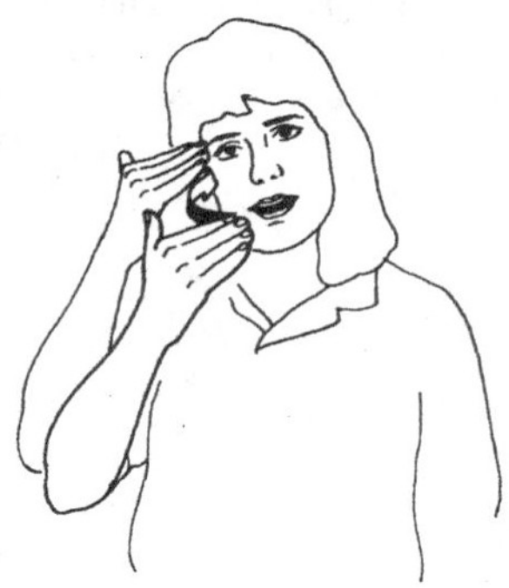

HEAD
Right flat hand, palm down, at chin. Move hand up face, touching temple.

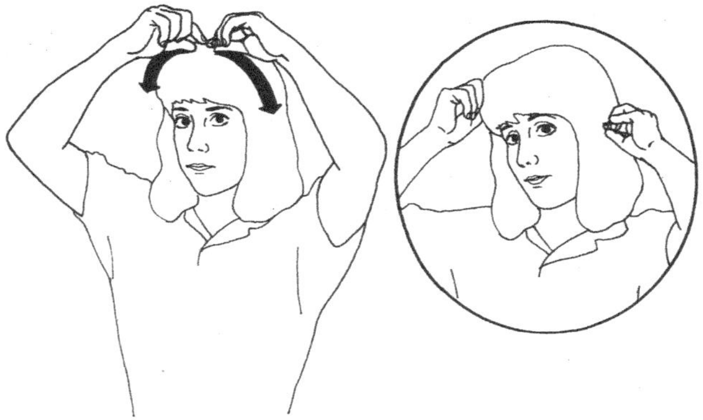

HEADBAND
O hands, palms down, on top of head. Move hands down toward ears.

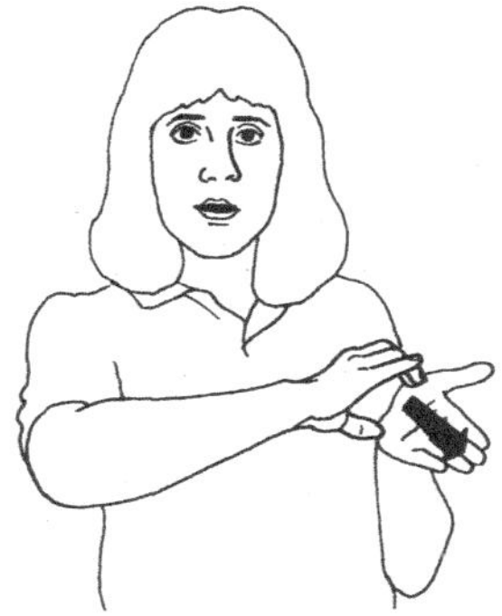

HEADLINE
Left flat hand, palm right, chest level. Right C hand, palm left, fingertips on base of left palm. Slide right hand over left palm ending at fingertips of left hand.

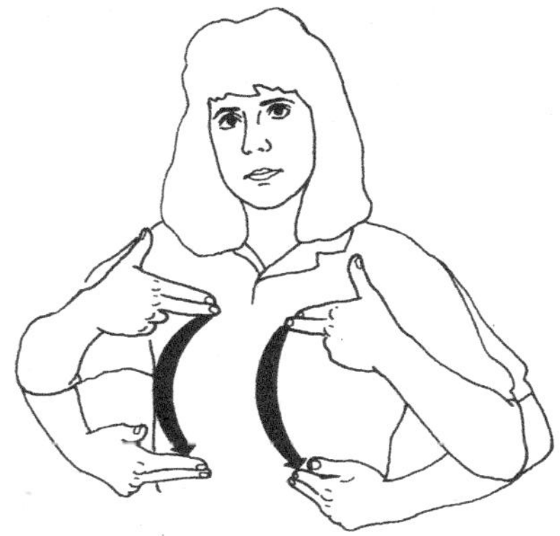

HEALTH
H hands, thumbs extended, palms in, H fingers touching chest. Move hands simultaneously to waist level.

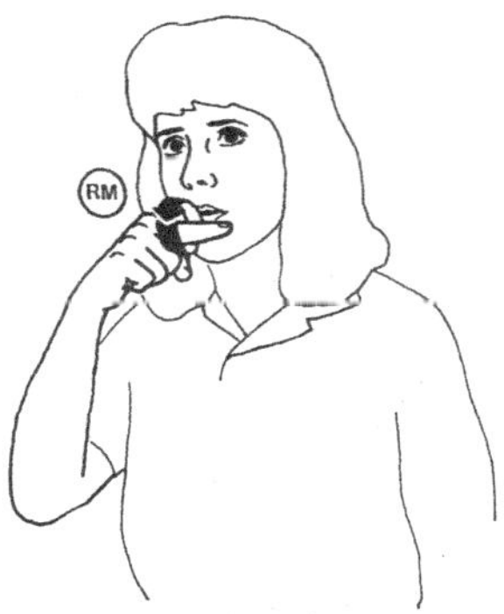

HEARING (person)/SAY
Right 1 hand, palm down, in front of mouth. Move hand in circle away from mouth.

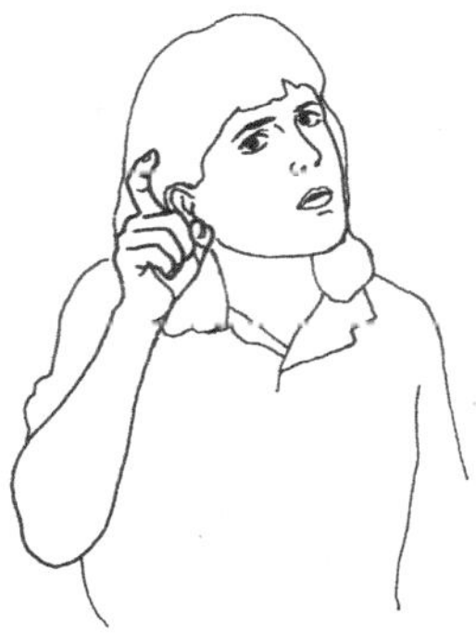

HEARING AID
Right X hand, palm out. Move behind right ear.
Clue: the shape or placement of an ear-level hearing aid.

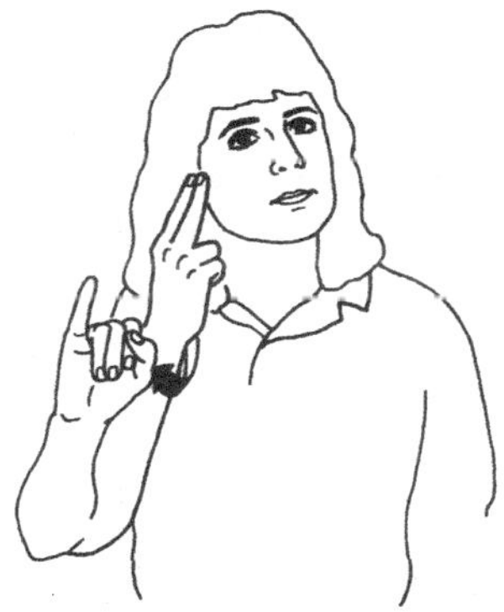

HEARING IMPAIRED
Right H hand, palm in, touching right ear. Move hand down to I shape, palm out.

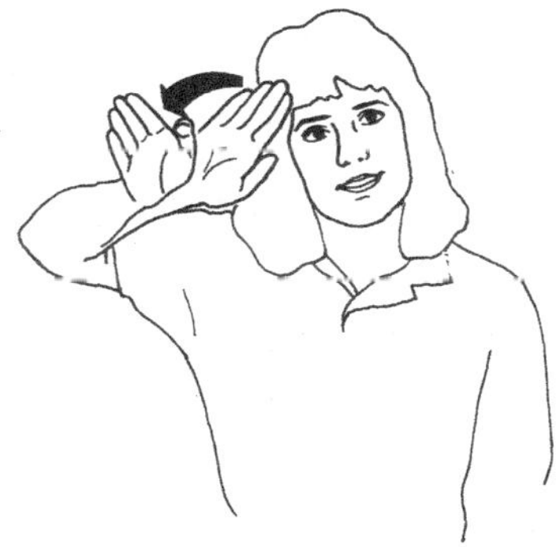

HELLO
Right 4 hand at side forehead. Bring hand out from body in quick snapping motion.

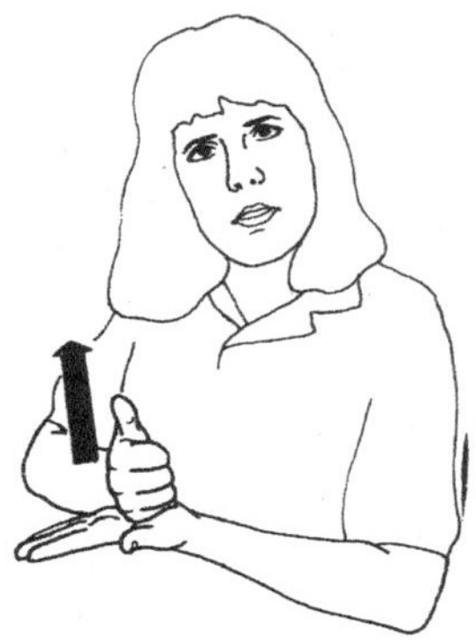

HELP
Right A hand, palm in. Left flat hand, palm up, waist level. Rest right hand on left palm. Move hands together in an upward motion.

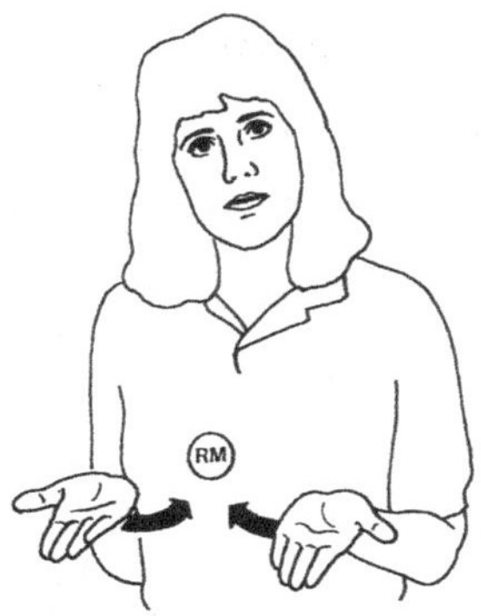

HERE
Flat hands, waist level, palms up. Lightly move hands back and forth in opposite direction.

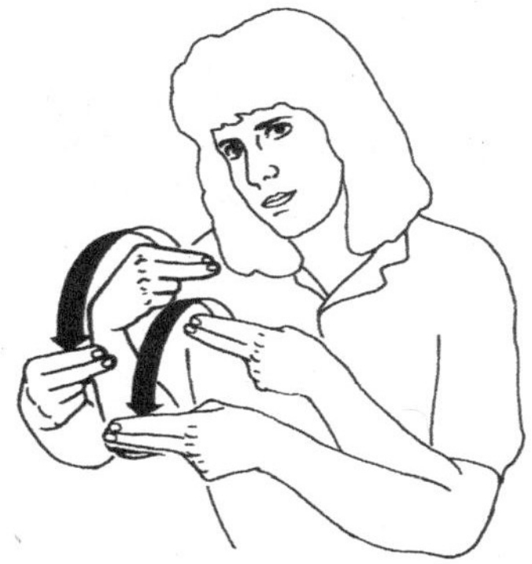

HEREDITARY
H hands, shoulder level, palms in, right hand touching shoulder, left hand in front. Bring right hand over left, left over right, followed by right over left.

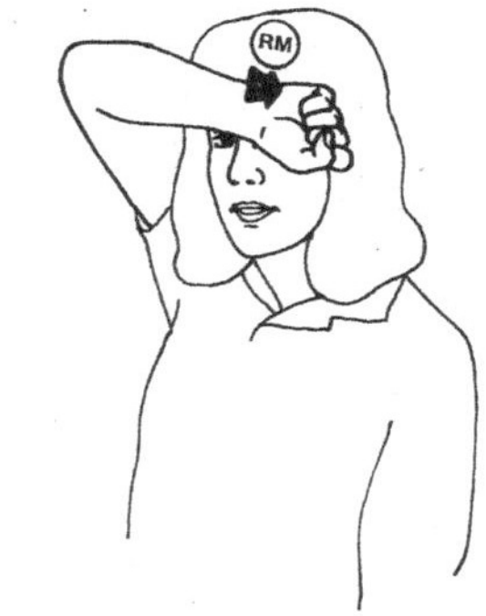

HIDE & SEEK
Right S hand, palm out, over eyes. Move head left-to-right, coming out from behind right hand.
Clue: peeking your head out.

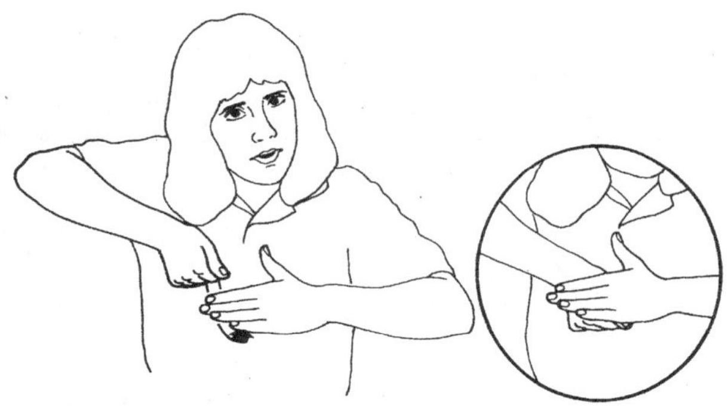

HIDE
Right A hand, palm left, chest level. Left flat hand, palm down, chest level. Move A under left hand and quickly tap up to hit left palm.

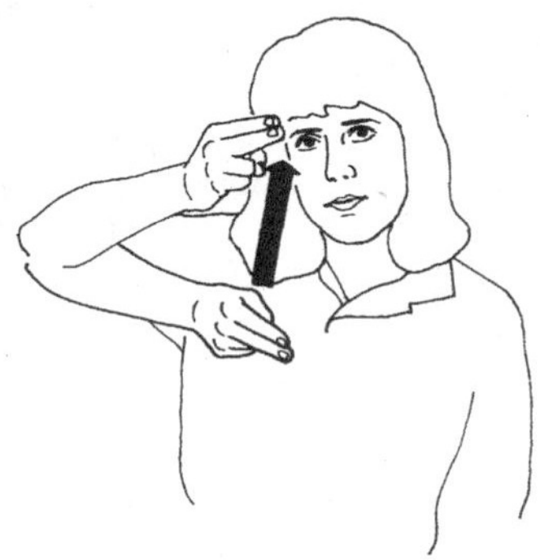

HIGH
Right H hand, chest level, palm in. Raise hand up to head level.

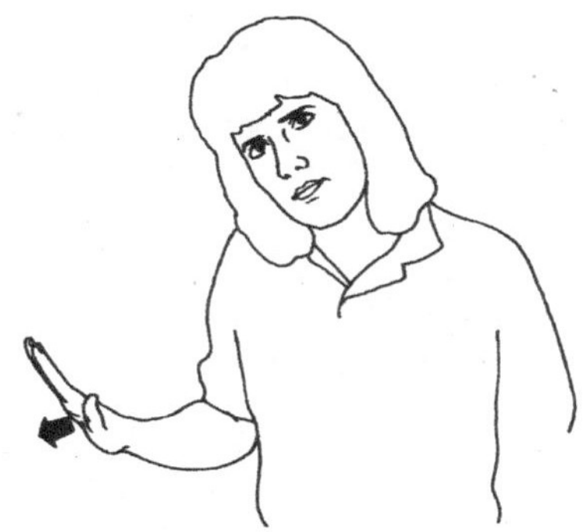

HIS/HER
Right flat hand, palm out, chest level. Move away from body in direction of referent.

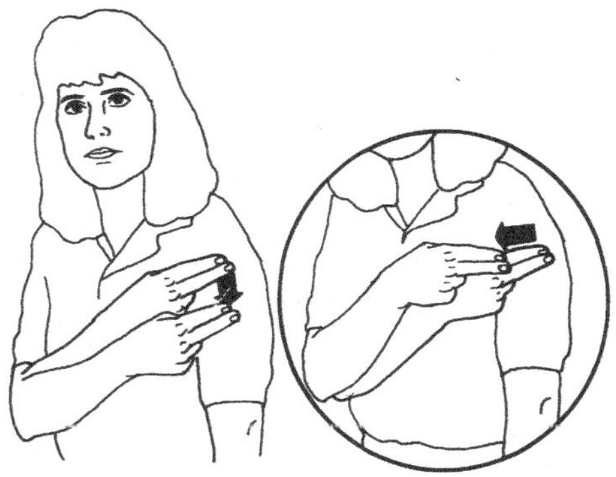

HOSPITAL
Right H hand, palm in, at left shoulder. Bring H down then across shoulder.
Clue: the Red Cross.

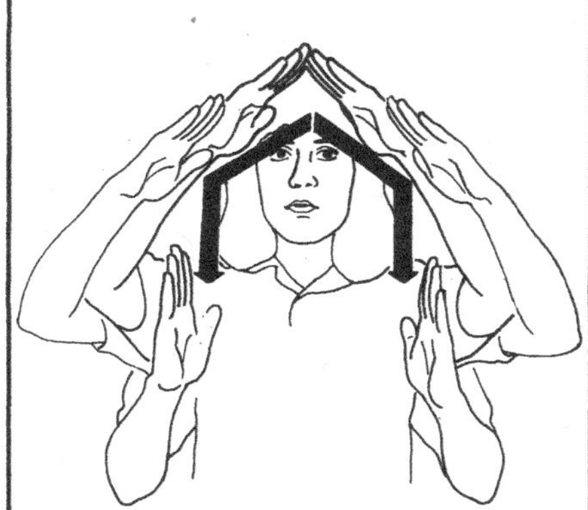

HOUSE
Flat hands, palms facing, fingertips touching, at forehead. Move hands simultaneously in the shape of a house.

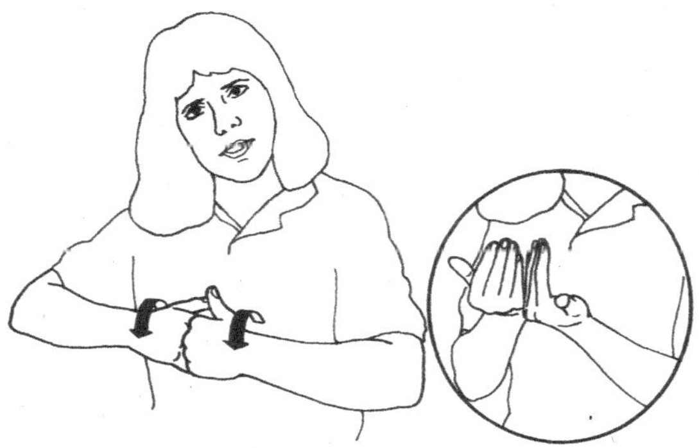

HOW
Cupped hands, palms in, chest level. Move at wrists simultaneously towards chest to flat hands, palms up.

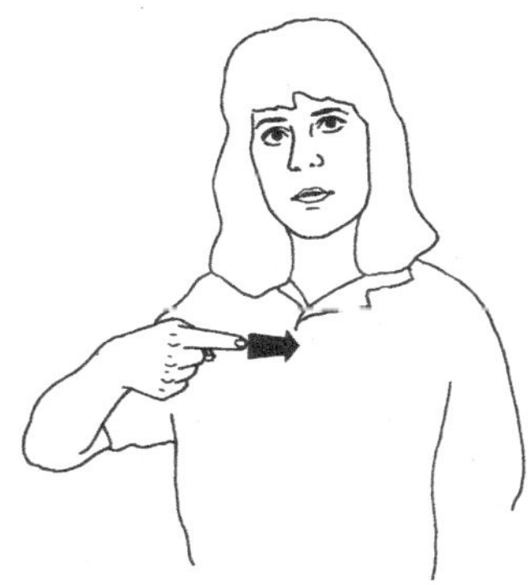

I
Right 1 points to and touches chest.

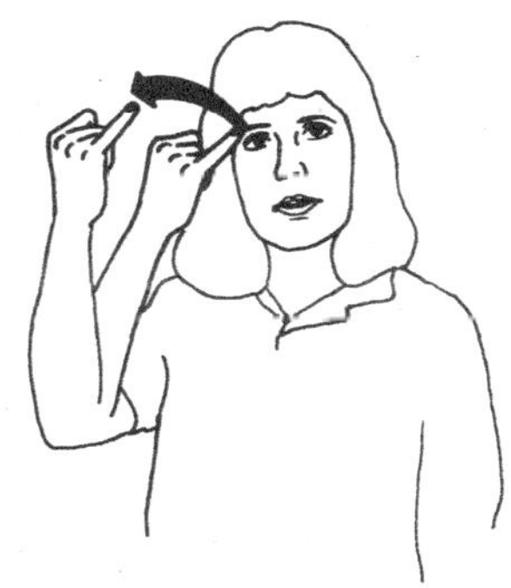

IDEA
Right I hand, palm in, I touching right temple. Quickly move hand away from head.

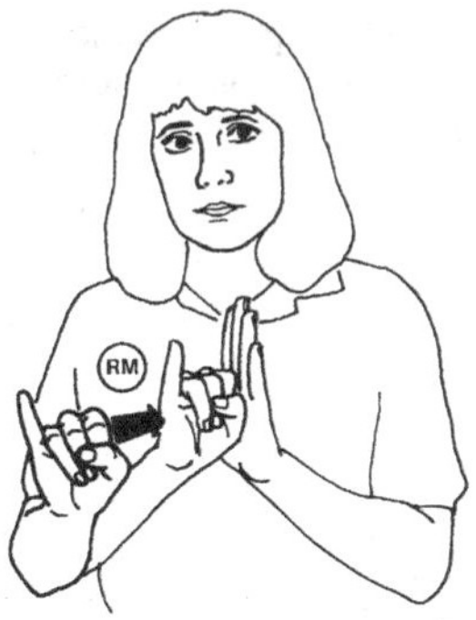

IDENTIFY
Left flat hand, chest level, palm right. Right I hand, palm out, thumb touching left palm. Bounce right hand into left.

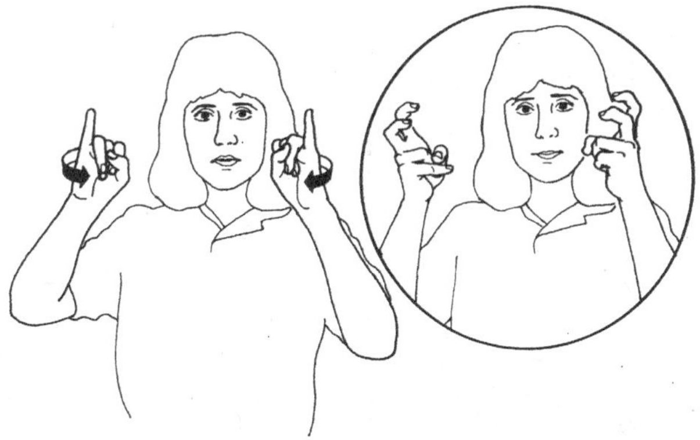

IDIOMS
I hands, palms out, head level. Simultaneously move hands in, towards body, changing to double X hands.
Clue: quotation marks around a phrase.

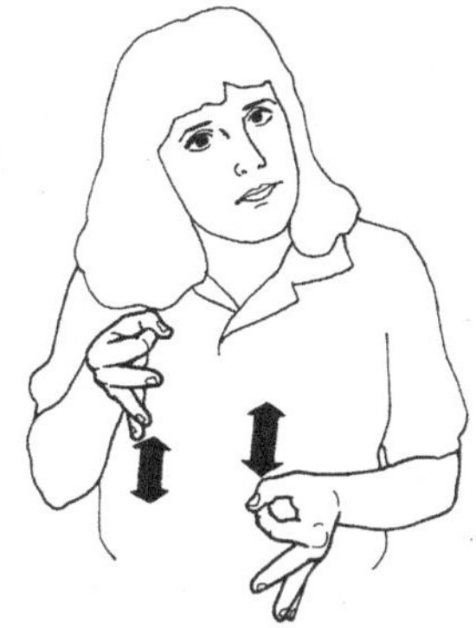

IF
F hands, palms facing each other, waist level. Move alternately up and down. Repeat.

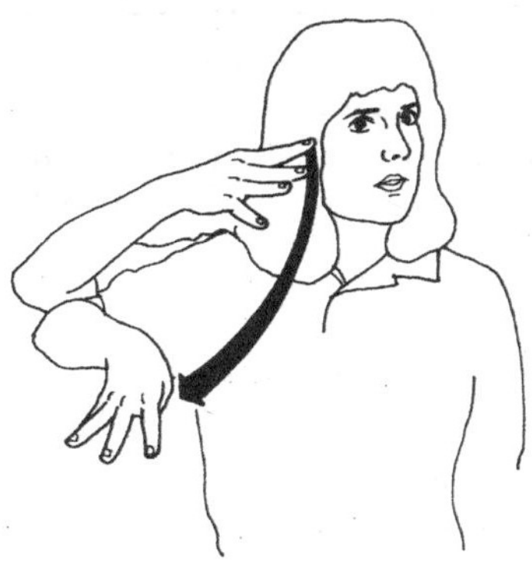

IGNORE
Right 4 hand, palm left, index finger at nose. In a quick sharp movement, move hand down and to the right.

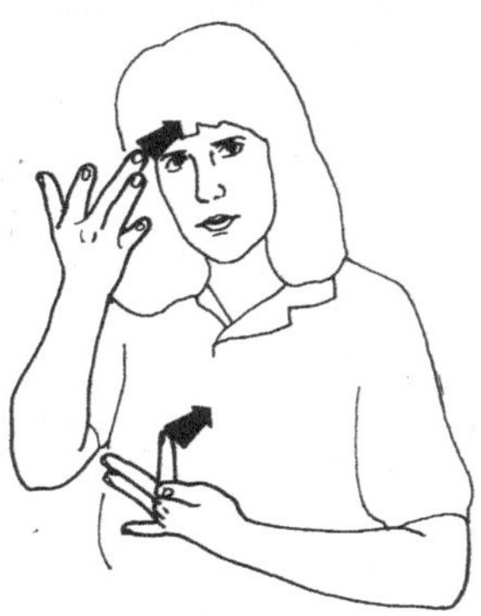

ILLNESS/SICK
5 hands, middle fingers turned in, palms in. Left hand at stomach, right hand at forehead. Simultaneously move hand in until middle fingertips touch body.

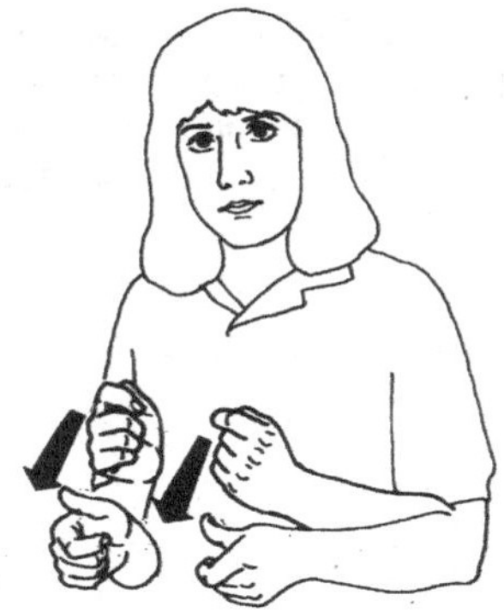

IMMEDIATELY
Closed hands, thumbs under index fingers, palms facing, chest level. Quickly, flick out thumbs.

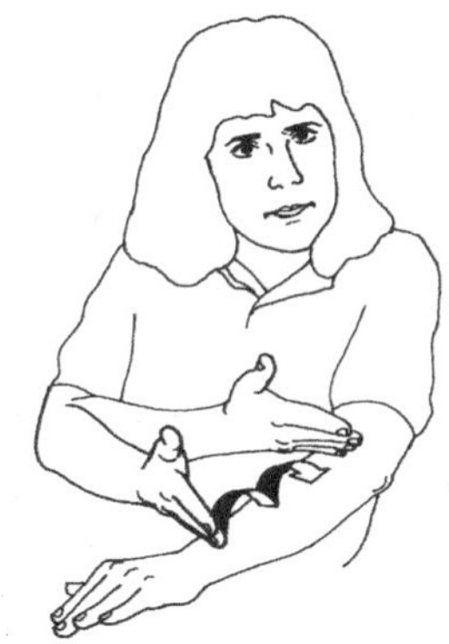

IMPROVE
Left arm extended, palm down, waist level. Right flat hand, palm in, on top of left hand. Bounce right hand up left arm, toward left shoulder.

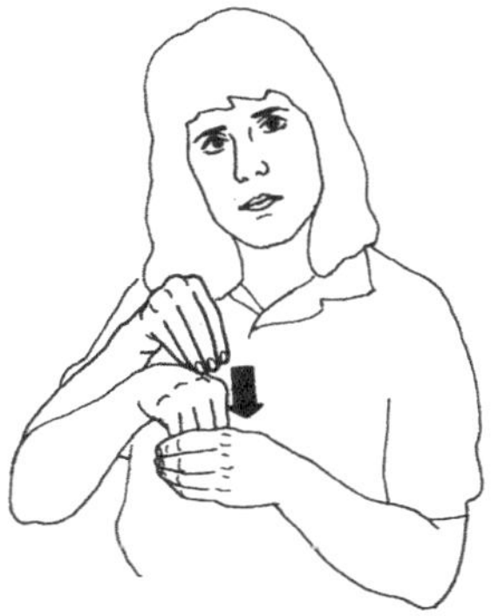

IN/INNER/INSIDE
Flat O hands, chest level, palms in. Put right hand inside left hand.

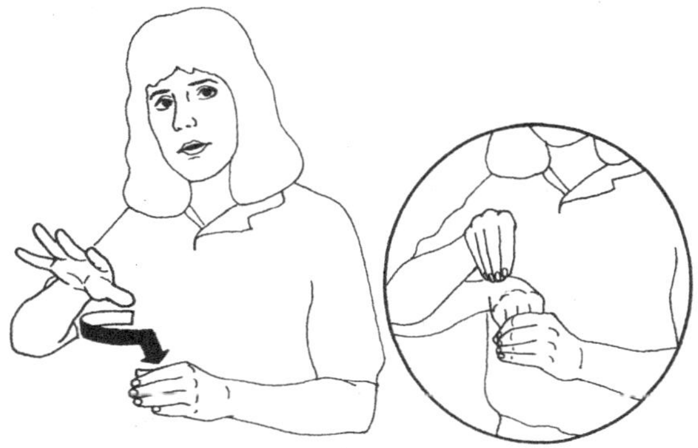

INCLUDE
Left O hand, at waist, palm in. Right 5 hand, palm down, chest level. Bring right hand in towards waist, closing to O hand and insert into left hand.

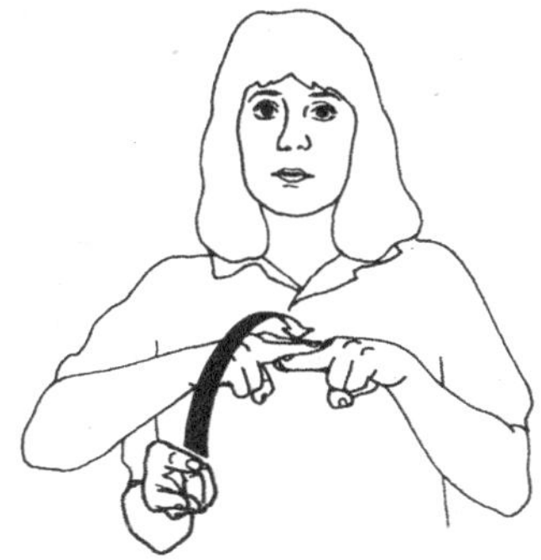

INCREASING
H hands, chest level, left palm down, right palm up. Bring right hand up and place on left fingers, palm down.

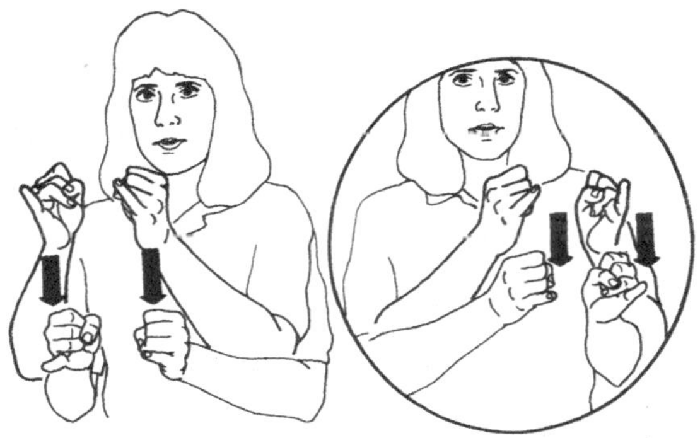

INDIVIDUALS
I hands, palms facing, chest level. Drop I hands down at wrists. Repeat movement to the right.

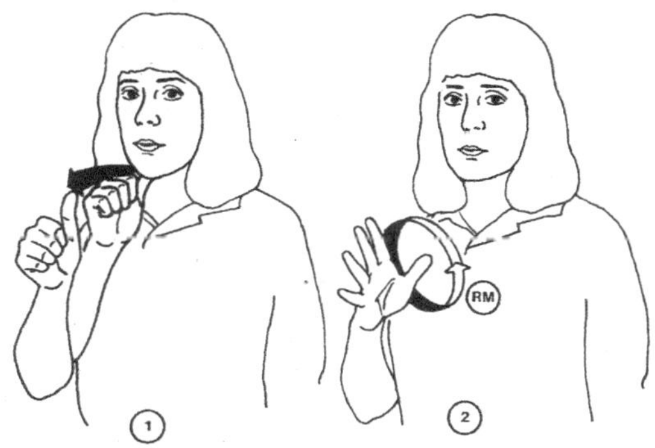

INFORMAL
Right A hand, palm left, thumb under chin. Quickly move A forward. Then change to 5 hand, palm left, thumb touching chest. Move hand in small clockwise circular motion, tapping chest with thumb.

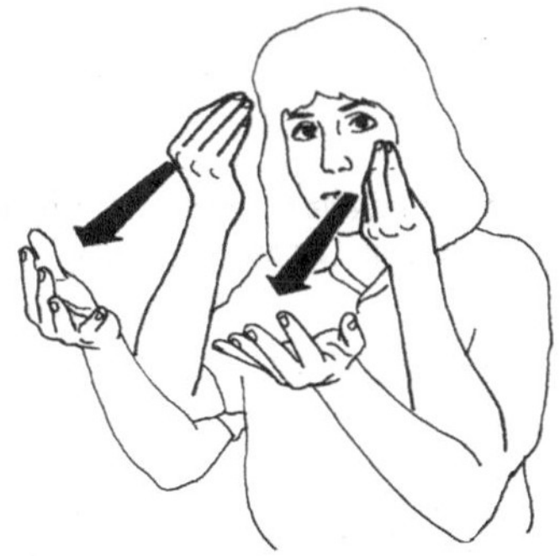

INFORMATION
O hands, palms in, right hand at forehead, left hand at eye level. Both hands move out from body, opening to 5 hands, palms up.
Clue: taking information from your brain and sharing it.

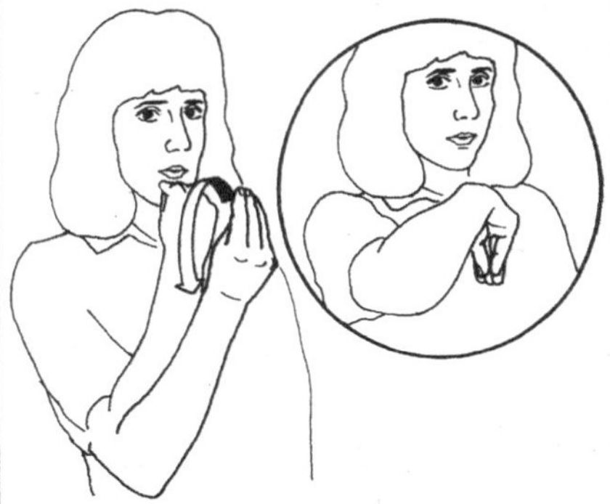

INGESTION
Right flat O hand, palm in, mouth level. Arc down to chest level, fingertips down.
Clue: simulates the act of swallowing from mouth to throat.

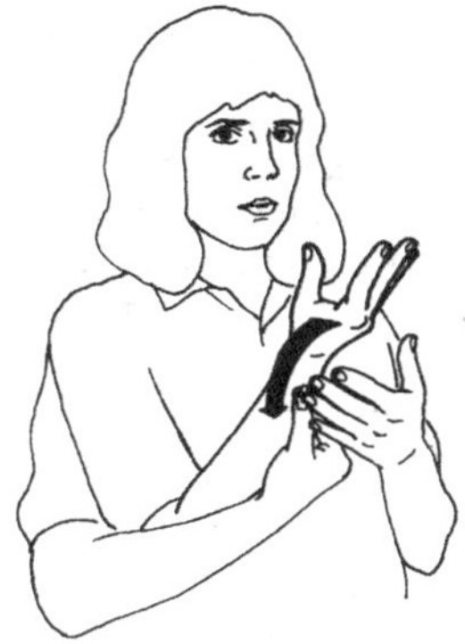

INHALATION
Left C hand, palm in, chest level. Right 5 hand, palm up, chin level. Bring right hand in towards body and down into left hand, closing right to O hand.
Clue: air coming into lungs.

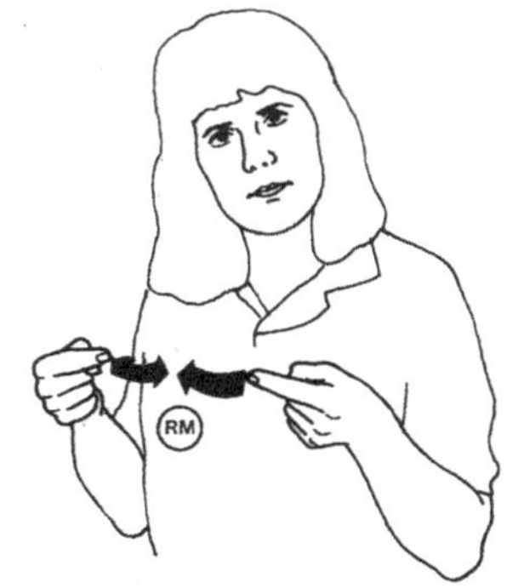

INJURY
1 hands, palms in, chest level, fingers pointing to each other. Move hands in and out from each other repeatedly.
Clue: placement of this sign changes depending on use; e.g., headache at temples, earache at ear.

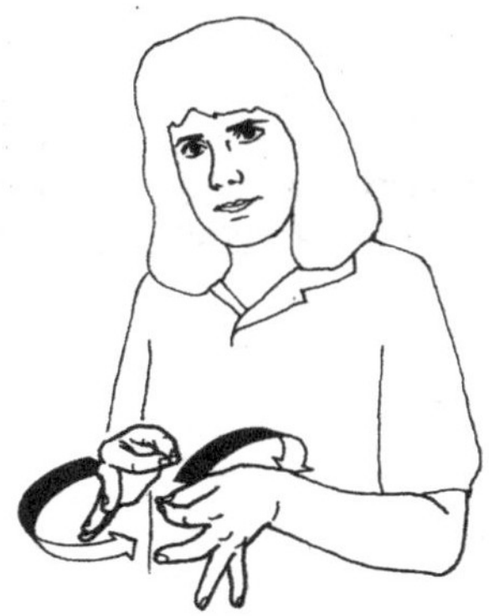

INSTEAD
F hands, right slightly in front of left, chest level, palms facing. Move right F under and behind left F while moving left F above and in front of right F.
Clue: to move something in place of something else.

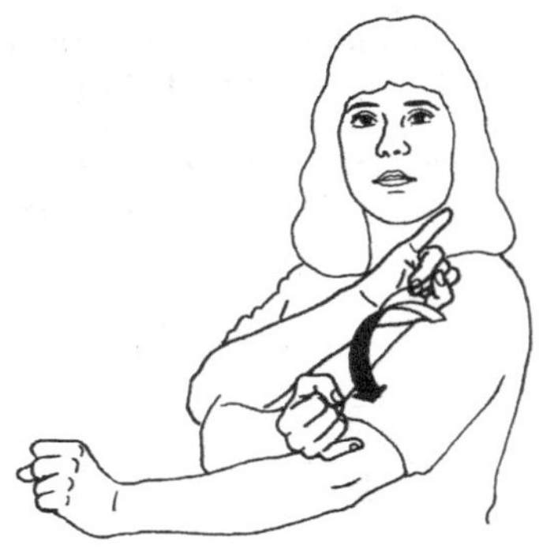

INTENSITY
Right I hand, palm left, thumb on top of left arm. Arc right hand over arm, ending with little finger near bend in elbow.

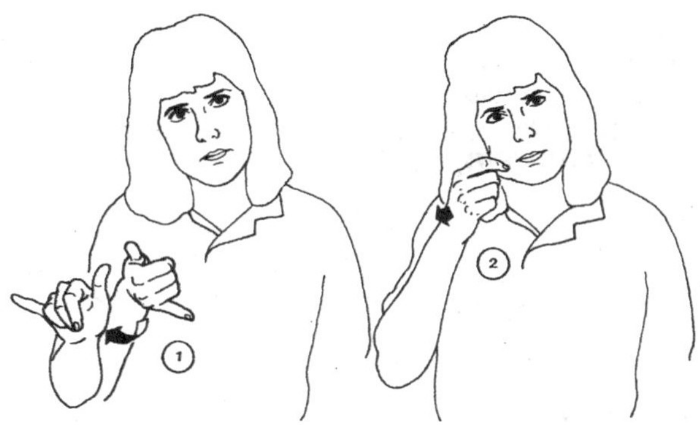

JAUNDICED
Right Y handshape, palm in, chest level. Shake palm away from body. Repeat. Use right hand to pinch right cheek and slightly shake.
Clue: yellow + skin.

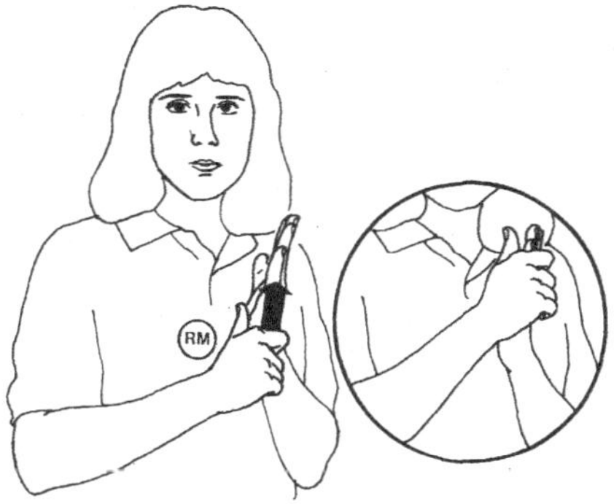

JOURNAL
Right A hand, palm left. Left flat hand, palm right and slightly tilted up, chest level. Pinch bottom of left hand with right A hand, between thumb and index finger. Slide A up hand. Repeat.

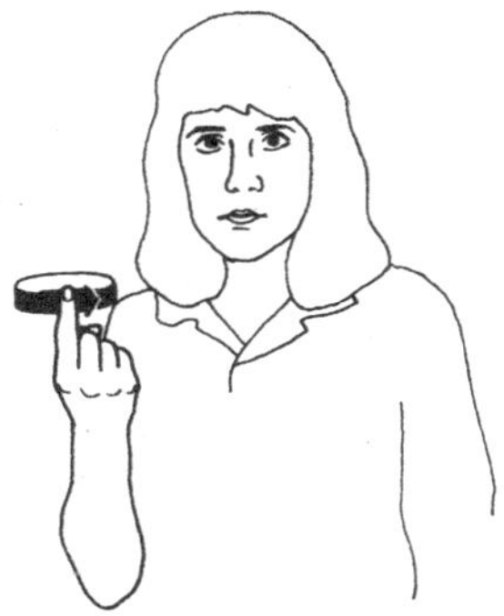

JUST/ONLY
Right 1 hand, chest level, palm in. Circle once in a small counterclockwise direction.

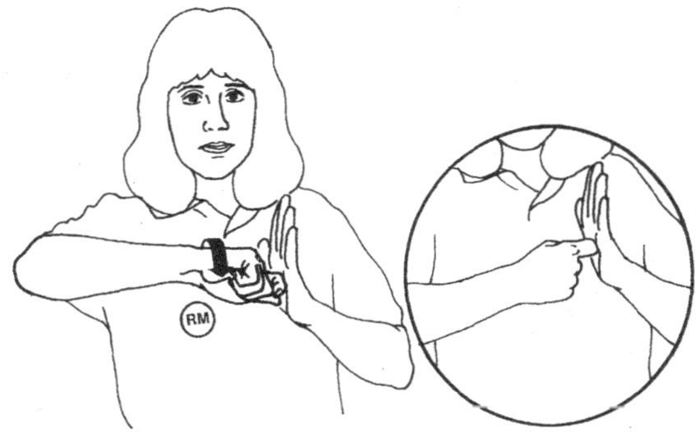

KEY
Left flat hand, palm right, chest level. Right X hand, palm in, X finger in the middle of left palm. Rotate right hand back and forth in palm.
Clue: starting a car.

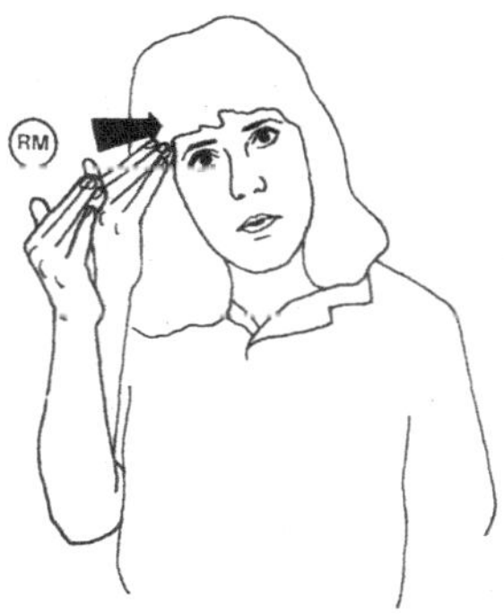

KNOW/AWARE/FAMILIAR
Right flat hand, palm down. Tap right temple with fingertips.

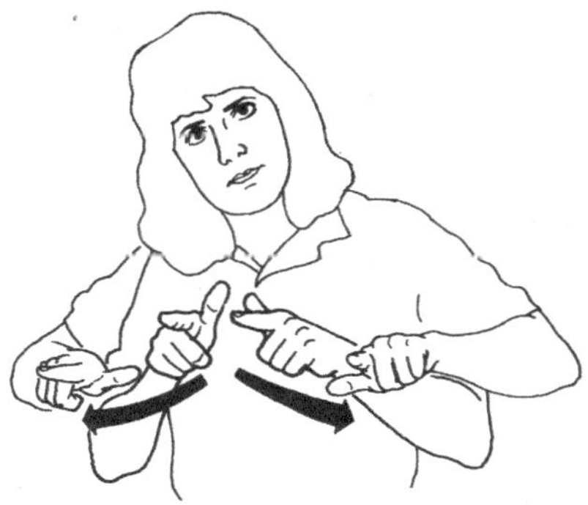

LANGUAGE
L hands, palms down, chest level, thumbs close together. Lightly move hands side to side.

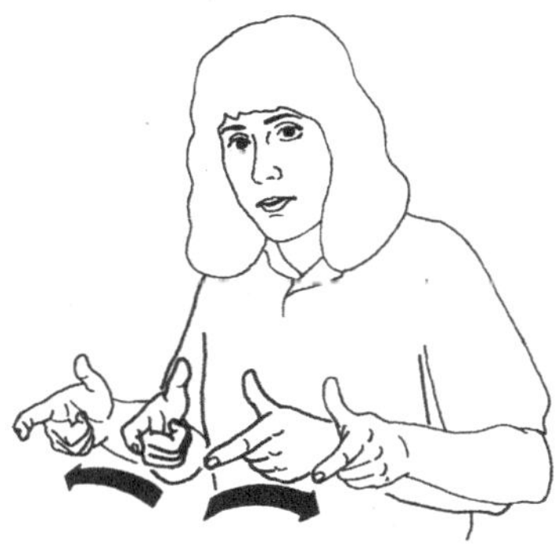

LARGE
L hands, palms facing, chest level. Move hands out to sides.

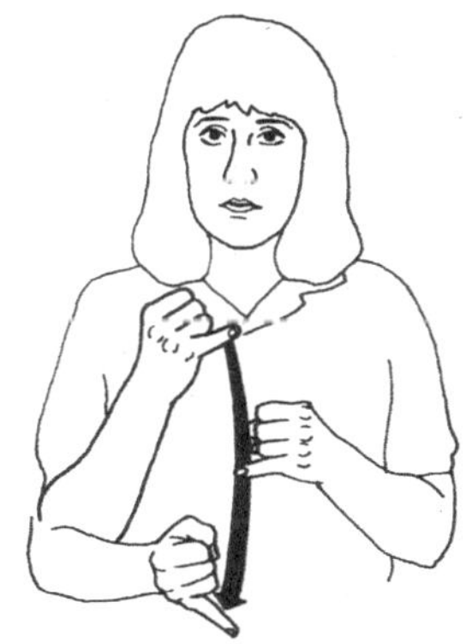

LAST/FINAL
I hands, palms facing, right hand above left. Bring right hand down, brushing left little finger.

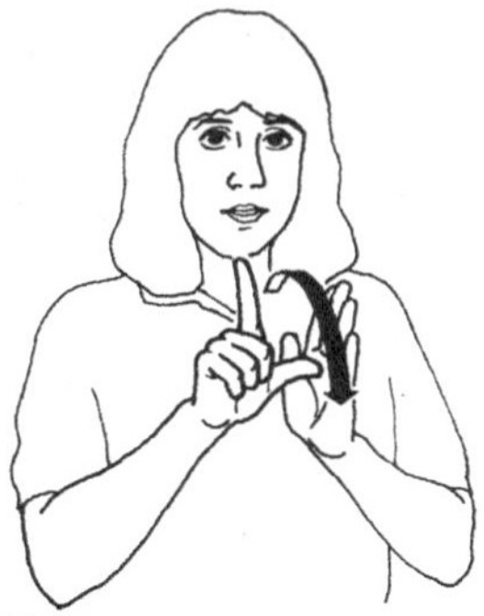

LATER
Flat left hand, chest level, palm right. Right L hand, palm out, thumb touching left palm. Rotate right wrist until index finger points out.

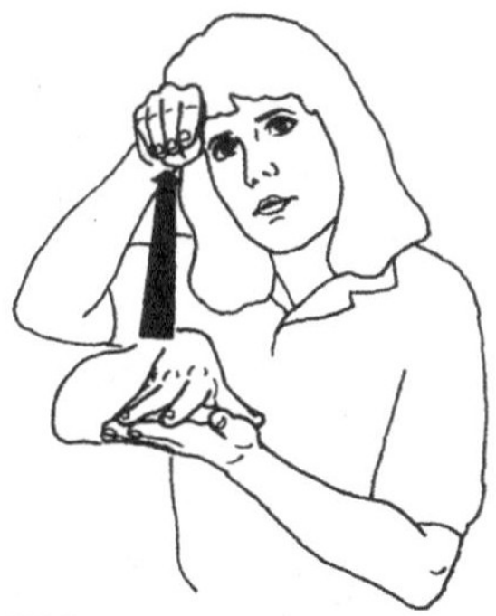

LEARN
Left flat hand, palm up, waist level. Right 5 hand, palm down, fingertips touching left palm. Right hand moves up to forehead, changing to flat O handshape.
Clue: putting knowledge into one's brain.

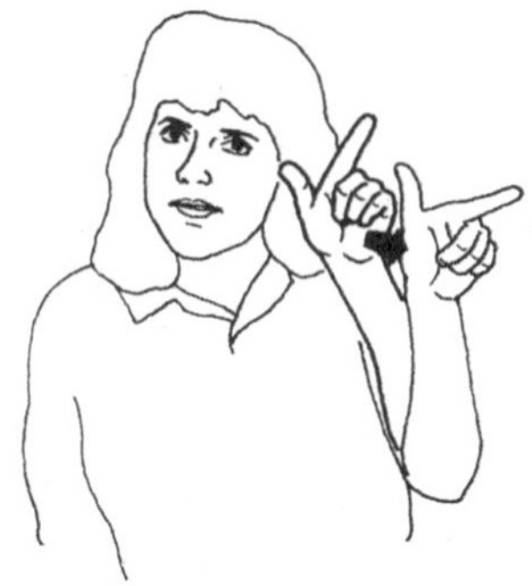

LEFT EAR
Left L hand, palm out, left ear level. Move away from ear.

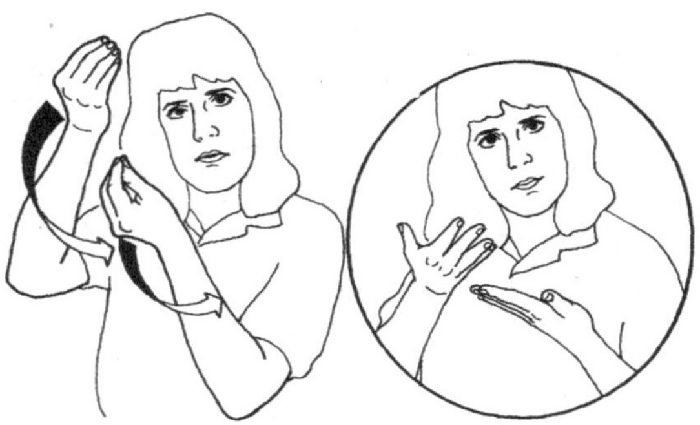

LET ME KNOW
Flat O hands, palms up, forehead level. Move hands down and towards chest opening to 5 handshapes.

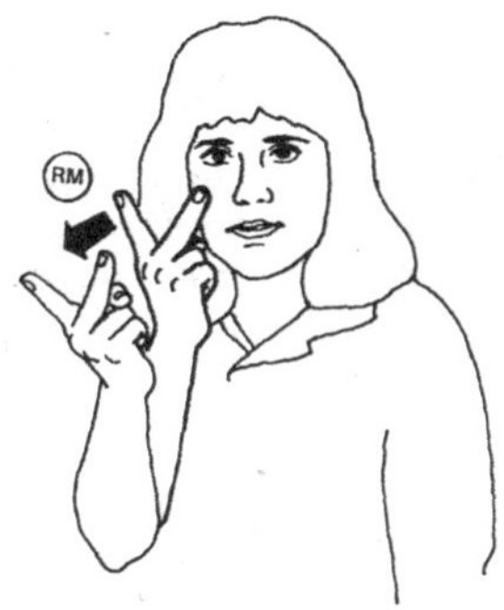

LET'S SEE
Right V hand, palm in, at corner of the eye. Hand bounces slightly.

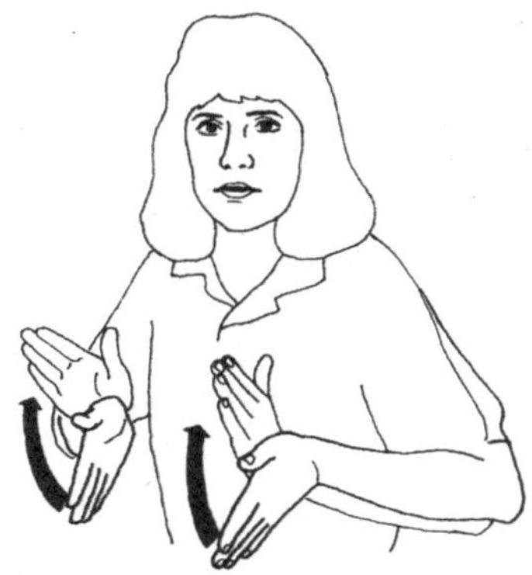

LET/ALLOW
Flat hands, at waist, palms facing, fingers pointing down. Bring hands up, fingers pointing up.

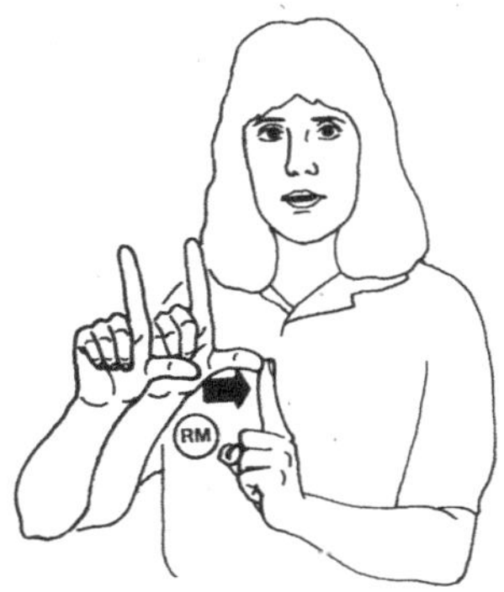

LETTER
Right L hand, palm out. Left 1 hand, palm right, chest level. Tap right L hand thumb on left index finger. Repeat.

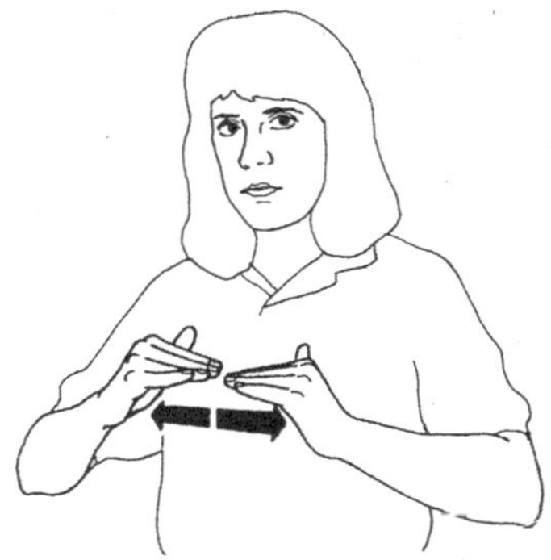

LEVEL
Bent hands, shoulder level, palms down, fingertips pointing to each other. Move fingertips close to each other.

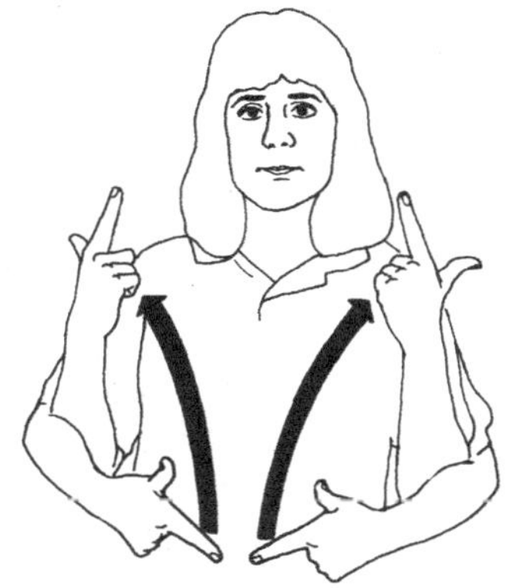

LIFE
L hands, palms in, at waist. Bring hands up body to chest level.

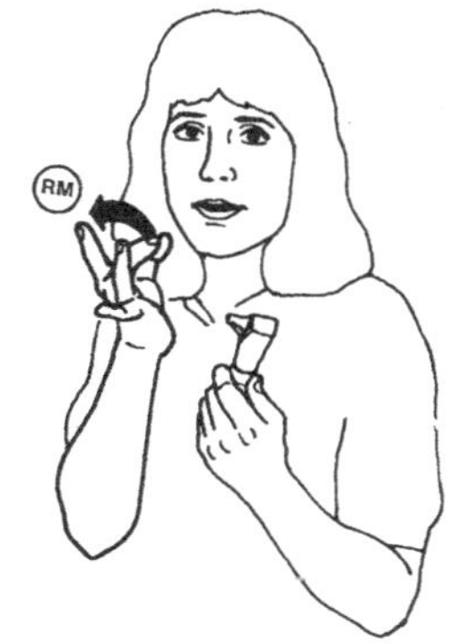

LIGHT
Right 8 hand, palm in, at chin level. Flick index finger off of thumb. Repeat. (Hold otoscope in left hand.)

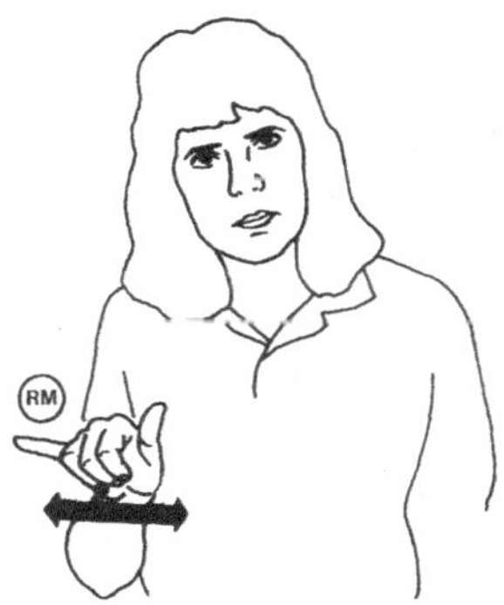

LIKE/SAME
Right Y hand, palm down, waist level. Move side to side repeatedly.

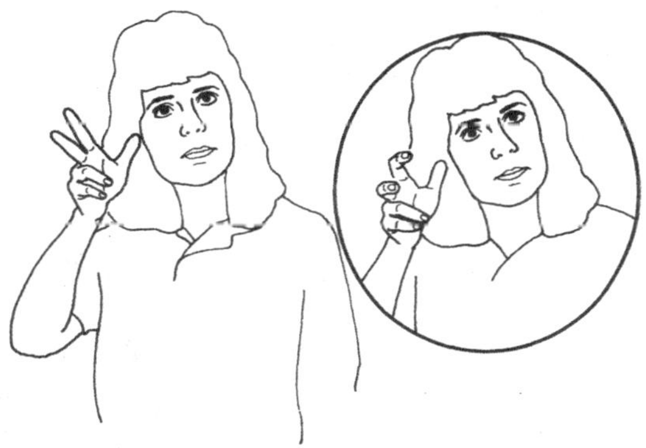

LISTEN
Right 3 hand, palm out, at ear. Repeatedly bend fingers.

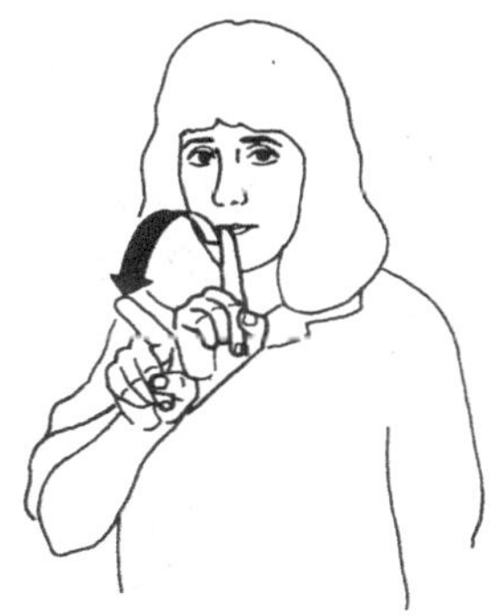

LITERAL/REAL
Right 1 hand, palm left, at mouth. Bring hand directly out from mouth.

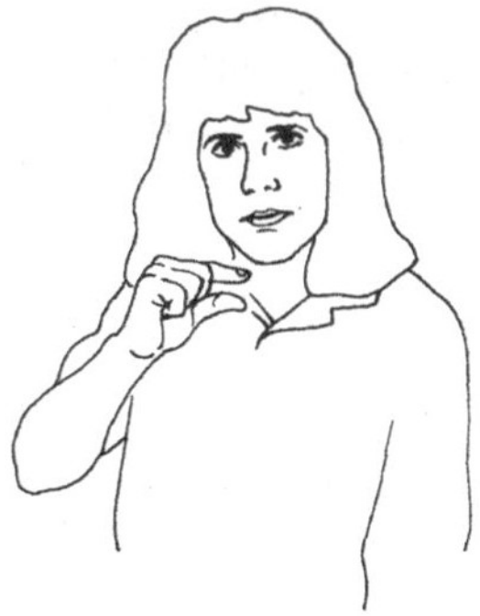

LITTLE
Right G hand, palm left, chest level. Close thumb and index finger slightly.

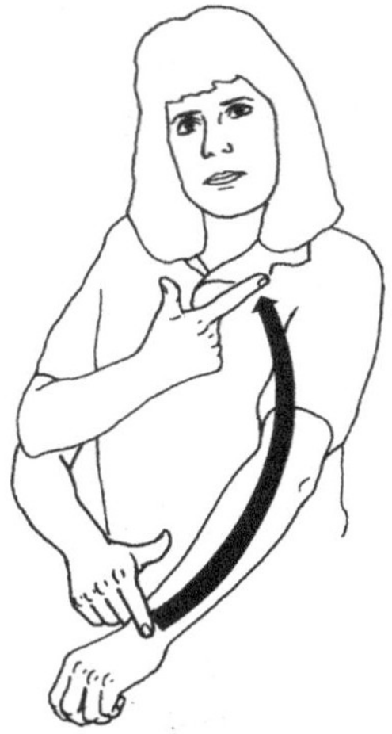

LONG
Left arm extended, palm down. Right L hand, palm down, at left wrist. Sweep L up arm to shoulder.

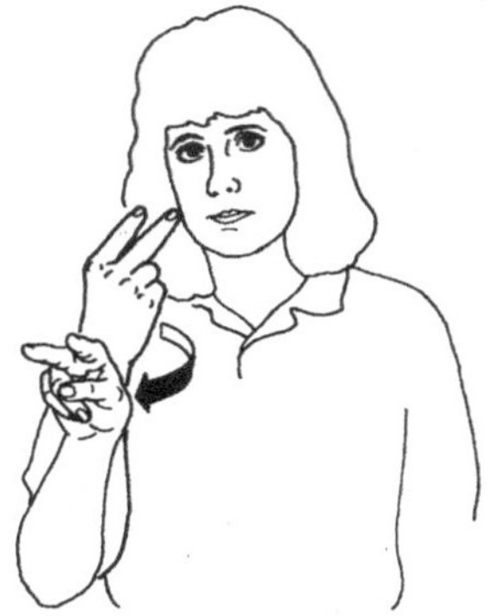

LOOK AT
Right V hand, palm out, below eye, pointing to person. Swing hand down towards the object the person should look at.
Clue: eyes focusing on something.

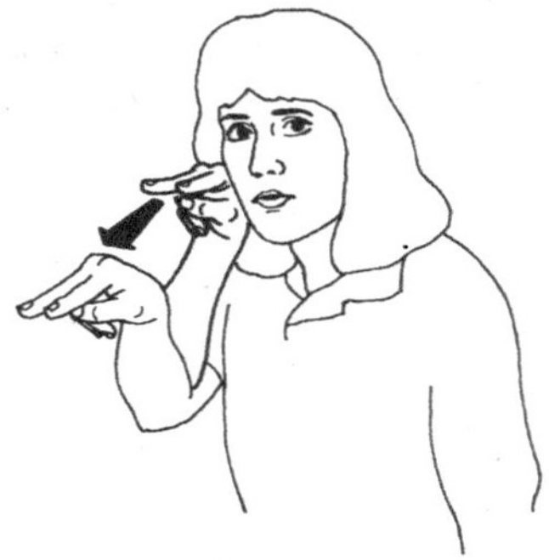

LOOK-AT-YOU
Right V hand, shoulder level, palm in. Sweep hand out, away from face so that fingers are pointing out.
Clue: eyes staring at a person.

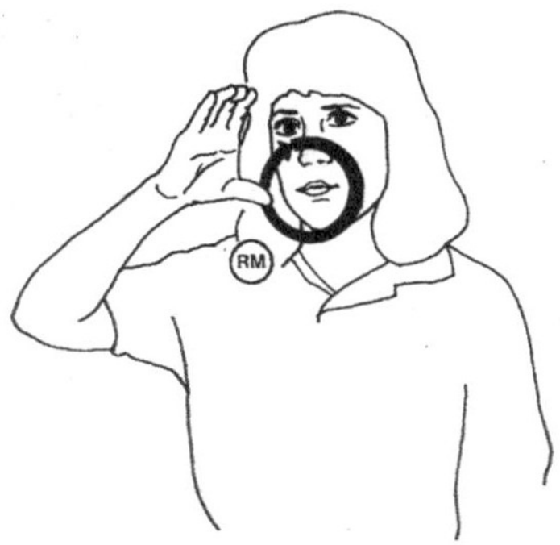

LOOK FOR
Right C hand, head level, palm left. Right hand circles in front of face repeatedly.

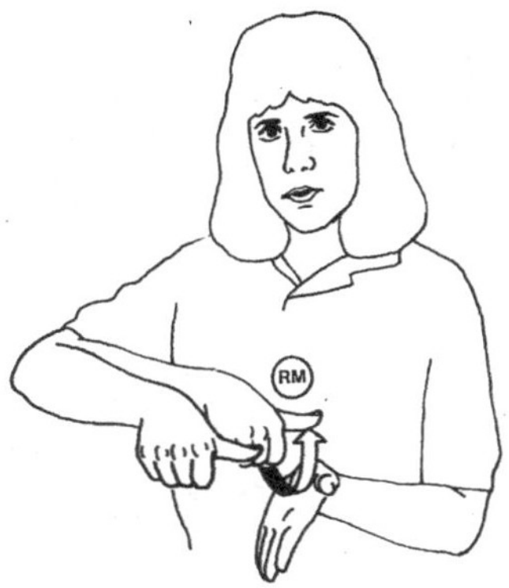

LOOK UP
Left flat hand, palm up, chest level. Right A hand, palm down, on left palm. Right thumb repeatedly brushes in towards body.
Clue: flipping through pages in a book.

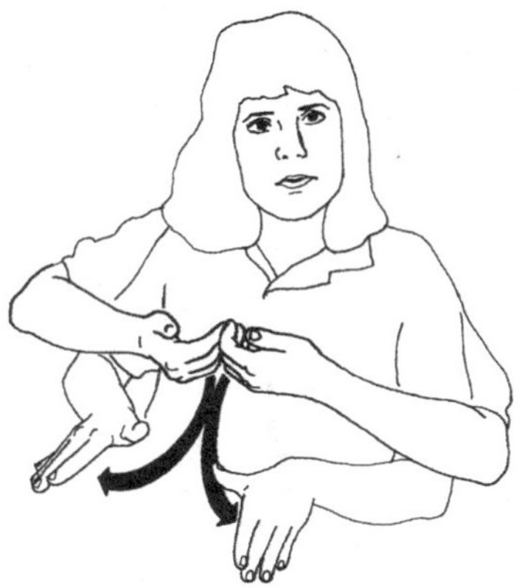

LOSS
C hands, chest level, palms up. While moving hands down sides, open to flat hands.
Clue: dropping something from your hands.

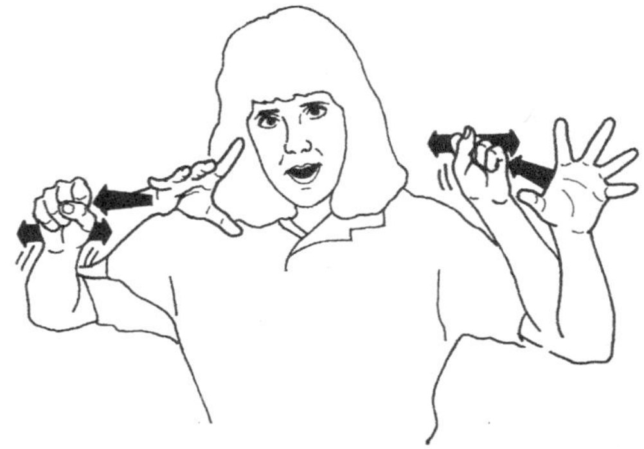

LOUD
Right 5 hand, palm out, near right ear. Left 5 hand, palm out, near left shoulder. Move right hand out, changing to S hand. Move left hand toward ear, changing to S hand. Shake S hands side to side.

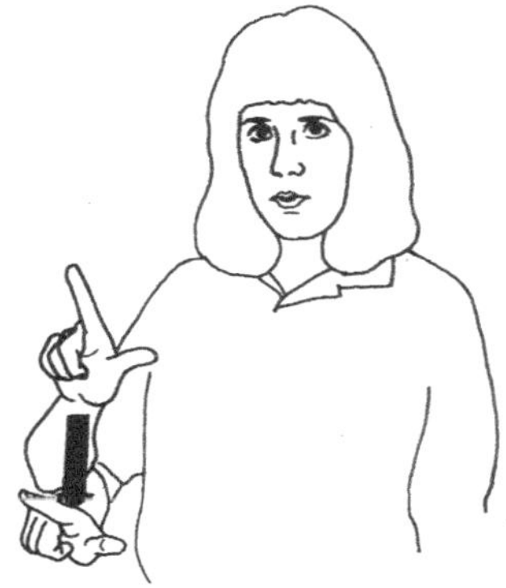

LOW
Right L hand, palm out, shoulder level. Move hand down, ending with palm down.

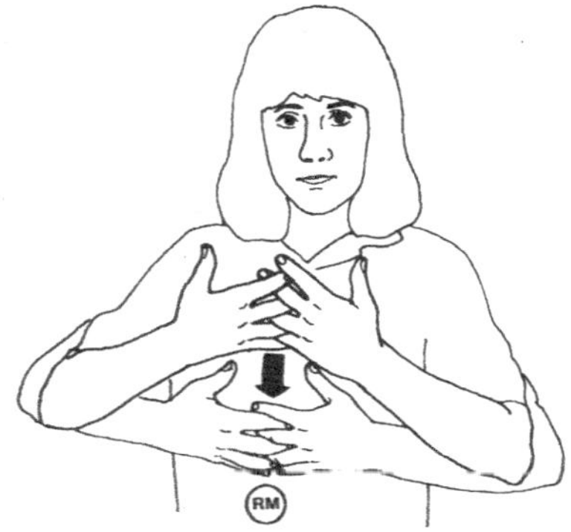

MACHINE
5 hands, palms in, chest level. Interlace fingers. Move both hands simultaneously up and down at wrists. Repeat.

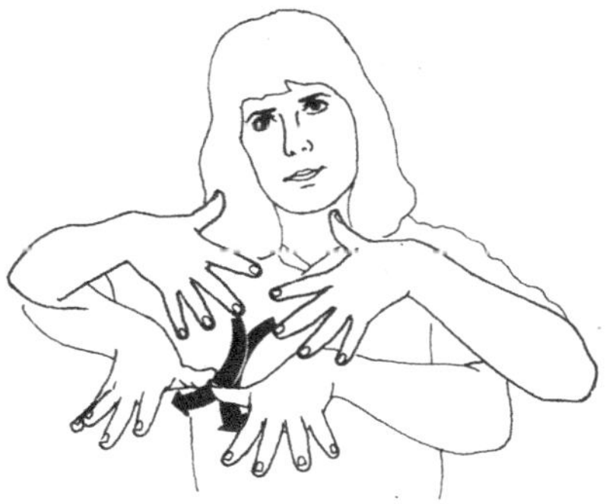

MAINSTREAM
5 hands, palms down, chest level, hands apart. Hands come together and move forward.
Clue: "blending" of children together.

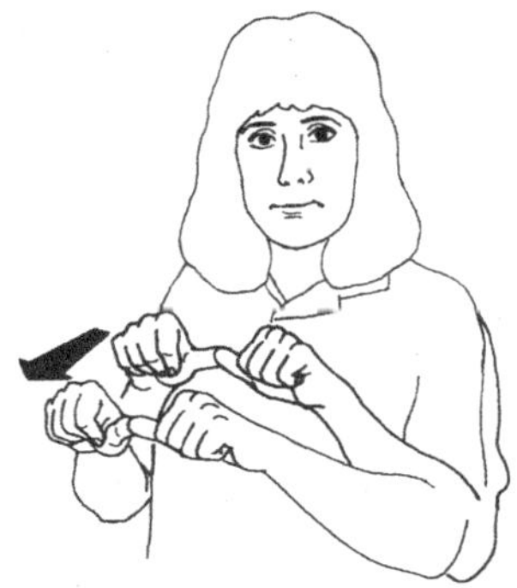

MAINTAIN
A hands, palms down, chest level, right thumb behind and touching left thumb. Simultaneously move hands out from body in a smooth movement.

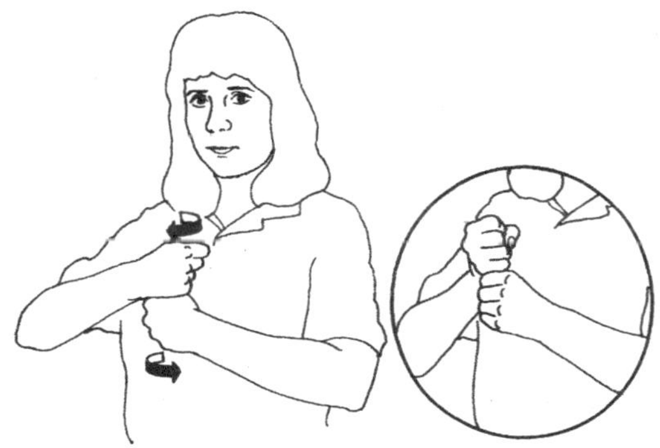

MAKE
S hands, waist level, right hand on top of left. Move hands 180 degrees in opposite directions.

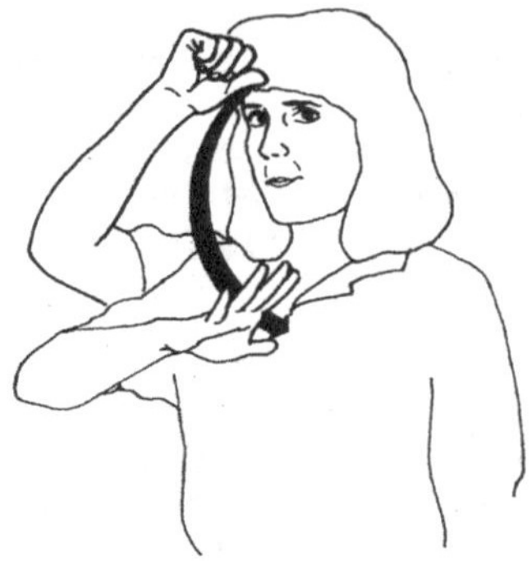

MAN
Right A hand, palm left, thumb at forehead. Bring hand down to chest, opening to 5 hands.

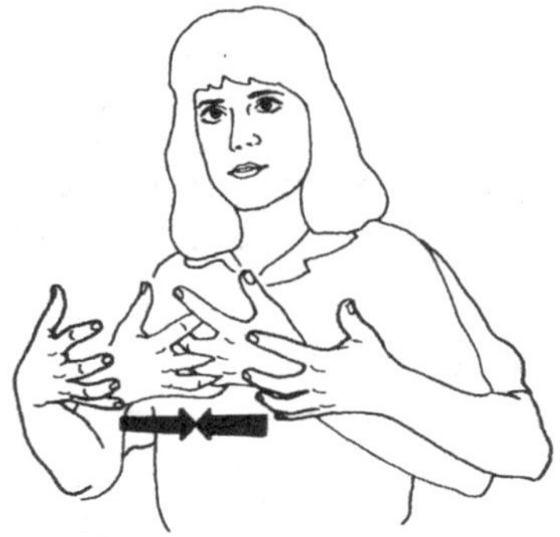

MATCH
5 hands, palms in, chest level. Begin at sides. Move hands together so fingers interlace.

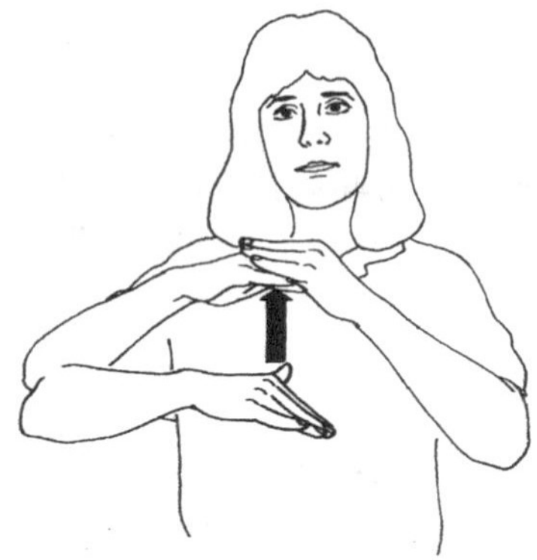

MAXIMUM
Flat hands, bent at knuckles, palms down. Right below left at chest level. Move right up to hit left.

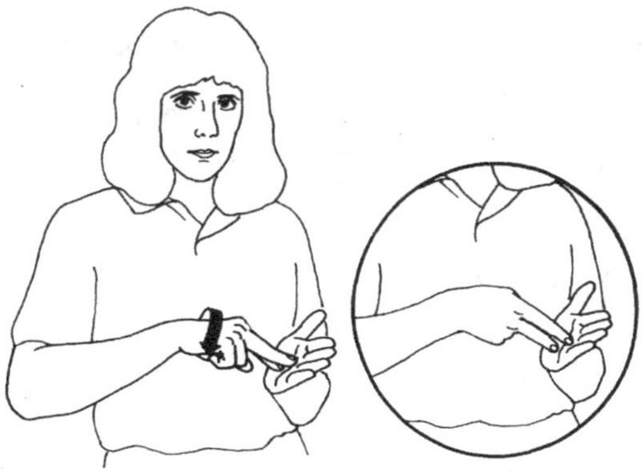

MEANING/MEAN (verb)
Left flat hand, palm right, chest level. Right V hand, palm down, fingertips on left palm. Rotate right hand in left palm.

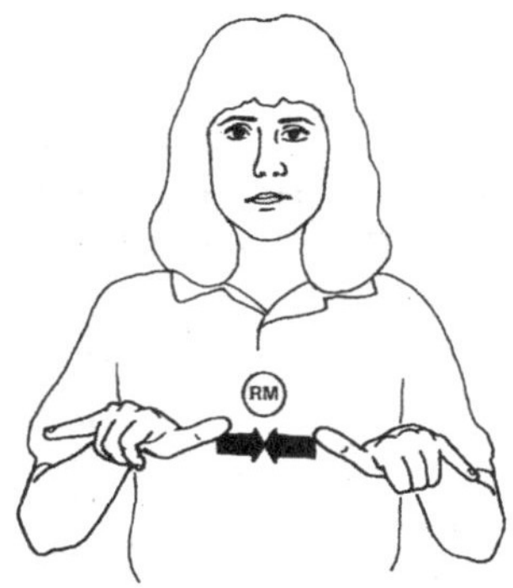

MEASURE
Y hands, palms down, waist level. Hands move towards each other so thumbs touch. Repeat.

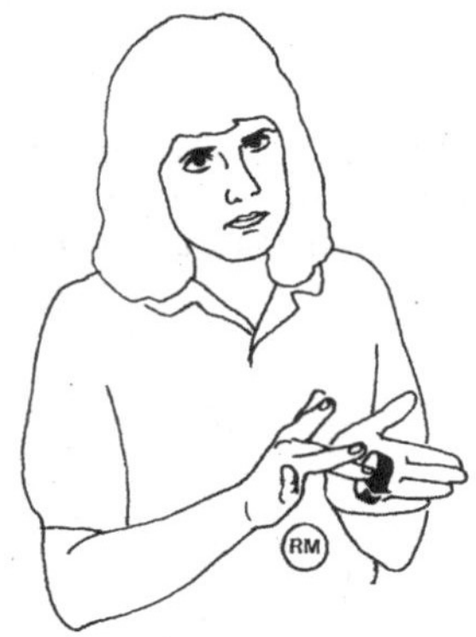

MEDICATION
Right 5 hand, middle finger down, palm down, waist level. Left flat hand, palm up, waist level. Touch right middle finger to left palm and shake right hand slightly.

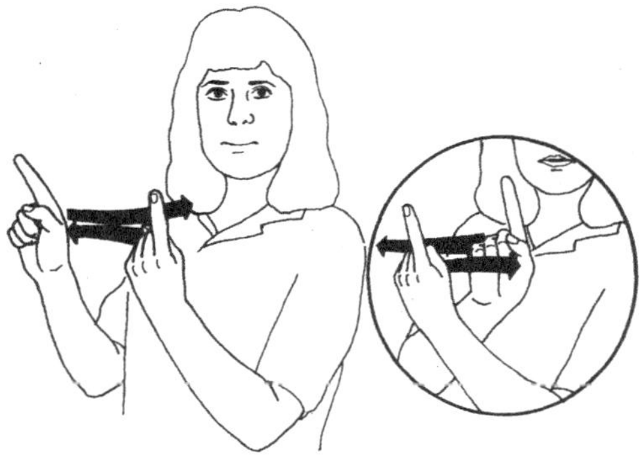

MEET
1 hands, palms facing each other, chest level. Move hands towards each other until wrists cross, then move apart.
Clue: two people "bumping into" each other.

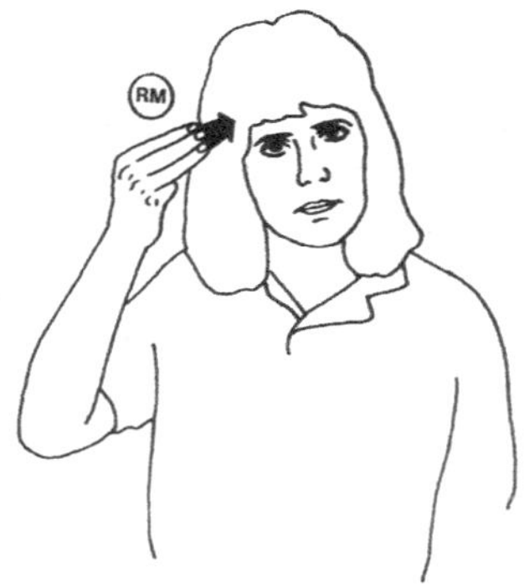

MENTAL
Right M hand, palm in, taps head at right temple. Repeat.

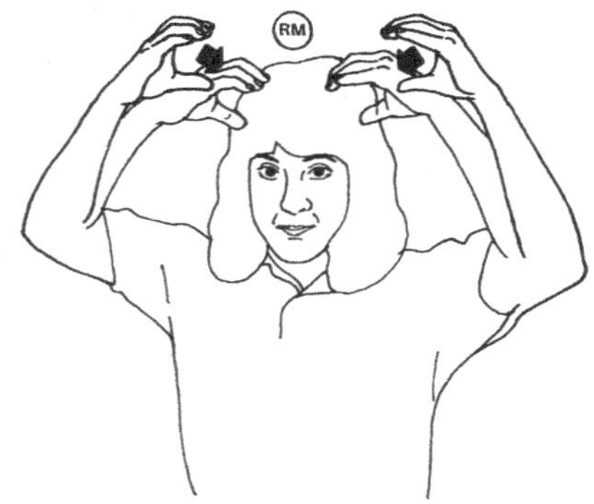

MICKEY MOUSE
C hands, palms down, repeatedly tap head.
Clue: simulates Mickey Mouse's ears.

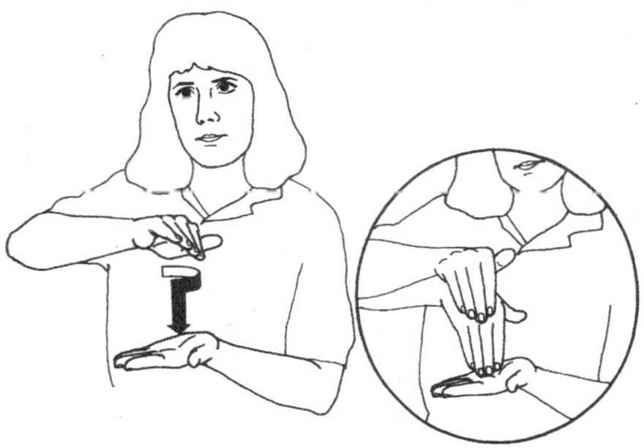

MIDDLE/CENTER
Left flat hand, palm up, waist level. Right flat hand, palm down, chest level. Right hand circles over left hand, ending with fingertips in center of left palm.

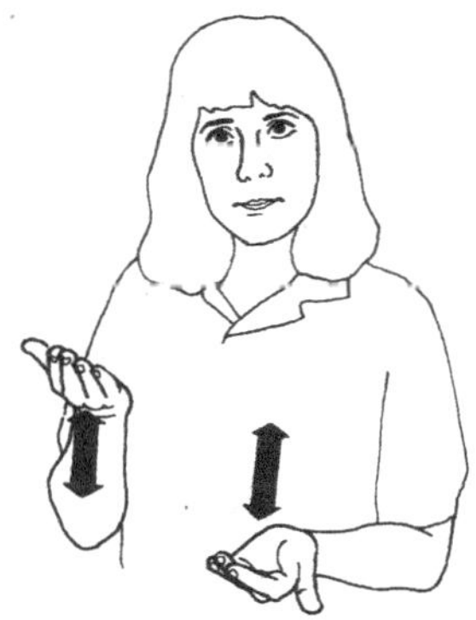

MIGHT/MAYBE
Slightly cupped flat hands, palms up, waist level. Move hands alternately up and down.

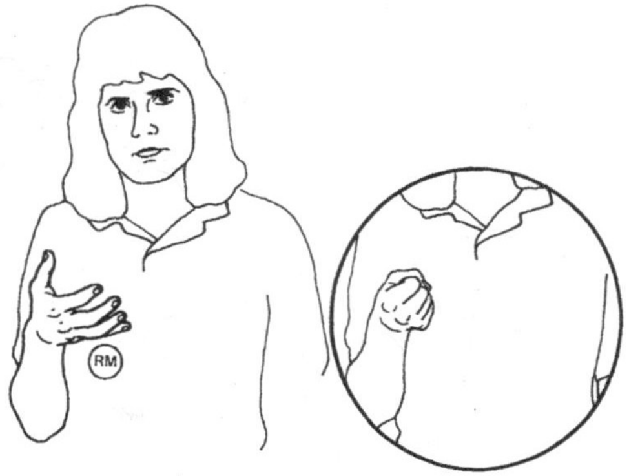

MILK
Right rounded 5 hand, chest level, palm to side. Open and close to S hand repeatedly.
Clue: milking a cow.

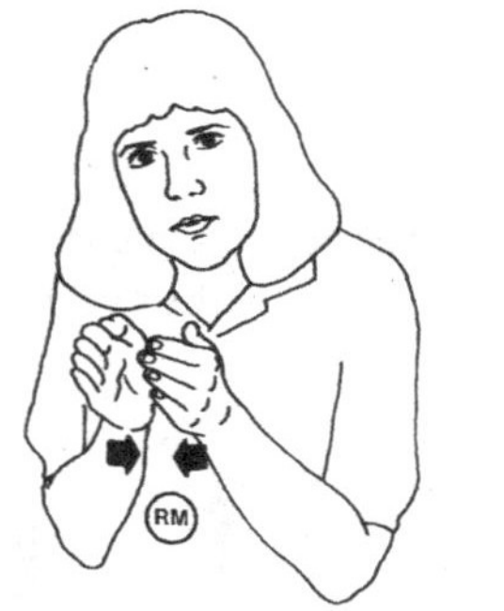

MINOR
Flat hands, palms facing each other, chest level. Hands move in slightly closer to each other.

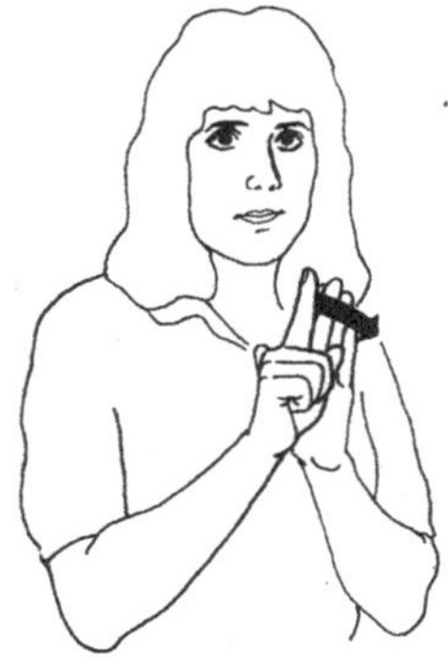

MINUTE
Left flat hand, chest level, palm to side. Right 1 hand touching left palm. Right hand moves back and forth.
Clue: minute hand on a clock.

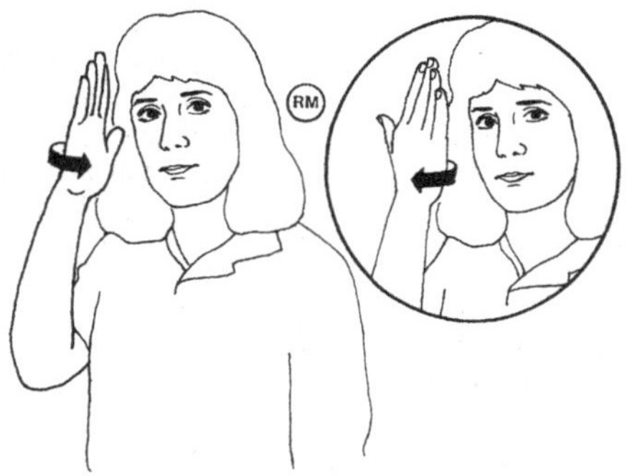

MIRROR
Right flat hand, palm left, head level. Hand moves slightly from left to right.

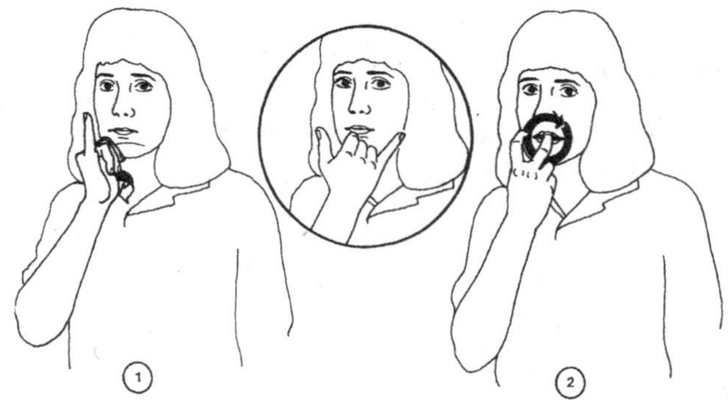

MISARTICULATION
Right Y hand, palm in at chin. Twist hand at wrist. Change to bent V hand, palm in, at mouth level. Circle clockwise in front of mouth.
Clue: wrong + speech.

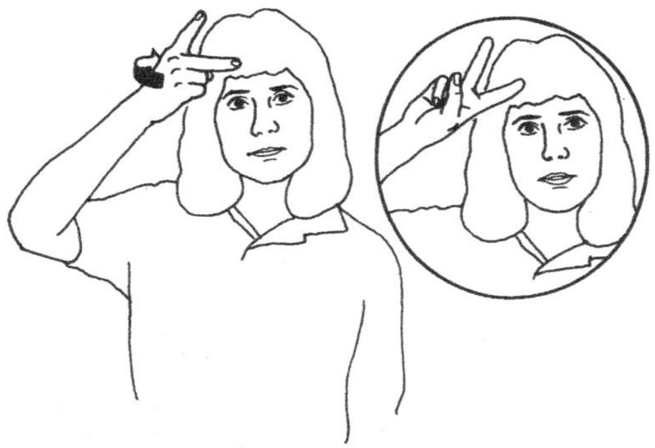

MISUNDERSTAND
Right V hand, palm out, index finger touching right temple. Rotate wrist so palm faces back and middle finger touches temple.

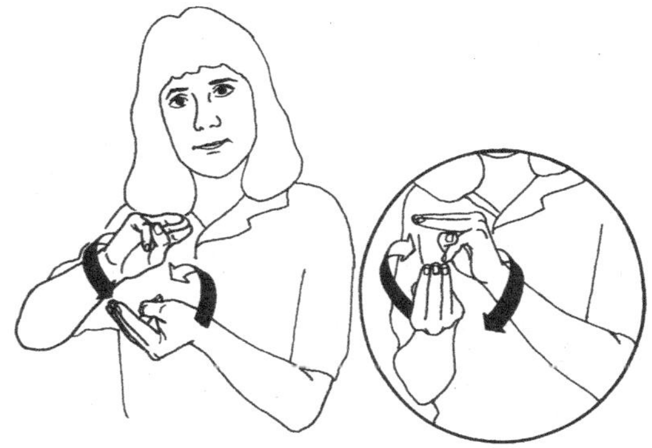

MODIFICATION
M hands, palms facing each other, right hand above left, chest level. Simultaneously twist hands 180 degrees in opposite directions.

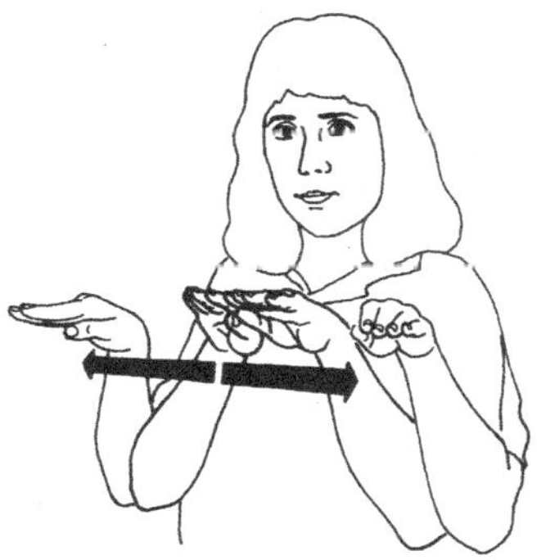

MONOTONE
B hands, palms down, chest level, hands touching. Bring hands apart.
Clue: showing a flat voice.

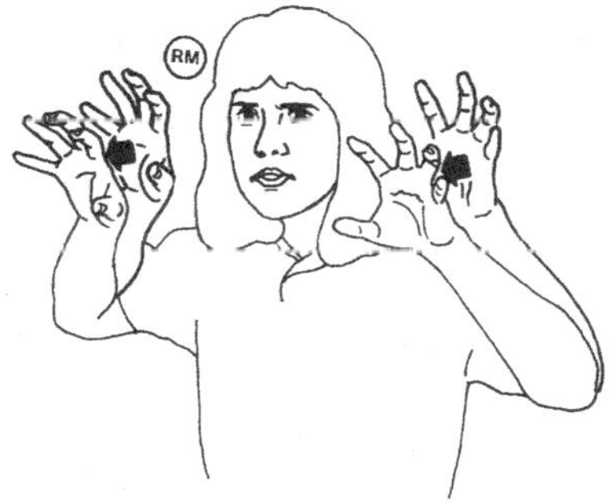

MONSTER
Claw hands, shoulder level, palms out. Tilt body forward while arching arms out.
Clue: a monster lunging forward.

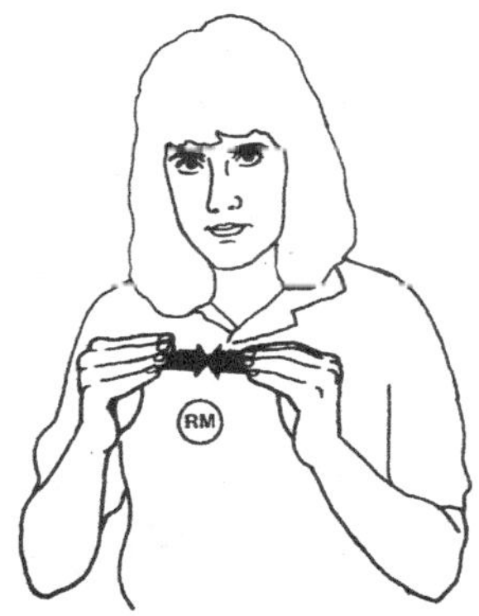

MORE
Flat O hands, palms facing each other, chest level. Tap fingertips of O hands.

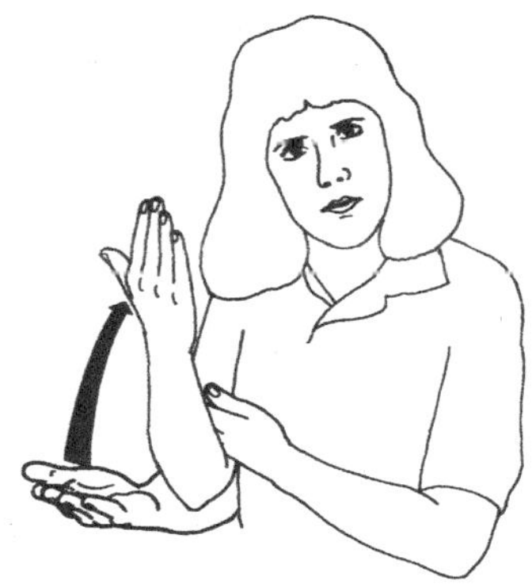

MORNING
Left arm folded at waist, palm up. Right flat hand, palm up, left hand resting in bend of right arm. Right arm moves up from below waist level straight up to right shoulder.

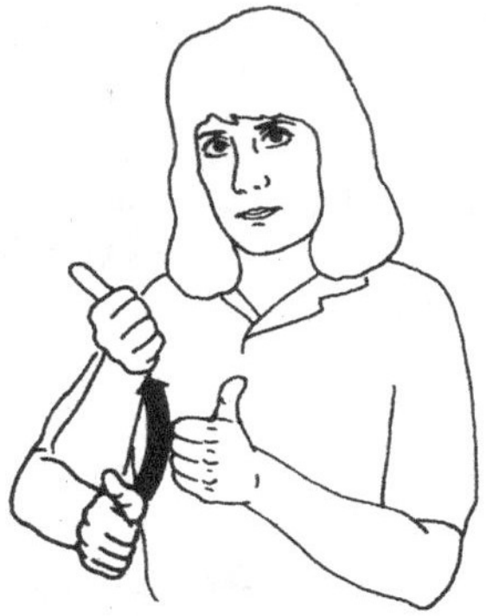

MOST
A hands, chest level, palms facing, right hand slightly below left. Right hand moves up left hand and stops at head level.

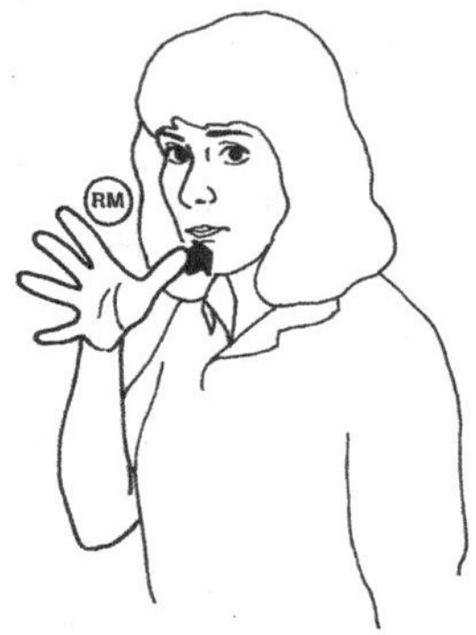

MOTHER
Right 5 hand, palm left, thumb touching chin. Bounce thumb against chin several times.

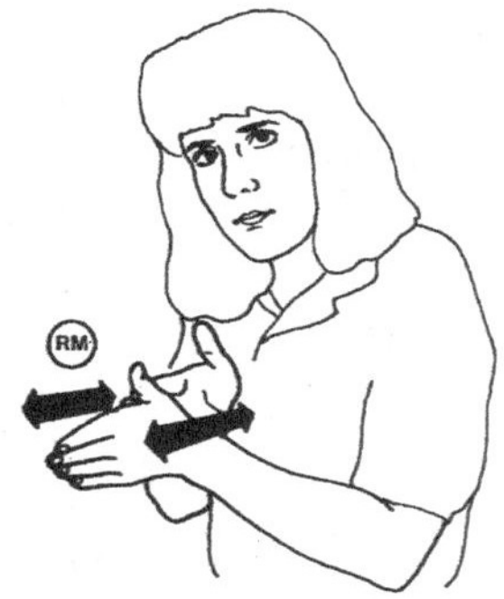

MOTIVATE
Flat hands, palms together, chest level. Rub hands repeatedly.

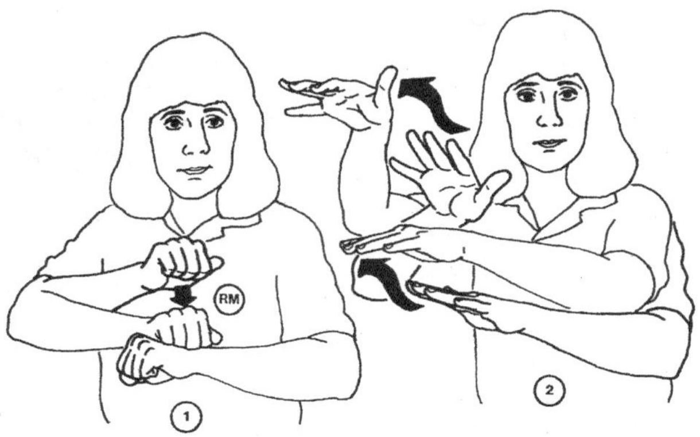

MOUNTAIN
A hands, palms down, chest level. Right A taps left A. Move up quickly to 5 hands, palms out.
Clue: rock + hill.

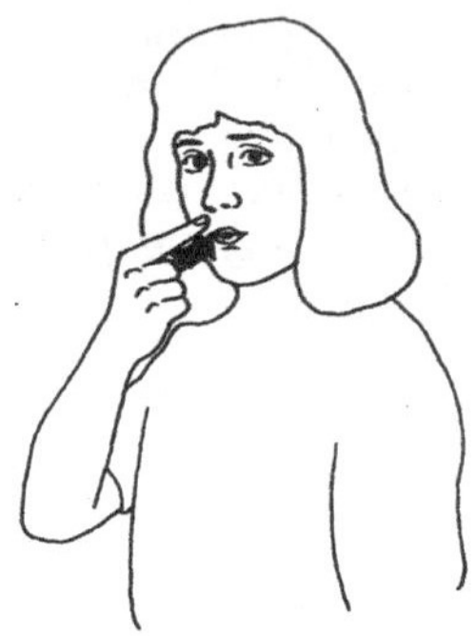

MOUTH
Right 1 hand, palm in. Point to mouth.

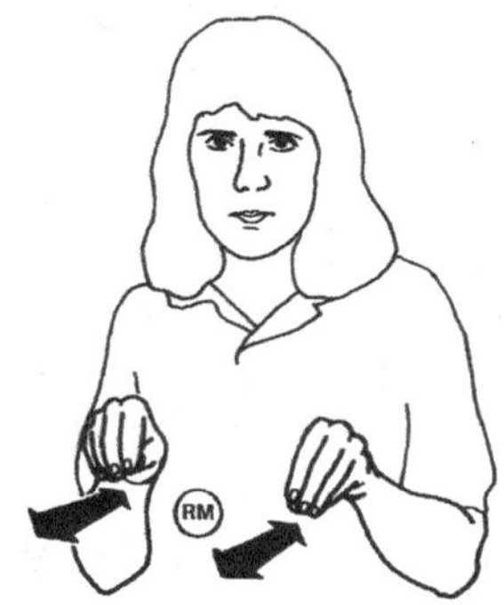

MOVE
Flat O hands, palms down, waist level. Simultaneously move hands to the right. Repeat.

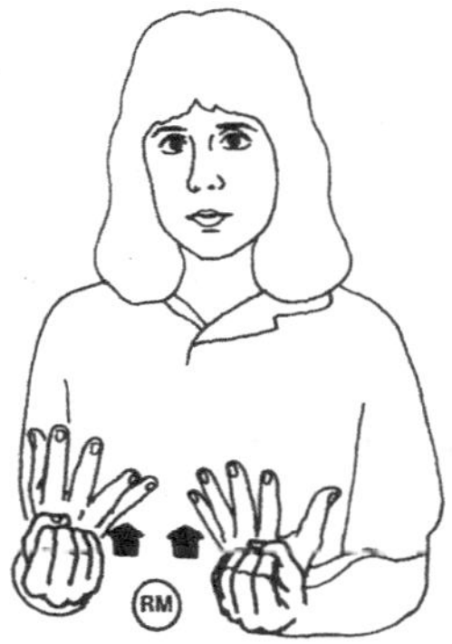

MULTI/MANY
S hands, palms up, chest level. Flick quickly to 5 hands.

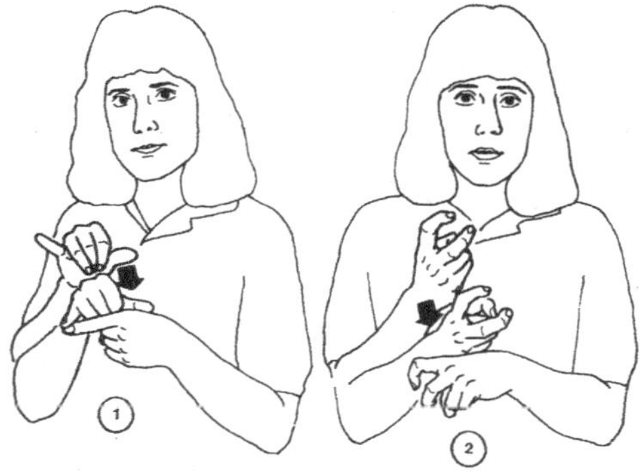

MULTISYLLABLE
Left 1 hand, palm in, chest level. Right Y hand, palm down, taps left index finger. Change to bent V hands. Right hand taps left.

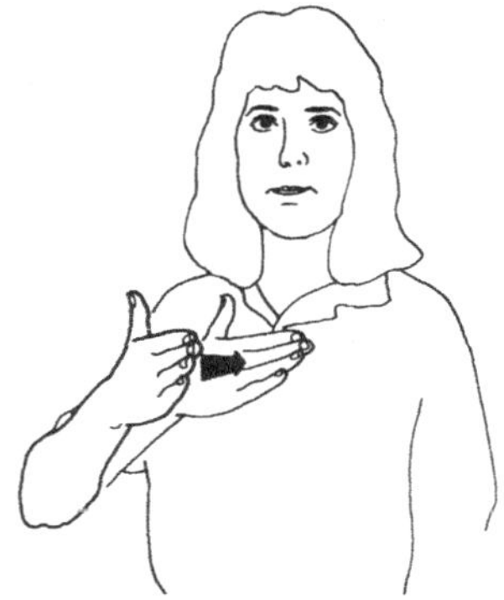

MY
Right flat hand touches chest repeatedly.

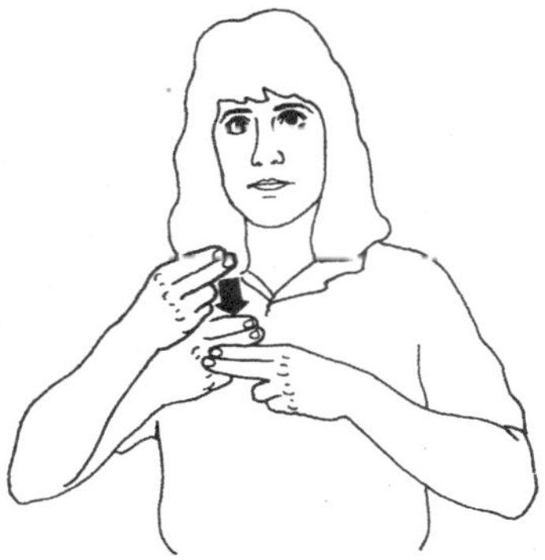

NAME
H hands, chest level, palms in. Right hand taps on top of left hand.

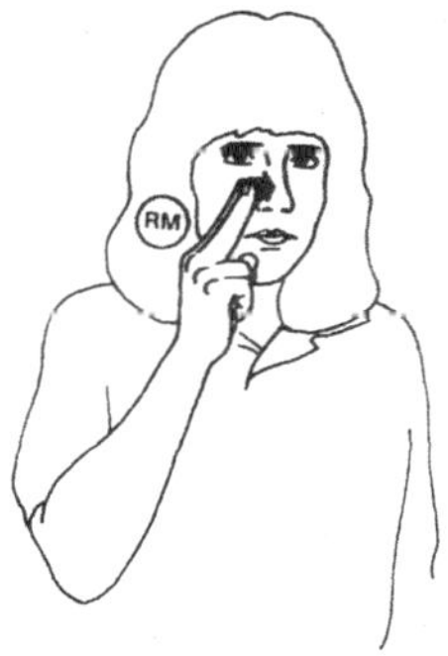

NASAL
Right U hand, palm in, repeatedly points to side of nose.

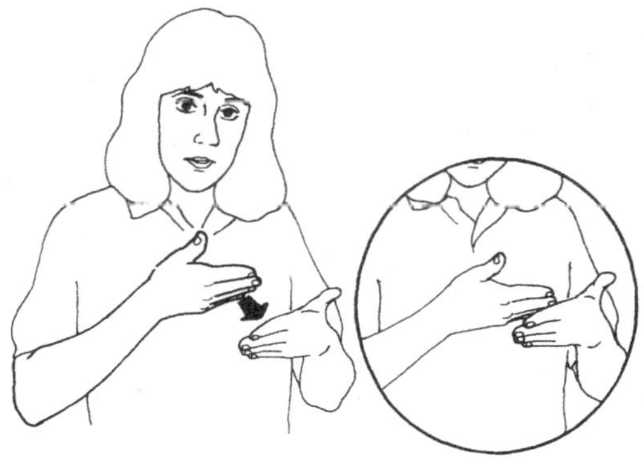

NEAR/CLOSE
Flat hands, palms in, chest level, left hand in front of right. Move right closer to left palm.

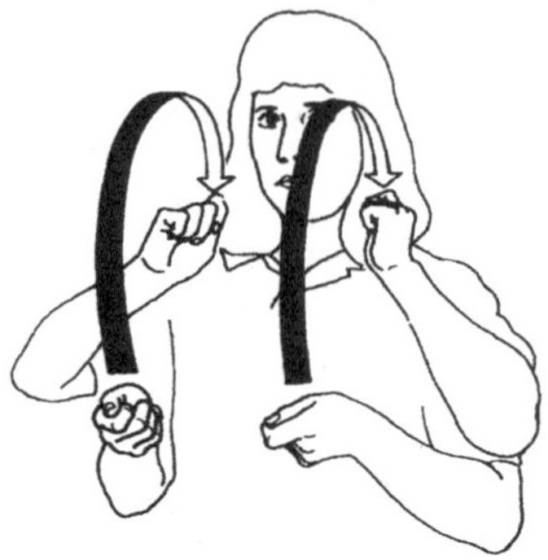

NECKLOOP
Closed hands, thumbs and index fingers touching, palms facing each other, chest level. Bring hands over head and down to neck level.
Clue: putting on a neck loop.

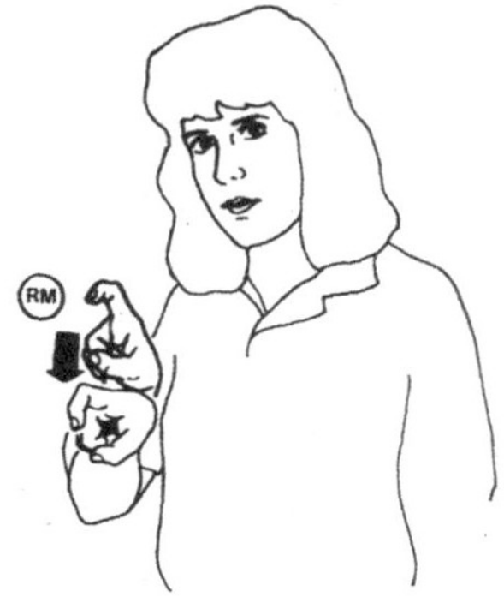

NEED
Right X hand, palm out, chest level. Move to palm down. Repeat.

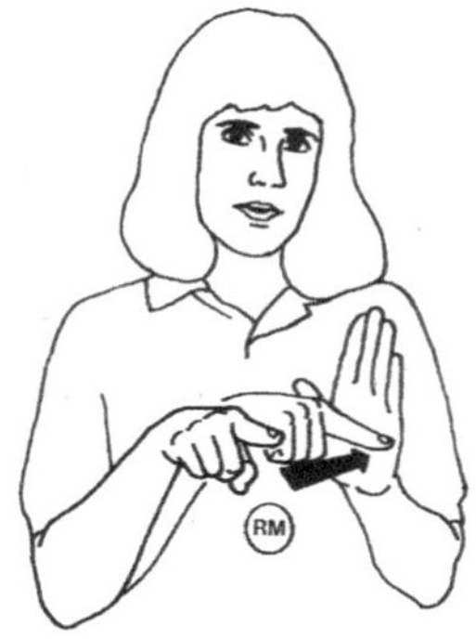

NEGATIVE
Left flat hand, palm out, chest level. Right 1 hand, palm down in middle of left palm. Right hand bounces in left palm.

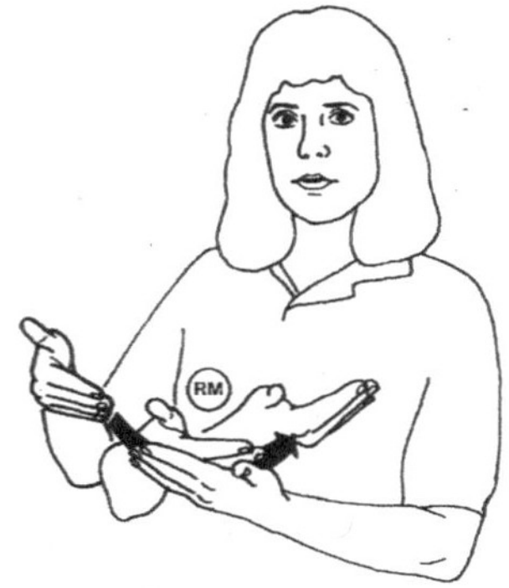

NEW
Right cupped hand, palm up, fingers left. Left flat hand, palm up, waist level. Swoop right hand to graze left palm.

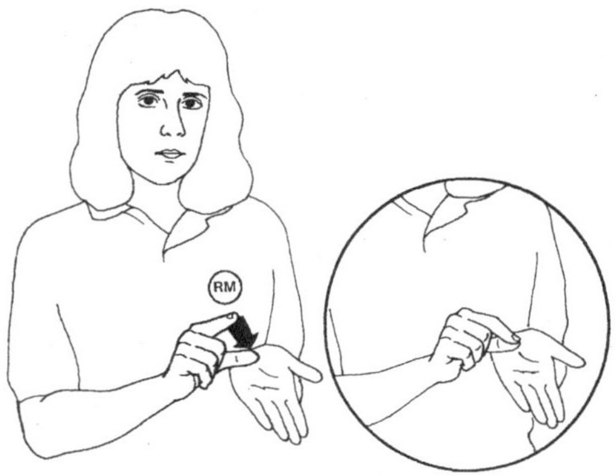

NEWSPAPER
Left flat hand, palm up, waist level. Right G hand, palm down, thumb in left palm. Move right index finger up and down (touching right thumb) repeatedly.

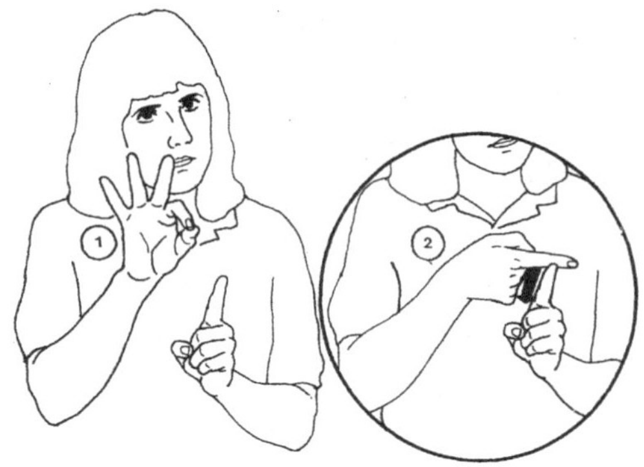

NINE-MONTH
Left 1 hand, palm right, chest level. Right 9 hand, palm out, chin level. Change to right 1 hand, palm in, finger pointing left. Move right index finger down left index finger.

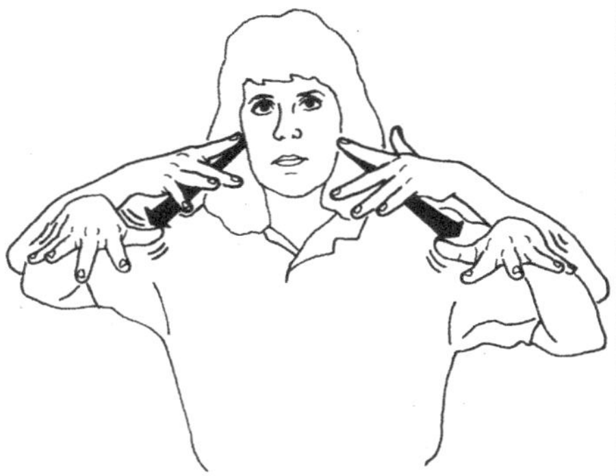

NOISE
5 hands at base of ears, palms down. Move hands to the side and shake.

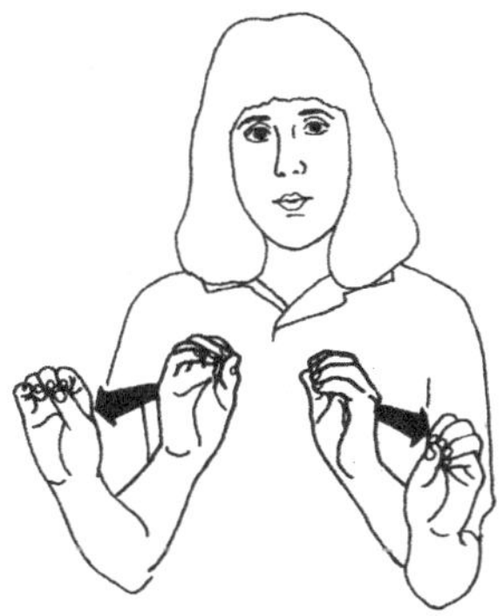

NONE
O hands, palms facing each other, chest level. Sharply move out and slightly apart from each other.

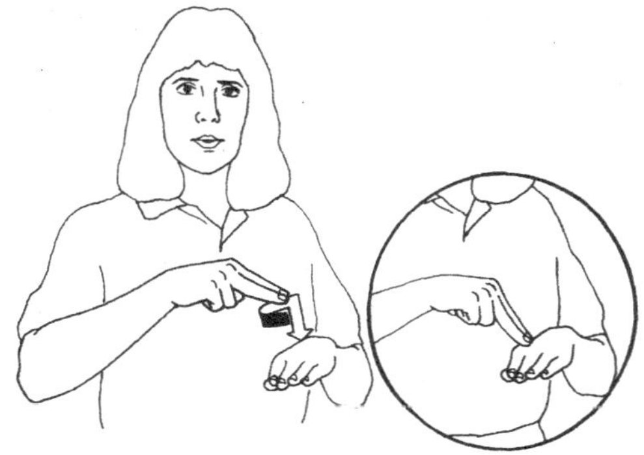

NORMAL
Right U hand, palm down. Left flat hand, chest level, palm down. Position right above left. Circle U in counterclockwise direction and tap left hand.

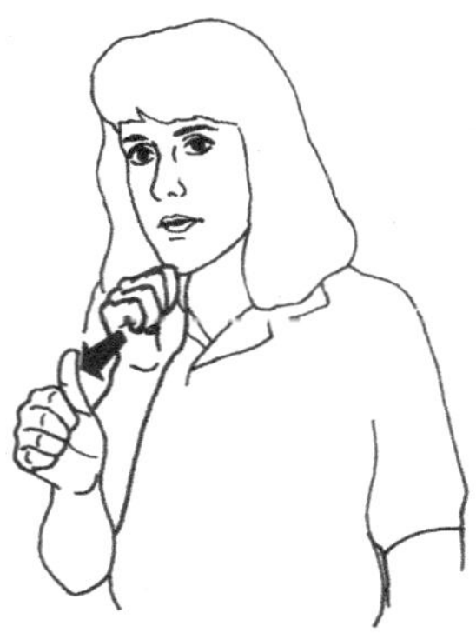

NOT
Right A hand, palm left, thumb under chin. Quickly move A forward, grazing chin with thumb.

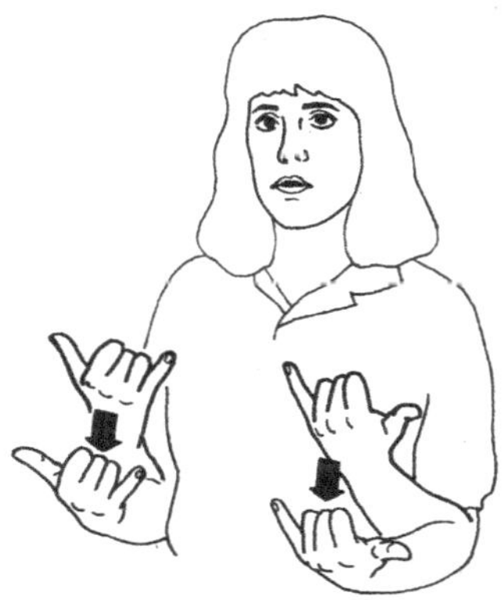

NOW
Y hands, palms up, chest level. Move simultaneously down to waist level.

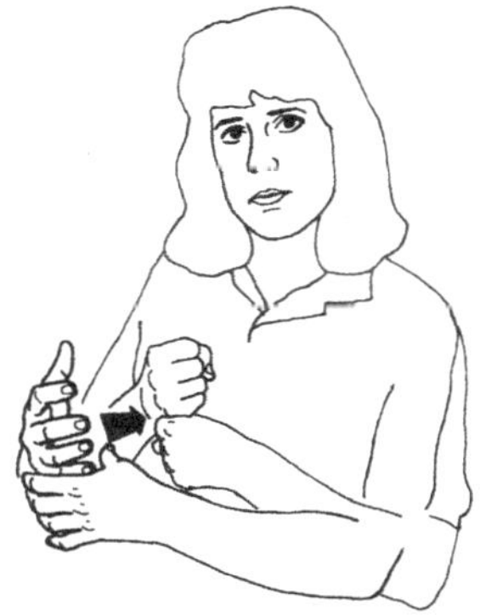

OBTAIN/GET/RECEIVE
Claw hands, palms facing, chest level, right hand on left index finger. Pull hands in towards body changing to S hands.

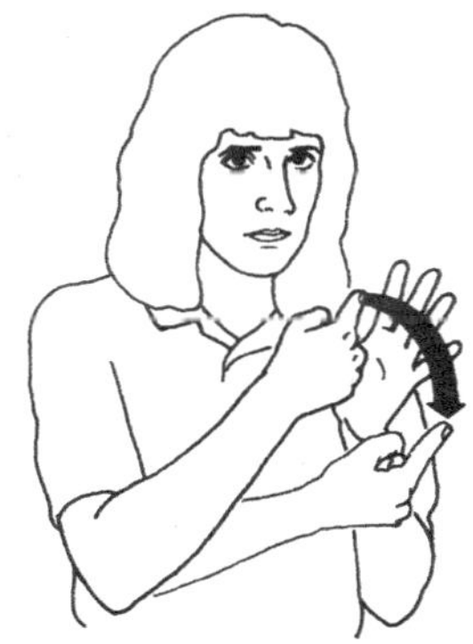

OF-THE-FOLLOWING/ OF-THESE
Left 5 hand, palm to side, chest level. Right 1 hand moves along left fingers, ending with little finger.
Clue: pointing to each item.

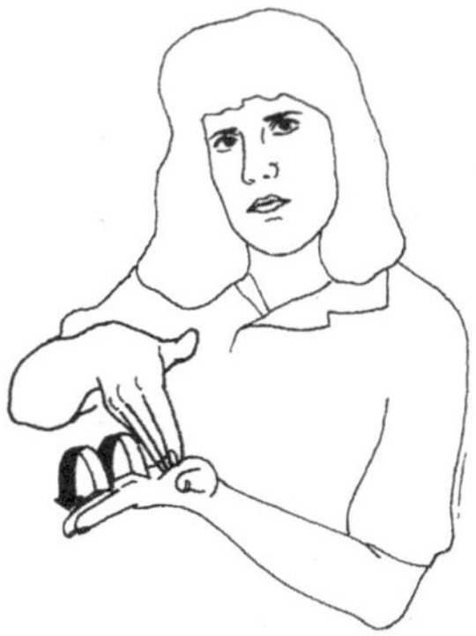

OFTEN/FREQUENT
Left flat hand, palm up, chest level. Right flat hand, palm in, repeatedly taps palm of left hand.

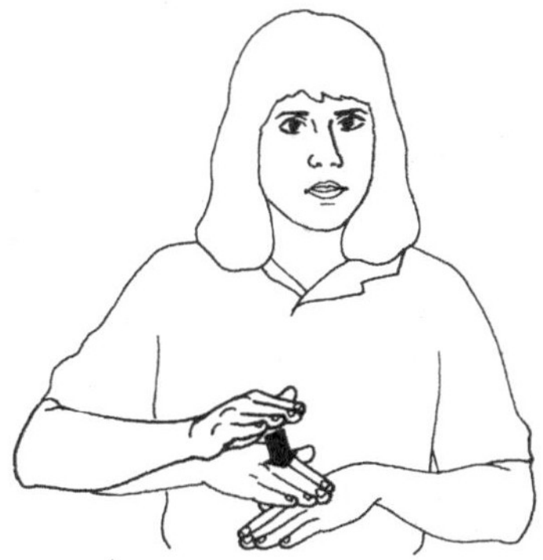

ON
Flat hands, waist level, palms down, right hand above left. Bring right hand down on top of left.
Clue: putting an object on a table.

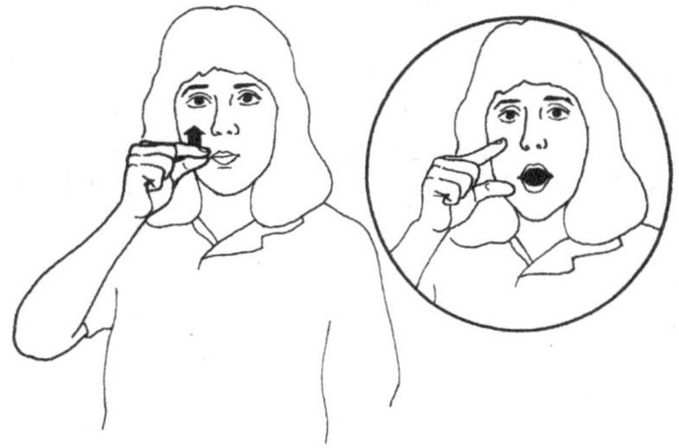

OPEN MOUTH
Right 20 hand, palm left, at right side of mouth. Move index finger and thumb apart, opening lips at the same time.

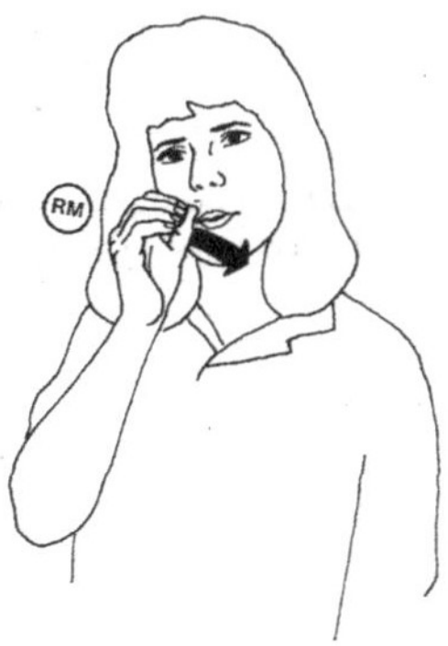

ORAL
Right O hand, palm to side at mouth. Move hand across mouth. Repeat.

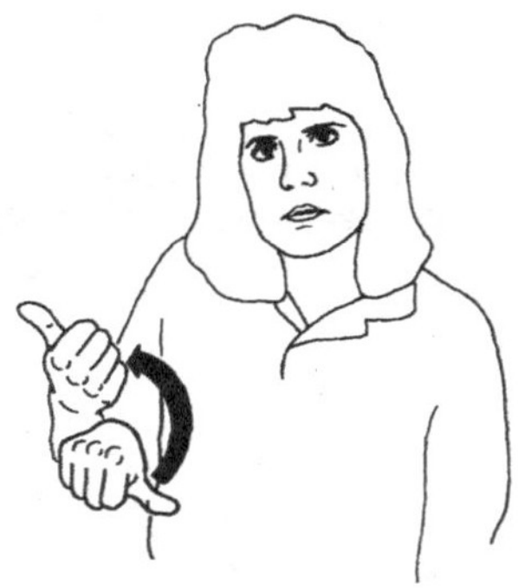

OTHER/ELSE
Right 10 hand, palm down, waist level. Sweep up to palm up.

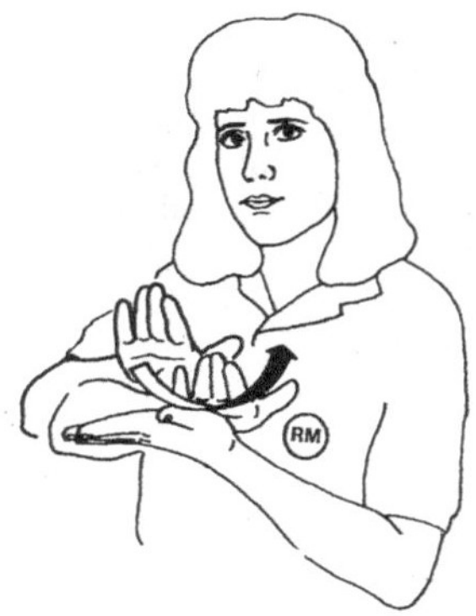

PAPER
Right flat hand, palm down, chest level. Left flat hand, palm up, chest level. Heel of right hand rests on heel of left hand. Bump heels of hands together repeatedly.

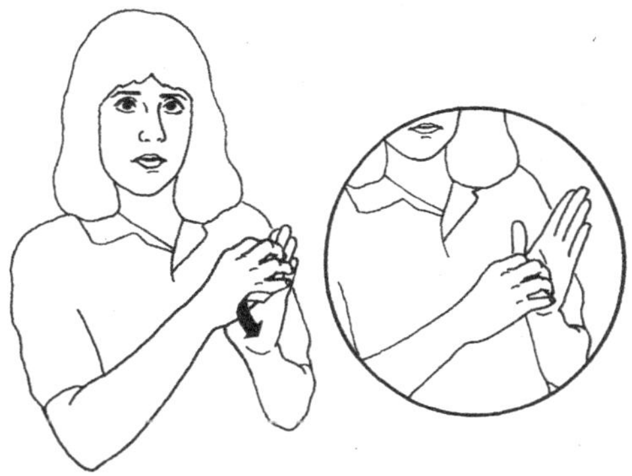

PARAGRAPH
Right C hand, palm left, chest level.
Left flat hand, palm right, chest level.
Place right C near top of left palm, then bounce C down once towards wrist.

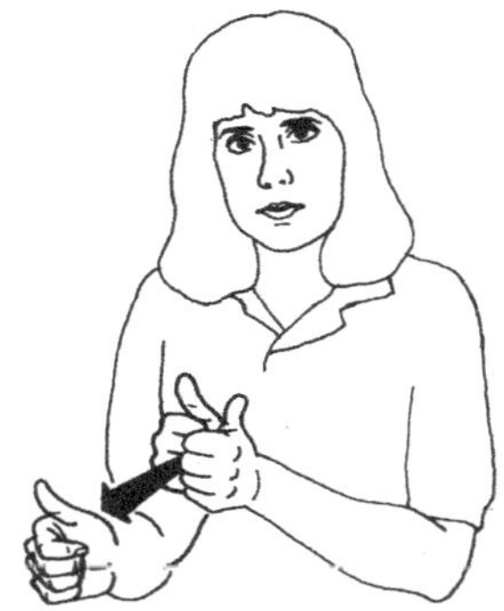

PASS
A hands, palms facing each other, chest level. Right A slightly behind left A. Move right A to graze and pass left A.

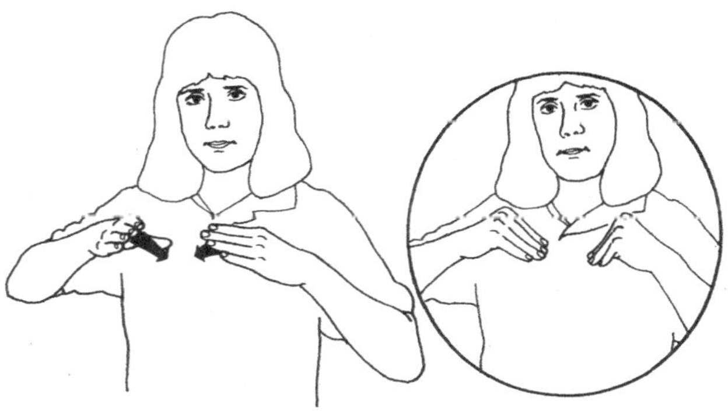

PASSIVE/ACCEPT
Flat hands, palms in, thumbs on chest.
Close hands to flat Os.

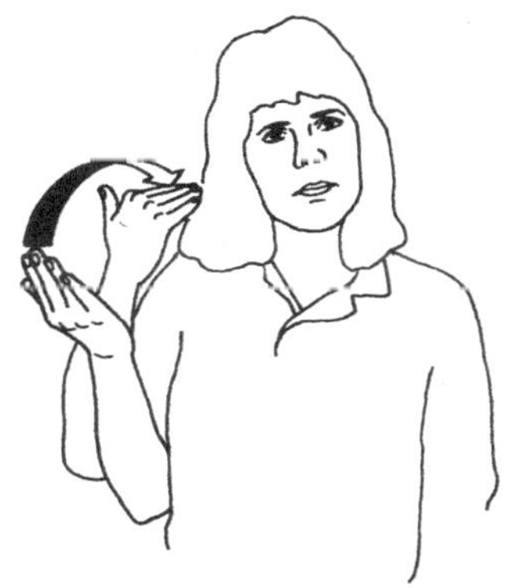

PAST
Right flat hand, at shoulder level, palm in. Wave hand over shoulder.
Clue: all signs related from the shoulder towards the back.

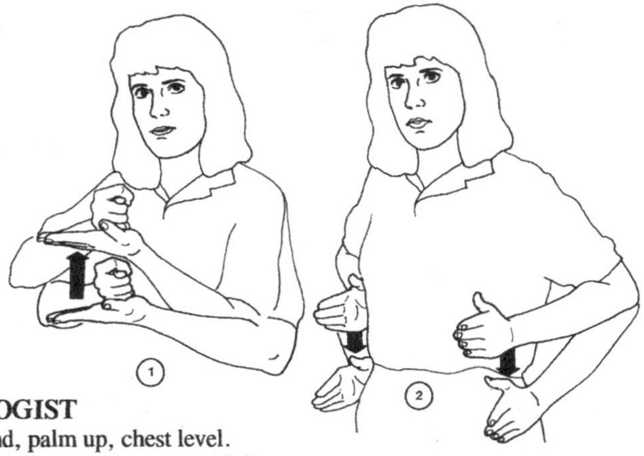

PATHOLOGIST
Left flat hand, palm up, chest level. Right T hand, thumb up, on top of left palm. Hands move up together and then change to flat hands, chest level, palms facing, and move down sides of body.

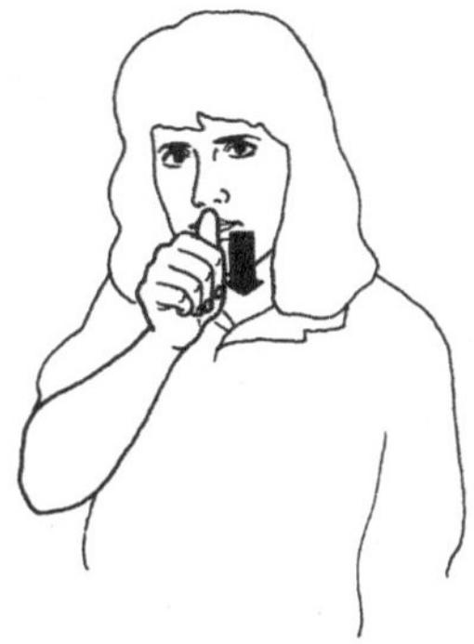

PATIENT
Right A hand, palm left, thumb resting on lips. Move thumb down to chin.

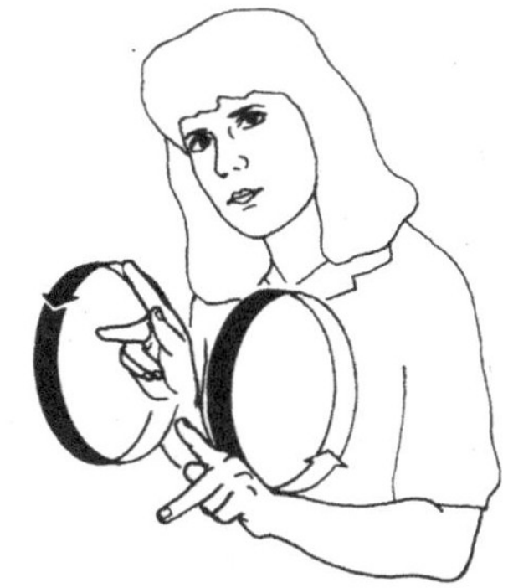

PEOPLE
P hands, palms out, waist level. Alternately circle hands out.

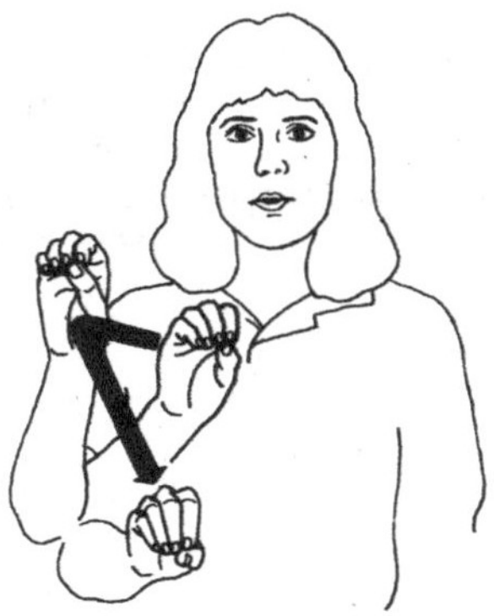

PERCENT
Right O hand, palm out, shoulder level. Move hand to the right and then down to the left in a quick movement.
Clue: drawing a percentage mark.

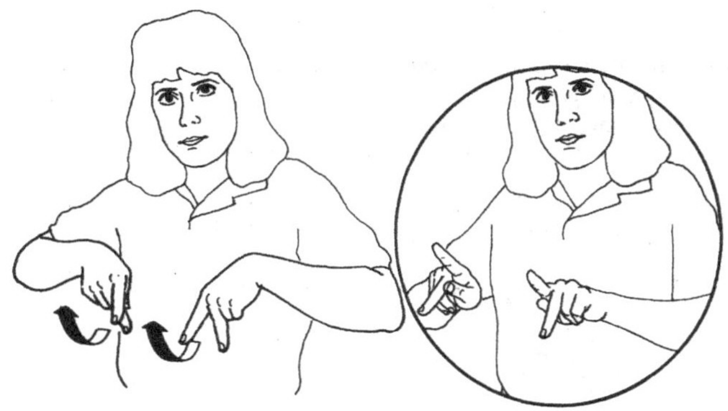

PERMISSION
P hands, palms down, waist level. Sweep up to palms out, chest level.

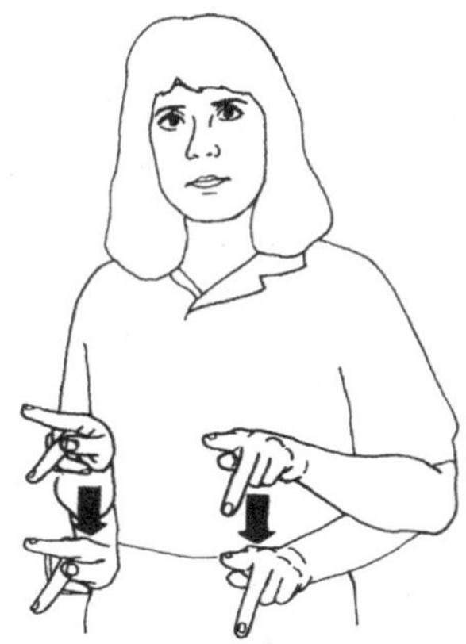

PERSON
P hands, chest level, palms down. Move hands down to waist.

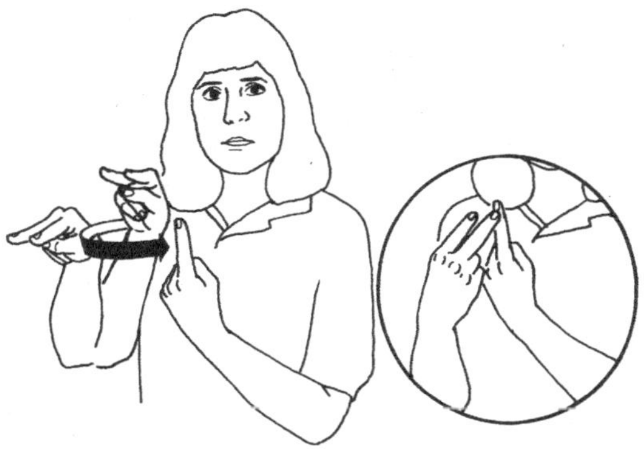

PERSPECTIVE
Right V hand, palm down, shoulder level. Left 1 hand, palm in, chest level. Move V around 1 so V fingertips face 1.
Clue: looking from the other's angle.

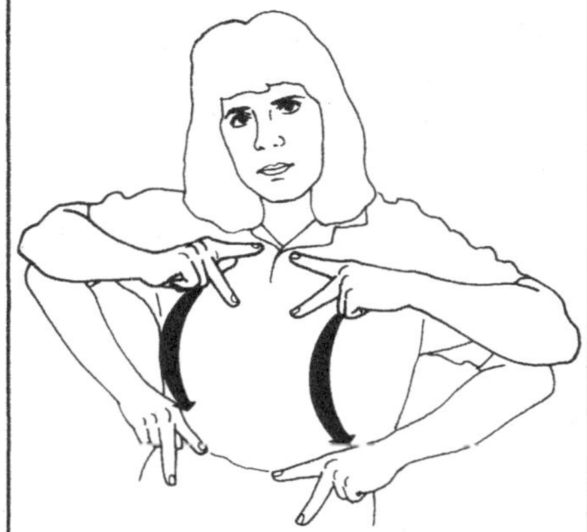

PHYSICAL
P hands, palms in, each hand on chest. Move hands simultaneously to waist level.

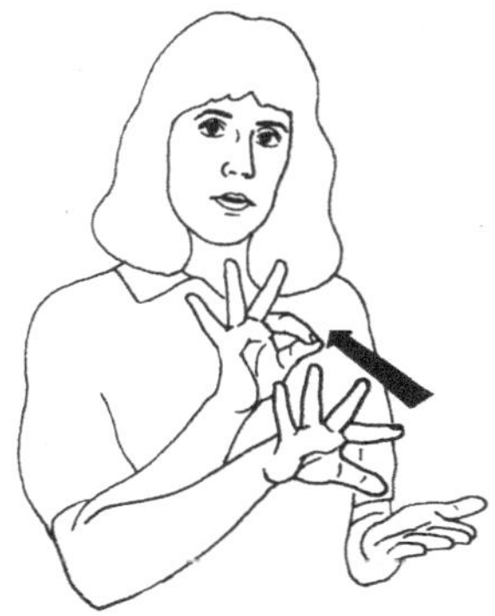

PICK OUT
Right 5 hand, palm down, chest level. Left flat hand, palm up, waist level. Right hand moves down to left palm, then up, changing to F hand.
Clue: picking something off the table.

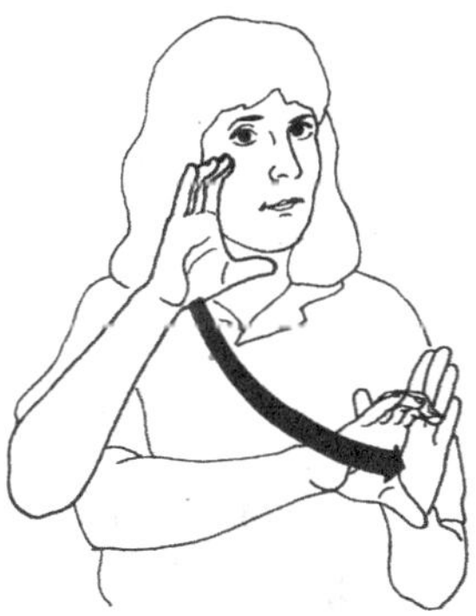

PICTURE
Left flat hand, chest level, palm right. Right C hand, palm out, on cheek. Move right hand down and place on left palm.

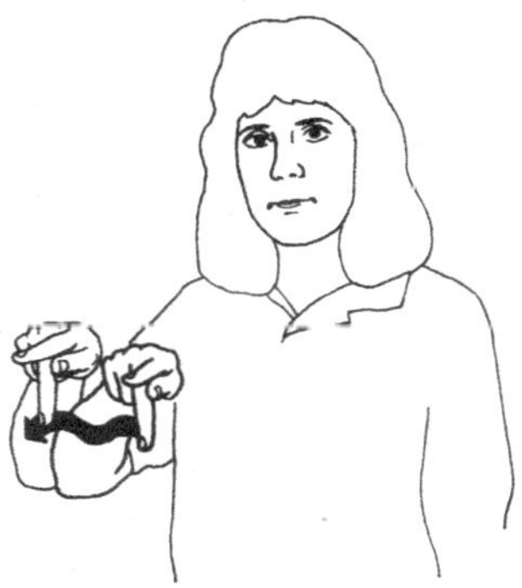

PITCH
Right P hand, palm down, chest level. Bounce hand while moving to the right.

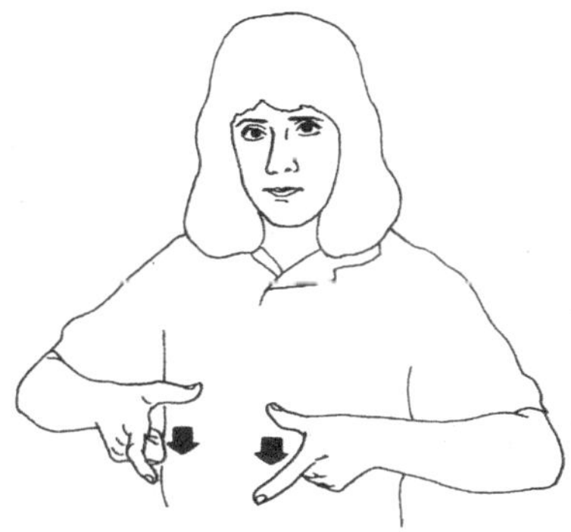

PLATE
Curved L hands, palms facing, chest level. Move sharply down at wrists.
Clue: the shape of a plate.

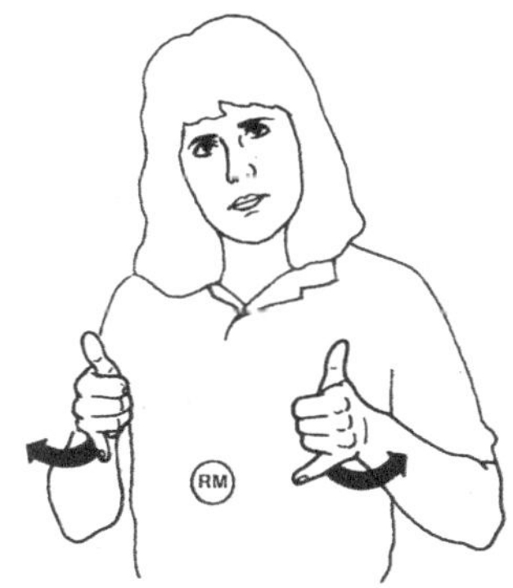

PLAY
Y hands, palms facing, chest level. Shake hands repeatedly.

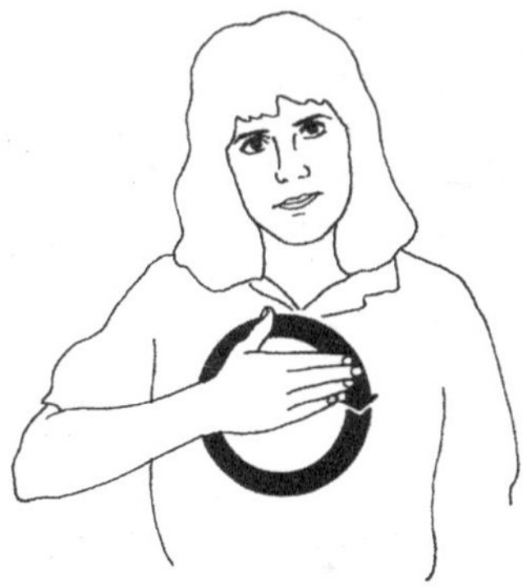

PLEASE
Right flat hand, palm on chest. Rub hand in clockwise direction.

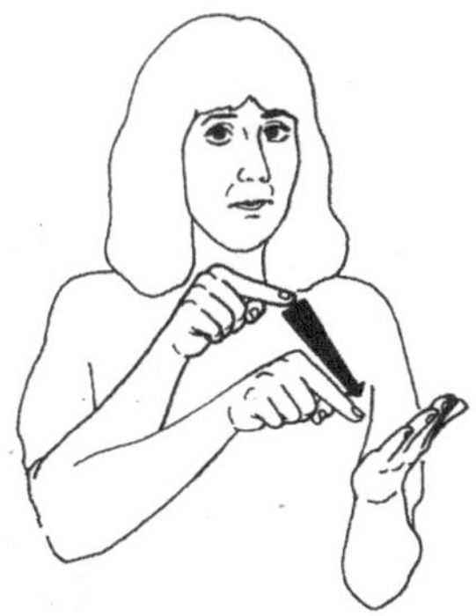

POINT
Right 1 hand, palm down, chest level. Left flat hand, palm in, chest level. Right hand moves down quickly towards left palm.
Clue: natural gesture.

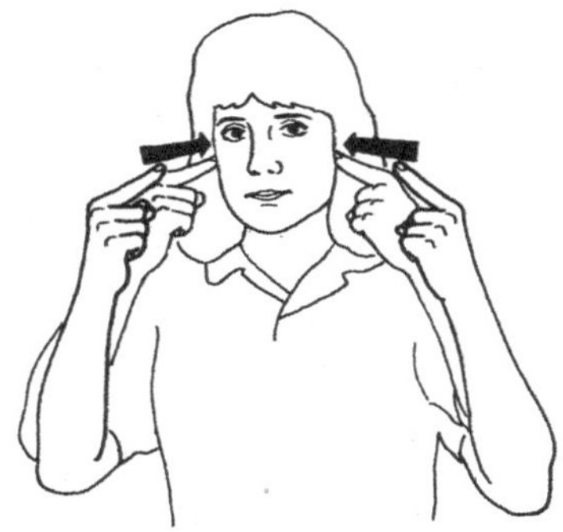

POINT-TO-EARS
1 hands, palms down, point to ears.

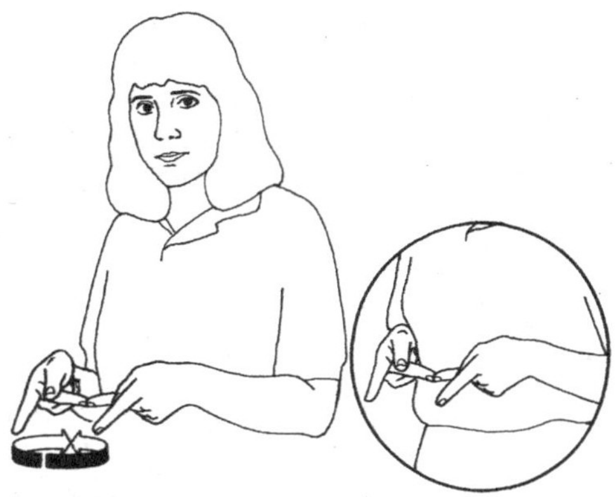

POSITION
P hands, palms facing each other, middle fingers touching, waist level. Simultaneously bring hands towards body in a circular motion until middle fingers are touching again.

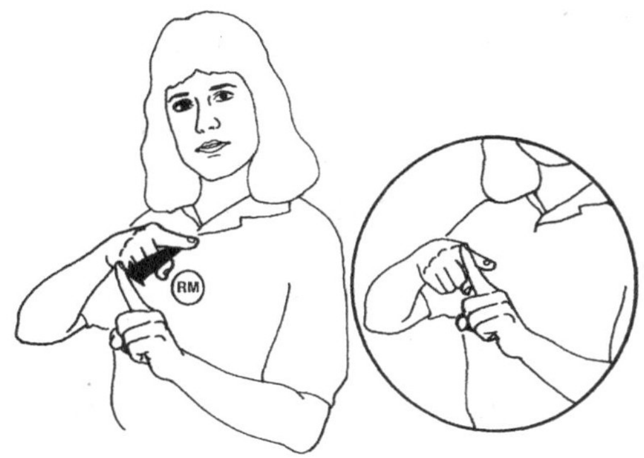

POSITIVE
1 hands, chest level. Left palm right, right palm down. Bounce right finger against the middle of left finger.
Clue: looks like the mathematical sign for positive.

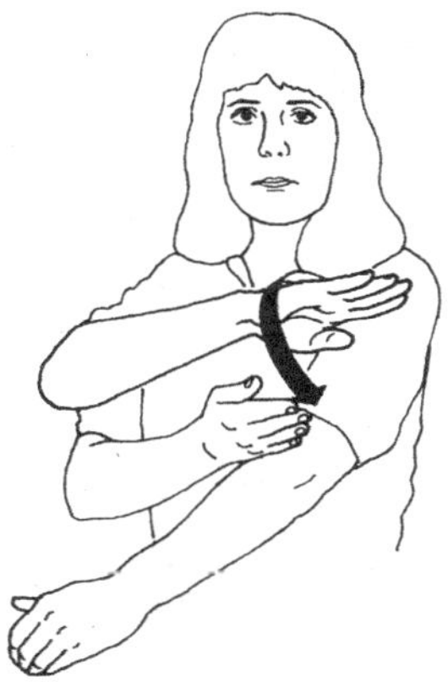

POWER
Right flat hand, thumb resting on left shoulder. Move hand in arc ending with side of right hand near left elbow.

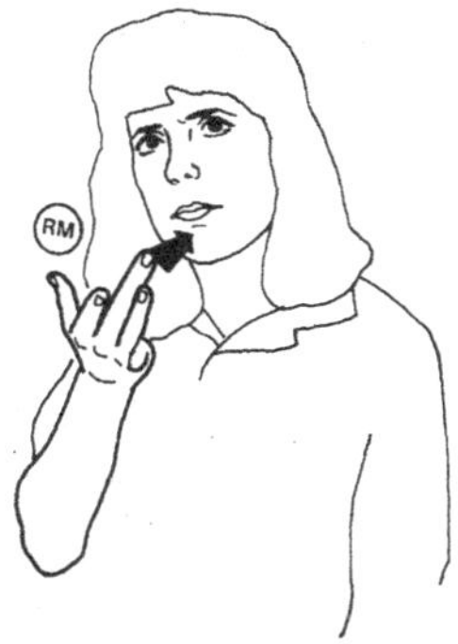

PREFER
Right 5 hand, palm in, near chin. Tap chin two or three times with middle finger.

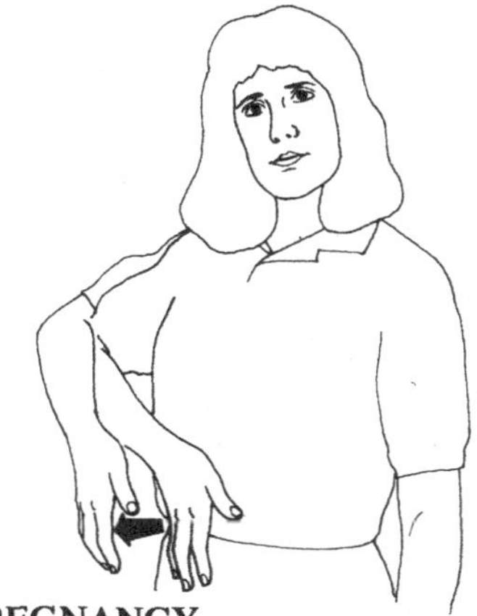

PREGNANCY
Right flat hand, palm on stomach, fingertips down. Move right hand away from body about six inches, changing to slightly curved hand.

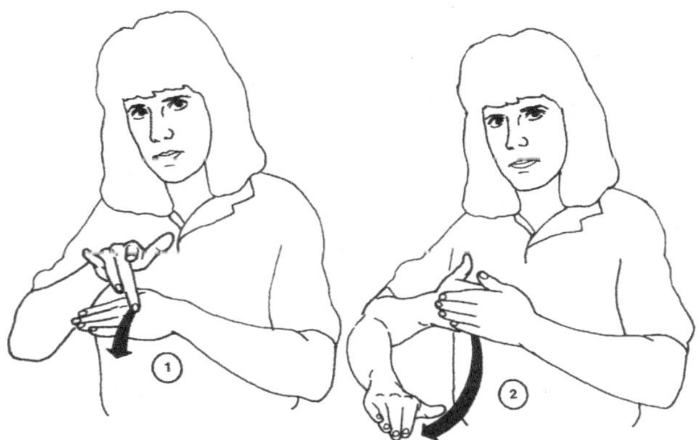

PREMATURITY
Right 5 hand, middle finger down, palm down, chest level. Left flat hand, palm down, chest level. Touch right, middle finger to top of left hand and move forward. Then change to flat hands, palms in, chest level, right hand inside left. Move right hand under and out from left.

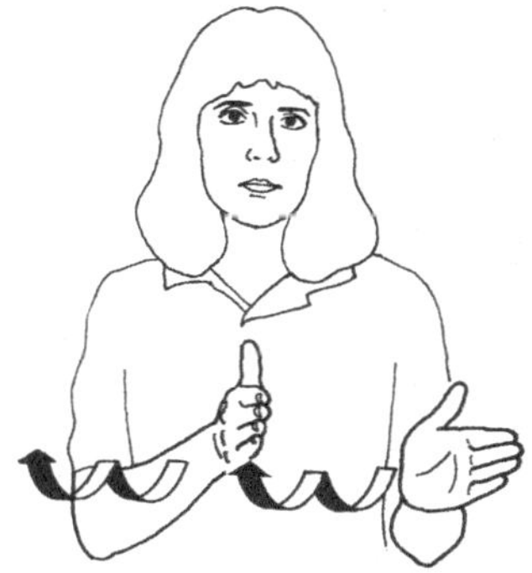

PREPARE
Flat hands, palms facing each other, chest level. Slide hands simultaneously to the right.

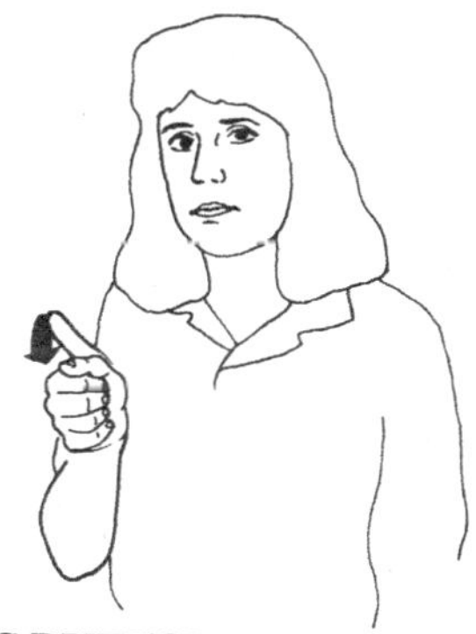

PRESS BUTTON
Right A hand, thumb slightly extended, palm left, chest level. Move thumb down to index finger.
Clue: natural gesture.

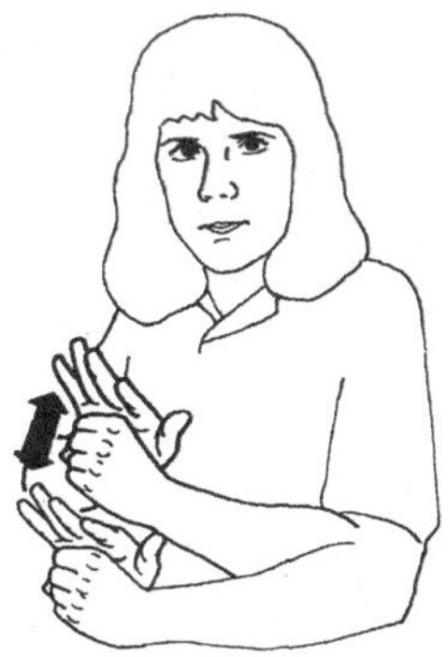

PRESSURE
Right flat hand, palm down, chest level. Left Ŝ hand against right palm. Right hand pushes down left hand. Repeat.

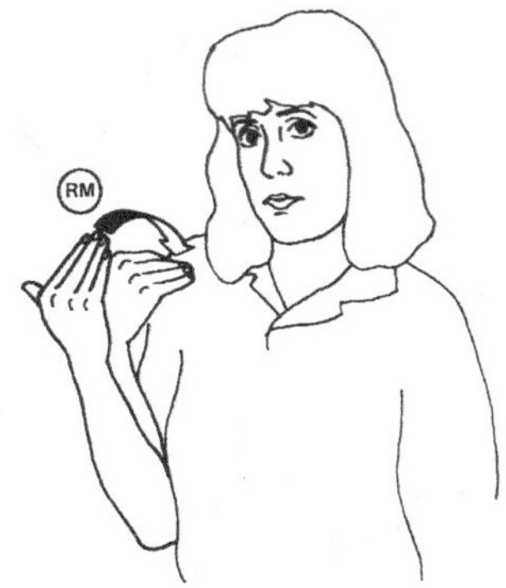

PREVIOUS
Right flat hand, palm in, near right shoulder. Move hand back and tap shoulder. Repeat.

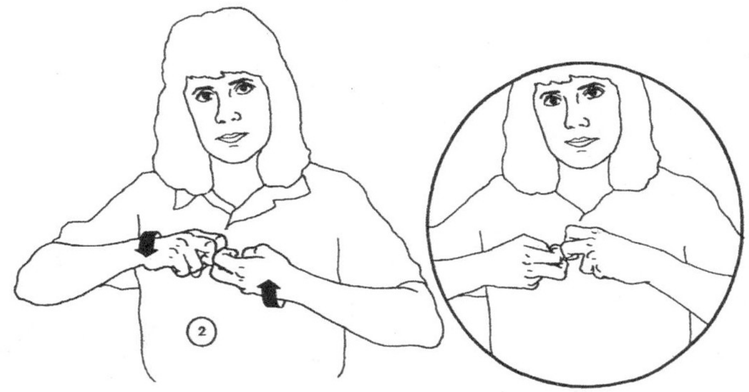

PROBLEM/DIFFICULT
Bent V hands, chest level, right fingertips on top of left fingertips, palms in. Rotate wrists 180 degrees in opposite directions. Repeat movement.

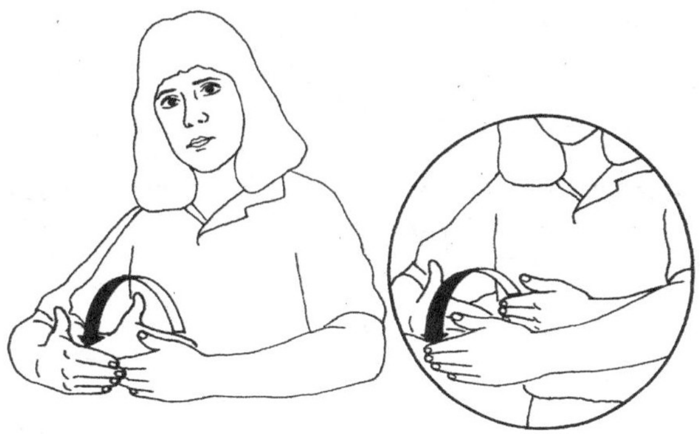

PROCESS/PROGRESS
Flat hands, palms in, chest level, left hand in front of right. Arc right hand over left, stopping in front of left hand. Continue alternating hands.

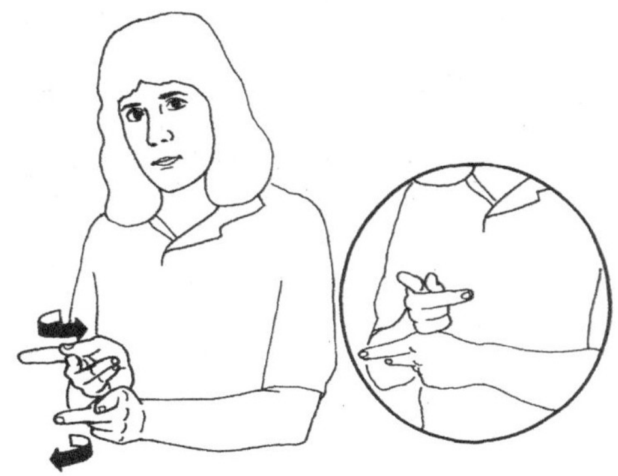

PRODUCE
P hands, palms in. Right hand on left at chest level. Move wrists simultaneously to palms facing sides. *Clue: initialized sign for "make."*

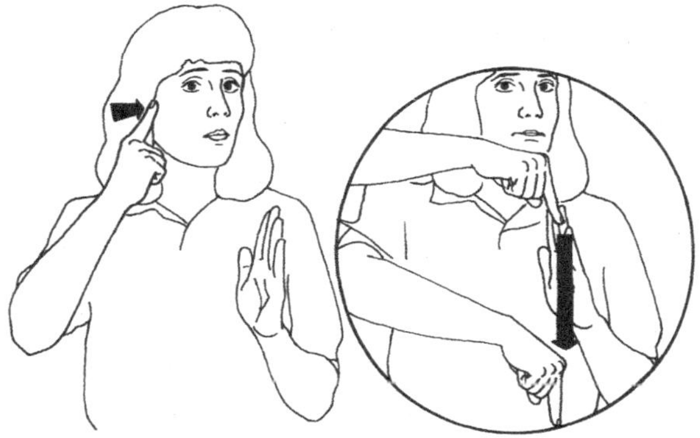

PROFOUND
Left flat hands, palm right, chest level. Right 1 hand, pointing to right ear. Bring right hand down in a sharp movement, brushing past left palm.

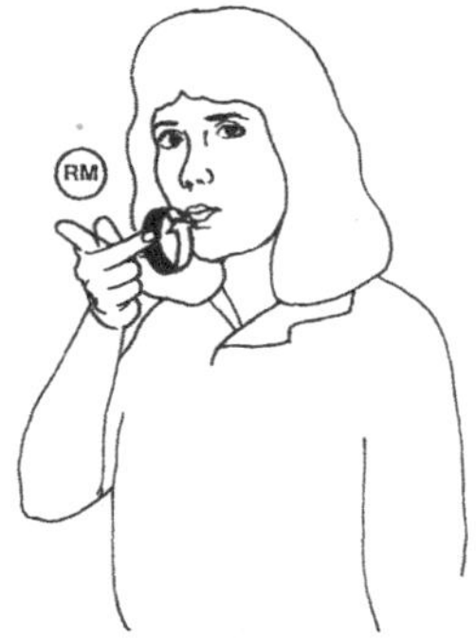

PRONOUNCE
Right P hand, palm in, middle finger at mouth level. Circle counterclockwise.

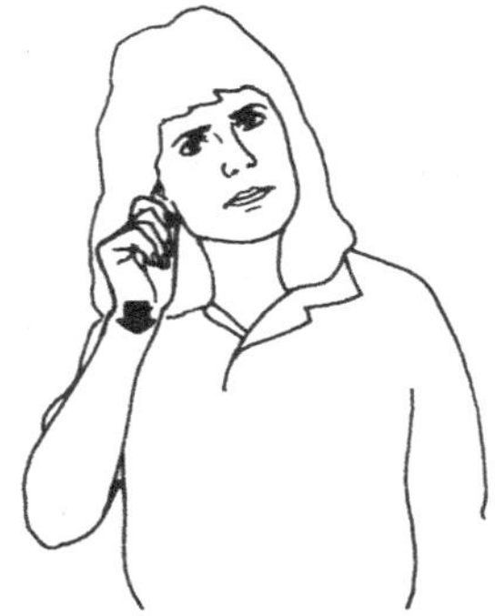

PULL EAR
Right A hand, palm left, thumb and index finger around ear lobe. Pull down slightly.
Clue: natural gesture.

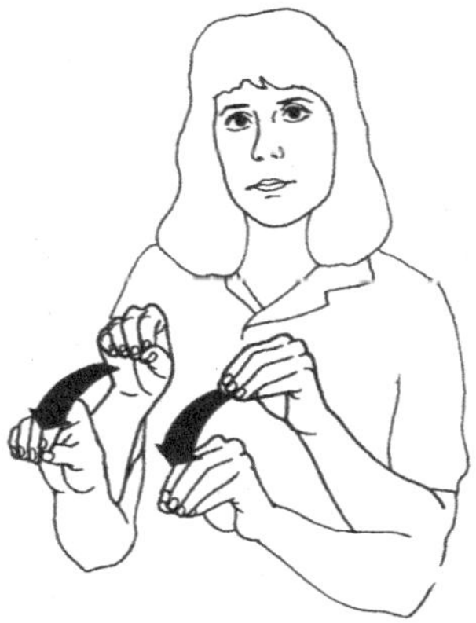

PUT
Flat O hands, palms down, chest level. Move hands forward simultaneously.

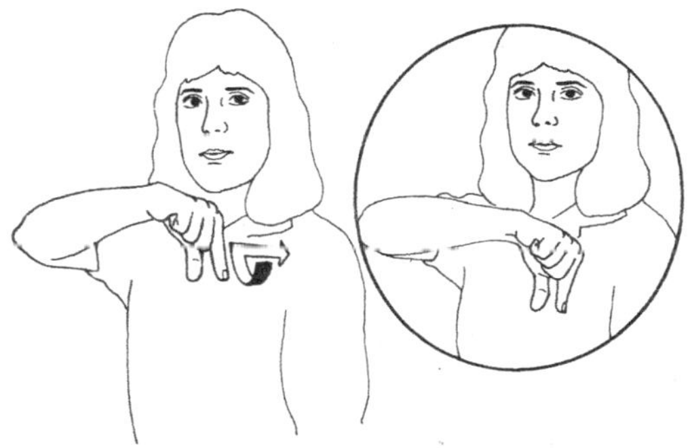

QUALITY
Right Q hand, palm down, left chest level. Circle in a clockwise direction while bringing hand to rest on upper left side of chest. .

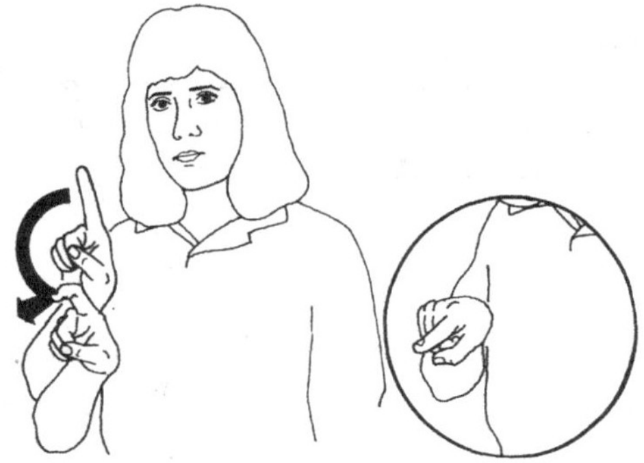

QUESTION
Right 1 hand, palm out, chest level. Move index finger in form of a question mark to palm down.

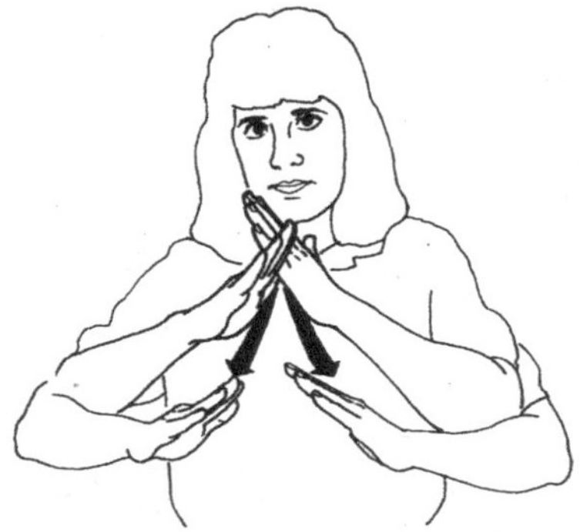

QUIET
Flat hands, palms down, hands crossed, right fingertips touching chin. Hands move down and apart.

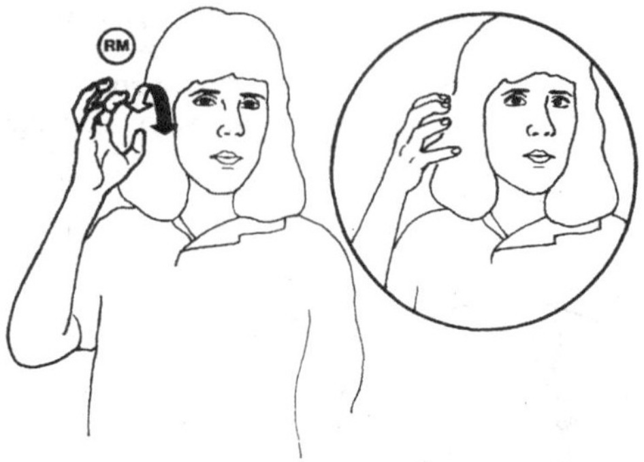

RADIO
Right claw hand, palm left, at right ear level. Shake hand slightly at wrist.

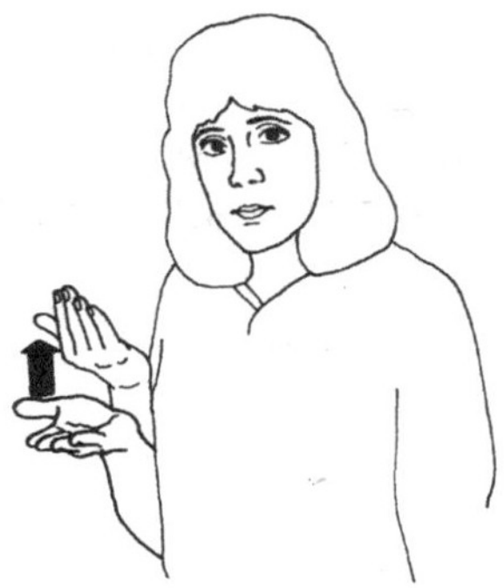

RAISE
Right 5 hand, palm up, waist level. Bring arm up to chest level.

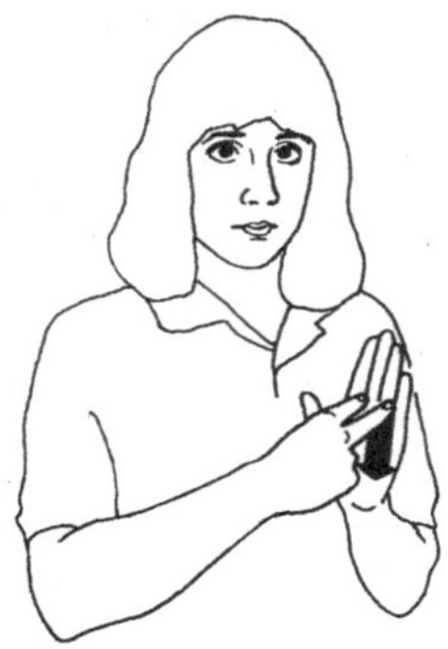

READ
Right V hand, palm down. Left flat hand, palm out, chest level. V fingertips start at left fingertips and move down left palm. Repeat.

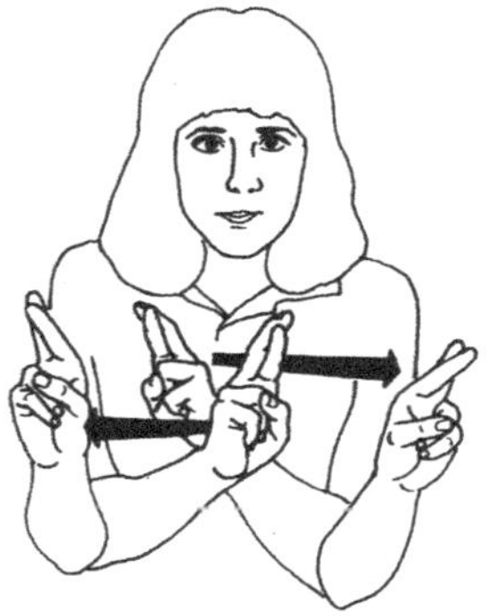

READY
R hands, chest level, palms out, hands crossed. In a quick movement, hands move to opposite sides.

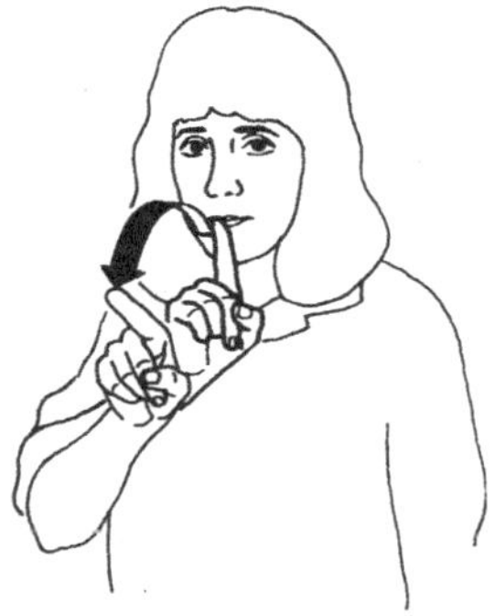

REAL
Right 1 hand, palm out, index finger on lips. Bring hand forward until index finger points out.

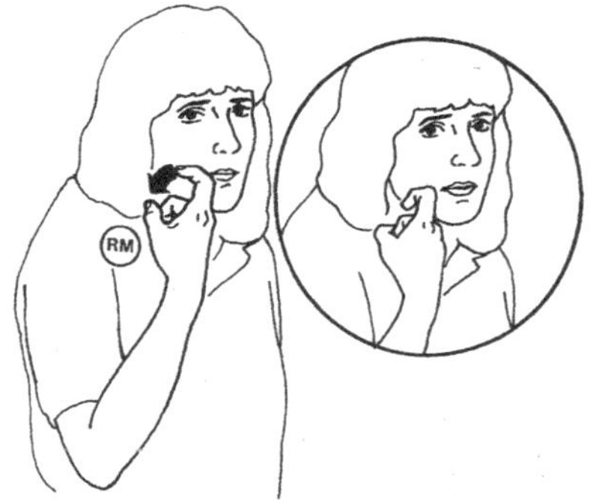

RECENT
Right X hand, palm facing back, at right cheek. Move index finger slightly up and down.

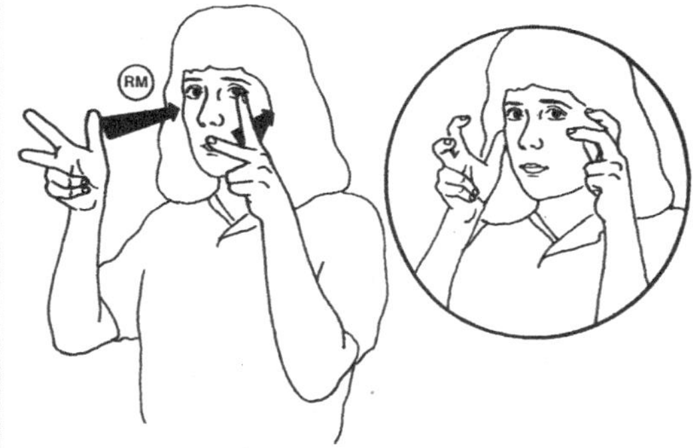

RECEPTIVE
3 hands, palms facing each other, thumbs at ear level. Move slightly back and bend all three fingers.
Clue: as if taking in information.

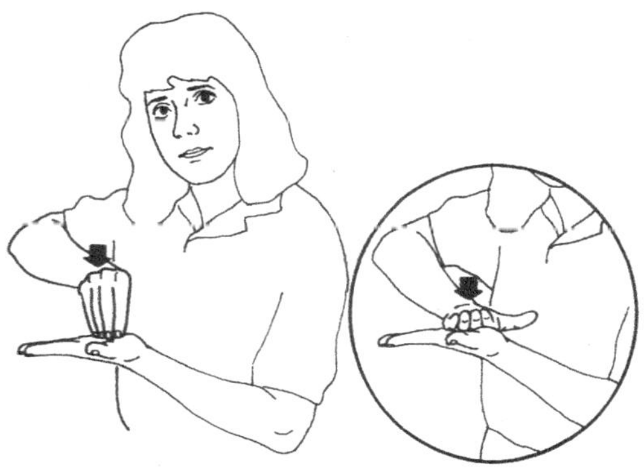

RECORD/PUT DOWN
Left flat hand, palm up, chest level. Right flat O hand, palm down, fingertips on left palm. Open right hand to 5 hand on left palm.
Clue: to write something down.

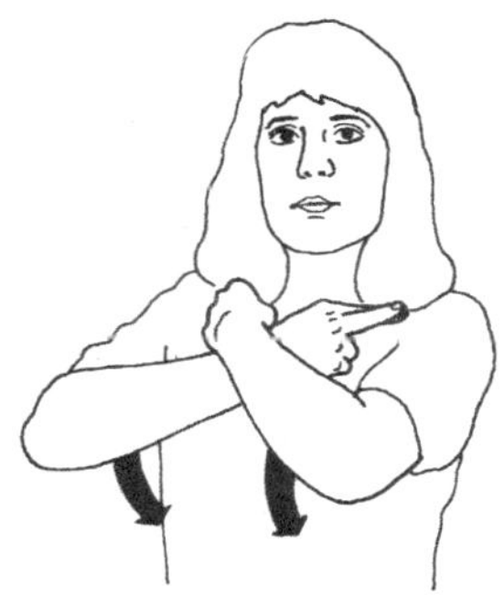

RELAX
R hands, crossed, fingertips resting on shoulders. Roll hands down until hands rest on chest.

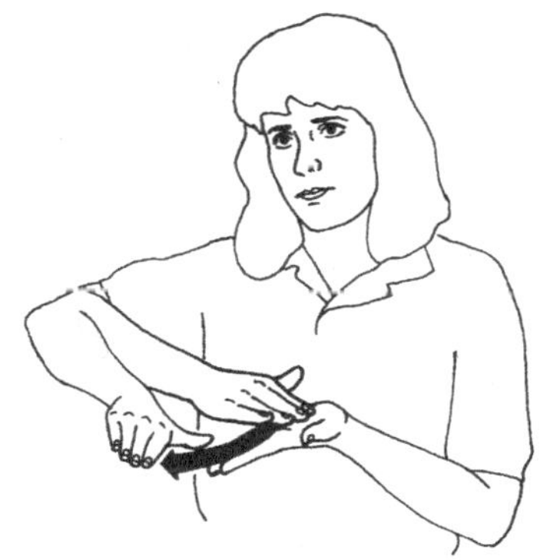

RELEASE, WAIVER
Right flat hand, palm down, chest level. Left flat hand, palm up, chest level. Right fingertips rest at base of left hand fingers. Move right hand forward, along fingers and out.

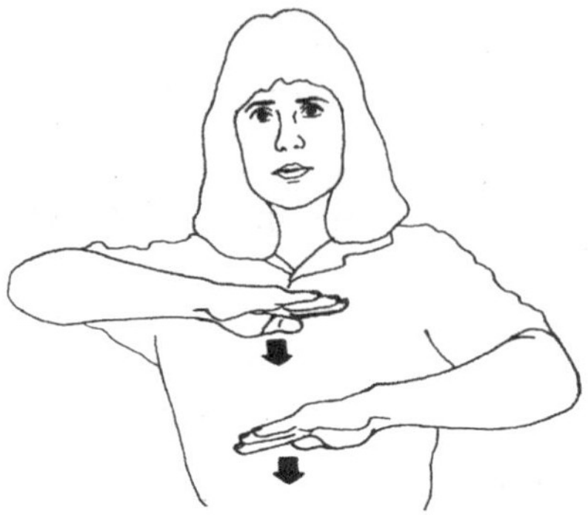

RELIEF
B hands, palms down, right hand at chest level, left hand at waist level. Simultaneously move hands down body.

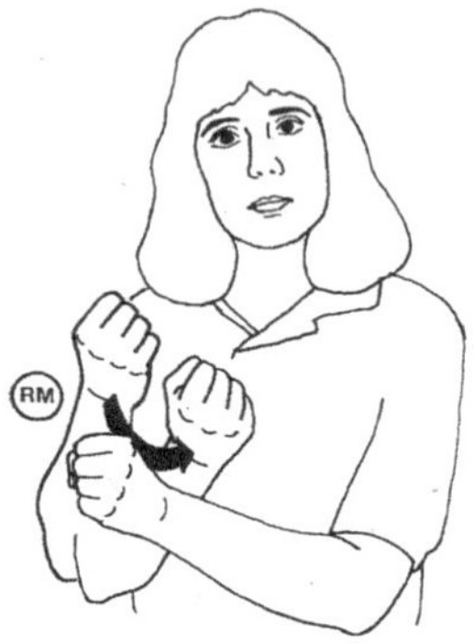

REPAIR
S hands, palms in, chest level, right hand on top of left. Right hand repeatedly brushes left hand.

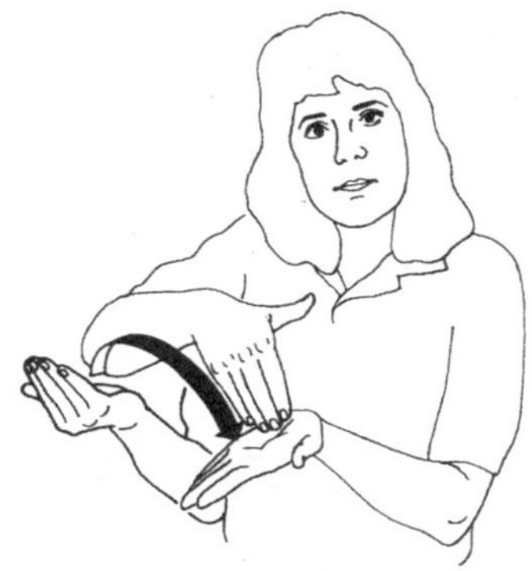

REPEAT/AGAIN
Right flat hand, palm up, chest level. Left flat hand, palm up, waist level. Move right hand to palm down, fingertips touching left palm.

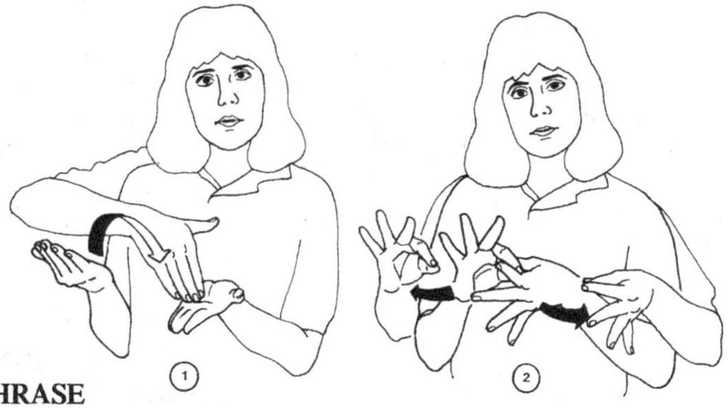

REPHRASE
Right flat hand, palm up, chest level. Left flat hand, palm up, waist level. Move right hand to palm down, fingertips touching left palm. Then change to F hands, chest level, thumbs and index fingers interlocked. Move hands apart in an up and down wavy motion.

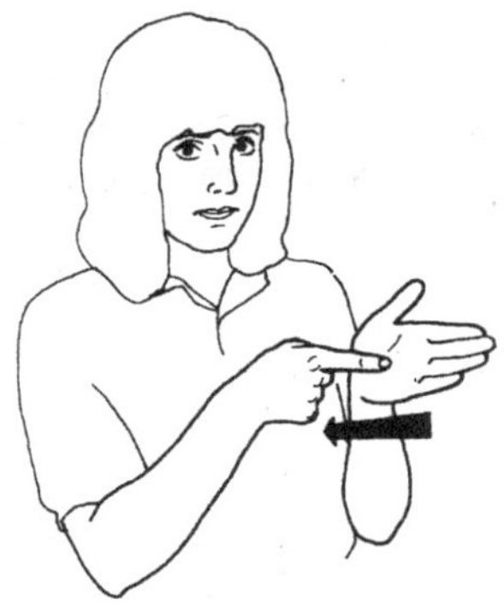

REQUIRE
Right 1 hand, palm in, chest level. Left flat hand, palm right, chest level, fingertips forward. Rest 1 fingertip on left palm. Move hands simultaneously towards chest.

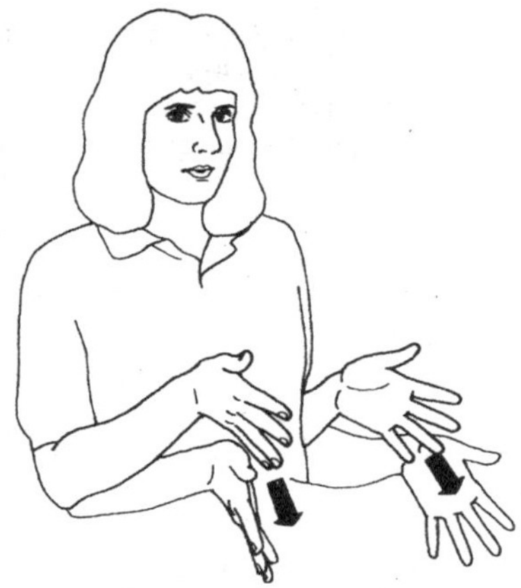

RESIDUAL
5 hands, palms facing, chest level. Drop hands down to waist level.

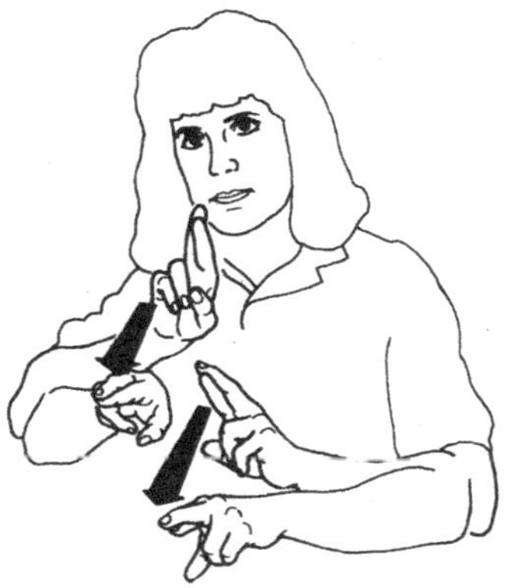

RESPOND/REPORT
R hands, chin level. Right hand fingertips touch chin, left hand in front. Move hands simultaneously to palms down.

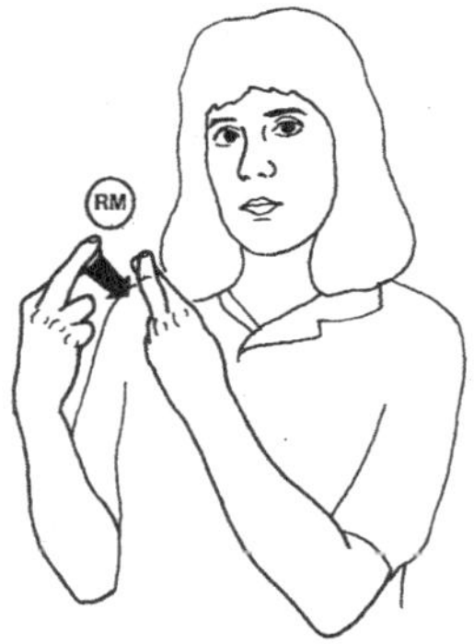

RESPONSIBILITY
R hands, palms in, at right shoulder. Repeatedly bounce hands on shoulder. *Clue: the burden/responsibility is on your shoulder.*

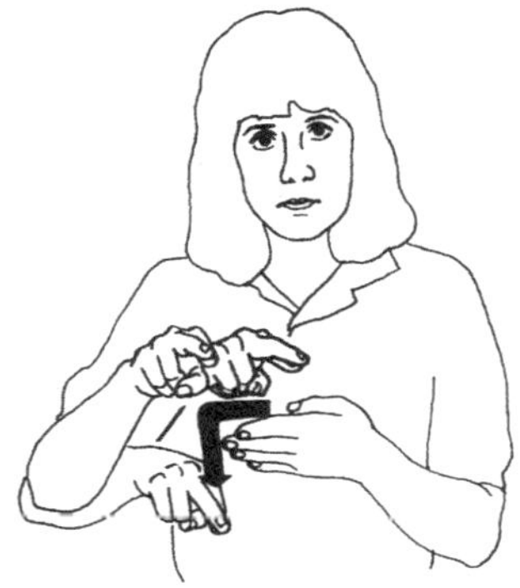

RESULT
Right R hand, palm down. Left flat hand, palm in, fingertips right, chest level. Move right R across left hand above left index finger and then over the edge of the hand and down.

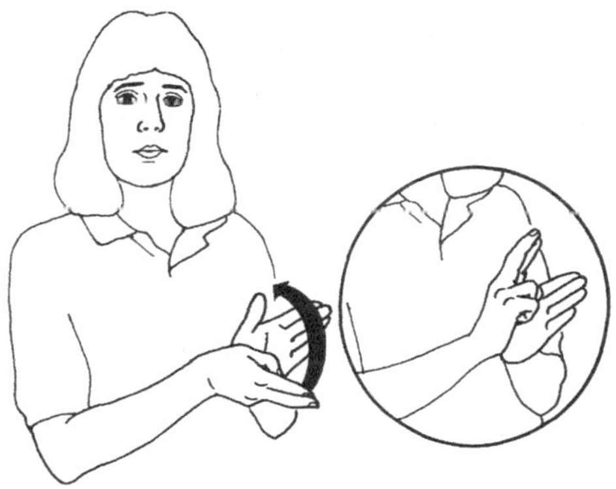

REVIEW
Left flat hand, palm right, chest level. Right R hand, palm left, touching base of left hand. Bring right hand up, brushing over left fingertips, ending with R on top of left thumb.

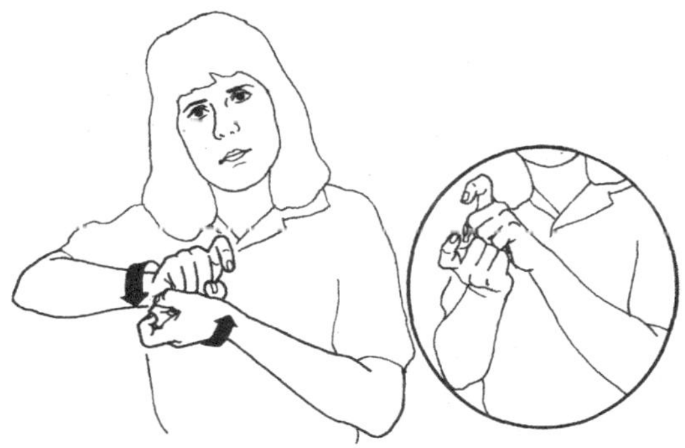

REVISE
X hands, left palm up, right palm down on left palm, chest level. Rotate hands 180 degrees in opposite directions, ending with left hand on top of right.

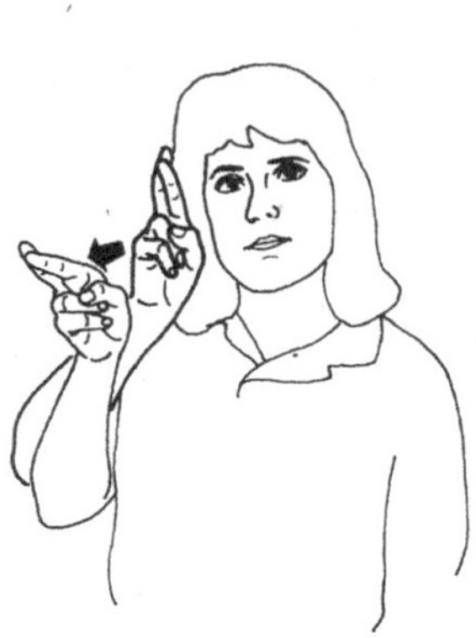

RIGHT
Right R hand, palm out, right ear level. Move away from ear.

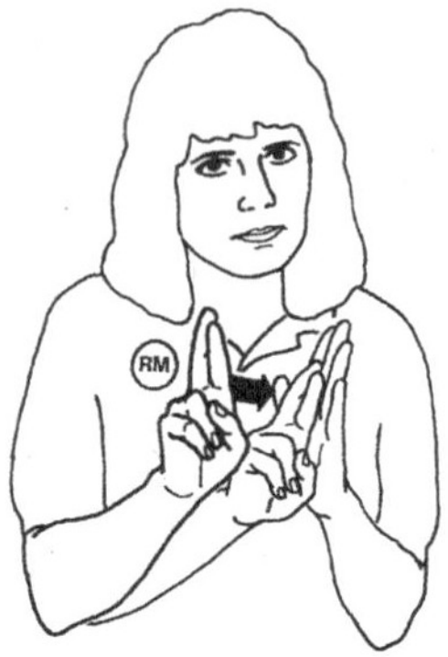

RING
Left flat hand, chest level, palm right. Right R hand repeatedly taps left palm.
Clue: movement represents the rhythm of the telephone ringing.

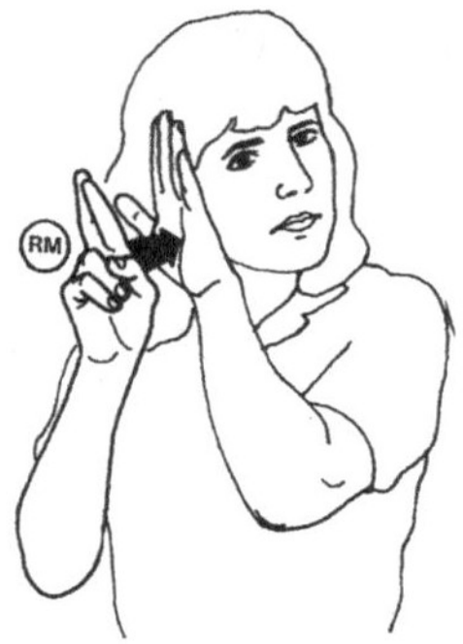

RINGING (IN EAR)
Left flat hand, palm out, ear level. Right R hand taps left palm repeatedly.

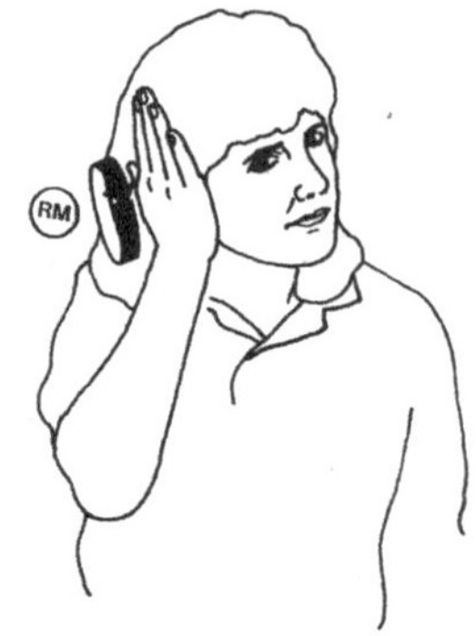

RUB
Right flat palm rubs ear.

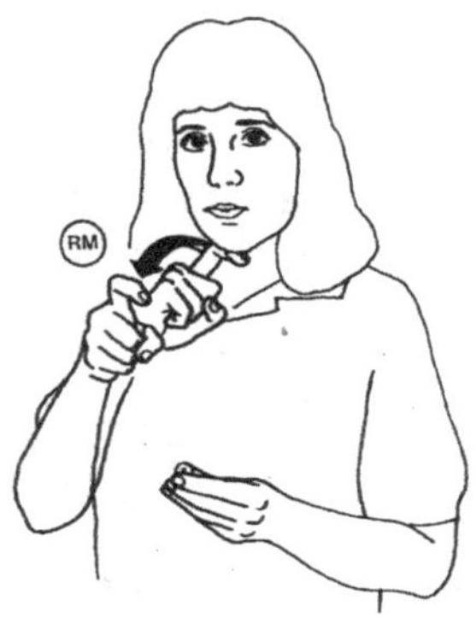

RUBBER
Right X hand, palm left, top of X under chin. Move out quickly from chin. Repeat.

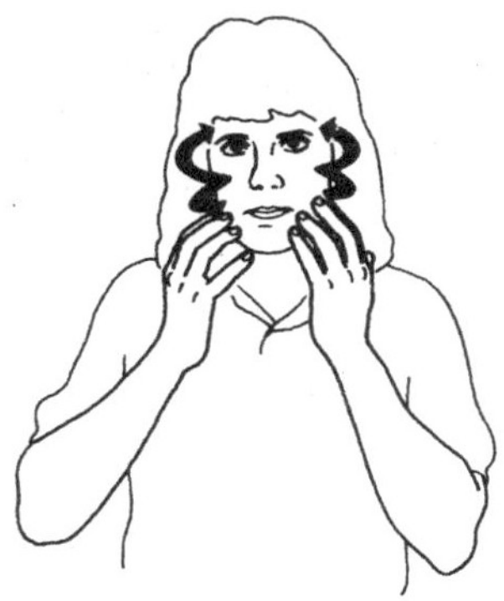

RUBELLA
Claw hands, palms in, at chin. Simultaneously bounce hands up the face, stopping at eyebrows.
Clue: the rash associated with measles.

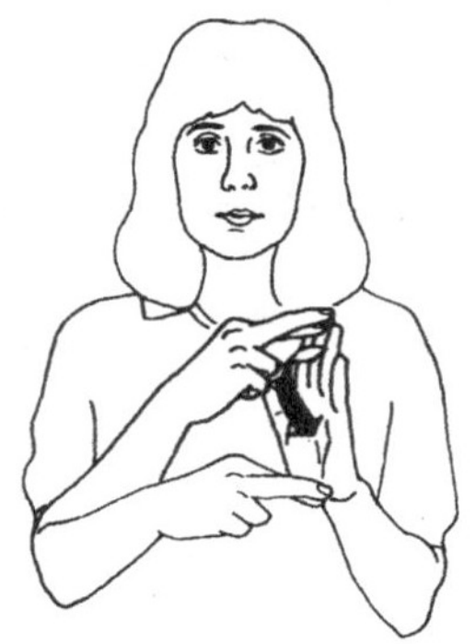

RULE
Right R hand, palm left. Left flat hand, palm right, chest level. Rest fingertips of R on fingertips of left hand. Bounce R down to heel of left hand.

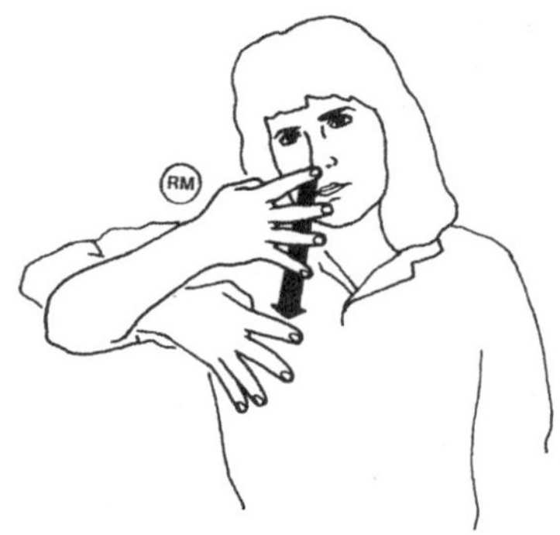

RUNNY NOSE
Right 4 hand, palm in, index finger on nose. Move hand up and down.
Clue: running nose.

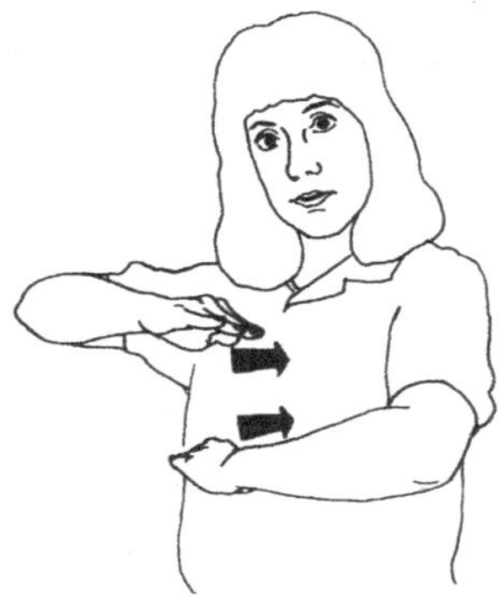

SATISFY
B hands, palms down, right hand chest level, left hand waist level. Simultaneously bring hands in towards body.

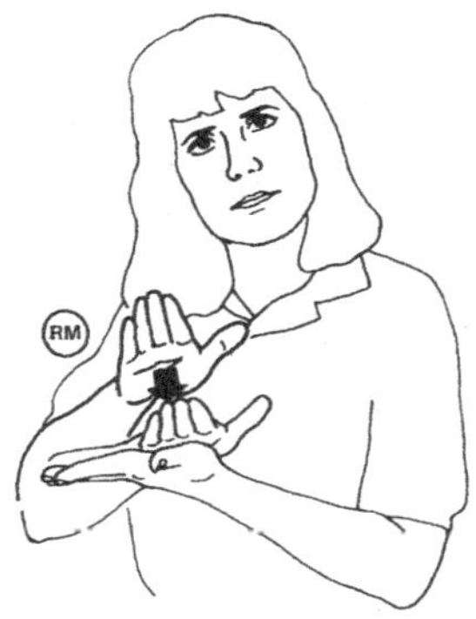

SCHOOL
Flat hands, chest level, left palm up, right palm down. Right hand comes down and claps on left hand repeatedly.
Clue: teacher getting the class's attention.

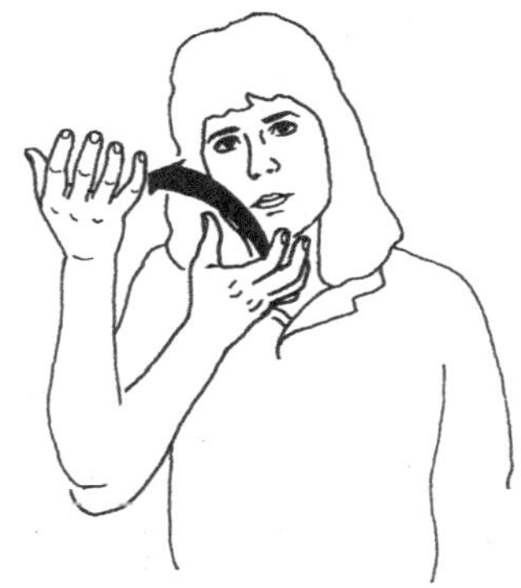

SCREAM/YELL
Right claw hand, palm up, chin level. Bring right hand up across face in a swift movement.
Clue: voice coming out of mouth.

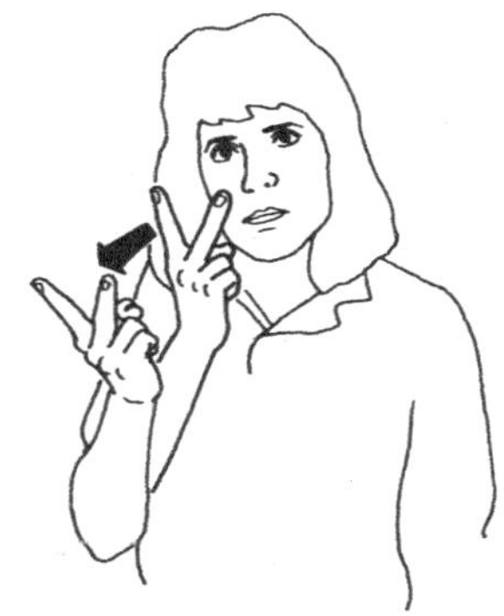

SEE
Right V hand, palm in, at right cheek. Move slightly away from face.

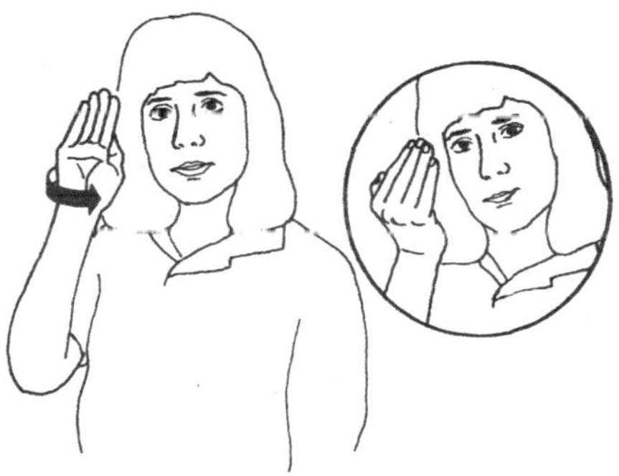

SEEM
Right flat hand, palm left, at right eye level. Slightly rotate hand at wrist so palm faces in.

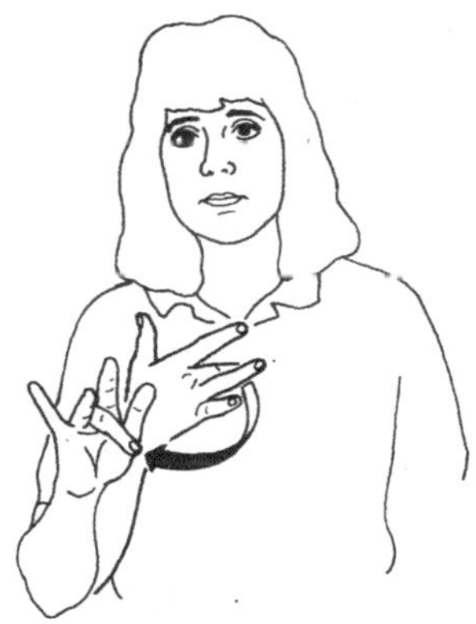

SENSITIVE
Right 5 hand, middle finger touching chest. Flick wrist out, turning palm out.

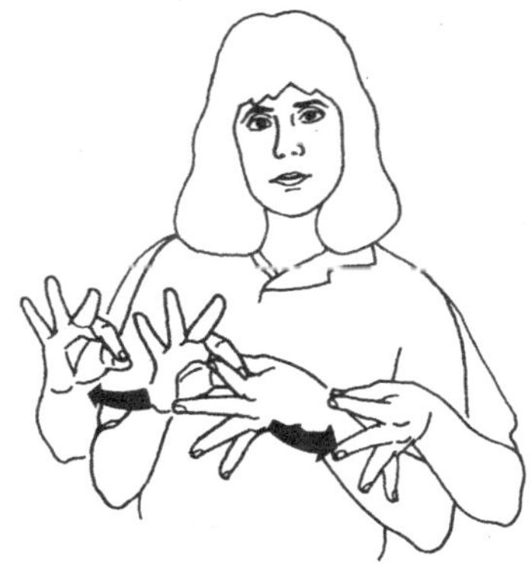

SENTENCE
F hands, chest level, thumbs and index fingers of both hands interlocked. Move hands apart in an up and down wavy motion.

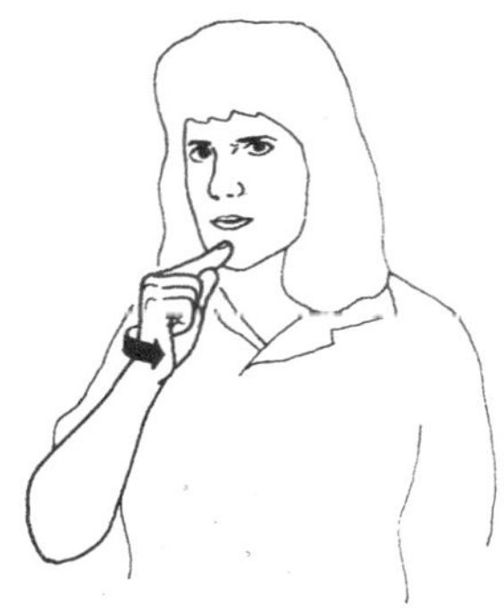

SERIOUS
Right 1 hand, palm in, at chin. Turn finger in a quick movement, on chin.

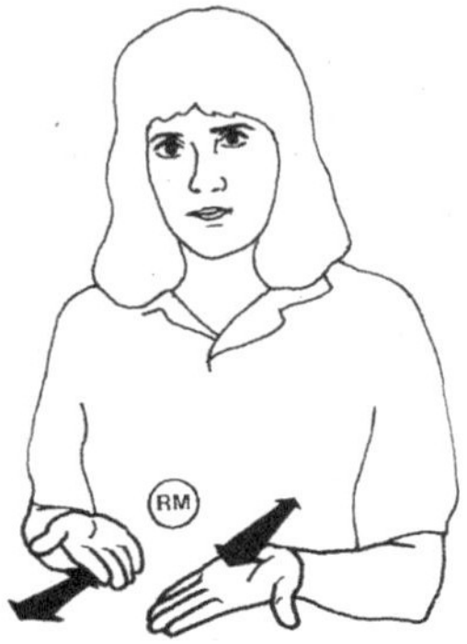

SERVICE
Flat hands, palms up, waist level. Move hands back and forth alternately.

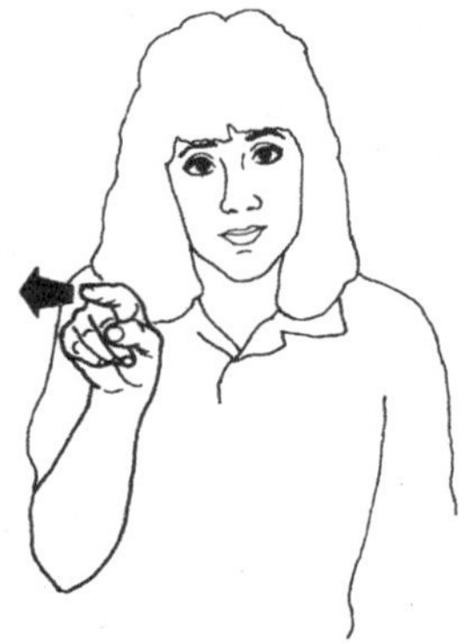

SHE/HE
Right 1 hand points in the direction of the person.

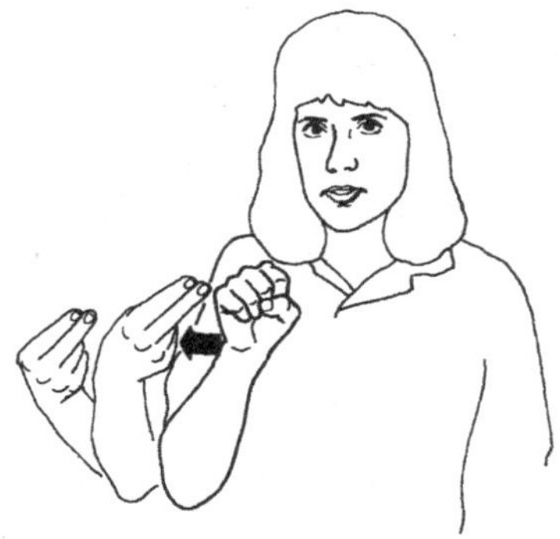

SHHHH
Right S hand, palm out, chest level. Change to H hand and move to the right.

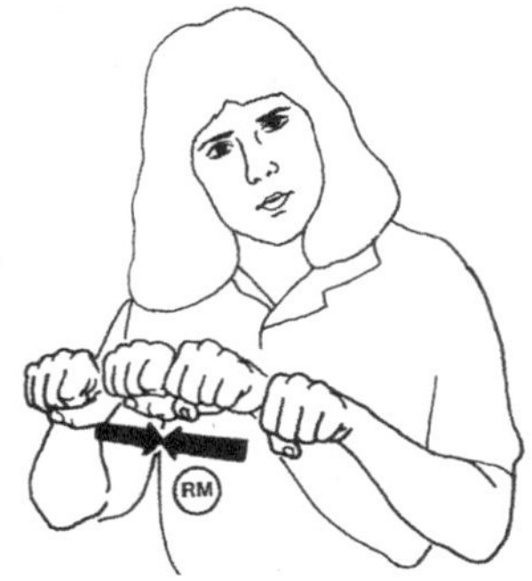

SHOES
S hands, palms down, chest level. Tap S hands together. Repeat.

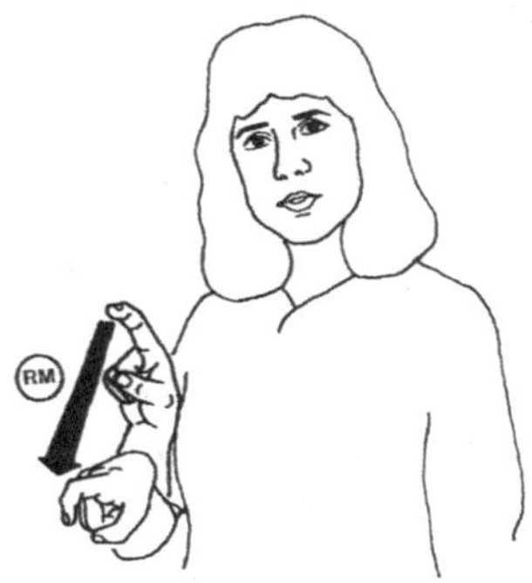

SHOULD
Right X hand, palm out, shoulder level. Right hand moves down in a short, sharp movement.

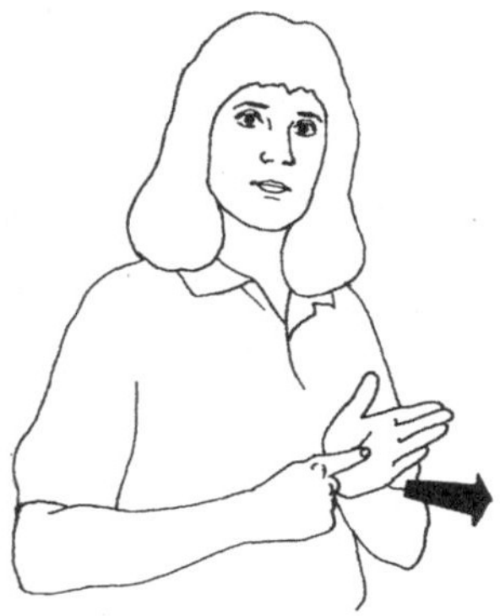

SHOW
Left flat hand, palm right, waist level. Right 1 hand, palm in, index finger on left palm. Simultaneously move hands forward.

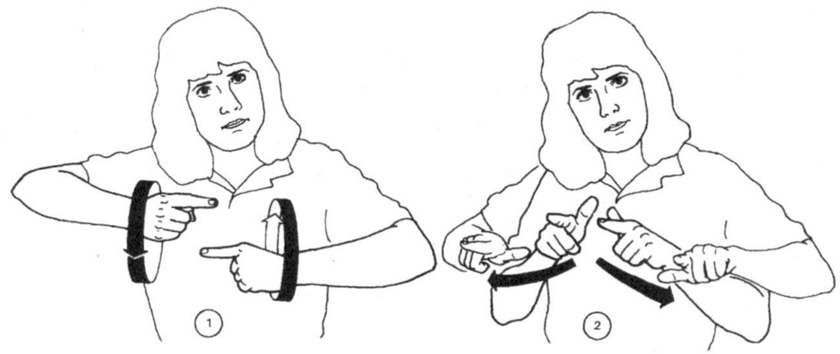

SIGN LANGUAGE
1 hands, palms in, chest level. Hands move alternately in a circular motion towards chest. Change to L hands, palms down, chest level. Hands move out to the sides in a shaking motion.
Clue: sign + language.

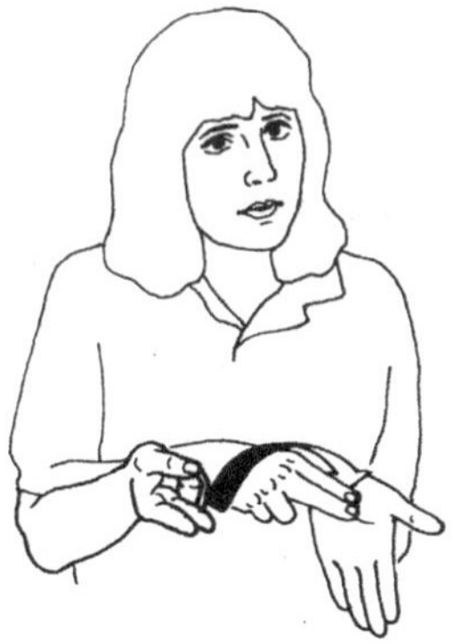

SIGN (signature)
Right U hand, palm up, chest level. Left flat hand, palm up, waist level. Right hand moves to palm down, U resting on left palm.

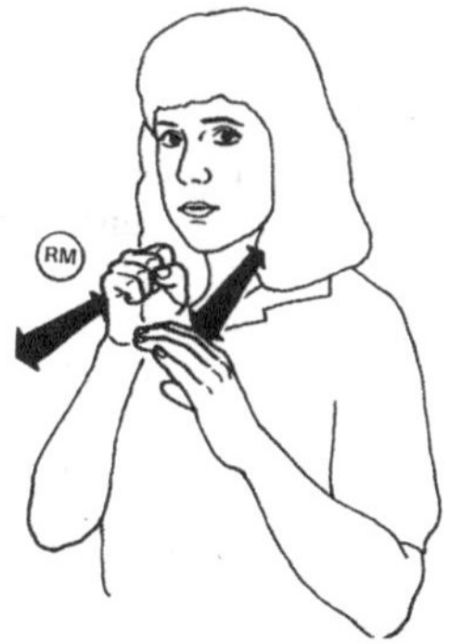

SIMULTANEOUS COMMUNICATION
Right S hand, palm left, mouth level. Left C hand, palm right, mouth level. Alternately move hands away from mouth. Repeat.

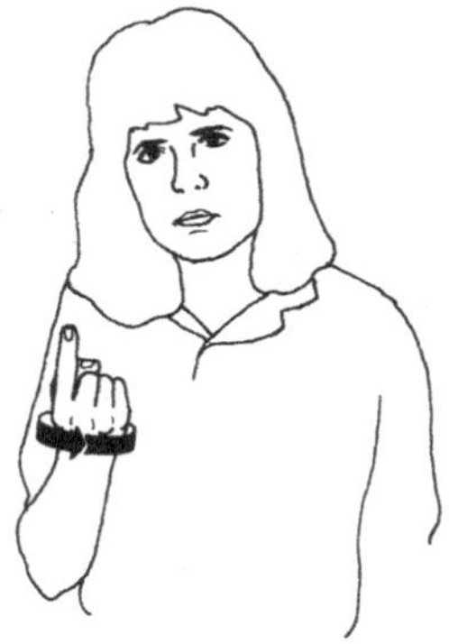

SINGLE
Right 1 hand, shoulder level, palm in. Circle once in a counterclockwise direction.

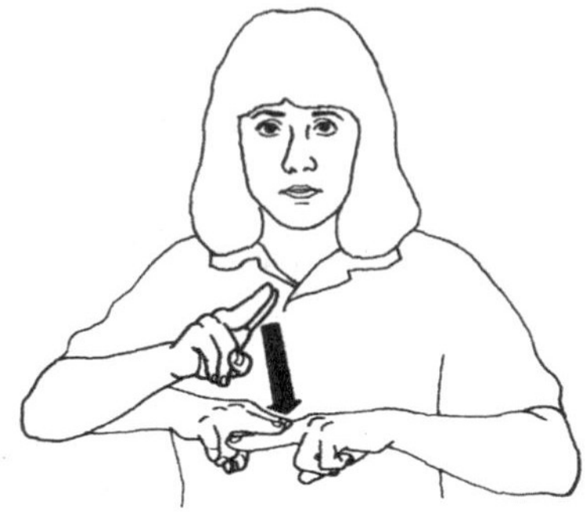

SIT
U hands, palms down, chest level. Right U taps left U twice.

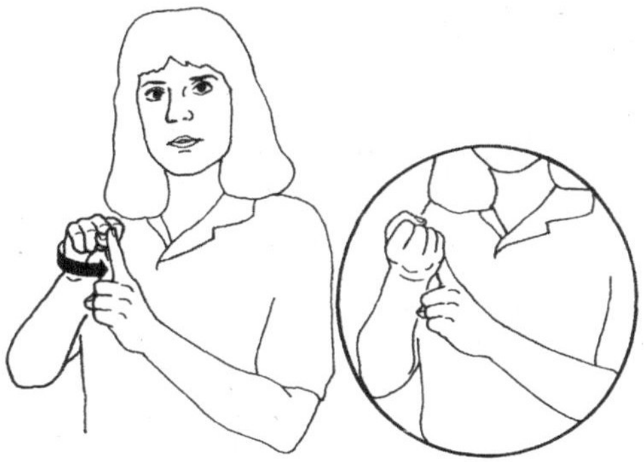

SITUATION
Left 1 hand, chest level, palm right. Right S hand, wrist touching thumb of left hand, circle right hand around left hand in counterclockwise direction.

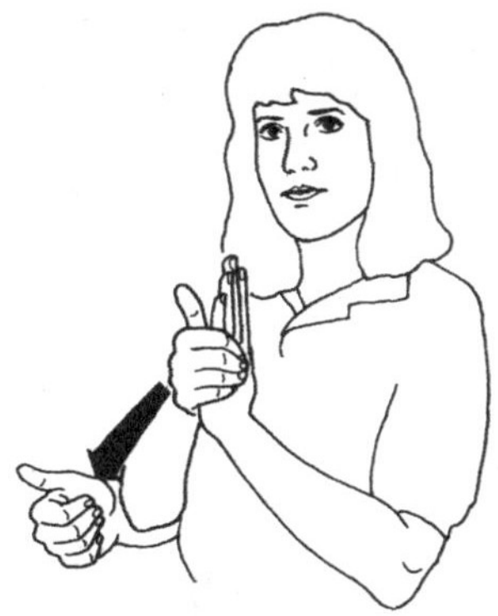

SKILL/TALENT
Left flat hand, palm right, chest level. Right hand grabs around bottom of left hand. Right hand moves down and closes.

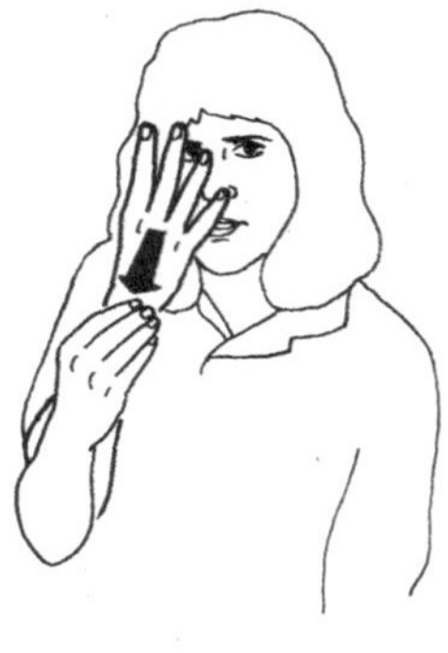

SLEEP
Right 5 hand, palm in, in front of face. Bring hand down face while closing hand. Eyes also close briefly.

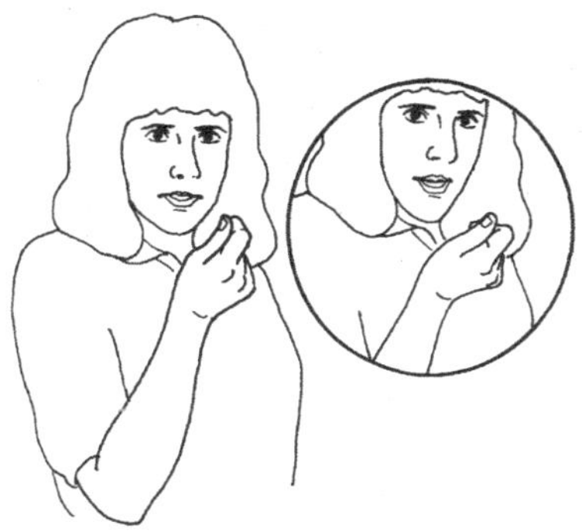

SLIGHTLY/LITTLE BIT
Right closed hand, thumb touching index finger, chest level, palm in. Lightly rub thumb against index finger.

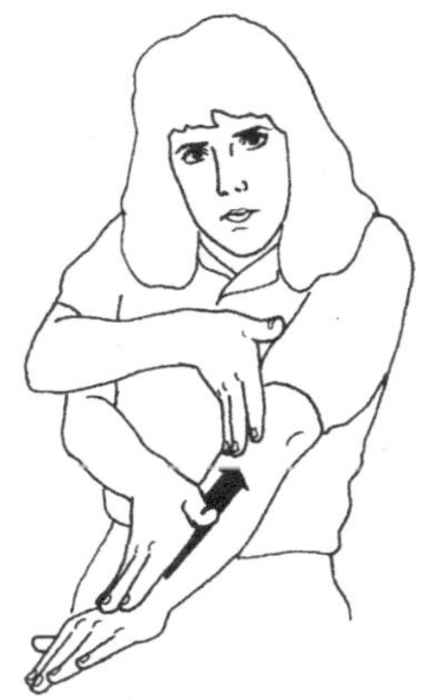

SLOW
Left flat hand, palm down, arm extended. Right flat hand, palm down, fingertips on back of left hand. Slide right hand slowly up left arm.

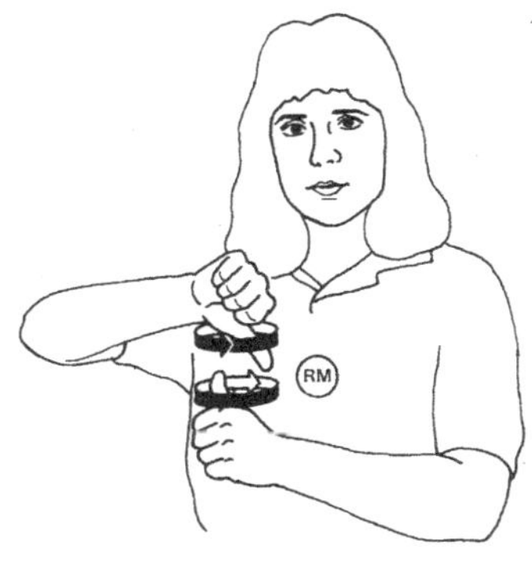

SOCIALIZE
A hands, left palm in, right palm out, thumb down, above left at chest level. Move A hands alternately in small clockwise circle.

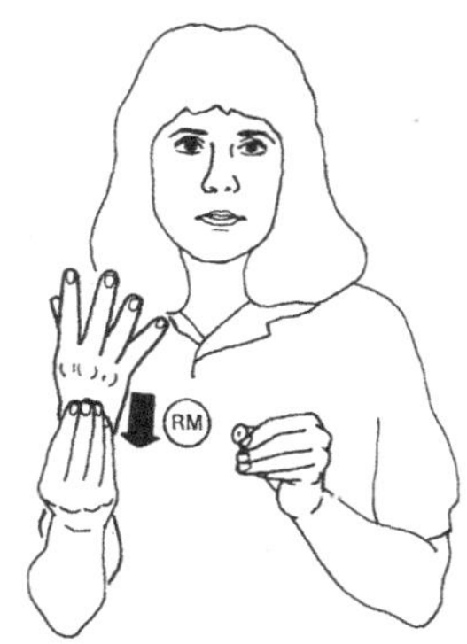

SOFT
Slightly open right flat O hand, palm up, chest level. Move hand down while closing to flat O. Repeat.

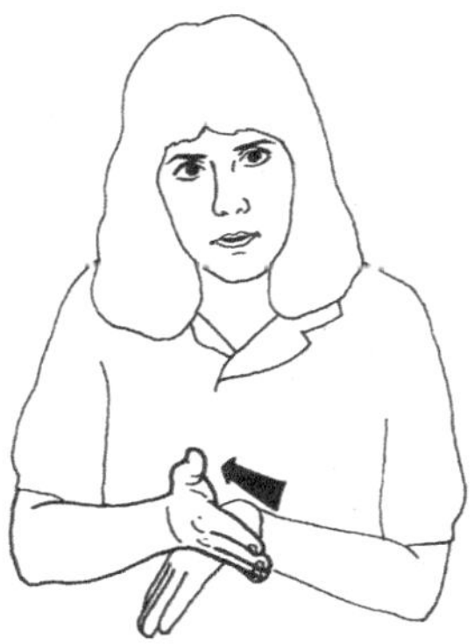

SOME/PART
Right flat hand, palm left. Left flat hand, palm up, chest level, right hand on left palm. Move right hand down across left palm.

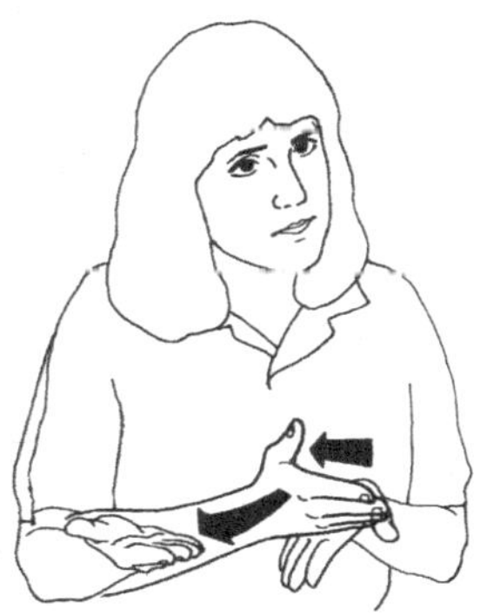

SOMETHING
Right flat hand, palm left. Left flat hand, palm up, chest level, right hand on left palm. Move right hand down across left palm. Change to right palm up and move to the right while left hand remains stationary.
Clue: some + thing.

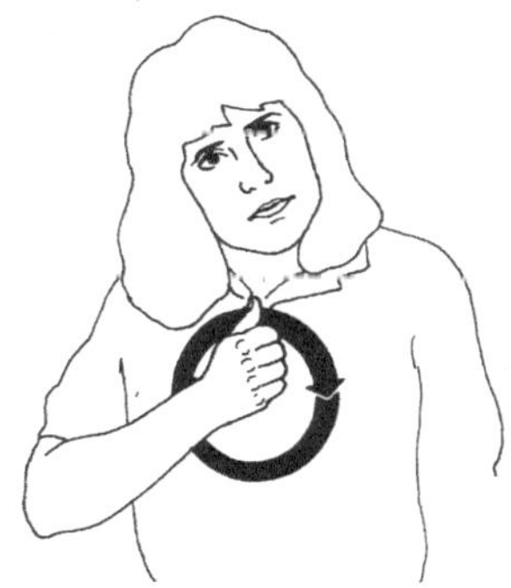

SORRY
Right A hand, palm in, resting on chest. Move in small counterclockwise motion.

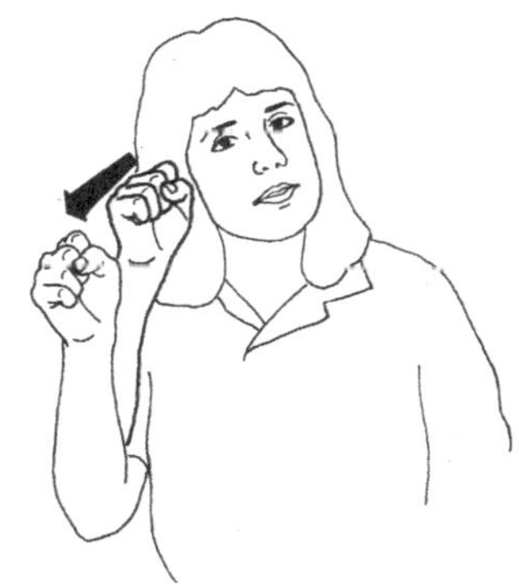

SOUND
Right S hand, palm left, at ear. Move hand out.

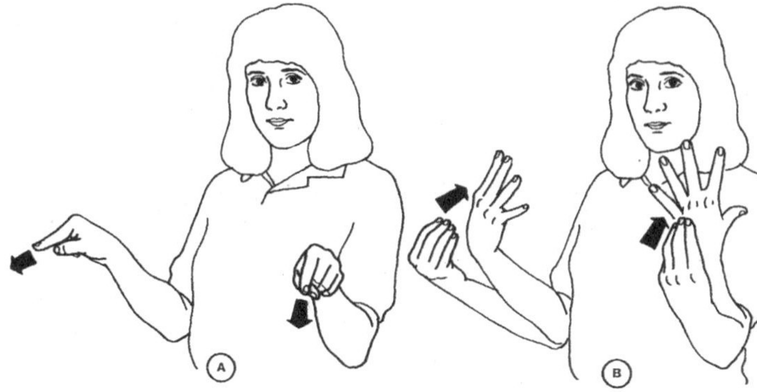

SPEAKER
1 hands, palms down, chest level. Point to imaginary speakers. Change to O hands, palms in. Move towards body simultaneously opening to 5 hands, palms in.

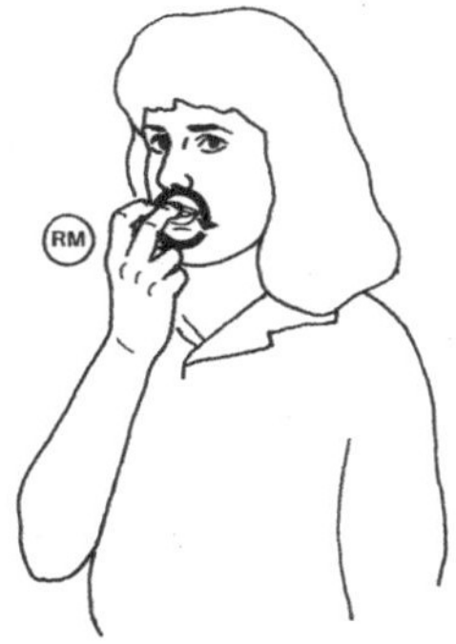

SPEECH
Right bent V hand, palm in, at mouth level. Circle clockwise in front of mouth.

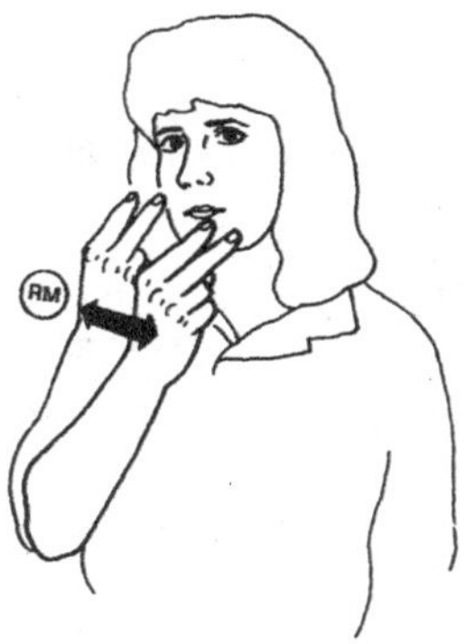

SPEECHREAD
Right 2 hand, palm in, fingertips at mouth. Move hand back and forth repeatedly in front of mouth.
Clue: eyes "reading" the lips.

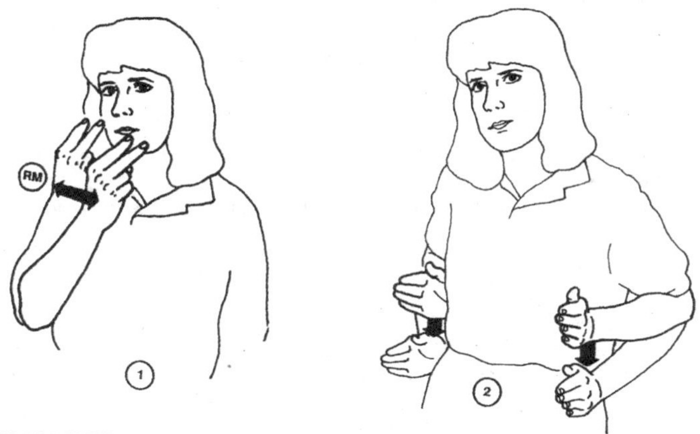

SPEECHREADER
Right 2 hand, palm in, fingertips at mouth. Move hand back and forth repeatedly in front of mouth. Change to flat hands, palms facing, at sides. Move down side of body.

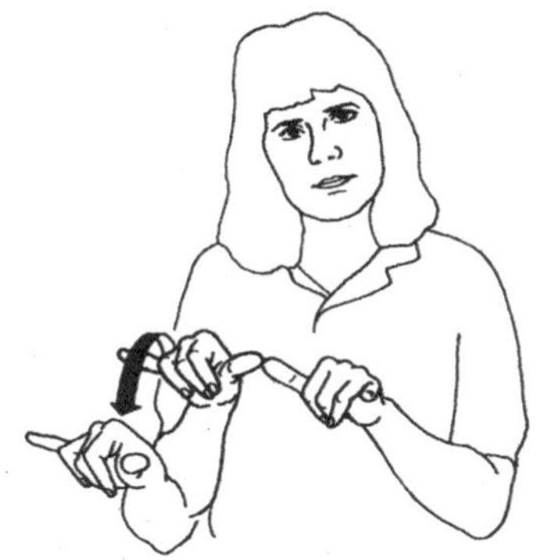

STAY
Y hands, palms down, thumbs touching at waist level. Move right Y forward.

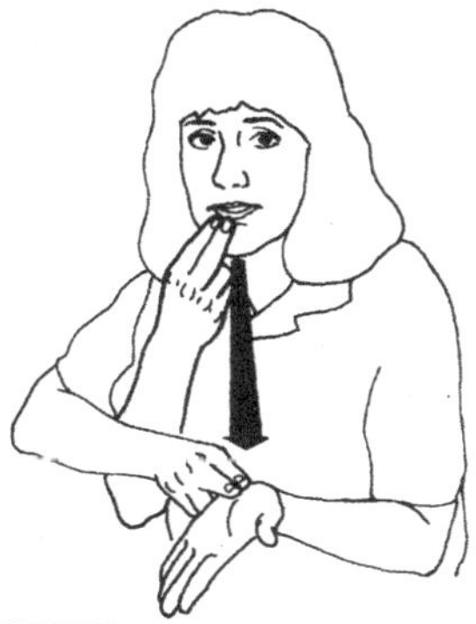

STICKER
Right U hand, palm in, on lips. Left flat hand, palm up, chest level. Move U to palm down. Smack left palm with U.
Clue: licking a sticker to put it on another object.

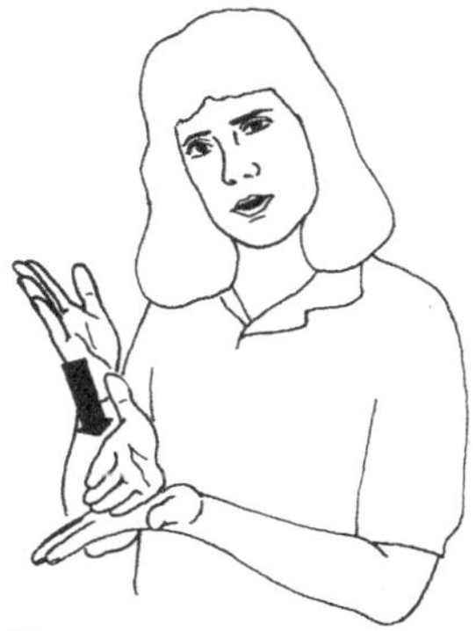

STOP
Flat hands, right palm left, at chest level, left at waist level, palm up. Quickly move right hand down to hit left palm.

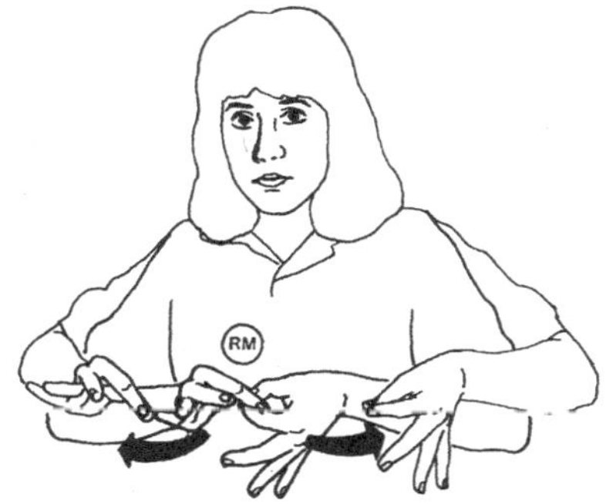

STORY
F hands, chest level, thumbs and index fingers interlocked. Move hands apart in an up and down wavy motion. Repeat.
Clue: similar to "sentence," but repeated to show longer length of a story.

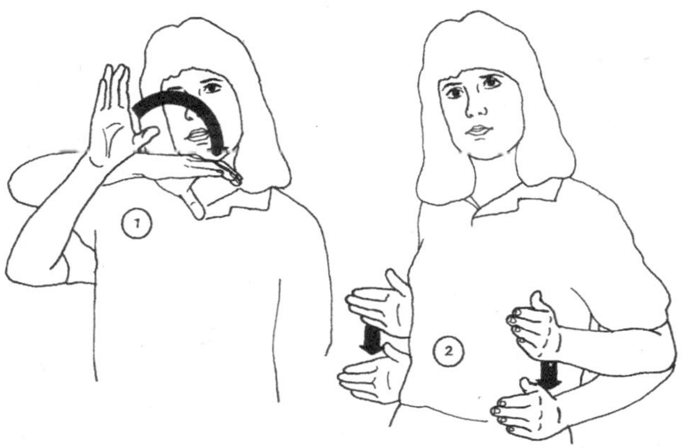

STRANGER
Right C hand, head level, palm right. Sweep hand across face, then change to flat hands, palms facing, at sides, move down side of body.

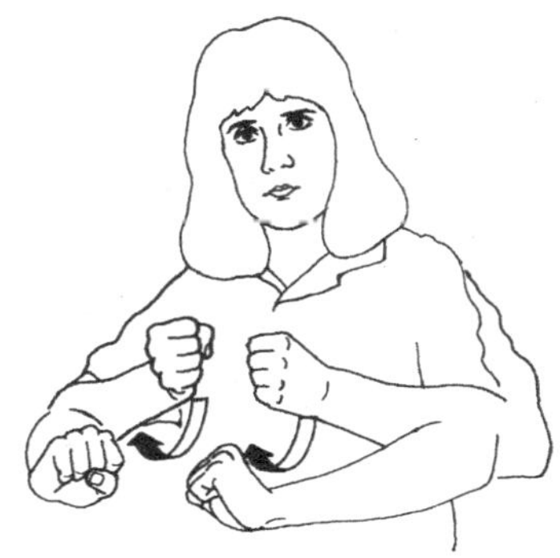

STRATEGIES
S hands, palms facing each other, chest level. Arch hands down and out simultaneously.

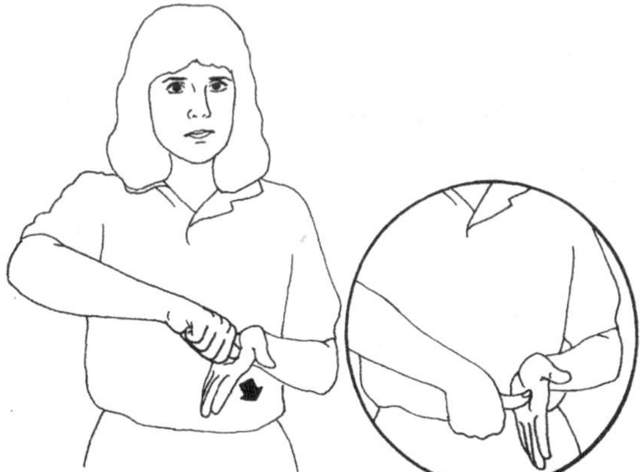

STRESS
Left flat hand, palm up, waist level. Right A hand, palm out, right thumb on left palm. Twist right hand, ending with palm in.

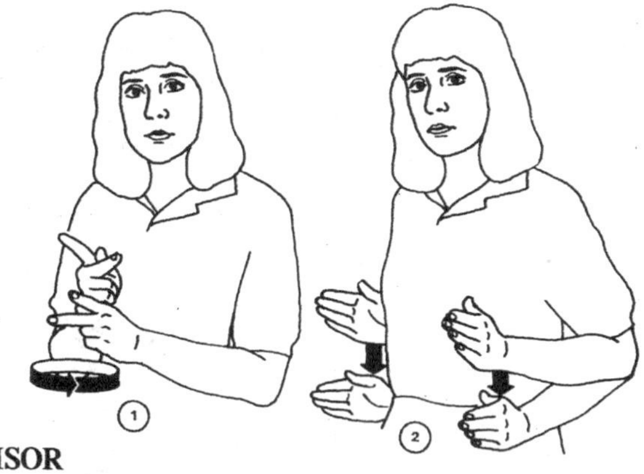

SUPERVISOR
V hands, waist level, palms to sides, right hand on top of left. Move in small clockwise circle twice. Change to flat hands, palms facing each other, chest level. Move simultaneously down to waist level.

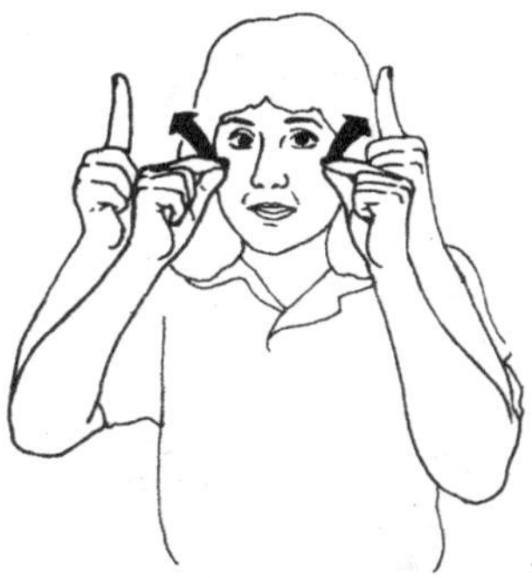

SURPRISE
Closed hands, index fingers and thumbs touching, hands below eyes, palms facing each other. Finger quickly snap open to 1 hands.
Clue: eyes opening in surprise.

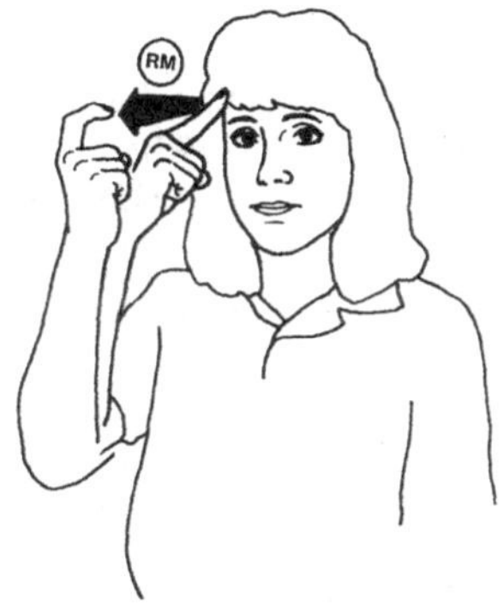

SUSPECT
Right 1 hand, palm in, at forehead. Bring right hand out from face while changing to X hand. Repeat.

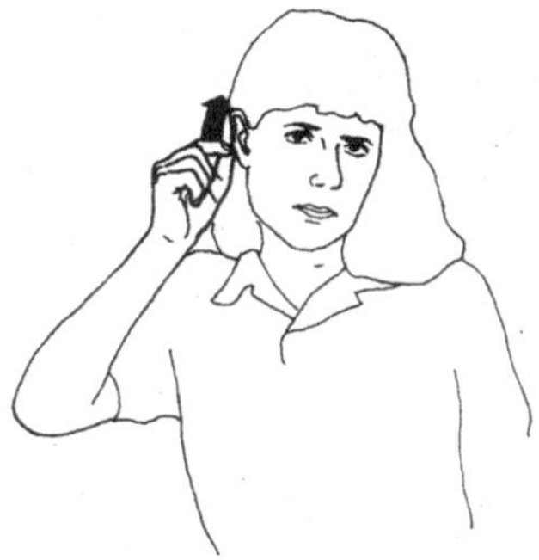

SWITCH
Right hand closed, thumb and index finger touching, behind right ear. Move hand up slightly.

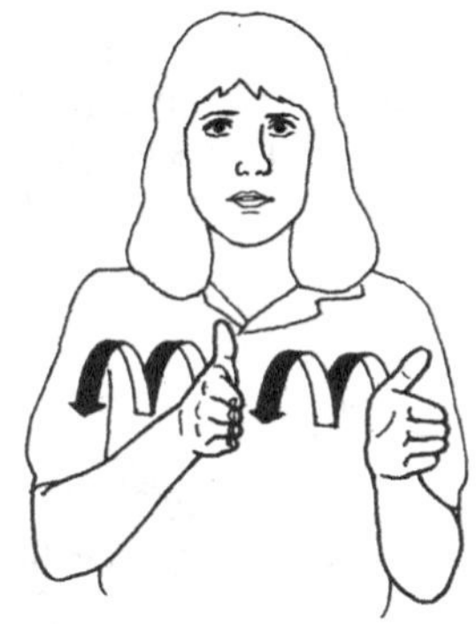

SYLLABLE
Flat hands, palms facing each other, chest level. Simultaneously bounce hands to the right.
Clue: the bounces represent syllables in a word.

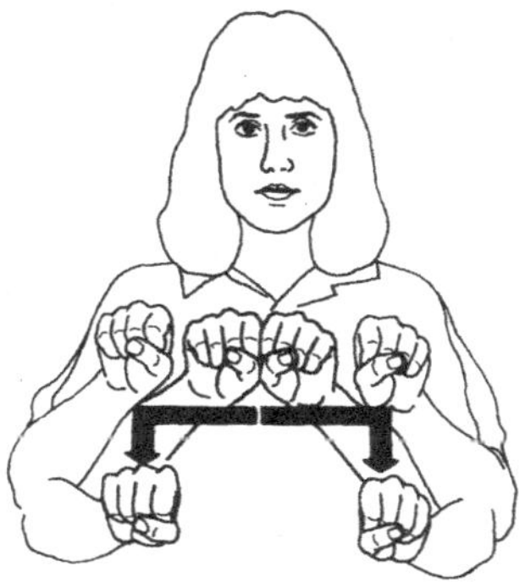

SYSTEM
S hands, palms out, hands touching, chest level. Move hands apart and down.

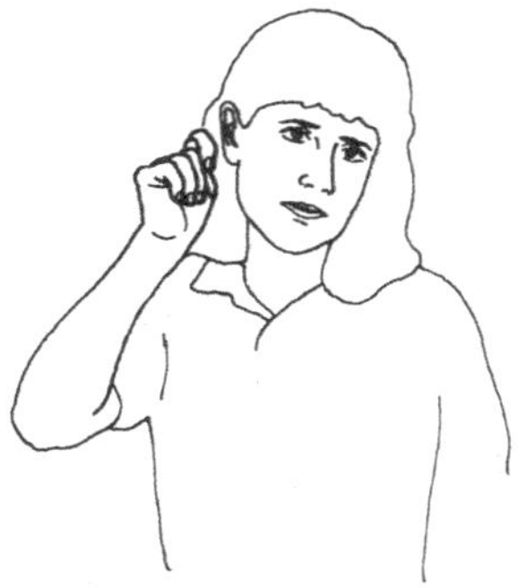

T SWITCH
Right T hand, palm out. Move up and down slightly behind right ear.

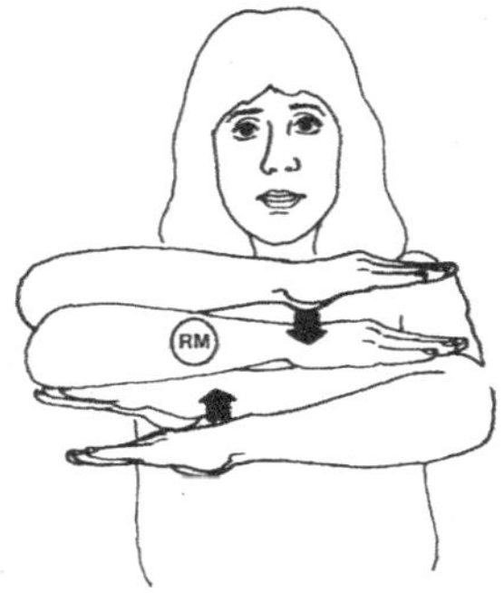

TABLE
Flat hands, palms down. Right lower arm rests on left lower arm at chest level. Repeatedly tap right arm on left.

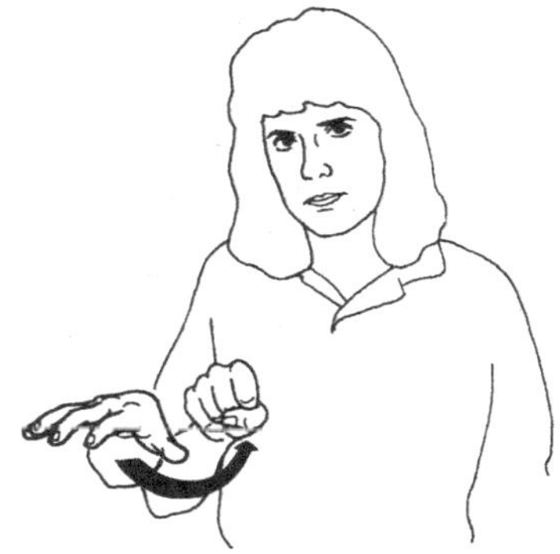

TAKE
Right rounded 5 hand, palm down, chest level. Move towards body quickly while changing to S hand.

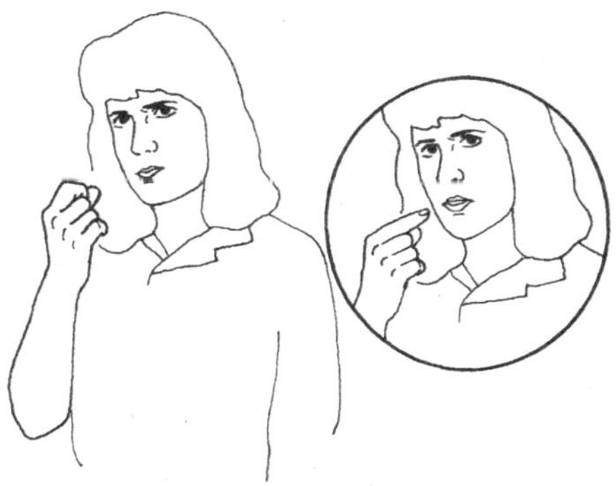

TAKE-A-PILL (orally)
Right closed hand, index finger and thumb touching, palm in, at mouth. Repeatedly flick fingers open.
Clue: action of popping a pill in your mouth.

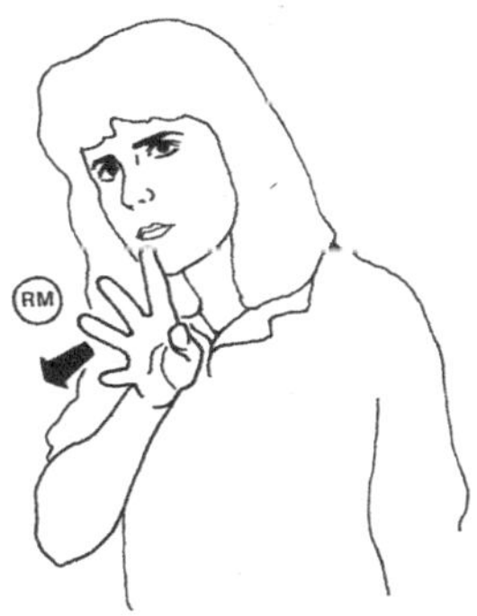

TALK
Right 4 hand, palm left, index finger touching chin. Repeatedly move hand out and back from mouth.
Clue: "words" coming out of mouth.

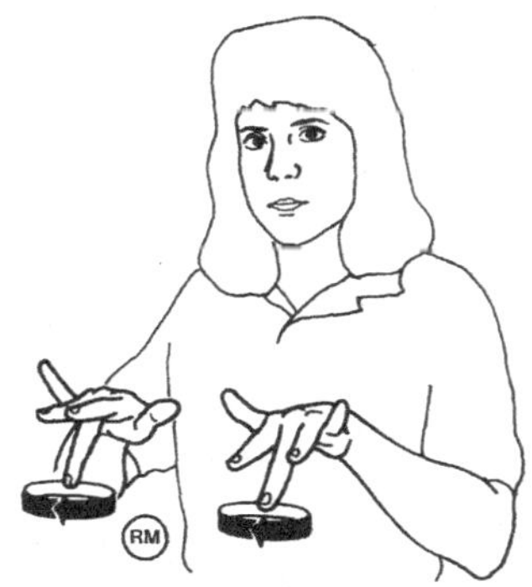

TAPE (recorder)
5 hands, palms down, waist level, with middle fingers pointing down. Simultaneously circle both hands in a clockwise direction.
Clue: cassette tape being played on a tape recorder.

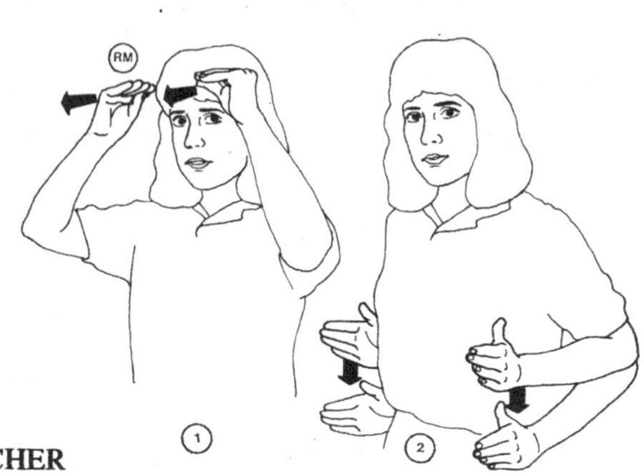

TEACHER
Flat O hands, palms facing each other, forehead level. Move hands simultaneously out. Change to flat hands, fingertips out, palms facing. Move down to waist level.
Clue: teach + person.

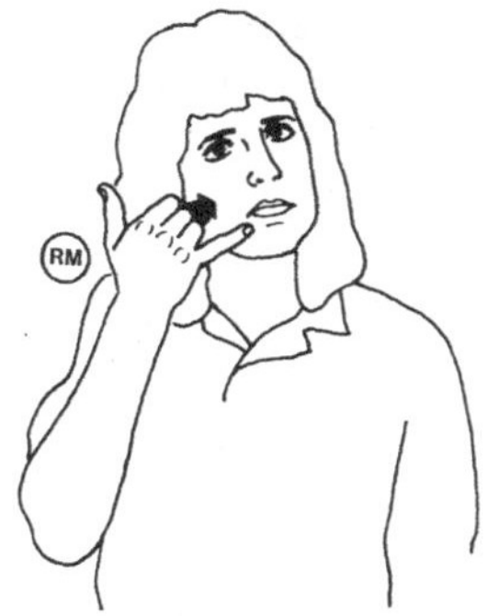

TELEPHONE
Right Y hand, at side of face, palm in.
Clue: telephone receiver.

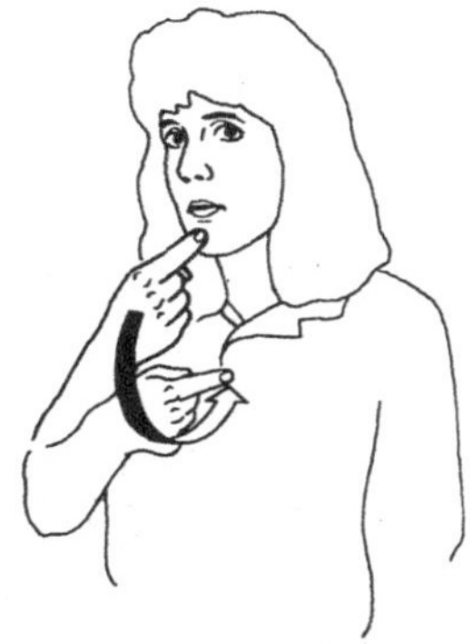

TELL-ME
Right 1 hand, chin level, palm in. Touch chin and then touch chest.

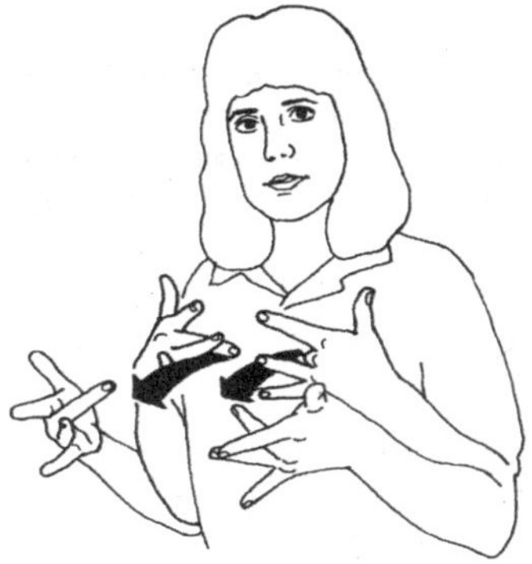

TEND
5 hands, palms in, middle fingers touching chest. Simultaneously bring hands out and slightly down from chest.

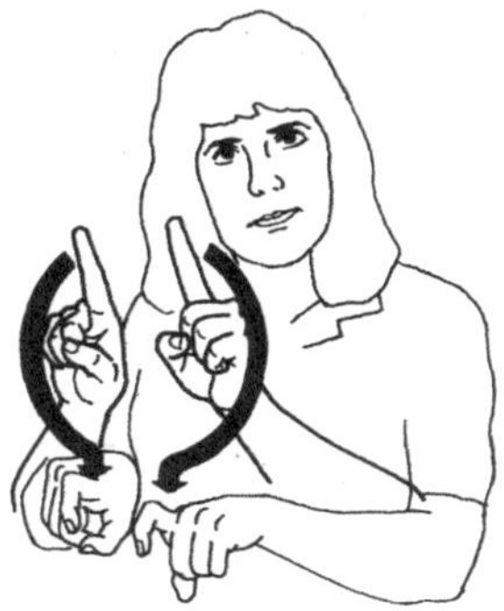

TEST
1 hands, shoulder level, palms out. Bring arms down while forming question marks with index fingers.
Clue: drawing many questions in the air.

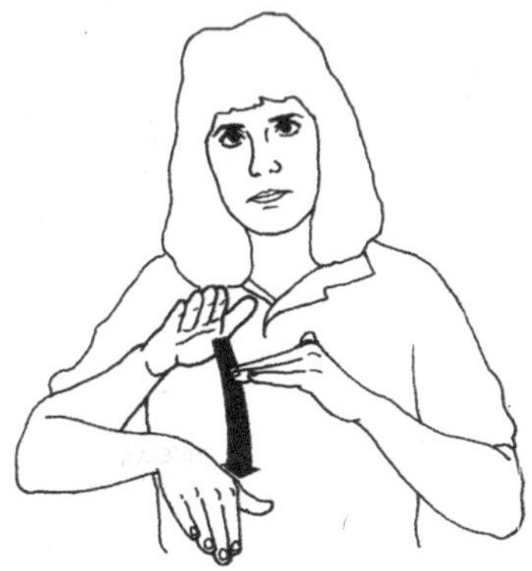

THAN
Flat hands, palms down, chest level, right hand above left. Right hand brushes past left hand.

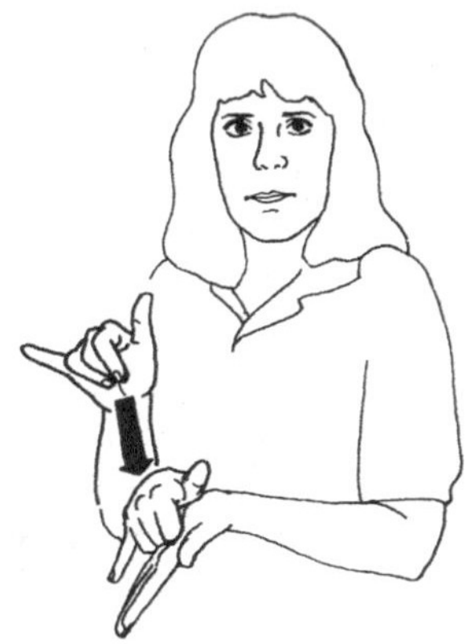

THAT
Right Y hand, palm down, chest level. Left flat hand, palm up, waist level. Bring right Y down on left palm.

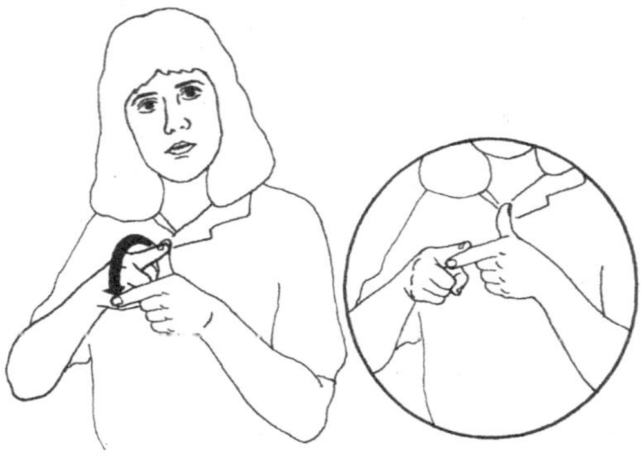

THEN
Left L hand, chest level, palm right. Right 1 hand, palm in, index finger touching left thumb. Right index finger then moves to left index finger.

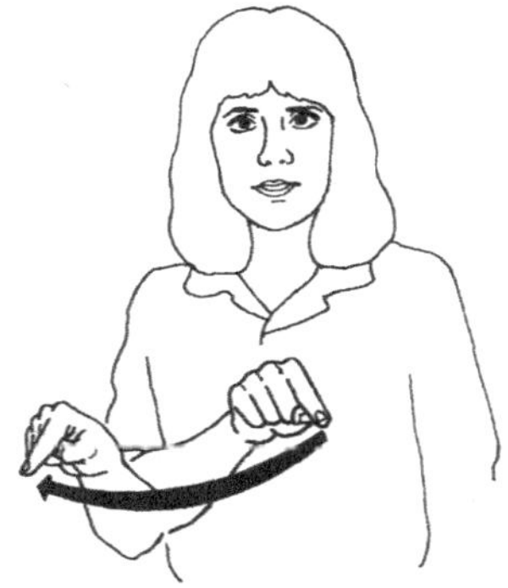

THESE
Right 1 hand, palm down, sweeps across referents.

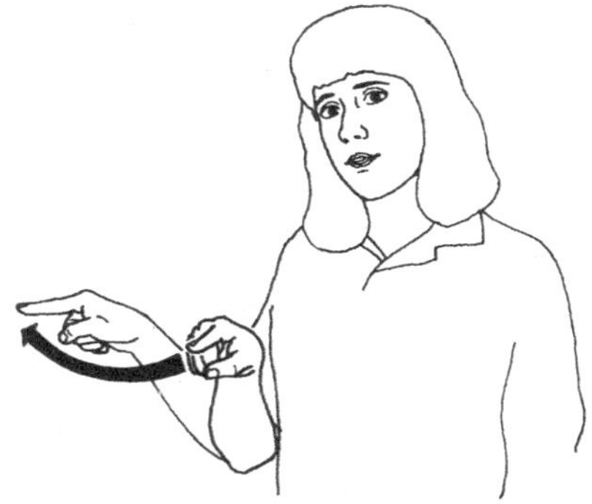

THEY
Right 1 hand, palm down, points in the direction of the people being addressed.

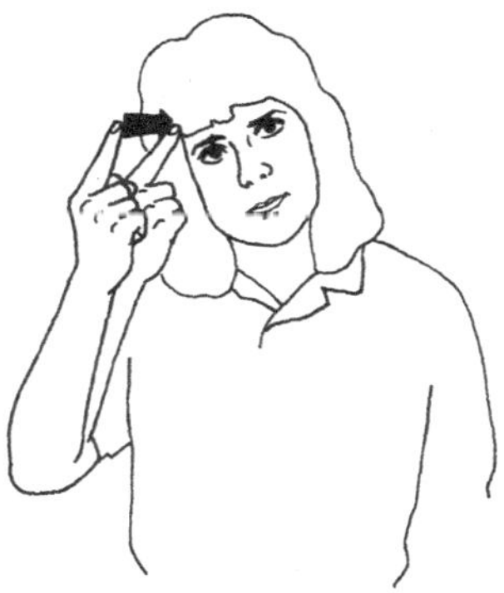

THINK
Right 1 hand, palm in, near forehead. Repeatedly touch side of forehead.

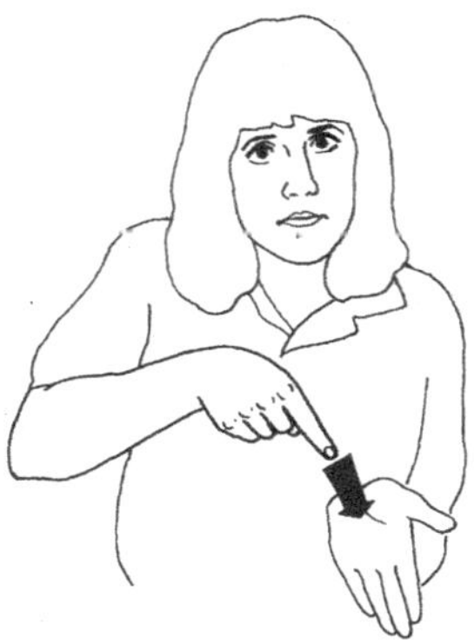

THIS
Right 1 hand, palm down, chest level. Left hand, palm up, waist level. Right fingertip touches left palm.

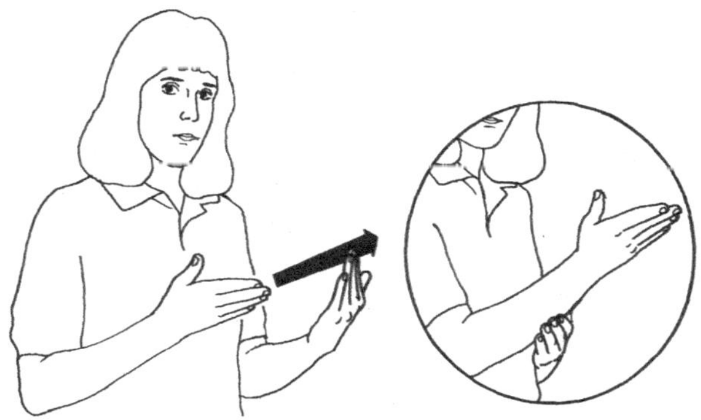

THROUGH
Left flat hand, palm in, chest level. Right flat hand, palm left. Right hand goes through left hand between the thumb and index fingers.

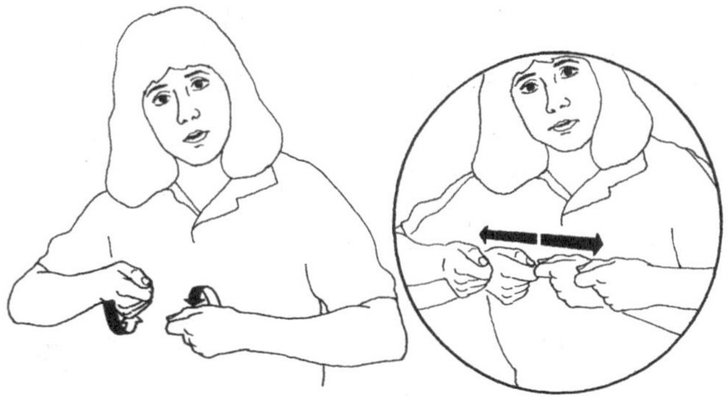

TIE
A hands, palms in, chest level. Right A slightly in front of left. Alternately circle A hands, ending with index fingers touching. Pull both hands quickly to sides.
Clue: act of tying a knot.

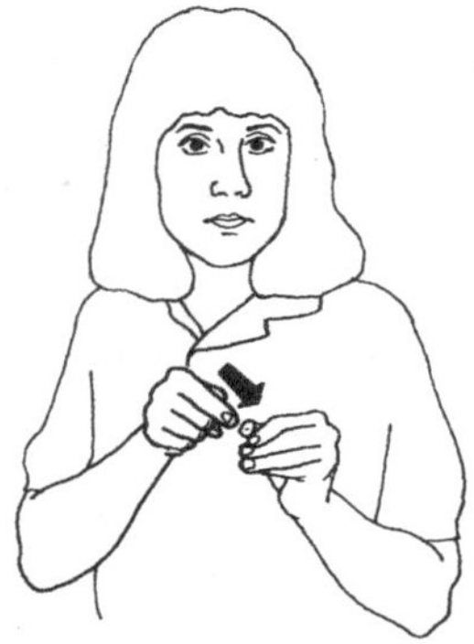

TIP
Right 1 hand points to the tip you hold in left hand.

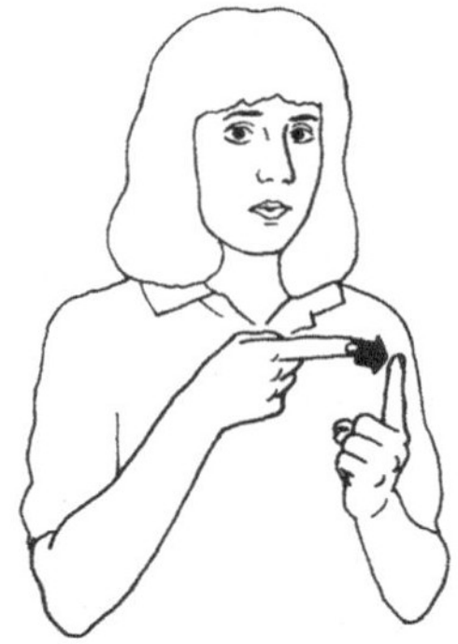

TO
1 hands, palms in, chest level, right 1 points left, left 1 points up. Move right 1 straight to touch left 1.

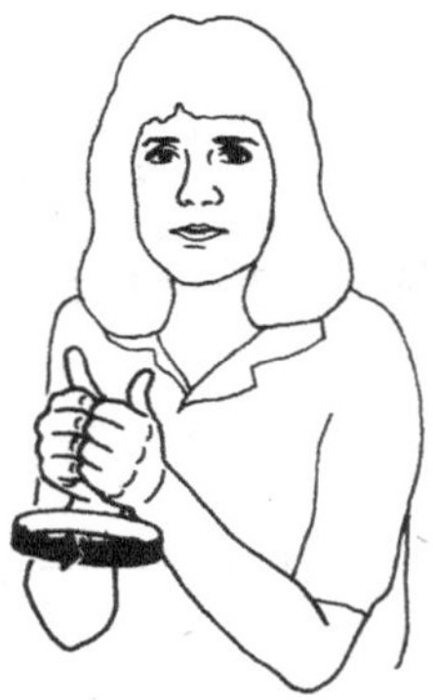

TOGETHER
A hands, chest level, palms facing. Hands come together, knuckles touching.

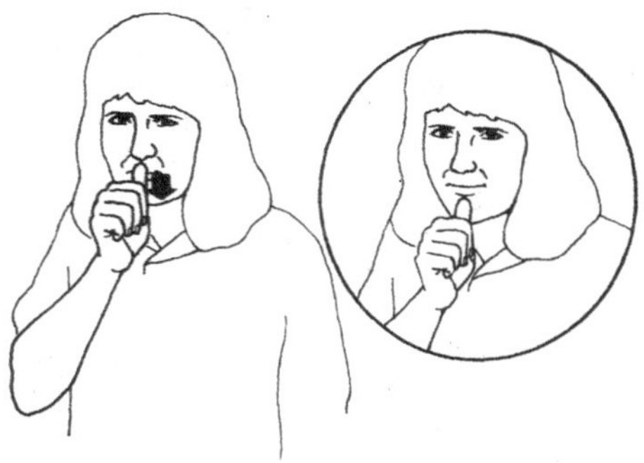

TOLERATE
Right A hand, palm left, thumb at lips. Slowly bring hand down lips to chin.

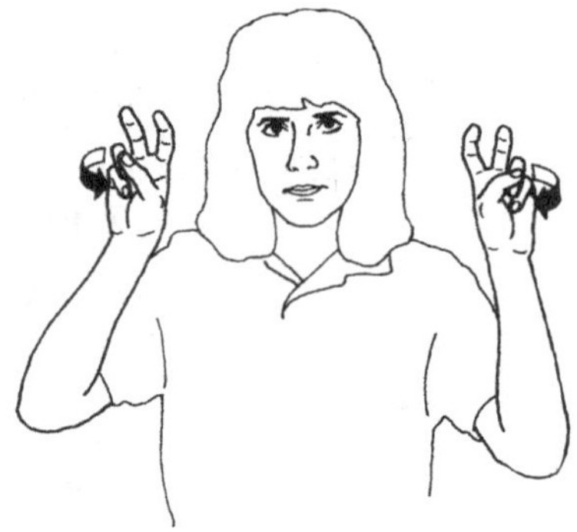

TOPIC/ISSUE
Bent V hands, palms out, head level. Rotate wrists from side to side.
Clue: looks like quotation marks.

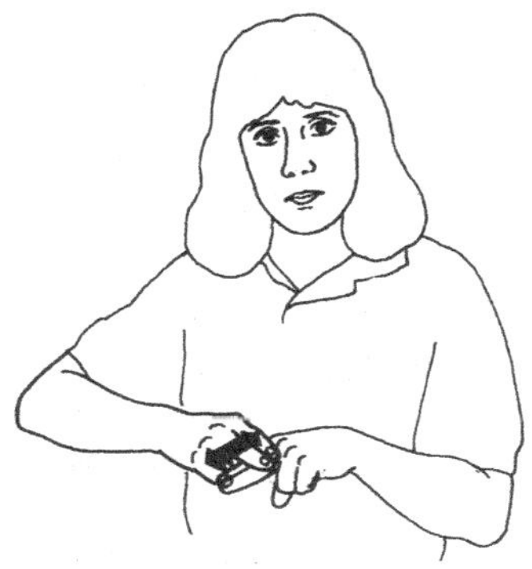

TRAIN (transportation)
U hands, palms down, chest level, right U on left U. Slide right U repeatedly back and forth on left U.

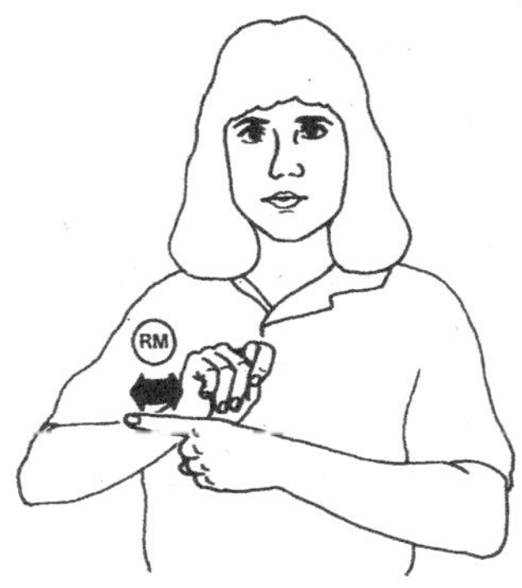

TRAIN (teach)
Left 1 hand, palm in, index finger pointing right, waist level. Right T hand, palm out, on top of left index finger. Right hand repeatedly moves back and forth over left index finger.

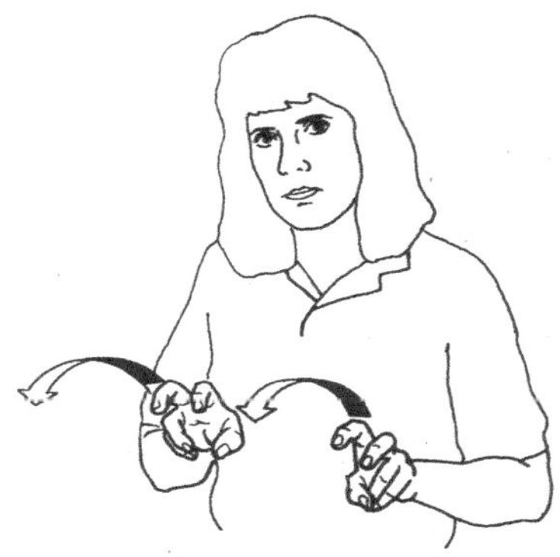

TRANSFUSION
Bent V hands, palms down, waist level. Sweep hands to the right simultaneously.

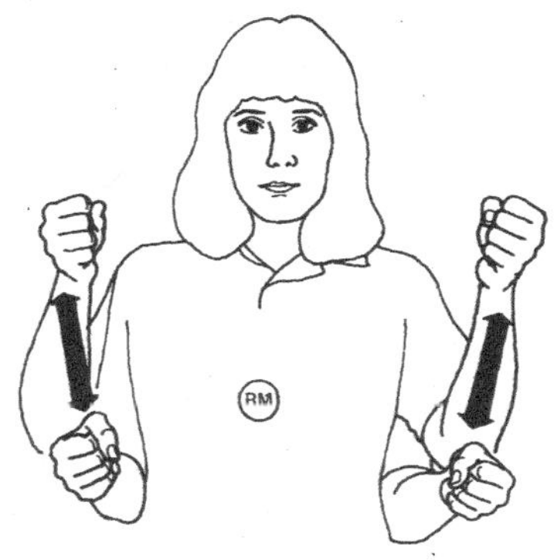

TRUCK
S hands, palms facing each other, shoulder level. Move hands up and down alternately.
Clue: holding and moving the steering wheel of a truck.

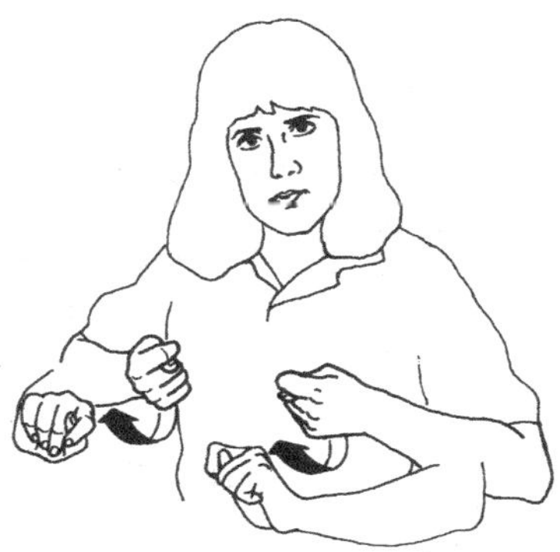

TRY
T hands, at chest, palms in. Simultaneously curve hands down slightly and out.

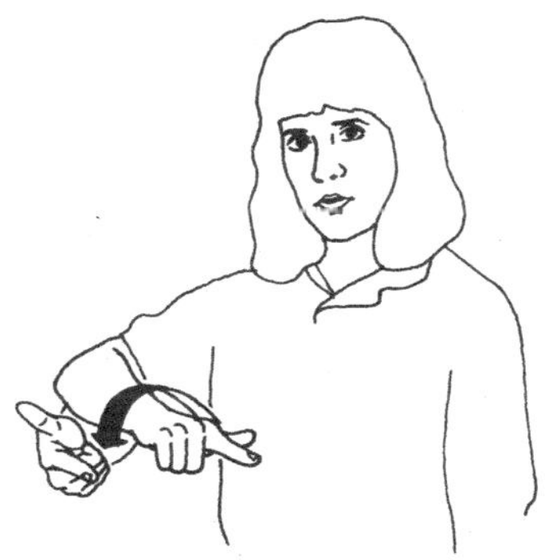

TURN
Right L hand, palm down, chest level. Rotate L at wrist to palm up.

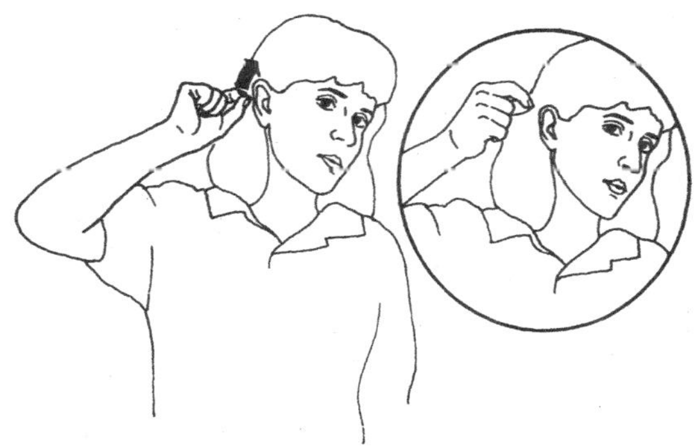

TURN VOLUME
Right closed hand, thumb and index finger touching, behind right ear. Move hand up slightly.

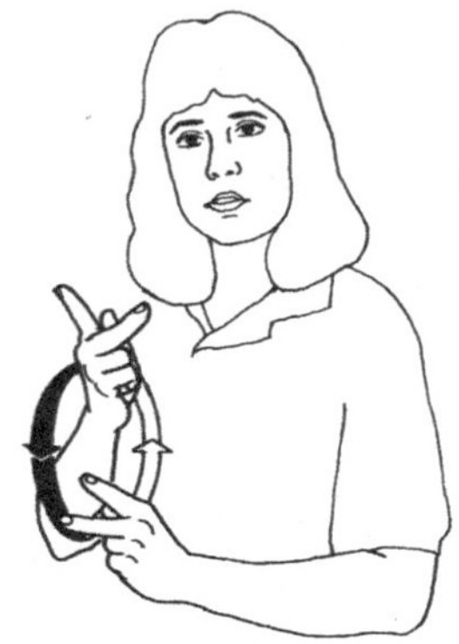

TYPE/KIND
K hands, palms to sides, waist level, right hand on top of left. Right hand circles out and around left hand.

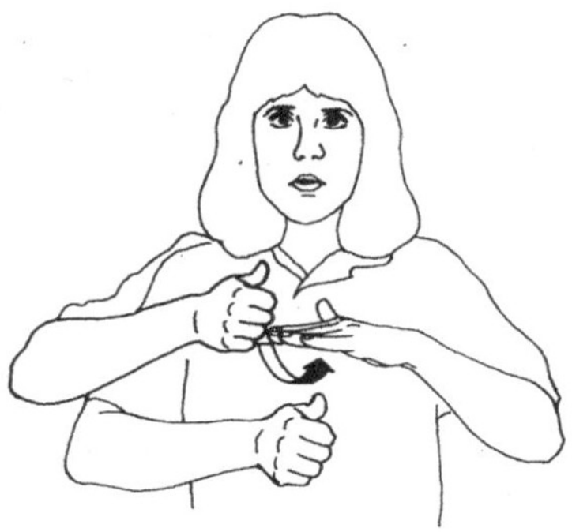

UNDER
Right A hand, palm left. Left flat hand, palm down, chest level. Move A under left hand.

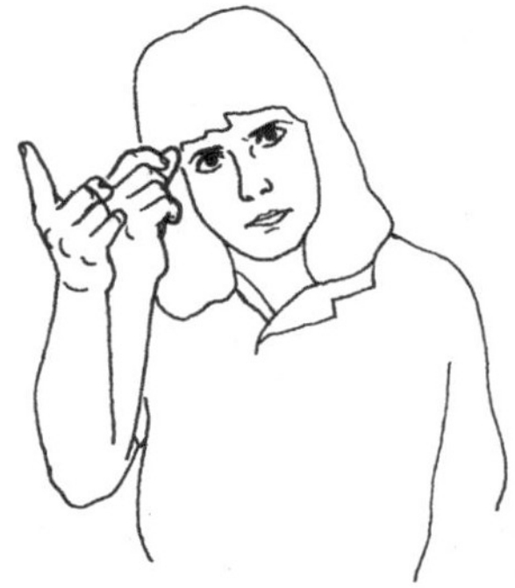

UNDERSTAND
Right S hand, palm in, at right side of forehead. Flick index finger up quickly to 1 handshape.

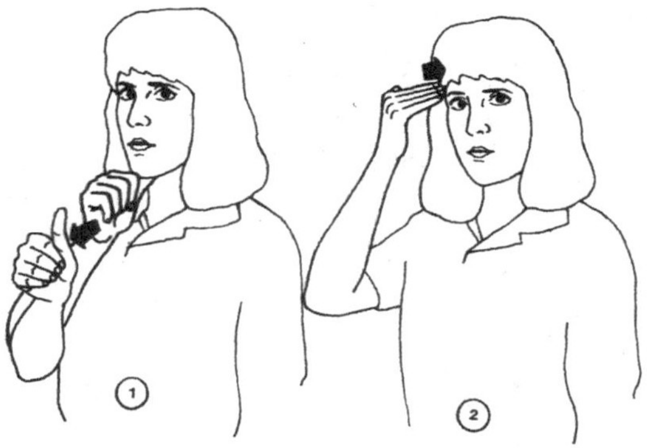

UNFAMILIAR
Right A hand, palm left, thumb under chin. Quickly move A forward, grazing chin with thumb. Change to right flat hand, palm in and touch fingertips to right temple.
Clue: not + know.

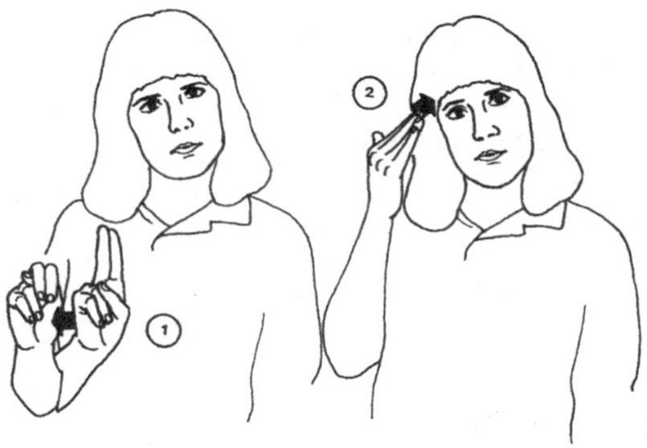

UNKNOWN
Fingerspell U-N. Right flat hand, palm in, forehead level. Touch fingertips to right side of forehead.

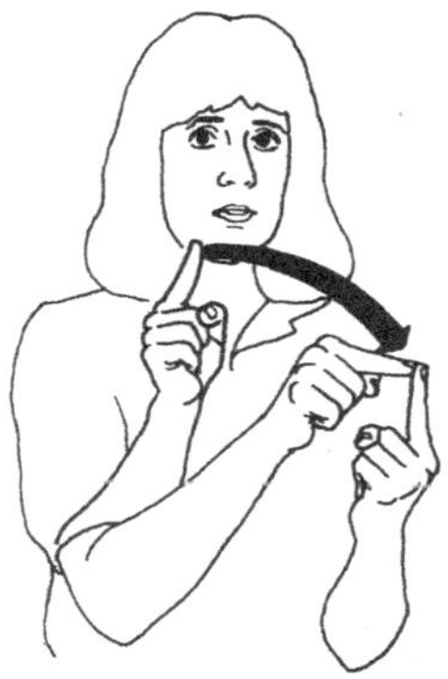

UNTIL
1 hands, palms facing, chest level. Arc right 1 to meet left 1.

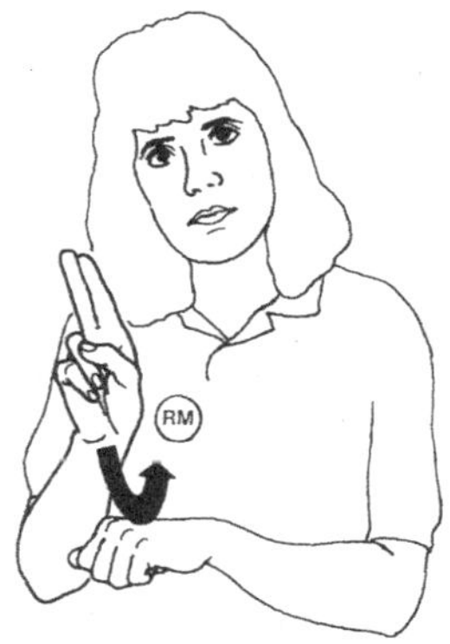

USE
Left A hand, waist level, palm down. Right U hand, palm out, rests on back of left hand and circles in a clockwise direction. Repeat movement.

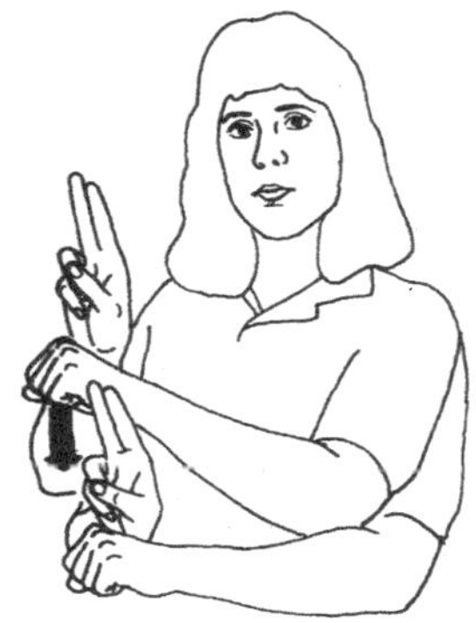

USED-TO
Left S hand, palm down, chest level. Right U hand, palm out, on back of left hand. Move hands down.

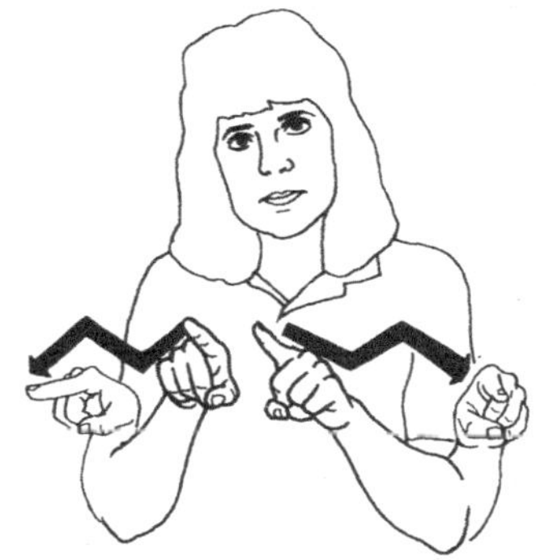

VARIOUS/ETC.
1 hands, chest level, palms down, fingers pointing out. Move hands apart, while fingers move up and down.

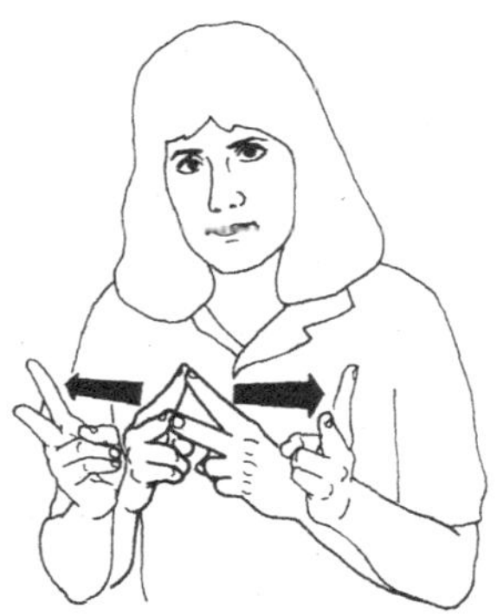

VERY
V hands, palms facing each other, fingertips touching, chest level. Move hands apart.

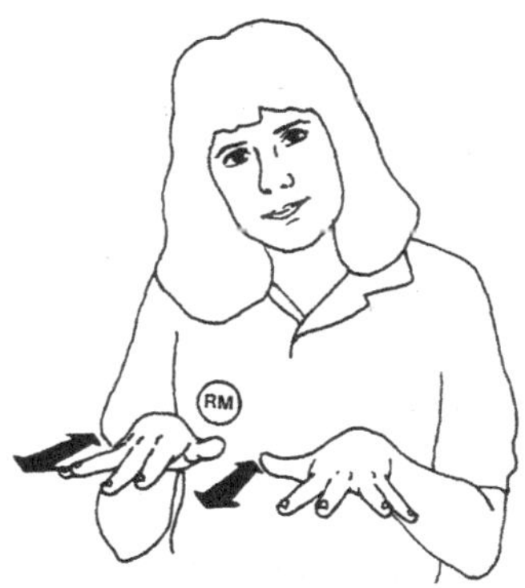

VIBRATION
5 hands, palms down, waist level. Shake hands from side to side. Repeat movement.
Clue: a floor vibrating.

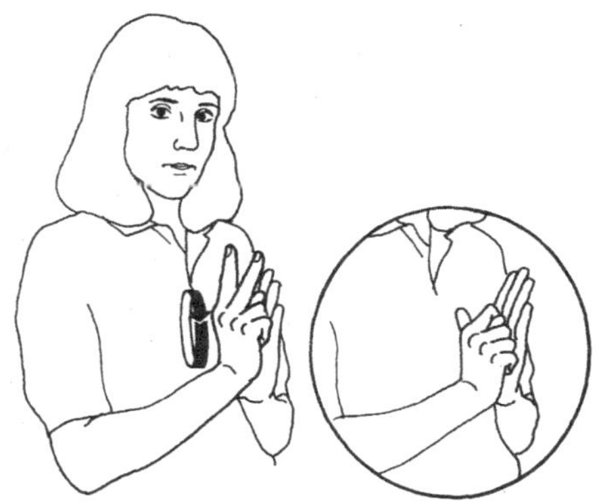

VIDEOTAPE
Left flat hand, palm right, chest level. Right V hand, palm left, on left palm. Circle right hand in a clockwise direction on left palm, changing to T hand, while completing circle.

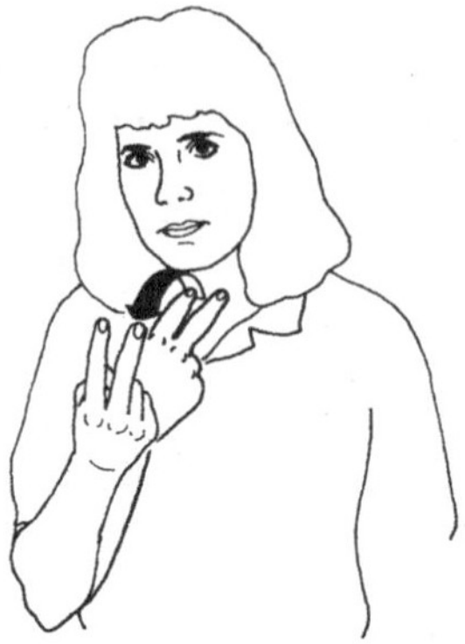

VOICE
Right V hand, palm in, at base of throat. Bring hand up to the top of throat and then out.

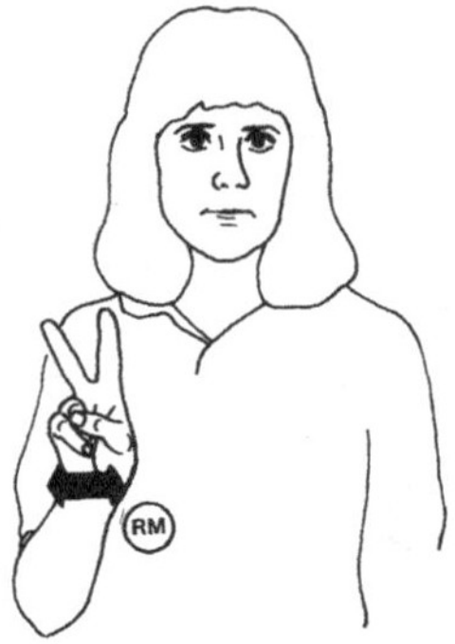

VOWEL
Right V hand, palm out, shoulder level. Shake hand from left to right.

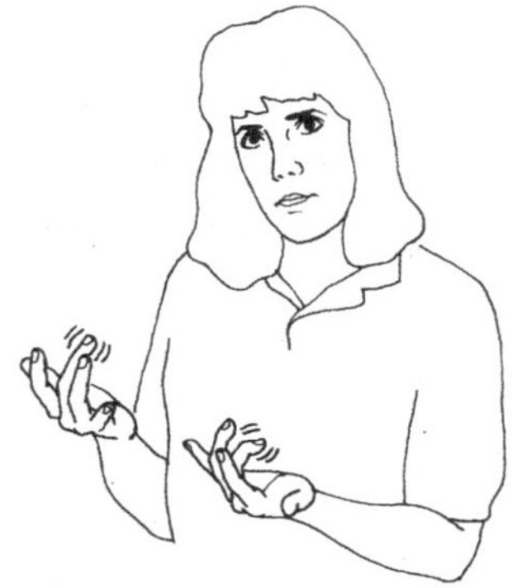

WAIT
5 hands, waist level, palms up, right hand closer to body. Wiggle fingers on both hands.

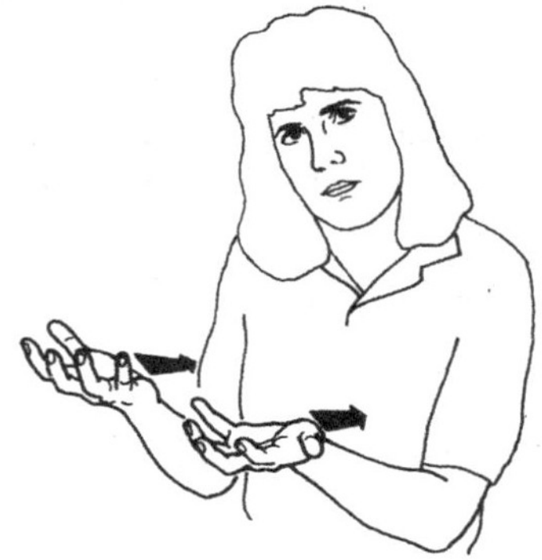

WANT
5 hands, chest level, palms up. Bring hands in, changing to claw position.

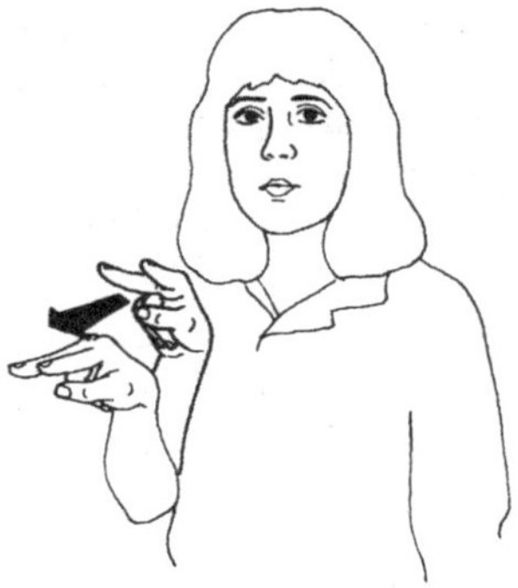

WATCH
Right V hand, palm out, eye level, points to referent.

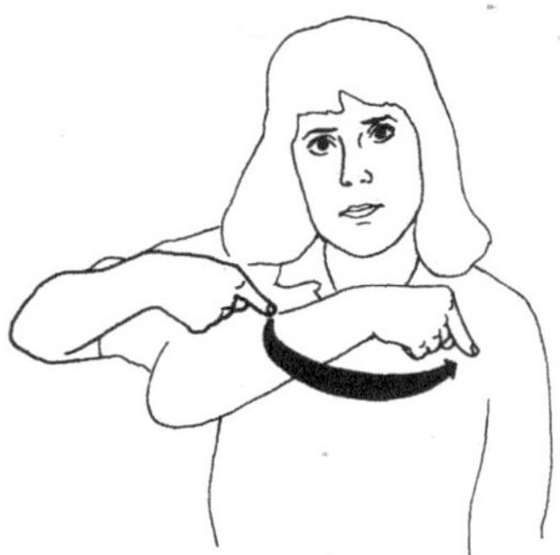

WE
Right 1 hand, palm down, on right shoulder. Move to touch left shoulder.

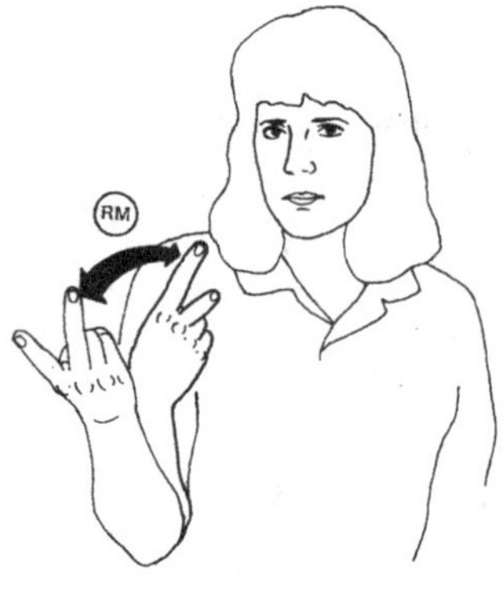

WE/TWO-OF-US
Right V hand, palm in, at right shoulder level. Rock hand back and forth in the direction of the other person.

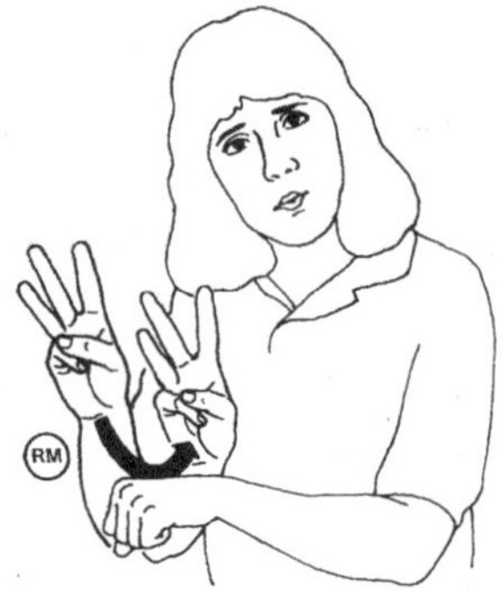

WEAR
Right W hand, palm out. Left S hand, palm down, chest level. Right wrist grazes left hand repeatedly.

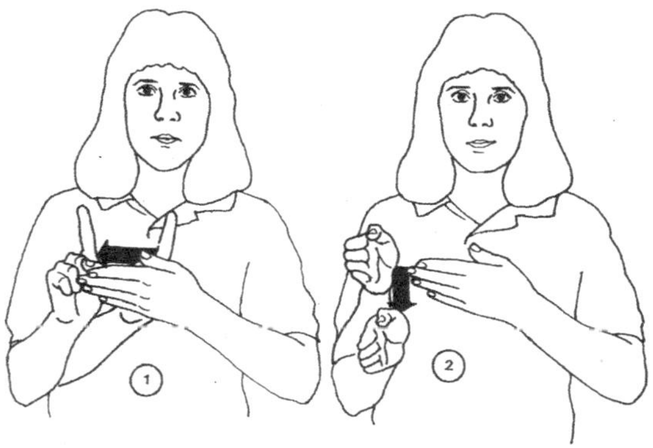

WEEKEND
Left flat hand, palm in, chest level. Right 1 hand, palm out, on base of left palm. Slide right hand down palm to end of hand, open to flat hand and brush down side of left hand.

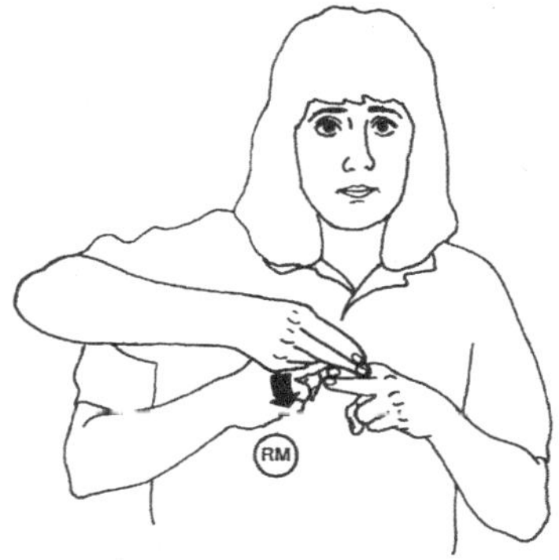

WEIGH
H hands, right H on left H, chest level. Rock right hand slightly at wrist. Repeat.

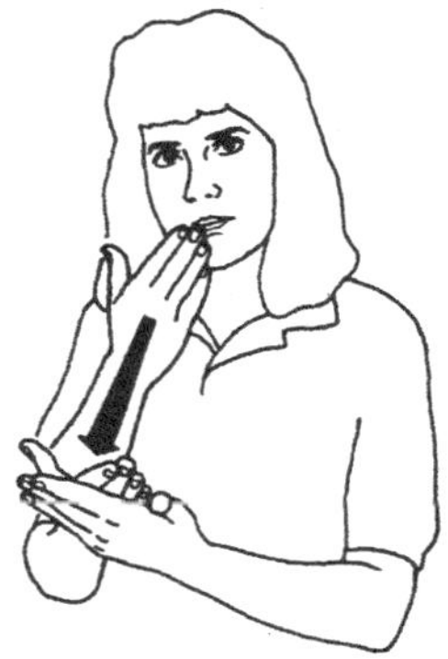

WELL/GOOD
Right flat hand, palm in, at chin. Left flat hand, palm up, at waist. Move right hand down to rest on left hand, palm up.

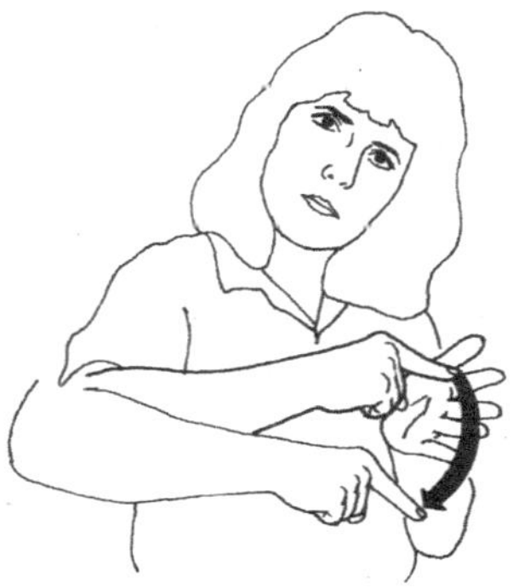

WHAT
Right 1 hand, palm in. Left 5 hand, palm left, waist level. Move right 1 down base of left fingers, beginning with the index finger.

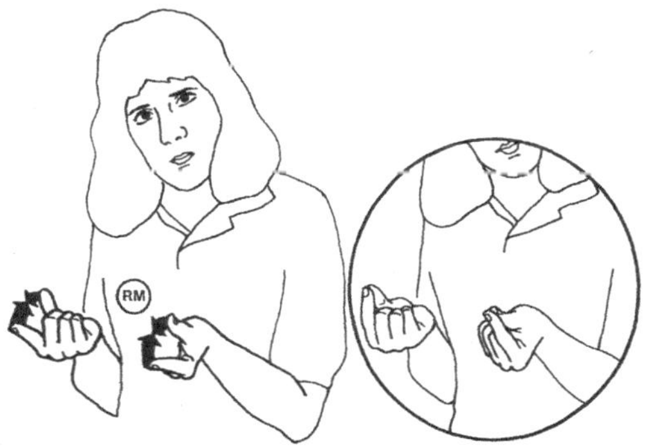

WHAT-DO
G hands, waist level, palms up. Repeatedly open and close index fingers and thumbs.

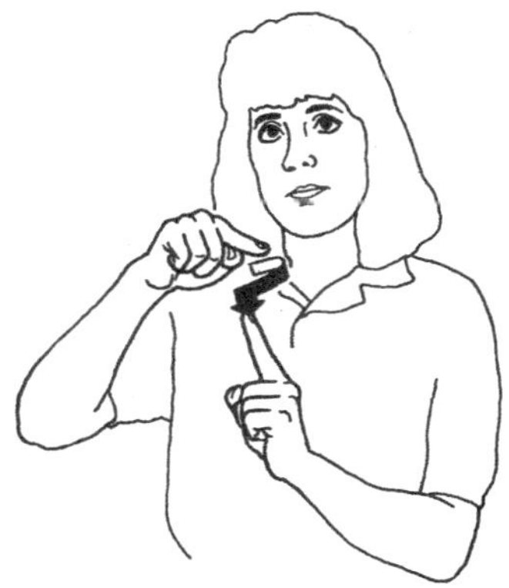

WHEN
1 hands, chest level, left palm right, right palm down. Right index finger circles over left finger in a clockwise direction.
Clue: the movement of a clock.

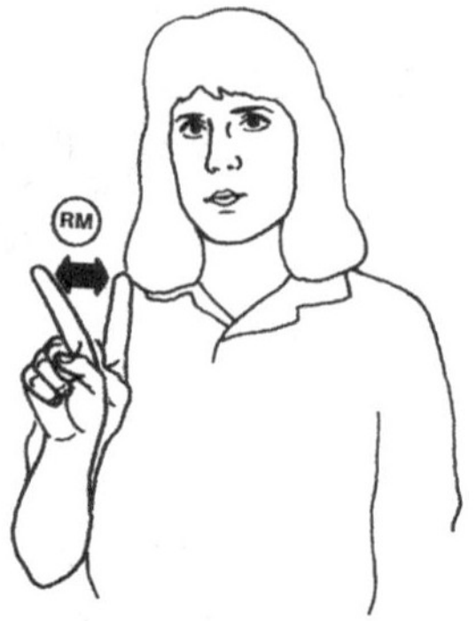

WHERE
Right 1 hand, palm out, shoulder level. Shake hand back and forth.

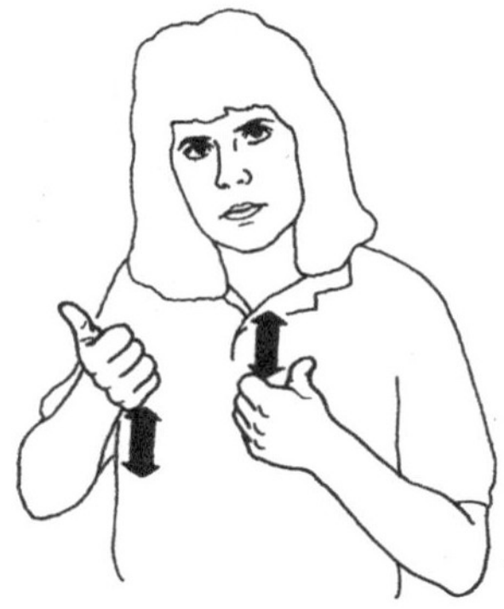

WHICH
A hands, palms in, chest level, thumbs up, hands slightly apart. Alternately move hands up and down.
Clue: tossing two things in the air, trying to decide which one you want.

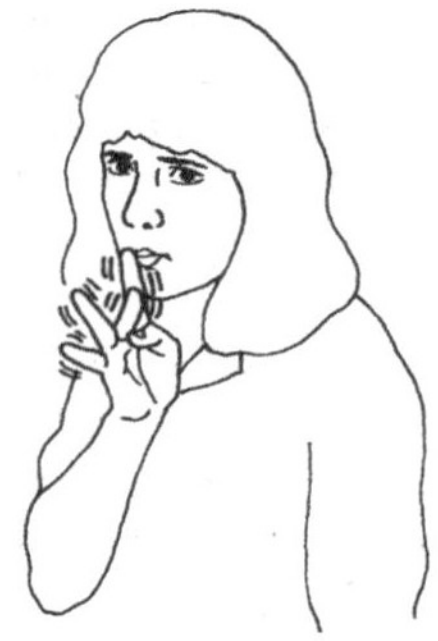

WHISPER
Right 4 hand, palm left, index finger on lower lip. Slightly wiggle fingers alternately.

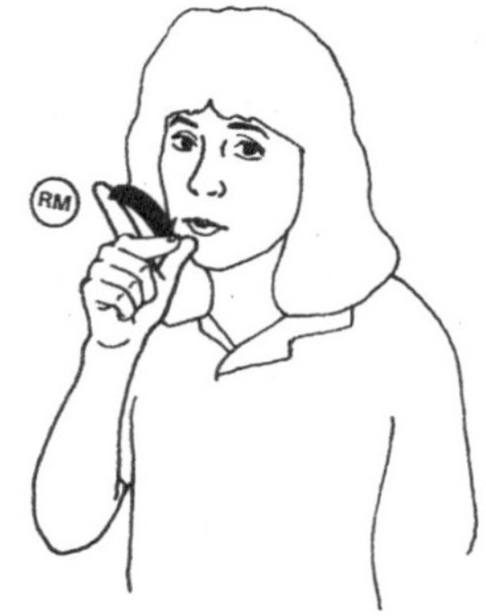

WHO
Right 1 hand, thumb on chin, palm left. Index finger moves up and down repeatedly.

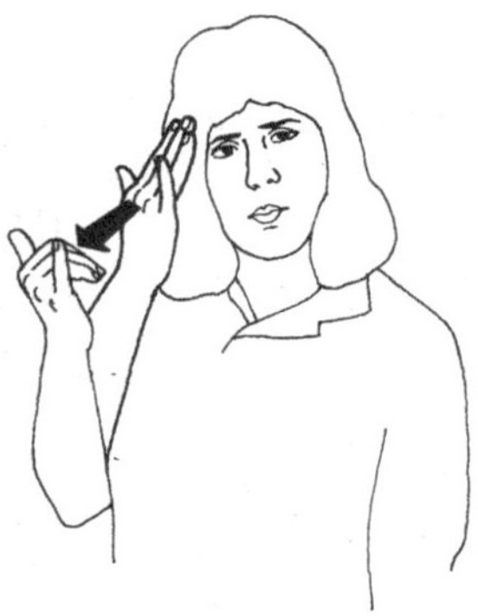

WHY
Right flat hand, palm in, at right temple. Pull hand away from face while changing to Y hand.

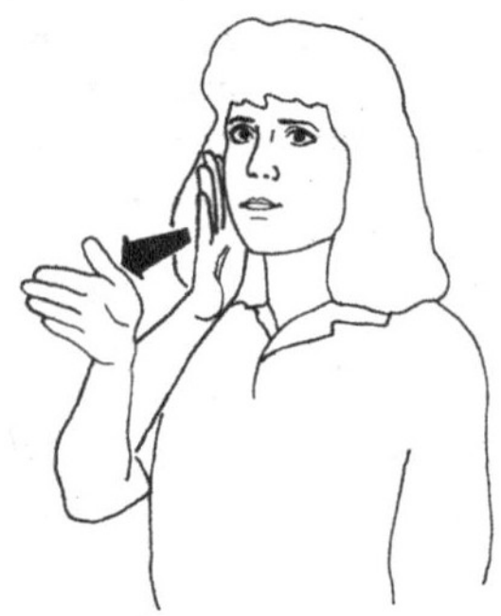

WILL
Right flat hand, palm left, ear level. Move forward.
Clue: future is forward.

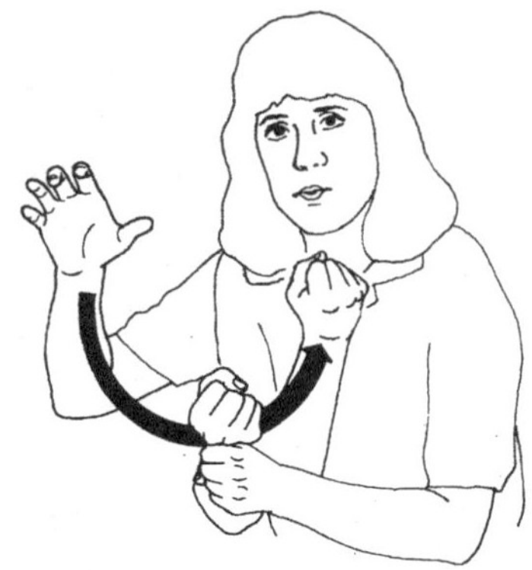

WIN
Right rounded 5 hand, palm out, shoulder level. Left S hand, palm in, waist level. Quickly bring right arm in, turning palm in, changing to S hand and brush past left hand.

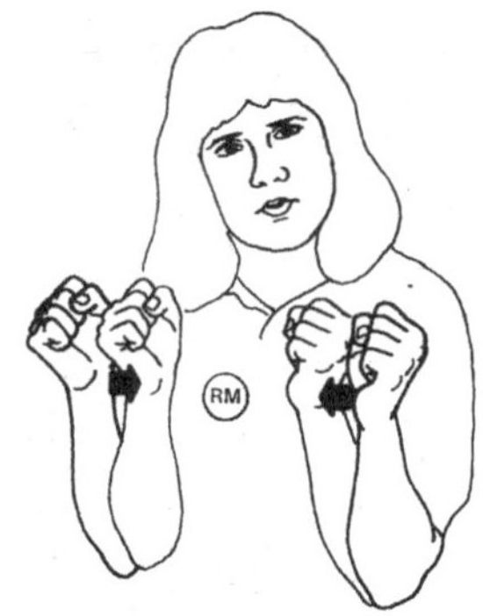

WINTER/COLD
S hands, palms facing each other, chest level. Hands slightly shake towards each other.

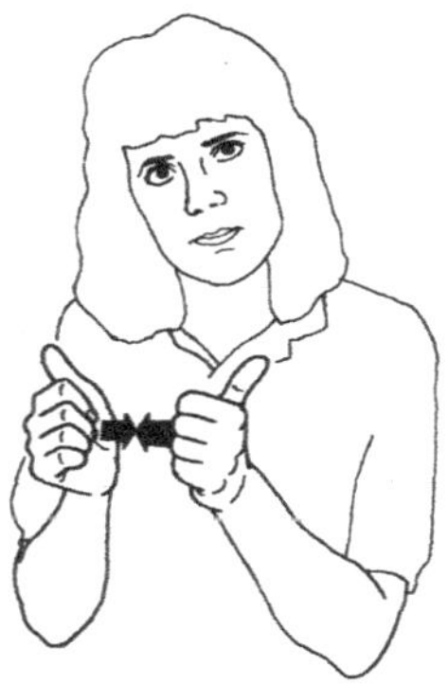

WITH
A hands, chest level, thumbs up, hands apart, palms facing. Bring hands together.

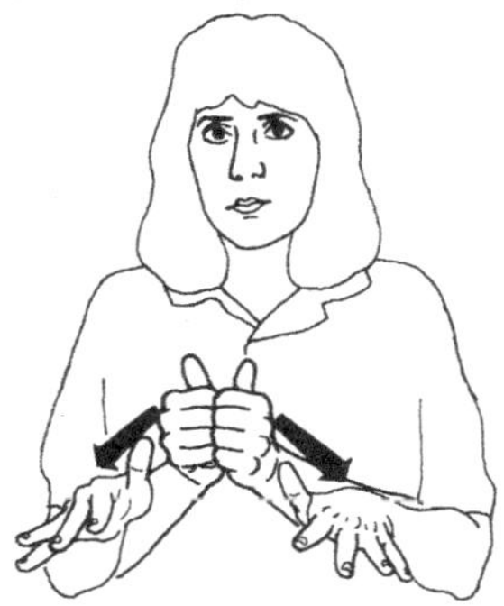

WITHOUT
A hands, palms facing each other, chest level, hands touching. Quickly move hands apart, changing to 5 hands, palms down, waist level.

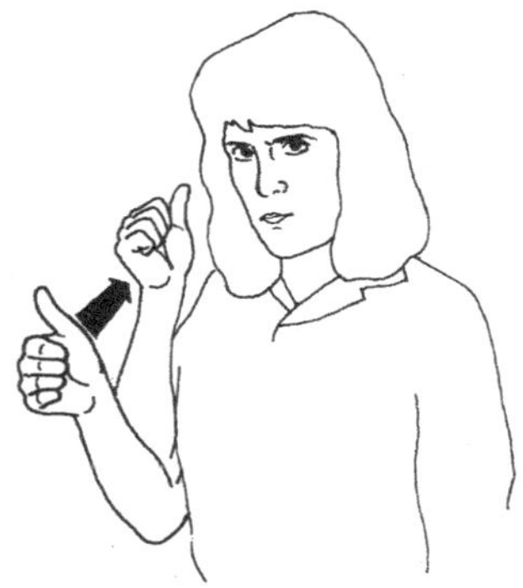

WON'T/REFUSE
Right A hand, chest level, palm left. Quickly bring arm back to shoulder.

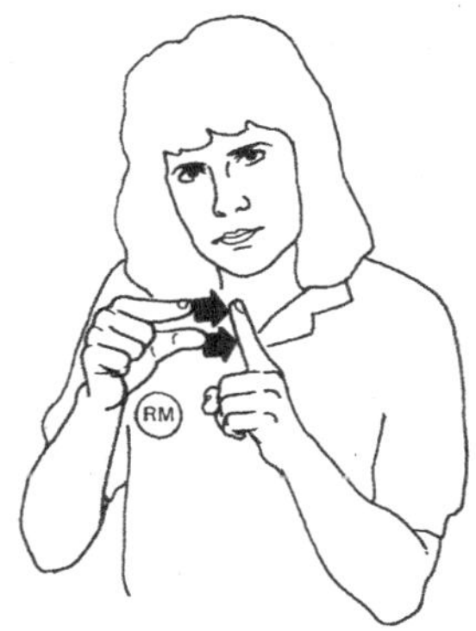

WORD
Left 1 hand, palm right, chest level. Right G, palm left. Right G fingertips repeatedly touch top of left index finger.

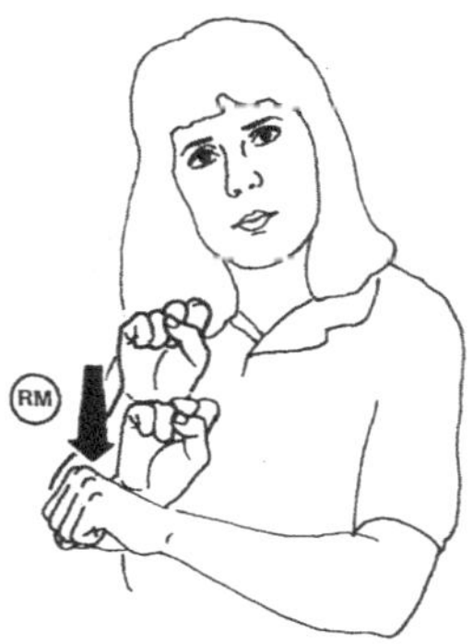

WORK
S hands, left palm down, waist level, right hand, palm out, on top of left. Bounce right hand repeatedly on top of left hand.

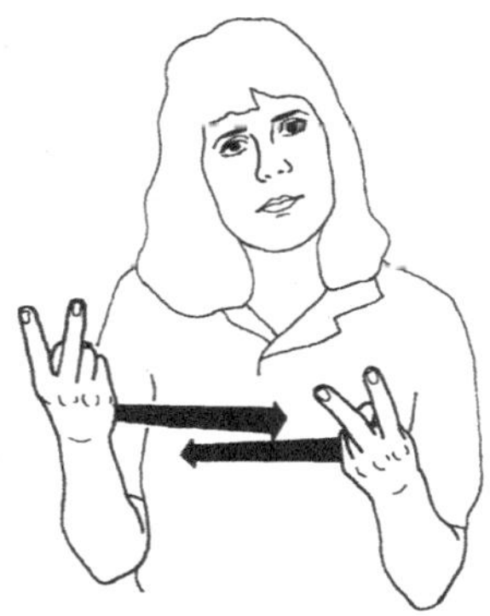

WORSE
V hands, palms in, shoulder level. Bring hands together, ending with right wrist crossed over left wrist.

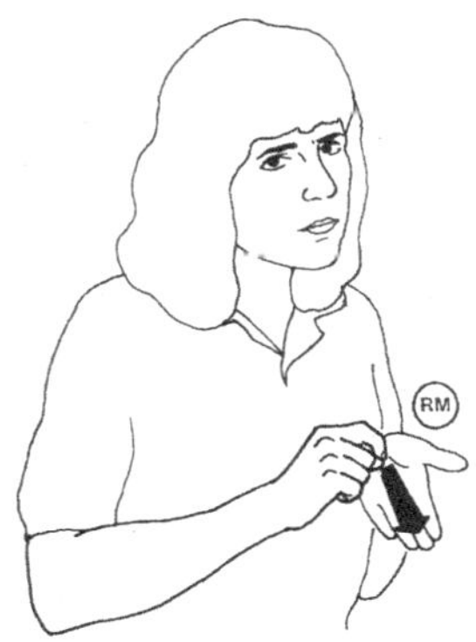

WRITE
Left flat hand, chest level, palm up. Right closed hand, thumb and index finger touching, "writes" on left palm. *Clue: writing on paper.*

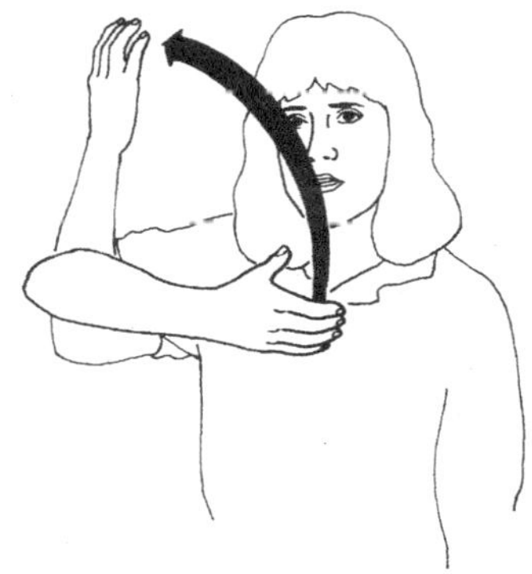

YELL
Right C hand, palm in, neck level. Sweep C up neck and across face.

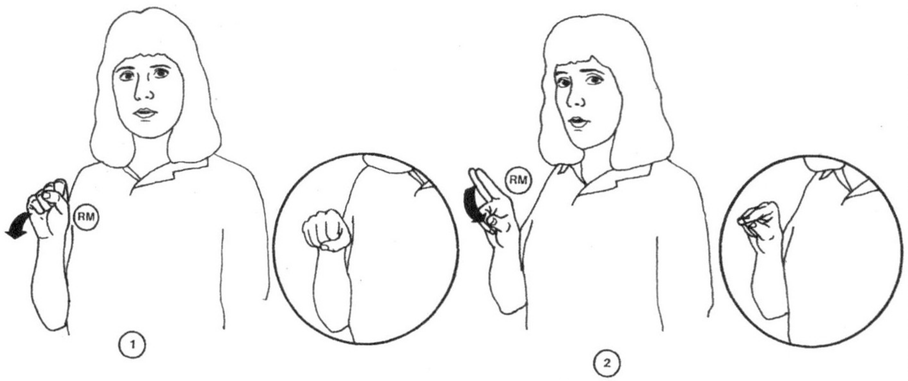

YES—NO
Right S hand, palm out, shoulder level. Move at wrist to palm down. While moving back to palm out, change handshape to U hand and tap thumb.

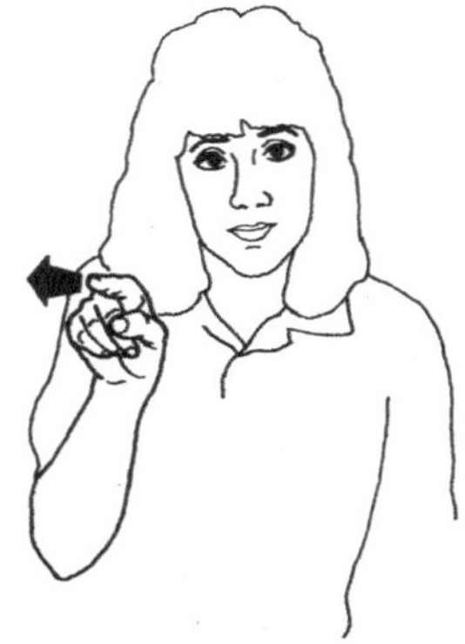

YOU
Right 1 hand, palm down, shoulder level. Point hand in the direction of the person you are addressing.
Clue: pointing at someone.

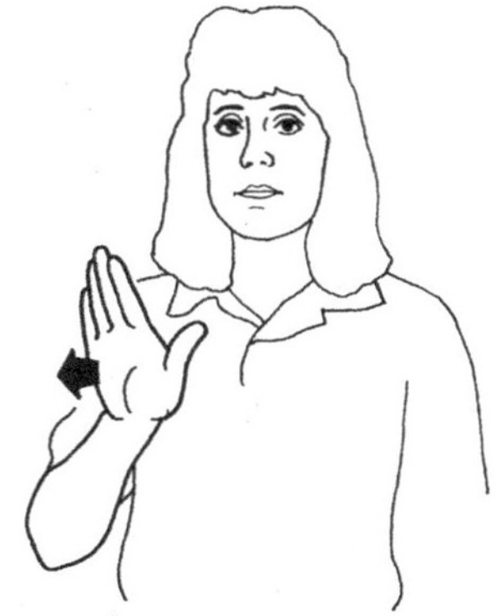

YOUR
Right flat hand, palm out, shoulder level. Move right hand forward in the direction of the person you are addressing.